The Nigerian Healthcare System

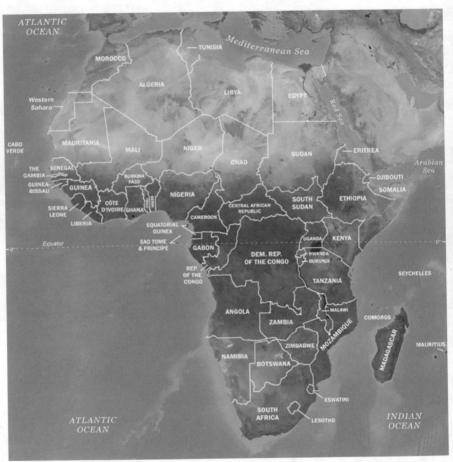

Source: (Africa Satellite. *The World Factbook 2021*. Washington, DC: Central Intelligence Agency, 2021. https://www.cia.gov/the-world-factbook/maps/)

Joseph Abiodun Balogun

The Nigerian Healthcare System

Pathway to Universal and High-Quality Health Care

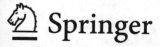 Springer

Joseph Abiodun Balogun
College of Health Sciences
Chicago State University
Chicago, IL, USA

ISBN 978-3-030-88865-7   ISBN 978-3-030-88863-3   (eBook)
https://doi.org/10.1007/978-3-030-88863-3

This Springer imprint is published by the registered company Springer Nature Switzerland AG
The registered company address is: Gewerbestrasse 11, 6330 Cham, Switzerland

This book is dedicated to my wife,
Dr. Adetutu Balogun, and our four children,
Omotade, Omotayo, Omotola, and
Omotoluwafe, for their steadfast support,
providing me the time and space that enabled
me to put in my best as a faculty and
university administrator for over
three decades

Foreword

My first contact with the author, Professor Joseph Abiodun Balogun, was at the University of Ibadan, Nigeria, where he studied physiotherapy from 1974 to 1977. I was then an academic staff in the Department of Economics at the University. He was one of the students from my hometown who frequently took a break from academic work rigors and visited my family on weekends. As a student, he showed great promise, so I remotely and keenly monitored his academic progress after relocating to the United States. In the last few years, we have maintained closer contact, exchanging publications, technical presentations, and opinions on Nigeria's health system development. He has been in the United States academy for over 30 years, 13 of which he served as the Dean of the College of Health Sciences at Chicago State University. His educational and professional experiences in Nigeria and the United States provided him a unique opportunity to write this book. Professor Balogun's academic and professional experiences also gave him a vantage position to share practical recommendations on improving the nation's healthcare system.

Indeed, this book is one of the very few comprehensive sources of information that I have come across on the Nigerian healthcare system, combined with the description of complementary and alternative medicine and the development of traditional medicine in Nigeria. In this 14-chapter book, Professor Balogun discusses the fundamental concepts of health care, the Nigerian healthcare system's evolution and developmental journey, and the Federal Ministry of Health's organizational structure. The book also analyses the contemporary challenges and past breakthroughs in the Nigerian health system.

The book discusses the plight of persons living with disabilities in Nigeria, including providing learning accommodation and campus architectural modifications on campus for students with physical disabilities. Professor Balogun also presents political and economic arguments for achieving a universal and high-quality health system in Nigeria, including practical recommendations to achieve the dual goals. This invaluable book would be handy to students of the various health disciplines; teachers of healthcare education; health practitioners and managers; regulators of the different health professions; policymakers in the ministries of health at the state and federal levels; and researchers on issues related to the various components of Nigeria's health system, especially human resources for health. I share the author's view that the book is ideal for several courses offered at diploma and degree levels in Nigerian universities.

The innovative book is well written and the contents are well sequenced to enhance the flow of information presented from the beginning to the end. Also noteworthy is that each chapter provides "Learning Objectives," which offer the readers an excellent tool for assessing the knowledge gained after reading the chapter. I strongly recommend this book to the categories of people mentioned above and to the public. I have learned a lot from reading the book, and you will, too, if you read it.

Eyitayo Lambo, PhD, FOR, FNES
Pioneer Lecturer in Operations Research, University of Ibadan, Ibadan, Nigeria, 1974–1982;
Foundation Professor of Economics and Management Sciences, Bendel State University, Ekpoma, Nigeria, 1982–1983;
Foundation Professor of Business Administration, University of Ilorin, Ilorin, Nigeria, 1984–1992;
Regional Advisor for Health Economics and Health Systems Research, WHO Regional Office for Africa, 1990–1999;
Minister of Health, Federal Republic of Nigeria, 2003–2007.
Abuja, Nigeria
October 2021

Preface

The Western-style healthcare system was imported into the region now known as Nigeria over 500 years ago, through the trans-Sahara trade routes by the European traders, explorers, colonial military and civilian administrators, and later the missionaries. The first national health plan in Nigeria was developed in 1947 by the colonial masters with the primary goal to provide universal health care to the citizens. To date, this goal remains an illusion. This preeminent book presents the roadmap needed to attain universal health care and offers a blueprint for achieving high-quality health care. In the last four decades, several articles have appeared in the literature on the Nigerian healthcare system's challenges. Still, there is currently no single authoritative source of information on the topic. This publication seeks to fill this gap in the literature.

Several challenges – human resources, leadership, financial, and infrastructures, including medication – plague the Nigerian health system that influenced affordable quality healthcare delivery. This classic book chronicles these vulnerabilities using the World Health Organization's six building blocks for health systems' evaluation. Six decades after independence, Nigeria has one of the world's worst health outcomes. Maternal mortality is extremely high, and underfive-mortality rates are 132 per 1000 live births, which means 1 in 8 Nigerian children never reach five years of age. These unacceptable health outcomes are due to the penurious health service delivery system compounded by limited preventive (screening for specific diseases and immunization) programs and the dismal health insurance coverage. Chapter 10 of this book identified and benchmarked six nations worldwide with stellar health systems that Nigeria can emulate to revitalize and invigorate its semi-comatose health system.

The book is illustrated in a reader-friendly format that can be read independently rather than predicated on material from a previous chapter. In other words, readers could begin with any section of their choice, unconstrained by any desire to start from the beginning. Overall, the publication is organized into 14 chapters, with behavioral learning objectives provided upfront that enable readers to evaluate the knowledge acquired after reading the chapter. Each chapter includes a case study at the end to allow the reader to contextualize the information presented. The contents are liberally supplemented by empirical data presented in tables or figures and subtitles inserted into the appropriate sections to enhance information retrieval.

The examples provided in this publication reflect contemporary and best practices drawn mainly from the United States because of its enormous educational and health systems achievements. This selection bias is not surprising, given prolonged socialization from my education, professional work experience, and extended residence in the country. On several occasions, this publication compared Nigeria's health system outcomes with many high-income countries worldwide to gauge high-quality performance, identify inefficiency, and how Nigeria can learn from best practices.

Several of the topical issues discussed and the recommendations prescribed may be controversial because they challenge the status quo and the entrenched dogma in Nigeria. I hope the comments will engender frank discussion and further dialogue that will improve interprofessional collaborations and achieve universal health care that has remained a pipe dream in the country.

General readers interested in the Nigerian healthcare system, aficionados, so to say, will find much in this comprehensive book to engage them. The extensive references provided may interest specialists or even general readers who seek in-depth exploration of any of the numerous topics presented. A conscious effort was made to avoid technical jargon that can impede comprehension of the material this work presents. The information and data shared were obtained from open access sources and references copiously cited to bolster the book's assertions. The omission of any pertinent evidence of fact or incorrect statement is regretted.

Although Nigeria is the secondary focus of this groundbreaking work, it contains precious resources applicable in many developing countries and underscores the publication's deliberate interdisciplinary framework. Therefore, it should strongly appeal to policy makers, health systems technocrats, and students from different health disciplines around the world. The book is ideal for adoption as a reference textbook in the health services administration, health policy management, health management and informatics, *introduction to complementary and alternative medicine*, healthcare delivery systems, and primary healthcare courses offered in Nigerian universities.

What sets this book apart is that, in addition to identifying the vulnerabilities of the Nigerian health system, it also sounds the urgency for reforms and provides concrete recommendations on how to achieve high-quality universal healthcare by 2030. Coincidentally, the release of this book co-occurred within the ongoing debates on health care reforms in Nigeria, climaxed most recently, in September

2021, with the formation of a Health Sector Reform Committee by the federal government. The Committee, chaired by Vice President Yemi Osinbajo and whose membership includes state governors, members of the National Assembly, and healthcare professional associations, was charged with reviewing all healthcare reforms adopted in the past 20 years under the Fourth Republic, including teachable lessons from those reforms. This compelling book is of significant contribution to that more extensive debate.

Chicago, IL, USA   Joseph Abiodun Balogun
Ondo City, Nigeria
Benin City, Nigeria
Tinley Park, IL, USA

Acknowledgments

My work experience at the Obafemi Awolowo University (OAU), Ile-Ife, Nigeria, between 1986 and 1991, and several visits to the country between 2015 and 2019 informed the opinions expressed in this book. I owe many people some gratitude that I would like to acknowledge in this space responsively. I am grateful to all my colleagues in the three institutions where I spent part of my sabbatical leave in 2019. Specifically, I appreciate the support provided by my colleagues at the University of Medical Sciences (UNIMED) Ondo City and the Center of Excellence in Reproductive Health Innovation at the University of Benin, and the Women's Health and Action Research Centre at Benin City. I am indebted to my iconic academic friend, Professor Friday Okonofua, pioneer vice chancellor of UNIMED and the hardest working academic I have met, for inviting me to present the Second Distinguished Guest Lecture in June 2017. A significant part of the materials in this book came from the speech.

Many individuals in my family deserve special recognition here. First and foremost are my dear wife, Dr. Adetutu Balogun, and our four children, to whom collectively I dedicate this work for their unwavering support of my academic career spanning more than three decades. I genuinely appreciate my esteemed colleague and research collaborator, Professor Philip Aka, to find time out of his exceedingly busy academic and university administrative work to read the initial draft of this work and provide extensive feedback. Also, I want to express my profound appreciation to my mentor, Professor Eyitayo Lambo, former Nigerian Minister of Health, for reading the first draft and providing many helpful references and comments used to improve the depth and clarity of this work. I owe sincere gratitude to all the authors whose work I cited and a heartfelt tribute to my publisher, Springer Nature, particularly Ms. Janet Kim, for working with me to meet the production deadline.

I am indebted to my brothers-in-law, Admiral Bamidele Daji and Admiral Olumuyiwa Olotu, and sister-in-law, Dr. Feyisayo Daji, for providing transportation and security protection during my many visits to Nigeria. I also want to express my most profound appreciation to Ms. Efe Mamuzo for compiling the information in Table 4.4 on the Ministers of Health profiles for 80 randomly selected World Health Organization member nations. I hereby acknowledge the support of my colleagues in Nigeria – Temitope Oluwatayo, Public Relations Officer at UNIMED, Col. (retired) Dr. Paschal Mogbo, Professor Babatunde Adegoke, and Professor Bamidele Ogbe Solomon – for providing the pictures in this book. No doubt, these photographs have added value to the information presented. I appreciate Professor Ade Oyeyemi for meticulously reading the galley proof and for deftly providing constructive feedback that ensures the accuracy of the information in this book.

Contents

1 Introduction 1
  Overview of the Nigerian State 1
    Geography and Politics 1
    Ethnicity 3
    Religion 4
    Economy 4
    Income Inequity 5
    Health System 6
  Overview of the Chapters 7
  Competition and Conclusion 10
  References 11

2 The Fundamentals of Health Care 15
  Introduction 16
  What Is Health? 16
  Determinants of Health 18
  Health Equity 19
  Health Disparities and Health Inequalities 19
  Health in All Policies 22
  Is Health a "Consumption Good" or an "Investment Good"? 23
  Relationship Between Health and Development 25
  United Nations Development Goals 25
  Global Access to Health Care 27
  Burden of Disease 28
  Life Expectancy 29
  Hand Hygiene in Healthcare Settings 30
  The Global Burden of Healthcare-Associated Infections 32
  Measuring Healthcare Outcomes 33
  Assessment of Quality of Health Care 35
  Framework for Monitoring Performance of Health Systems 36
  Recent Advances and Innovations in Health Care 38

Healthcare Financing Models........................... 40
Conclusion 42
References... 43

**3 The Evolutionary Developments, Threats
and Opportunities Within the Nigerian Healthcare System**........ 47
Introduction... 47
Critical Milestones in the Development of Western-Style
Healthcare System (1472–2019)........................... 48
The Current State of the Nigerian Health System (2019–2021)....... 56
Health Outcome Indicators.............................. 61
The National Health Insurance Scheme Debacle 62
Present and Future Threats to the Health System................. 67
Opportunities Within the Health System 74
Performance of Health System in African Countries 75
Conclusion 79
References... 80

**4 The Organizational Structure and Leadership
of the Nigerian Healthcare System** 87
Introduction... 87
Operational Definitions................................. 88
Organization Structure of the Federal Ministry of Health 89
Healthcare System Structure.............................. 93
Impact of the Private Sector in Health Service Delivery 96
Conventional Medicine Private Health Care................... 96
Traditional Medicine Private Health Care 98
Management and Leadership of the Health Departments............. 99
Leadership of the Federal Ministry of Health................... 100
The Functions of the Health Minister and Skills Needed
to Be Successful 110
The Controversy Over the Surgeon General Position............... 110
Conclusion 112
References... 113

5 The Vulnerabilities of the Nigerian Healthcare System........... 117
Introduction... 117
Methodology... 118
Health System Vulnerabilities............................. 119
Vulnerability #1: Poor Governance and Ineffective Leadership..... 119
Vulnerability #2: Low-Quality Health Service Delivery 120
Vulnerability #3: Shortage of Healthcare Workforce 124
Vulnerability #4: Paltry Health Systems Financing 127
Vulnerability #5: Limited Access to Essential Medicines
and Vaccines 130
Vulnerability #6: Weak Health Information Systems 133

Major Achievements and Contributions of Nigeria
to Global Health 135
Genesis of Primary Health Care and Itinerant/Community-Based
Physiotherapy Systems 136
Community Health Workers 137
Medical and Surgical Discoveries. 139
How Nigeria Effectively Contained the Spread of Ebola 141
Recent Improvements in Health Outcomes 143
Conclusion 143
References. 144

6　The Spectrum of Complementary and Alternative Medicine 153
Introduction. 153
Classification of Complementary and Alternative
Medicine Systems 154
Distinction Between Complementary and Alternative
Medicine and Integrative Medicine 157
Differences in Treatment Philosophy Between Mainstream
Medicine (Standard Care) and Complementary and Alternative
Medicine 157
　　Complementary Medical Systems 158
　　Alternative Medical Systems 169
Global Demand for the Use of CAM 193
CAM Utilization in the United States. 195
Conclusion 197
Appendix. 198
References. 204

7　Complementary and Alternative Medical Practice in Nigeria 213
Introduction. 213
The Evolution of Complementary and Alternative Medical
Systems in Nigeria 214
Utilization of Complementary and Alternative Medicine
Treatments in Nigeria 217
Acupuncture 220
Chiropractic. 221
Osteopathy 221
Traditional Chinese Medicine. 222
Ayurveda. 223
Naturopathy. 223
Homeopathy 223
Aromatherapy 224
Spirituality. 224
Herbal Medicine 226
Conclusion 228
References. 230

**8   Emerging Developments in Traditional Medicine
      Practice in Nigeria**.   235
      Introduction.   235
      Genesis of Traditional Medicine.   237
      The World Health Organization's Role in Promoting
      Traditional Medicine.   238
      Common Medicinal Plants in Nigeria.   240
      Therapeutic Values of Wild Animal Species.   249
      Major Milestones in the Development of Traditional
      Medicine in Nigeria   251
          Nigerian Traditional Medicine Policy.   251
          National Agency for Food and Drug Administration
          and Control   253
          Nigerian Herbal Pharmacopoeia.   254
          Regulation and Practice of Traditional Medicine in Nigeria   254
      Traditional Medicine Occupations in Nigeria.   256
      Indications for Traditional Medicine   260
      Traditional Medicine Treatment Philosophies   261
      Treatment Approach Utilized by Traditional Medical
      Practitioners in Nigeria.   261
      Challenges in the Development of Traditional Medicine
      in Nigeria   262
      Emerging Training and Practice Trends and the Future
      of Traditional Medicine in Nigeria.   263
      Breakthroughs in Pharmaceutical Products Development   264
      Efficacy of African Traditional Medicine.   266
      Safety of African Traditional Medicine   268
      Conclusion   270
      Referenccs.   270

**9   The Plight of Persons Living with Disabilities:
      The Visible Invisibles in Nigeria**   277
      Introduction.   277
      Types of Disabilities   278
      Classification and Consequences of Disease   279
      Causes of Disabilities   281
      Dimensions and Scope of Disability.   281
      The Burden of Disability in Nigeria.   284
      Challenges of Living with Disabilities in Nigeria   284
      Global Effort to Enhance the Quality of Life of People
      Living with Disabilities.   286
      The Rights of People Living with Disabilities
      and Relevant Protection Laws.   288
      Recommendations to Improve the Quality of Life
      of People Living with Disabilities   289

National Disability Strategy and Action Plan 289
Address Stigma Against PLWDs 289
Address the Barriers in Buildings 290
Address the Barriers of Roads 290
National Policy on Educating Children with Disability 291
Independent Living, Healthcare Access,
and Vocational Training 291
Health System Reforms 292
Training of Healthcare Professionals 292
Overcoming Barriers and Provision of Accommodation
for Adult Students with Learning Disabilities 293
Conclusion 293
References 295

10 A Comparative Analysis of the Health System
of Nigeria and Six Selected Nations Around the World 299
Introduction 299
Operational Definitions 300
Health Systems Performance Indicators 301
Workforce Supply 303
United States 304
United Kingdom 310
South Korea 313
Singapore 315
Taiwan 318
Cuba 321
Comparative Analyses 325
Health Outcome Indices 325
Health Insurance Coverage 329
Health Expenditure 330
Philanthropy 332
Cost of Health Service Delivery 333
Manpower Shortage 335
Health Worker Remuneration 336
Conclusion 337
References 338

11 A Qualitative Investigation of the Barriers to the Delivery
of High-Quality Healthcare Services in Nigeria 345
Introduction 345
Methodology 347
Results 348
Ineffective Leadership 348
Corruption 349
Migration of Professionals Abroad 350

Inadequate Financing 350
Archaic Infrastructures 351
Adulterated Medications...................................... 351
Interprofessional Disputes and Industrial Strikes 352
Discussion.. 353
Conclusion 356
References 357

**12   The Political and Economic Reforms Needed to Achieve
      Universal and High-Quality Health Care in Nigeria**.............. 361
Introduction 362
Developmental Challenges and Budget Priorities 364
Evolution of States in Nigeria 365
Evolution of the Local Government System 369
The Politics of Population Census and Revenue
Allocation Formula... 371
The State of the Nigerian Nation 373
History of Nigeria's Sudden Wealth and the Aftermath
Economic Woes 374
Wasteful Spending and Corruption: Barriers to Universal
and High-Quality Health Care 375
Assets of Wealthy Nigerian Presidents.......................... 381
Who Is Nigeria's Greatest President?............................ 382
The Political Reforms Needed to Achieve Universal
and High-Quality Health Care 384
Authority and Roles of the Federal and State Governments
in the New Dispensation....................................... 385
Economic Reforms Needed to Achieve Universal
and High-Quality Health Care 387
Salaries of the Highest-Paid Heads of Government
and Judiciary Around the World................................ 391
Cost Analysis of the Proposed Economic and Political Reforms...... 392
Lessons from Other Countries 395
Conclusion 396
References 397

**13   Reimagining the Nigerian Healthcare System to Achieve Universal
      and High-Quality Health Care by 2030** 407
Introduction 407
The Pathway to Universal Health Care in Nigeria................. 410
Elect Leaders Committed to Universal Health Care.............. 411
Stifle Corruption 412
Demand for the Implementation of the 2001 Abuja Declaration
Pledge, Supplemented by Innovative Financing Schemes 415
Reform the Informal Sector Economy 419
Eradicate Extreme Poverty 420

The Blueprint for High-Quality Health Care in Nigeria   422
    Merge the University Teaching Hospitals, Federal Medical
    Centers, and Specialist Hospitals in All States..................   423
    Train all Health Care Administrators in Conflict Resolution
    Strategies..   424
    Invest in Electricity and Clean Water   425
    Promote Telehealth and Mobile Health Van for Health
    Services Delivery   426
    Address the High Maternal and Perinatal Death................   426
    Invest in Resources for People Living with Disabilities...........   427
    Slow Down Population Growth   427
    Curtail Industrial Strikes in the Health Sector   428
    Enhance Retention and Tracking of Healthcare Professionals......   429
    Improve Work Conditions....................................   430
    Foster Partnership with Nigerian Healthcare Professionals
    in the Diaspora   435
    Promote the Production of Locally Produced Medical
    Equipment and Pharmaceuticals.............................   436
    Invest in Medical Intelligence and Surveillance Systems
    to Improve Health Information Systems.......................   437
    Update the Curricula of Healthcare Education Academic
    Programs..   438
    Promote Transformative Research to Address Nigeria's
    Unresolved Developmental Health Challenges   439
    Expand Access to Essential Medicines and Vaccines.............   441
    Conclusion   444
    References   445

14 **Nigeria's Health System Response to the COVID-19
    Pandemic and Lessons from Other Countries**....................   455
    Introduction   456
    Assessment of Patient Satisfaction with the Healthcare System   457
        Global   457
        Nigeria..   458
    Management of COVID-19 Crisis in Nigeria: Evaluation
    of Physical Resources and Human Capacity   460
    Nigeria's Health System Response to the COVID-19 Pandemic......   461
    Healthcare Workers at the Frontline of the COVID-19 Crisis   463
    COVID-19 Social Welfare Assistance Program...................   464
    Comparative Analyses   465
        COVID-19 Diagnostic Testing Per Capita
        (1 Million/Population)   465
    COVID-19 Cases and Deaths.................................   465
    The Top Five Countries that Handled the Coronavirus
    Crisis the Best...   468

The Bottom Five Countries that Handled the Coronavirus
Crisis the Worst.   470
COVID-19 Vaccine Development and Therapeutics   475
Conclusion   477
References   478

Index.   483

About the Author

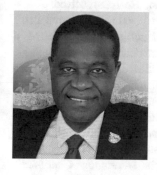 **Joseph Abiodun Balogun, PT, PhD, FACSM, FNSP, FAS, FIMC, FRSPH, FAcadMedS,** is the former dean and retired distinguished professor in the College of Health Sciences at Chicago State University (CSU), Chicago, Illinois, USA. He is also an emeritus professor of physiotherapy; associate director of research development and innovation at the University of Medical Sciences, Ondo City, Nigeria; and visiting professor/program consultant at the Centre of Excellence in Reproductive Health Innovation, University of Benin, Nigeria. Professor Balogun is the founder and president/chief executive officer of Joseph Rehabilitation Center, a social service organization at Tinley Park, Illinois, USA, that provides community-integrated living arrangement services for adults with disabilities.

Professor Balogun obtained his Bachelor of Science (Honors) degree in physiotherapy in 1977 from the University of Ibadan, Nigeria. And earned his master's degree in orthopedic and sports physical therapy (1981) and PhD in exercise physiology (cardiac rehabilitation) with a minor in research methodology from the University of Pittsburgh, Pennsylvania in 1985. He has held full-time and visiting faculty and administrative positions at various universities around the world – Russell Sage College, Troy, New York; Obafemi Awolowo University (OAU), Ile-Ife, Nigeria; University of Florida, Gainesville; Texas Woman's University, Houston; State University of New York Health Science Center at Brooklyn (SUNY-HSCB); Barry University, Florida; and King Saud University, Saudi Arabia. He served for 13 years (1999–2012) at CSU as dean of the College of Health Sciences. He established seven academic programs and the HIV/AIDS Research and Policy Institute to address the disproportionate incidence and complex burdens of HIV/AIDS in minority populations. He also served for six years as chairman of the physical therapy program (1993–1999) and associate dean for student academic affairs (1994–1999) at SUNY-HSCB, consultant physiotherapist (1988–1991), and vice-dean in the Faculty of Health Sciences at OAU (1990–1991).

Professor Balogun has contributed to physical therapy, cardiovascular epidemiology, ergonomics, and HIV behavioral research. He has authored six books, 18 book chapters, monographs, technical compendia, 170 full articles, and 24 peer-reviewed conference abstracts and proceedings. In 2015, he delivered Christopher Ajao's keynote speech at the 55th Annual Conference of the Nigeria Society of Physiotherapy. In 2017, he presented the second Distinguished University Guest Lecture at the University of Medical Sciences, Ondo City, Nigeria, and in 2021 delivered the keynote speech at the inaugural conference of the International Association of Nigerian Physical Therapists.

Professor Balogun is the deputy editor of the *African Journal of Reproductive Health* and serves on the editorial board of the *International Journal of Physiotherapy Theory and Practice*, *Journal of the Nigeria Society of Physiotherapy*, *Kanem Journal of Medical Sciences*, and *International University of Sarajevo (IUS) Law Journal*. He also serves as a consultant and advisory board member at the Women's Health and Action Research Centre (WHARC), Benin City, Nigeria. He has received over a dozen major academic and service awards. In 2003, he received the J. Warren Perry Distinguished Author's Award by the *Journal of Allied Health* and was conferred in 2018 with the Distinguished Decorated Affiliate of the American Health Council. He is a Fellow of the Academy of Medicine Specialties (FAcadMedS), Royal Society for Public Health (FRSPH), Institute of Management Consultants (FIMC), Academy of Science (FAS), Nigeria Society of Physiotherapy (FNSP), and the American College of Sports Medicine (FACSM). Professor Balogun's most recent books include *Healthcare Education in Nigeria: Evolutions and Emerging Paradigms* (Routledge, 2020), *Healthcare Professions in Nigeria: An Interdisciplinary Analysis* (Palgrave Macmillan, 2021), and *Contemporary Obstetrics and Gynecology for Developing Countries -* Co-authored with Okonofua, Odunsi and Chilaka (Springer Nature, 2021).

Abbreviations

ACA	Affordable Care Act
ADL	Activities of Daily Living
AIDS	Acquired Immunodeficiency Syndrome
ART	Antiretroviral Therapy
ARV	Antiretroviral
BHSS	Basic Health Services Scheme
BOD	Burden of Disease
CAGR	Compound Annual Growth Rate
CAM	Complementary and Alternative Medicine
CDC	Centers for Disease Control and Prevention (USA)
CEO	Chief Executive Officer
CHEWs	Community Health Extension Workers
CHF	Congestive Heart Failure
CIA	Central Intelligence Agency (USA)
CMD	Chief Medical Director
COVID-19	Coronavirus Disease 2019
DALY	Disability-Adjusted Life Year
DNA	Deoxyribonucleic Acid
DO	Doctor of Osteopathy
DPT	Doctor of Physiotherapy
ECWA	Evangelical Church of West Africa
EFCC	Economic and Financial Crimes Commission
EIND	Emergency Investigational New Drug
EMRS	Electronic Medical Record Systems
EOCs	Emergency Operation Centers
EUA	Emergency Use Authorization
EVD	Ebola Virus Disease
FDA	Food and Drug Administration (USA)
FMCs	Federal Medical Centers
FMH	Federal Ministry of Health
GBD	Global Burden of Disease

HCAI	Healthcare-Associated Infection
HCPs	Healthcare Professionals
HCWs	Healthcare Workers
HIV	Human Immunodeficiency Virus
HMO	Health Maintenance Organization
HPO	Health Practitioners' Offices
ICIDH	International Classification of Impairments, Disabilities and Handicaps
ICT	Information and Communication Technology
ICUs	Intensive Care Units
IHME	Institute for Health Metrics and Evaluation
IHP	InterCEDD Health Products
IL-6	Interleukin-6
InterCEDD	International Centre for Ethnomedicine and Drug Development
IV	Intravenous
JCHEWs	Junior Community Health Extension Workers
JOHESU	Joint Health Sector Unions
LBP	Low Back Pain
LGAs	Local Government Authorities
LUTH	Lagos University Teaching Hospital
MABs	Monoclonal Antibodies
MD	Doctor of Medicine
MDCAN	Medical and Dental Consultants' Association of Nigeria
MDCN	Medical and Dental Council of Nigeria
MDGs	Millennium Development Goals
MPH	Meritocracy, Pragmatism, and Honesty
MRTB	Medical Rehabilitation Therapists (Registration) Board of Nigeria
NAFDAC	National Agency for Food and Drug Administration and Control
NANTMP	National Association of Nigeria Traditional Medicine Practitioners
NATO	North Atlantic Treaty Organization
NCCIH	National Center for Complementary and Integrative Health
NCDC	Nigeria Centre for Disease Control
NDLEA	National Drug Law Enforcement Agency
NHIS	National Health Insurance Scheme
NHMIS	National Health Management Information System
NIH	National Institutes of Health
NSHDP-II	National Strategic Health Development Plan
NSIA	Nigerian Sovereign Investment Authority
NSP	Nigeria Society of Physiotherapy
NUC	National Universities Commission
OECD	Organisation for Economic Co-operation and Development
OMT	Osteopathic Manipulative Treatment
PHC	Primary Healthcare Center
PLWDs	People Living with Disabilities
POMS	Profile of Mood States

QOL	Quality of Life
RCT	Randomized Controlled Trial
SDGs	Sustainable Development Goals
TB	Tuberculosis
TCM	Traditional Chinese Medicine
TMPs	Traditional Medical Practitioners
UCH	University College Hospital
UDUTH	Usmanu Danfodiyo University Teaching Hospital Sokoto
UHC	Universal Health Care
UNDP	United Nations Development Programme
UNICEF	United Nations Children's Emergency Fund
UNIMED	University of Medical Sciences
UNTH	University of Nigeria Teaching Hospital
USAID	United States Agency for International Development
UTH	University Teaching Hospital
VC	Vice Chancellor
YLD	Years Lived with Disability
YLL	Years of Life Lost

Chapter 1
Introduction

Learning Objectives

After reading this chapter, the learner should be able to:

1. Describe the geography, ethnicity, and dominant religion in Nigeria
2. Discuss income inequality, population growth, and recent economic reforms in Nigeria
3. Contextualize Nigeria's healthcare system
4. Discuss the primary causes of death in Nigeria
5. Articulate the primary issues covered in each of the 14 chapters of this book

Overview of the Nigerian State

Geography and Politics

The Nigerian nation is the secondary focus of the information presented in this pioneering book; therefore, it is appropriate to describe here the topography and current political developments in the country briefly. Nigeria, located in the Gulf of Guinea on the West Coast of Africa, has a landmass of 910,768 km^2, making it twice as large as California in the United States and four times the size of the United Kingdom. It is the most populous country in Africa, and one of every 43 people in the world is Nigerian. Nigeria has a three-tier government (federal, state, and local) constitutionally established, and each tier is autonomous with executive and legislative arms. The federal, state and local governments collectively mobilize and deploy health care resources to their respective jurisdictions. Given its large population and

J. A. Balogun, *The Nigerian Healthcare System*,
https://doi.org/10.1007/978-3-030-88863-3_1

sudden wealth from oil, Nigeria acquired the nickname "the Giant of Africa" under General Yakubu Gowon's administration in the 1970s (Peter, 1987; Ojieh, 2016). Arguably, Nigeria is no longer the "Giant of Africa" but the laughingstock of the world. The most tragic paradox of our time is that Nigeria, in some circles, is considered a failed nation like the Democratic Republic of the Congo, Central African Republic, and Myanmar (National Pivot, 2021, Beaumont, 2021, Campbell & Rotberg, 2021, Kinnan et al., 2011). John Campbell, the former American Ambassador to Nigeria, in a joint article published with political scientist Robert Rotberg in the May 31 2021 edition of *Foreign Affairs* now considers Nigeria a failed state. They opined, "If a state's first obligation to those it governs is to provide for their security and maintain a monopoly on the use of violence, then Nigeria has failed, even if some other aspects of the state still function. Criminals, separatists, and Islamist insurgents increasingly threaten the government's grip on power, as do rampant corruption, economic malaise, and rising poverty". They warned about the long-term negative impact of Nigeria's failure on the neighboring West African countries (Campbell & Rotberg, 2021).

Nigeria has witnessed several kidnappings of innocent citizens in the past decade, particularly in the northern states. For example, on February 26, 2021, armed men abducted 317 girls from the Government Girls Secondary School in Jangebe, in Zamfara state, and killed one police officer during the attack. This particular incident was the second mass abduction within weeks and part of an alarming incident going back to 2014 when Boko Haram - a violent extremist group - abducted 276 girls from a secondary school in Chibok, Borno state. The school was supposedly under the protection of the Nigerian military. The kidnapping is no longer just Boko Haram carrying out the abductions but organized criminal gangs (locally known as bandits) and Fulani herders throughout the country. The government's inability to protect citizens, schools, sea, and land borders, especially in the north, is part of a growing list of government security failures. Inter-ethnic violence is also on the rise. For instance, five people were killed in Ibadan following an altercation in a market between Yorubas and Hausas. The incident sparked a riot, and the market was looted and burned down. The Indigenous Peoples of Biafra, a primarily Christian and Igbo separatist movement, formed an armed militant wing. Similarly, the Eastern Security Network has an ongoing feud with the Buhari government. They claimed the government favors Muslims and against the Muslim Fulani people, whom they accused of attacking the Igbo people. The constant political and economic stresses, lack of progress in the education and health sectors, multiple violent conflicts and insecurity, and the escalated divisive rhetoric by politicians have shifted the political debate from restructuring the nation to the demand for the Biafra Republic and new agitation to create the Oduduwa and the Kwararafa Republics (Ajeluorou, 2020; SaharaReporters, 2021). The multiple campaigns for self-determination reignite the most significant tension and instability of the Nigerian state since independence.

The recent storm in the teapot is the ban of Twitter by the Nigerian government (Blankenship & Golubski, 2021) and the uproar on the barbaric and tyrannical raiding of Sunday Adeyemo Igboho's house, killing several of his aides and destroying properties by federal security agents (Akinkuotu et al. 2021). Both acts taken by President Muhammadu Buhari's administration arose from criticism of his government. Mr. Igboho is a human rights activist, a Yoruba self-determination activist agitating for the freedom of the Southwest region, and a vociferous critic of the Buhari's government. Although criticism is one of the cardinal tenets of democracy, and civil rights organizations worldwide believe the right thing to do is criticize one's country by pointing out its flaws to make it a better place for all citizens. Along this line of thinking, Howard Zinn contends that "dissent is the highest form of patriotism" (Zinn, n.d.). That said, in Nigeria, critics are considered the enemy of the state. President Buhari, in his second term, has two more years before his party faces thevoters again. It's unlikely his government will solve the insecurity issue and the multiple challenges confronting the nation in the short amount of time left in his presidency. The government cannot solve all the problems, but a functioning and accountable security service are critically needed to keep Nigeria stable and growing. After Buhari, the next civilian administration has their job cut out for returning Nigeria back to the glory days. Myprimary goal in this book, particularly in Chaps. 12 and 13, is to critically analyze Nigeria's health system and offer practical recommendations that will invigorate its operations. Hopefully, the government will receive my analysis and critique with good intentions. If policymakers implement many of the prescribed recommendations, they will undoubtedly jump-start the dying healthcare system.

Ethnicity

The sheer size and ethnic complexity of Nigeria present considerable challenges to health policymakers. The population is diverse, with nearly 300 ethnic groups speaking over 500 languages and two primary religious groups (Islam and Christianity).

Almost 70% of the Nigerian population belongs to the four largest ethnic groups – Hausa, Fulani, Yoruba, and Igbo. The Hausa and Fulani people are located primarily in Northern Nigeria and Southern Niger and make up the largest ethnic groups in West Africa. The Hausa language is spoken by around 40 million people, more than any other language in sub-Saharan Africa. The Fulanis are nomads who rear cattle and inhabit many West African countries, including Senegal, Mali, and Burkina Faso – they are a minority in each country they inhabit, except Guinea, where they represent about 40% of the population. The Hausa-Fulani account for about 30% of the Nigerian people. The Yoruba occupy the Southwest and the Southern portion of neighboring Benin and make up about 20% of the Nigerian population. The Yoruba territory was one of Africa's most significant slave-exporting regions during the 1800s, with the largest concentration transported to Cuba, Trinidad, and Brazil. The Yoruba and Igbo peoples from the Bights of Benin and Biafra constituted about one-third of all enslaved Africans in the Americas. The

Igbo people, with a population of about 30 million, live primarily in the Southeast and Cameroon, Sierra Leone, and Equatorial Guinea. In the United States, many of the slaves in Virginia and Maryland were Igbo, and till today constitute a large proportion of the African American population in the region (Ancestry, 2021).

Religion

Apart from Benin and Warri, which came in contact with Christianity through the Portuguese as early as the fifteenth century, most missionaries arrived in the nineteenth century by sea. The Roman Catholics and Anglicans established contact in the Southern region. After World War I, the Church of the Brethren (*Ekklesiyar Yan'uwaa* Nigeria), Seventh-Day Adventists, and others worked in interstitial areas, not to compete directly with other missions. In the nineteenth century, African-American churches engaged in missionary work in Nigeria that lasted well into the colonial period.

Nigeria has the largest number of Muslims and Christians in sub-Saharan Africa; over 80 million Nigerians are Christians. About 50% of Nigerians are Muslim, 40% Christians, and 10% adhere to traditional beliefs. It is estimated that by year 2060, people of the Muslim faith will account for 60% of the country. Presently, Islam dominates the Northern states, and the Yoruba tribe in the Southwest practice Islam, Christianity, and the traditional religions. The Igbo tribe in the Southeast and the Ijaw in the South-south are predominantly Christians (Catholics) and practitioners of traditional religions. The Middle Belt, which contains mostly minority ethnic groups, are mostly Christians, traditional doctrine followers with few Muslim converts.

Economy

Nigeria is regarded as the African powerhouse, arguably the largest economy on the continent. Its gross domestic product (GDP) is worth $410 billion, and the value represents 0.34% of the world economy (Trading Economics, 2020; World Population Review, 2020; The World Bank Group, 2020). As of 2010, agriculture was an essential component of the economy employing about 30% of the population and transformed by commercialization at the small, medium, and large-scale enterprise levels. The major crops include beans, rice, sesame, cashew nuts, cassava, bananas, yams, cocoa beans, groundnuts, gum arabic, palm kernels, palm oil, plantains, kola nut, corn, melon, millet, rice, rubber, sorghum, soybeans. Before the Nigerian civil war, the country was self-sufficient in food until after 1973 but currently does not produce enough food to feed its citizens. A decade ago, groundnut and palm kernel oil were significant agricultural exports, but the shipping of these products to other countries has reduced over the years. A few years back, local companies exported groundnuts, cashew nuts, sesame seeds, moringa seeds, ginger, cocoa, but this trend has also decreased. Bread made from American wheat replaced domestic crops as the cheapest staple food. Between 1980 and 2016, yam production increased from more than five million tons to 44 million tons.

Deterred by years of corruption and mismanagement, the past decade witnessed economic reforms in Nigeria that put the country on track towards achieving its full economic potential. The economy is a middle-income, mixed economy with an emerging market and expanding manufacturing, financial, service, communications, technology, and entertainment sectors. As the dominant economy in Africa, its re-emergent manufacturing sector became the largest on the continent in 2013. It produced the necessary amount of goods and services for the West African region.

Petroleum contributes 75% of Nigeria's revenues, but the production accounts for only about 3% of the global supply compared to Saudi Arabia and Russia, which produces 13%, and the United States which provides 9%. Although government revenues still rely heavily on oil, it remains a small part of the country's overall economy, as it only contributes about 9% to the GDP. In 2011, Citi economist Willem Buiter projected that Nigeria will have the highest average GDP growth globally between 2010 and 2050 and will be one of two African nations among 11 global growth generator countries (Weisenthal, 2011). These projections in 2021 may no longer be realistic given the mismanagement of the country's resources.

In 2018, Nigeria's GDP was $398,186 million, an increase of 1.9% compared to 2017. The absolute value of the GDP rose by $21,825 million compared to 2017. In the same year, the GDP per capita was $2033, $61 less than in 2016, when it was $1972. Over the 10 years from 2008 to 2018, the highest GDP was in 2014 ($568,496 million), and the lowest was in 2009 ($297,458 million). Nigeria's GDP ranked 31st among the top 196 countries globally, and the GDP per capita ranked 147th; the population of Nigeria has a low level of affluence compared to the 196 countries.

Income Inequity

Income inequality is one of Nigeria's most pressing but least discussed challenges. The minimum yearly income required to sustain a healthy living in Nigeria is about $1000 per year in urban areas and about $700 in rural areas – 74% of the citizens live below this yearly income level (Abeeda, 2018). About 86 million live in extreme poverty, while the richest man in the country, Aliko Dangote, earns 8000 times more each day than a poor worker would spend on their basic needs in a year (Akinwotu & Olukoya, 2017).

A study by Oxfam and Development Finance International in 2017 produced a "global index" that placed Nigeria last among 157 countries rated on their commitment to reducing inequality (Oxfam, 2017). Following an analysis of government spending on health, education, and social protection, the report asserts that Nigeria is "shamefully low" and reflected in very poor social outcomes for its citizens. Some technocrats lament that the disparity between the rich and poor in Nigeria, more than poverty itself, generates anti-government sentiment and potentially could fuel civil unrest in the future (Akinwotu & Olukoya, 2017).

Health System

The health system is the primary focus of this book and an overview of the Nigeria's healthcare system will be presented here. Because of its geographical location, malaria is a risk for 97% of the Nigerian population and accounts for more deaths than in any other country in the world. Each year, about 100 million malaria cases and over 300,000 deaths are reported in Nigeria Malaria also contributes to 11% of maternal mortality in the country. The horrific malaria statistics compare with the 215,000 deaths per year from HIV/AIDS. The maternal mortality rate in Nigeria is 814 per 100,000 live birth, which compares with that of Chad (856), Central African Republic (882), and Sierra Leone (1360). It is disheartening that the maternal mortality indices for war-torn Somalia and the Democratic Republic of Congo outperformed Nigeria's. More depressing, Botswana and Mauritius have 100% births attended by skilled practitioners. Nigeria only has 35% which competes with Eritrea, Ethiopia, South Sudan, and Chad in the number of deliveries performed by qualified practitioners. The statistics worsen for every 1000 births in Nigeria; 108 infants (and children) die before five, which is the worst in Africa (United States Embassy in Nigeria, 2011).

Nigeria's population complexity is mirrored by the different health outcomes and health services across the country's six geopolitical zones. The federal government assigns health system responsibilities to the three government levels, each of which is primarily autonomous in management and financing despite national policies that provide a certain standardization measure. Most importantly, poverty—one of the determinants of health outcomes and health service utilization—is widespread. Health inequalities—significant urban-rural disparities and regional equalities— loom large, translating into poor health outcomes and limited access to health services. Weak governance has been a barrier to improving services within the healthcare system. However, over the years, successive governments, both military, and democratic, have developed ineffective healthcare policy plans. The high dependency on oil revenue, poor economic management, and waste have produced volatility and a lack of confidence in public establishments, including the healthcare system (World Bank, 2005).

For decades, Nigeria's health system is inefficient and has one of the worst health outcomes in the world (World Health Organization - WHO - 2000, 2020). Sadly, healthcare spending has never risen to 10% of the gross domestic product, and over 95% of Nigerians have no health insurance (NOIPolls, 2017). Sixty-one years after independence, Nigeria is yet to achieve universal health care (UHC). The health system is weak, and the services are of low quality with inequitable distribution and insufficient infrastructure (WHO, 2000, 2006, 2010, 2015, 2016, 2017). Furthermore, the health system is still confronted with many challenges, including counterfeit medications, medical clinics in hot sweltering conditions without air conditioners, and lack of state-of-the-art medical equipment, among other problems.

The health system is enduring the "double burden" of infectious diseases and non-communicable conditions. Life-threatening contagious diseases have reduced substantially in the last decade, and performance on key health indices slightly improved. Yet, Nigeria failed in 2015 to meet the United Nations' eight Millennium Development Goals (MDGs), ranging from having extreme poverty to halting the spread of HIV/AIDS and providing free primary education by 2015. In January 2016, after the MDGs' successes globally, the United Nations set in motion the 17 sustainable development goals (SDGs) to end poverty by 2030 and ensure that the global community protects the planet and enjoys peace and prosperity.

The 17 SDGs incorporated new interconnected ideas on economic inequality, innovation, climate change, peace, justice, and sustainable consumption; the first goal is eradicating extreme poverty in the world. Regrettably, due to a lack of political will, Nigeria is one of the countries in the world that did not achieve the eight MDGs and has made little or no progress on the 17 SDGs. As a result, poverty in the country is at an all-time high, and malnutrition is still prevalent, with a 43.6% stunting rate. The challenge is complicated further by the environmental pollution and climate challenges that are on the ascendant.

In the last decade, Nigeria's health system has deteriorated further. Sadly, solutions to the disease burden are not in sight as the successive governments have no coherent national health policy. In 2016, President Muhammadu Buhari's government launched a plan to achieve 30% health insurance coverage by 2020. Unfortunately, this goal did not materialize, and the health system is presently on life support. The overwhelming consensus of health analysts and scholars is that the system is in a crisis state and needs urgent intervention. Given the above inadequacies, Nigeria is unlikely to meet the SDGs by 2030 unless some drastic interventions are taken to address these critical challenges.

Overview of the Chapters

The United Nation's sustainable development goal number three *(SDG 3)* sets an aspiration to achieve UHC for all men and women worldwide by 2030. In addition to UHC, *SDG 3* proposes, among other things, to end the preventable death of newborns, infants, and children under five (child mortality) and end epidemics (UN, 2015; Global Compact, 2021). This book provides a blueprint on how Nigeria can achieve UHC by 2030 as recommended by the *United Nations*.

This groundbreaking publication begins with an introductory section that provides an overview of the contents of the book. Chapter 2 lays the foundation for the various topical issues addressed and examines the primary determinants of good health and the differences between health equity, health disparities, or inequities. The chapter also discusses the causes of health inequalities, appraises Grossman's health demand model, describes the relationship between health and development, the global burden of healthcare-associated infection, and the new guidelines for healthcare workers' hand hygiene. It concludes by describing the outcome indicators used for evaluating health systems' performance and recent advances and innovations in health care.

Chapter 3 describes the critical milestones in developing a Western-style health system in Nigeria from 1472 to the contemporary era, including why UHC has been elusive for over 60 years. The chapter also identifies the present and future threats and opportunities within the health system and compared the Nigerian health system's performance with other African countries. Chapter 4 analyses the organizational structure of the Federal Ministry of Health vis-à-vis the health system structure, the impact of the private sector in health services delivery, and the health system's leadership, including the debate surrounding the Surgeon General's position. The chapter also investigated the widely held perception that physicians and men dominate the health system's leadership worldwide, including Nigeria.

Chapter 5 examines the factors that make universal health care unattainable in Nigeria. Secondly, it discusses the challenges facing the effective delivery of high-quality health care in the country. The analyses identified five key factors that forestall the implementation of universal health care: Despite the health system's vulnerabilities, it is not all doom and gloom, as Nigeria has meaningfully contributed to global health in several areas. This chapter also discusses these historical contributions in primary health care, itinerant/community-based physiotherapy services, containment of the Ebola virus, and medical and surgical discoveries.

During the past decade, interest in complementary and alternative medicine has surged, and the global public attitude about these modalities has been positive. The clinical effectiveness of these methods remain controversial because advocates make several claims; however, researchers do not know how safe they are and how well they work. Chapter 6 introduces the primary complementary and alternative medicine modalities, which are currently gaining popularity worldwide. The chapter also discusses the origin, treatment philosophy, therapeutic efficacy, and safety of acupuncture, chiropractic, osteopathy, traditional Chinese medicine, Ayurveda, naturopathy, homeopathy, aromatherapy, and spirituality.

Chapter 7 traces the origin of complementary and alternative medical practices within the Nigerian health system. It also describes the evolving developments of three complementary medical systems—acupuncture, chiropractic, and osteopathy—and seven alternative medical systems such as traditional Chinese medicine, Ayurveda, naturopathy, homeopathy, aromatherapy, spirituality, and African traditional medicine.

Some scholars argued that the process of modernization in Africa is intrinsically linked to Europeans' arrival, particularly in the areas of health care and democracy. Chapter 8 chronicles the origin and evolutionary developments and challenges associated with traditional medicine in Nigeria. The chapter also examines the traditional medicine occupations, including their treatment philosophies and treatment approaches. Finally, the chapter analyses the emerging trends and future of traditional medicine in Nigeria, including breakthroughs in pharmaceutical product development, efficacy, and safety of traditional medical practice.

Disability is a component of the human condition, and many disabilities are not visible. In Nigeria, people living with disabilities are often stigmatized and excluded from the larger society's social, economic, and political affairs. In describing the unsatisfactory situation, one analyst referred to persons with disabilities in Nigeria as "visible but invisible people." Chapter 9 explores the challenges of living with disabilities in Nigeria, the relevant protection laws, the global effort to enhance the quality of life of people living with disabilities, including learning accommodation for students with disabilities.

Chapter 10 identifies the nations with stellar health systems worldwide that Nigeria can emulate to revitalize its dying health system. After an exhaustive review of the literature, six countries—United States, United Kingdom, Singapore, South Korea, Taiwan, and Cuba—were identified for in-depth evaluation and comparative analysis on several health outcomes. The exposition revealed Cuba's health system is the best adaptable and fit to improve Nigeria's health system.

Many reviews and critique articles on the Nigerian healthcare system have been published, but there is limited research on the system's challenges. A qualitative investigation presented in Chap. 11 uncovered the barriers to delivering affordable and high-quality healthcare services. The recurrent shared views expressed by 15 healthcare professionals interviewed include ineffective leadership, corruption, lack of modern infrastructure, adulterated medications, inadequate funding, migration of professionals abroad, interprofessional disputes, and industrial strikes.

Chapter 12 provides the political and economic reforms needed to achieve universal and high-quality health care. Chapter 13 presents the roadmap for universal health insurance coverage and offers a blueprint for attaining high-quality health care. The recommendations are in two parts. Part I proposes the reforms needed to achieve universal health care, and Part II discusses the blueprint to achieve the goal.

The year 2020 started peacefully in many parts of the world, except in the Republic of China. Suddenly, on March 11, 2020, the World Health Organization (WHO) characterizes coronavirus disease 2019 (COVID-19) as a pandemic (WHO, 2020). Then, suddenly the COVID-19 crisis exposes the weaknesses and fragilities of the global health systems. Eleven months into the COVID-19 pandemic, many nations' health systems were overwhelmed and their leaders mismanaged the situation. The writing of this book was near completion when the COVID-19 pandemic struck. The manuscript concluded on January 17, 2021, at the pandemic's peak worldwide. On that date, there were 94,759,289 COVID-19 cases and 2,026,617 deaths globally. Many of the countries with stellar health systems did not manage the crisis effectively.

Chapter 14 sets out to determine the lessons Nigeria can learn from other countries worldwide that managed the COVID-19 crisis effectively. The chapter analyses the literature on patient satisfaction with healthcare systems worldwide and in Nigeria and identified the top five countries with the lowest and highest number of fatalities from coronavirus, and examined their COVID-19 preventive strategies. Additionally, the chapter examines the surveillance and laboratory testing capabilities available in the country to curb emerging diseases, the health system response to the COVID-19 pandemic, the challenges facing healthcare workers at the front-line of the crisis, and the Nigerian government's social welfare assistance programs. Finally, the chapter discusses COVID-19 vaccine developments and therapeutics.

Competition and Conclusion

Twelve books on the Nigerian healthcare system have been published within the last decade. However, none focus on universal and high-quality health care, which is the primary theme of this work. Five of the 12 books were published by non-peer-reviewed vanity presses. Two of them were on Nigerian health system challenges (Mcdikkoh, 2010 – *Xlibris.com*; Brown, 2018 – *Ola Brown*), and the others were on the infrastructure challenges within the Nigerian health system (Nnadi, n.d. – *Xlibris.com*), history of dentistry (Ogunbodede, 2015 – *Foundation for Dental Education Museums and Archives*) and primary health care (Chimezie, 2015 – *Outskirts Press*).

Additionally, seven existing books on Nigeria's health system were released by highly reputable peer-reviewed academic publishers (see publishers ranking list in The Education, 2021). They include Nigeria's health care education (Balogun, 2020 – *Routledge*) and interdisciplinary analysis of the health professions (Balogun, 2021 – *Palgrave Macmillan*), contemporary obstetrics and gynecology practice (Okonofua et al., 2021 – *Springer Nature*), health care and economic restructuring (Aka & Balogun, 2022, 2021 – *Palgrave Macmillan*), Nigerian medicinal plants and their therapeutic values (Adodo & Iwu, 2020 – *Routledge*), Nigeria's health system outcomes compared with several other countries around the world (Johnson et al., 2018 – *Jones & Bartlett Learning*), and evaluation of primary healthcare programs in four Nigerian states (World Bank, 2010 – *World Bank Publications*). This seminal treatise published by Springer Nature discusses several of the aforementioned topics and more – thus, it exemplifies the book's comprehensiveness and innovation.

Case Study
1. What is the stated mission of your Health Institution/Faculty/College?
2. Investigate the history of your Health Institution/Faculty/College and discuss its contributions to your community, state, and the nation.
3. What is the current ranking of your university nationally and internationally?
4. What is the current ranking of your Health Institution/Faculty/College with peer institutions nationally?
5. What poses an existential threat to the future of your Health Institution/Faculty/College?

References

Abeeda. (2018). *Nigeria's wealth disparity situation is only getting worse.* [online]. Available at: http://affinitymagazine.us/2018/05/16/nigerias-wealth-disparity-situation-is-only-getting-worse/. Accessed 14 July 2021.

Adodo, A., & Iwu, M. M. (2020). Healing plants of Nigeria: Ethnomedicine and therapeutic applications. *Routledge.* [online]. Available at: https://www.routledge.com/Healing-Plants-of-Nigeria-Ethnomedicine-and-Therapeutic-Applications/Adodo-Iwu/p/book/9781138339828. Accessed 18 May 2021.

Aka, P., & Balogun, J. A. (2021). *Healthcare and economic restructuring: Nigeria in comparative perspective.* Palgrave Macmillan.

Akinwotu, E., & Olukoya, S. (2017). *Shameful Nigeria: A country that doesn't care about inequality.* [online]. Available at: https://www.theguardian.com/inequality/2017/jul/18/shameful-nigeria-doesnt-care-about-inequality-corruption. Accessed 14 July 2021.

Ancestry. (2021). *Discover your ethnic origins with one simple test.* [online]. Available at: https://www.ancestry.com/dna/ethnicity/nigeria. Accessed 14 July 2021.

Balogun, J. A. (2020). Healthcare education in Nigeria: Evolutions and emerging paradigms. *Routledge.* [online]. Available at: https://www.routledge.com/Healthcare-Education-in-Nigeria-Evolutions-and-Emerging-Paradigms/Balogun/p/book/9780367482091. Accessed 18 May 2021.

Balogun, J. A. (2021). Health professions in Nigeria: An interdisciplinary analysis. *Palgrave Macmillan.* [online]. Available at: https://www.palgrave.com/gp/book/9789811633102. Accessed 14 July 2021.

Brown, O. (2018). Fixing healthcare in Nigeria: A guide to some of the key policy decisions that will provide better healthcare to all Nigerians. *Ola Brown – Vanity Press.* [online]. Available at: https://www.dropbox.com/s/g8a2m2n49wlavui/Fixing%20Nigeria%20(2). Accessed 18 May 2021.

Chimezie, R. O. (2015). Primary healthcare in Nigeria: Overview, challenges, and prospects. *Outskirts Press – Vanity Press.* [online]. Available at: https://www.amazon.com/Primary-Healthcare-Nigeria-Challenges-Prospects/dp/1478743689. Accessed 18 May 2021.

Global Compact. (2021). *UHC2030's mission is to create a movement for accelerating equitable and sustainable progress towards universal health coverage (UHC).* [online]. Available at: https://www.uhc2030.org/our-mission/; https://www.uhc2030.org/fileadmin/uploads/uhc2030/Documents/About_UHC2030/mgt_arrangemts___docs/UHC2030_Official_documents/UHC2030_Global_Compact_WEB.pdf. Accessed 27 May 2021.

Johnson, J. A., Stoskopf, C., & Shi, L. (2018). Comparative health system (2nd ed). *Jones & Bartlett Learning.* [online]. Available at: https://www.jblearning.com/catalog/productdetails/9781284111736?%20utm_term=&utm_campaign=All%20Strategic%20Products%20(HI)%20-%20NTV&utm_source=adwords&utm_medium=ppc&hsa_acc=6959852188&hsa_cam=12449043532&hsa_grp=115744959982&hsa_ad=501771825996&hsa_src=g&hsa_tgt=pla898606414745&hsa_kw=&hsa_mt=&hsa_net=adwords&hsa_ver=3&gclid=CjwKCAjw1uiEBhBzEiwAO9B_HQqz46Z_2adieVVtIJLNf6nyTLAQeXnBke2RpxwQvtiYkkP6ItE53xoCEF8QAvD_BwE. Accessed 18 May 2021.

Mcdikkoh, D. M. N. (2010). The Nigerian health system's debacle and failure! *Xlibris Corporation. www.Xlibris.com – Vanity Press* [online]. Available at: https://www.amazon.com/Nigerian-Health-Systems-Debacle-Failure/dp/1450021042?asin=1450021042&revisionId=&format=4&depth=1. Accessed 17 July 2021.

Nnadi, A. O. (n.d.). Distribution of resources in the Nigerian health care system: Ethical considerations and proposals applying Catholic social teaching. *www.Xlibris.com – Vanity Press* [online]. Available at: https://books.apple.com/gb/book/distribution-resources-in-nigerian-health-care-system/id1495761184. Accessed 20 May 2021.

NOIPolls. (2017). *Emigration of Nigerian medical doctors: Survey report.* [online]. Available at: https://noi-polls.com/2018/wp-content/uploads/2019/06/Emigration-of-Doctors-Press-Release-July-2018-Survey-Report.pdf; https://noi-polls.com/new-survey-reveals-8-in-10-nigerian-doctors-are-seeking-work-opportunities-abroad/. Accessed 10 Oct 2020.

Ojieh, C. O. (2016). *Extraneous considerations to the personality variables in foreign policy decision-making: Evidence from Nigeria.* [online]. Available at: https://escholarship.org/content/qt4pt5j44w/qt4pt5j44w_noSplash_3c8081fdb56a996ade1cf16fbb323c69.pdf. Accessed 18 Jan 2021.

Ogunbodede, E. O. (2015). History of dentistry in Nigeria. *Foundation for Dental Education Museums and Archives – Vanity Press,* Ilesa Road, Ife Bus stop, PMB 011, OAU Post-office, Ife.

Okonofua, F. E., Balogun, J. A., Odunsi, K., & Chilaka, V. N. (2021). Contemporary obstetrics and gynecology for developing countries. *Springer Nature.* [online]. Available at: https://www.springer.com/gp/book/9783030753849. Accessed 14 July 2021.

Oxfam. (2017). *What is your country doing to fight inequity? The commitment to reducing inequality (CRI) index.* [online]. Available at: https://www.inequalityindex.org/#/. Accessed 14 July 2021.

Peter, H. (1987). *Nigeria giant of Africa.* London: Swallow Editions. 1987and 1985. [online]. Available at: https://www.worldcat.org/title/nigeria-giant-of-africa/oclc/19060960. Accessed 20 May 2021.

The Education. (2021). *Ranking list of academic book publishers.* [online]. Available at: https://studylib.net/doc/18373359/ranking-list-of-academic-book-publishers. Accessed 20 May 2021.

Trading Economics. (2020). *Nigeria GDP: 1960–2019 Data | 2020–2022 Forecast | Historical | Chart | News.* [online]. Available at: https://tradingeconomics.com/nigeria/gdp. Accessed 23 Jan 2020.

UN. (2015). *The 17 sustainable development goals (SDGs) Department of Economic and Social Affairs Sustainable Development).* [online]. Available at: https://sdgs.un.org/goals. Accessed 27 May 2021.

United States Embassy in Nigeria. (2011). *Nigeria malaria fact sheet.* [online]. Available at:https://photos.state.gov/libraries/nigeria/231771/Public/December-MalariaFactSheet2.pdf. Accessed 4 April 2021.

Weisenthal, J. (2011). *Forget the BRICS: Citi's Willem Buiter presents the 11 "3G" countries that will win in the future.* [online]. Available at: https://www.businessinsider.com/willem-buiter-3g-countries-2011-2?slop=1https://en.wikipedia.org/wiki/Economy_of_Nigeria. Accessed 23 Jan 2020.

World Bank. (2005). Nigeria: Health, nutrition, and population, country status report, Volume 2, Main Report. Washington, DC. *World Bank Publications.* [online]. Available at: http://hdl.handle.net/10986/8804. Accessed 23 Jan 2020.

World Bank. (2010). Improving primary health care delivery in Nigeria: Evidence from four states. World Bank Africa Region Health Systems for Outcomes Program. *World Bank Publications.* [online]. Available at: https://play.google.com/store/books/details/World_Bank_Improving_Primary_Health_Care_Delivery?id=_IL8M5Ems38C. Accessed 18 May 2021.

WHO. (2000). *The world health organization's ranking of the world's health systems, by rank.* [online]. Available at: https://photius.com/rankings/world_health_systems.html. Accessed 10 Oct 2020.

WHO. (2006). The world health report. In *Working Together for Health* (pp. 1–15). World Health Organization.

WHO. (2010). *Monitoring the building blocks of health systems: A handbook of indicators and their measurement strategies.* [online]. Available at: https://www.who.int/healthinfo/systems/monitoring/en/. Accessed 10 Oct 2020.

WHO. (2015). *World health statistics. Part I: Global health indicators.* [online]. Available at: https://www.who.int/gho/publications/world_health_statistics/EN_WHS2015_Part2.pdf. Accessed 10 Oct 2020.

WHO. (2016). *Global health observatory (GHO) data: World health statistics 2016: Monitoring health for the SDGs.* [online]. Available at: https://www.who.int/gho/publications/world_health_statistics/2016/en/. Accessed 10 Oct 2020.

WHO. (2017). *World Bank and WHO: Half the world lacks access to essential health services, 100 million still pushed into extreme poverty because of health expenses.* [online]. Available at: https://www.who.int/news-room/detail/13-12-2017-world-bank-and-who-half-the-world-lacks-access-to-essential-health-services-100-million-still-pushed-into-extreme-poverty-because-of-health-expenses. Accessed 10 Oct 2020.

WHO. (2020). *Rolling updates on coronavirus disease (COVID-19)*. [online]. Available at: https://www.who.int/emergencies/diseases/novel-coronavirus-2019/events-as-theyhappen. Accessed 18 Jan 2021.

World Population Review. (2020). *Nigeria Population 2020*. [online]. Available at: [online]. Available at: https://worldpopulationreview.com/countries/nigeria-population/. Accessed 23 Jan 2020.

The World Bank Group. (2020). *Nigeria*. [online]. Available at: https://data.worldbank.org/country/nigeria. Accessed 10 Oct 2020.

Chapter 2
The Fundamentals of Health Care

Learning Objectives

After reading this chapter, the learner should be able to:

1. Explain the meaning of health
2. Discuss the primary determinants of good health
3. Discern the differences between health equity, health disparities, or inequities
4. Argue the causes of inequalities in health
5. Appraise Grossman's model of health demand and Donabedian model for quality of health care
6. Describe the relationship between health and development
7. Discuss the global access to health care
8. Analyze the Health in All Policies advocated by the World Health Organization (WHO)
9. Compare and contrast life expectancy in Nigeria and the United States
10. Explain the concept of burden of disease and the global burden of healthcare-associated infections
11. Articulate why hand hygiene is critical to minimize nosocomial healthcare-associated infections in the COVID-19 era and discuss the strategies to improve adherence to institutional guidelines
12. Appraise the WHO's framework for evaluating the performance of health systems
13. Describe recent advances and innovations in health care
14. Discuss the different healthcare financing methods

© The Author(s), under exclusive license to Springer Nature Switzerland AG 2021
J. A. Balogun, *The Nigerian Healthcare System*,
https://doi.org/10.1007/978-3-030-88863-3_2

Introduction

Health care promotes health through diagnosis, treatment, and prevention of diseases and individuals' impairments across the life span. Healthcare professionals and supportive occupations deliver healthcare services in primary, secondary, and tertiary care settings. Social and economic conditions influence individual access to health care and are determined by national policies on insurance coverage, transportation, and paid time off work privileges. Consequently, they vary across nations, communities, and geographical locations. Limitations to healthcare services negatively affect medical and rehabilitation services, treatments' efficacy, and overall health outcomes such as morbidity and mortality rates.

This chapter lays the foundation for the various topical issues discussed in this book focused on the Nigerian healthcare system. First, it examines the meaning of health, differences between health equity, health disparities, and health inequities, including the primary determinants of good health. Second, the chapter appraises Grossman's health demand model, Donabedian model for quality of health care, Health in All Policies advocated by the World Health Organization, and the United Nations' developmental goals. Third, the chapter introduces the disease burden concept and discusses the global burden of healthcare-associated infections, hand hygiene, and the new guidelines for healthcare workers' hand hygiene. The chapter also compares life expectancy in Nigeria with the United States. Finally, it discusses the healthcare outcome indicators, the World Health Organization's framework for evaluating health systems performance, healthcare financing methods, and recent advances and innovations in health care.

What Is Health?

Health is the most critical of all things and the foundation of all happiness surrounding human beings. The importance of good health cannot be overemphasized because it is a crucial determinant of an individual's socioeconomic development, and therefore the discussion of healthcare is blighted with politics. Nigeria's healthcare system has been in turmoil for decades; therefore, it is not surprising that it has not attained its full economic potential. At the cellular level, health is the level of metabolic efficiency of a living organism. At the functional or practical level, the World Health Organization (WHO) defined health as the "state of complete physical, mental, and social well-being and not merely the absence of disease or infirmity" (WHO Constitution, 1948). This definition has been criticized for lacking operational value and for using the word "complete." An alternate definition that correlates health and personal satisfaction has been proposed. The new definition considers health as the individual's or community's ability to adapt and self-manage when facing physical, mental, or social challenges.

Good health is central to human existence and the ability to handle stress and live a long and productive life. Good health consists of seven major components:

physical, emotional, social, mental, spiritual, environmental, and reproductive (Sampson & Felman, 2020; Institute for Integrative Nutrition, 2021). *Physical health* refers to the ways and means of pursuing a healthy lifestyle that will decrease the risk of chronic lifestyle diseases, maintain physical fitness, eat a balanced diet, and avoid drug and alcohol use (Fig. 2.1). *Emotional health* entails expressing one's emotions in a constructive, nondestructive way. An emotionally healthy person can cope well with unpleasant feelings and stresses and not get overwhelmed by them. *Social health* is the quality of a person's relationship and support from friends, family, peers, supervisors, and other people within the community: respect other people, express the need to other people, have supportive relationships, and stay away from individuals who are condescending and intolerant.

Mental health is the ability to be in tune with reality and cope with daily life stressors, free of mental disease (e.g., phobia). *Spiritual health* maintains cordial relationships with peers and lives according to morality, religion, ethics, and strong values and ideals. Environmental health is the capacity to keep the air and water clean, food, and land around safe. *Reproductive health* implies having satisfying and safe sex life vis-à-vis the rights to make crucial choices about family welfare, procreative decisions, and being able to set future conceptive goals.

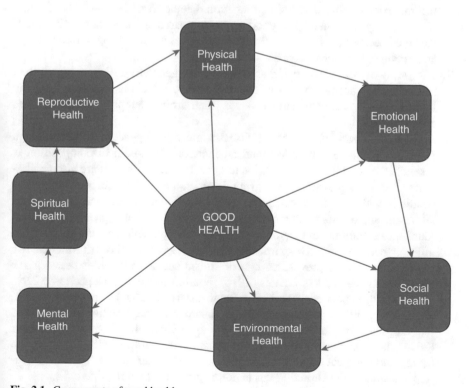

Fig. 2.1 Components of good health

Determinants of Health

Health and education have a synergistic effect on one another. Adults with higher education tend to live healthier and have higher life expectancy than their less-educated peers. In addition, education is the most impactful of the many social determinants of health (geography and demographic factors such as age, gender, and race ethnicity). Studies have shown that educational attainment (particularly of the mother) is a significant predictor of health outcomes in developing countries. Moreover, in high-income countries, economic trends have intensified the relationship between education and health (Zimmerman & Woolf, 2014).

Health is an essential component of being human, and the ability to thrive as a nation is intricately linked to citizens' overall health. Sound health is a central determinant of human happiness, and well-being and good health contribute to economic progress. Effective health systems are a marker of a fair and just society, and in many countries, the health sector is the top employer of labor (American Medical Association, 2015). The following critical factors are determinants of good health for an individual:

1. *Social and economic factors*: They are reflected by social support and positive relationship networks, education, literacy, employment/working conditions, income, social status, and resident location. People from the upper social strata of the society are generally in good health compared to the economically disadvantaged because they have the financial resources to provide optimum nutrition and obtain the best health care.
2. The *physical environment*: Urban dwellers are generally in better health than rural dwellers because they are less exposed to infectious diseases from the immediate environment and because their water supply is usually less contaminated.
3. *Biological characteristics*: Many diseases are linked genetically and pass on from generation to generation, and an individual's biological composition is essential for good health. In addition to genetics, many diseases are also gender-linked. For example, autism spectrum disorder, a complex neurodevelopmental condition with lifelong impacts, has been attributed to genetic and environmental factors and occurs in all racial, ethnic, and socioeconomic groups. It is about four times commoner among boys than girls are. Epidemiological research from different parts of the world, particularly in Asia, Europe, and North America, has reported an average prevalence rate of autism spectrum disorder between 1% and 2%. Chinawa and associates (2016) reported autism prevalence to be 2.9% among children between 3 and 18 in Southeastern Nigeria. In the United States, one in every 59 children has an autism disorder. Some scientists now contend that the scheduling of vaccines may have unanticipated consequences. Hooker (2014) attributes the high incidence of autism in the United States, in part, to the timing and compact duration of immunization (Hooker, 2014). The immunization schedule in the United States is more aggressive than in Nigeria.

4. *Lifestyle and behaviors*: Personal health practices, cultural beliefs, and coping skills are predictive of many debilitating chronic diseases such as obesity, diabetes, and heart disease. For example, a healthy balanced diet high in fiber but low in cholesterol with moderate physical activity or exercise will prevent many of the aforementioned chronic diseases. In addition, managing stress levels, getting 7–9 hours of sleep per night, reducing alcohol intake, and avoiding smoking are essential lifestyle behaviors that determine good health.
5. *Healthy child development*: Children born with a developmental disability ranging from mild disabilities, such as speech and language impairments, to severe disabilities, intellectual retardation, cerebral palsy, and autism, can live a productive life in an environment where medical rehabilitation services are readily available, but their quality of life is substantially impaired even in the best of circumstances.
6. *Access to quality health care: The opportunity* to have annual screening for diseases can lead to early detection and better treatment outcomes.

Health Equity

Health equity implies that every person in the population has a fair opportunity to live a long, healthy life and has equal access and the right to affordable health care. It is morally vital that citizens' health is not compromised or disadvantaged because of social, economic, and environmental factors. Achieving health equity requires creating fair opportunities and eliminating gaps in health outcomes between different social groups. Attainment of health equity status also needs addressing challenges outside of the healthcare system to improve and create opportunities for an excellent school system, efficient transportation, housing, and agriculture sectors.

Equal healthcare access for every citizen in need requires both economic and political input. Moreover, any nation's economic power plays a crucial role in financing the health system and detecting diseases. Screening programs, research funding, provision of adequate, updated infrastructure, and access to these facilities are necessary for a comprehensive health system. Inadequate healthcare financing is a crucial hurdle in providing universal healthcare coverage (UHC) to citizens in developing countries, including Nigeria.

Health Disparities and Health Inequalities

Health disparities are the differences observed between population groups in the presence of disease, health outcomes, or access to health care. Conversely, health inequities are unfair health differences that adversely affect groups of people and are often linked closely to social, economic, or environmental disadvantages. Health inequities are the observable differences in health that are avoidable, unfair, and unjust.

Health inequities are rooted in social injustices that make some population groups more vulnerable to poor health than other groups. Knowing what causes health differences among people from different social and economic backgrounds is essential to understand health inequity. Social inequality occurs when people are treated unequally based on race, gender, class, sexual orientation, and immigration status. Institutions such as corporations and schools have the power to create different opportunities based on social status. Unequal opportunities can cause poor educational outcomes with fewer job opportunities and economic (income) disadvantages. In addition, the location and environment where we live is a determinant of unequal health. For example, living in a neighborhood polluted with chemical hazards, radiation from a power plant, high crime and violence rate, and limited access to healthy nutrition (natural food/vegetables) will hurt a person's life.

In the United States, male babies are heavier at birth than females. This situation is a case of health disparity. While birth weight between female and male babies may vary, the difference is unavoidable and rooted in genetics. On the contrary, children of mothers from low socioeconomic backgrounds and rural dwellers in their first year of life are more likely to die than children of wealthy mothers or affluent urbanites. Poverty is responsible for some of the differences. A higher percentage of rural dweller mothers in Nigeria are impoverished and face unnecessary hardships that can affect their health.

Socioeconomic factors are a strong determinant of health. For example, the poor often lack proper education, which invariably affects their ability to make a sound judgment about health treatment and the choices about where they live. In addition, they find themselves in squalid living and working environments, which breed various disease vectors that affect mental health. For these reasons, poor people are needier and far more prone to produce higher healthcare costs (Adeyanju et al., 2017).

In sub-Saharan Africa, health outcomes and access to critical health services are uneven across the different countries and ethnic groups in each nation. Poverty and access to healthcare services are substantial development challenges on the continent. Health has a considerable impact on earning capacity and productivity; it affects educational performance, determines employment prospects, and is fundamental to life quality.

The combined wealth of the five richest Nigerians—tagged at $29.9 billion—is large enough to end extreme poverty in the country, yet five million face pangs of hunger. More than 112 million Nigerians live in poverty, and the wealthiest Nigerian would have to spend about $one million a day for the next 42 years to exhaust his fortune. The amount of money he earns annually from his wealth is sufficient to uplift two million people out of poverty for 1 year. Nigerian women represent 60–79% of the rural labor force but are five times less likely than men to own land and estates. Besides, women are less likely to have a decent education. Over 75% of the poorest women have never been to school, and 94% are illiterate (Oxfam International, 2020). Women and children from socioeconomically disadvantaged backgrounds have higher morbidity and mortality rates and lower health coverage than wealthier upbringing.

The travel distance impacts healthcare access to a health facility, but socioeconomic and cultural factors are more dominant in access to service delivery for individuals and within nations (Chukwudozie, 2015). For example, in Nigeria, 56% of Nigerian women in 2017 had some financial barriers in accessing the healthcare system, while 33% had a physical challenge (Adeyanju et al., 2017). Similarly, in the United States, the health of black and white mothers and babies of mothers from the same socioeconomic background are different. Many scientists attribute the difference in health status to racism experienced by black women. Racism creates stress, and a high level of pressure and fear creates a risk for mothers and babies. This situation is health inequity because the difference between the groups is unfair, avoidable, and rooted in social injustice. Healthcare and public health policies directly affect health services, health insurance, and prevention (screening for specific diseases and immunization) programs.

In contrast, social policies may indirectly affect health by influencing social or economic outcomes (including income, education, employment, housing, marriage). Since social and economic factors are also causes of health, they, in turn, can affect health. Osypuk and associates (2014) assert that the extent to which social policies influence health is an empirical question. Equity in health care occurs when *resources are provided according to the population's needs,* irrespective of social status or a more significant disease burden. Equal access to health care for everyone in need requires both economic and political input. The economic power of any nation plays a crucial role in financing the health system and detecting diseases. Screening programs, research funding, provision of adequate, updated infrastructure and access to these facilities are necessary for a comprehensive health system. Inadequate health financing is one of the crucial obstacles in the eradication of diseases in developing countries.

Socioeconomic factors are a strong determinant of health. The economically disadvantaged often lack proper education, which invariably affects their ability to make a sound judgment about health treatment and the choices about where they live. They find themselves in squalid living and working environments, which breed an assortment of disease vectors and impact mental health. For these reasons, poor people are needier and far more prone to produce higher healthcare costs. In most nations around the world, there is an income disparity. For example, the wealthiest 10% of South Africans have 47% of all income, while the lowest 10% have 0.2% of all income, one of the world's most exceptional income disparity levels (Ranchod, 2016).

In 2010, 62% of Nigerians lived on less than $1.25 a day, and most Nigerians live under the global poverty level (WHO, 2007). The inability to access health care under this social condition is problematic and a significant public health problem. Ichoku and associates (2013) put these alarming statistics into stark reality when they revealed that, on average, it costs $10 to treat an episode of malaria, a very commonplace scourge in West Africa. Health financing is an essential bridge in closing inequality gaps within any economy, and a functional health insurance system is critical to ensuring access to health services within the population (Adeyanju et al., 2017).

Health in All Policies

The need for an inter-sectoral approach or collaboration is vital to improve the health of the population. The Health in All Policies advocated by WHO and approved in 2013 in Helsinki, Finland, is an approach to developing public policies across sectors by systematically considering the health implications of decisions, seeking synergies, and improving population health and health equity to avoid harmful health impacts. As a concept, the Health in All Policies promotes transparency, access to information, sustainability, participation, and collaboration across the private sectors (WHO, 2017a). Similarly, the government should promote the program and bear responsibility for citizens' and health authorities' health. Thus, they should actively seek partnerships with donor organizations (multilateral, bilateral, regional, etc.) to provide significant support for health and development outcomes.

The impact of the Health in All Policies has several dimensions and stakeholders. One in eight deaths is associated with air pollution exposure – mostly from heart and lung disease and stroke. To address air pollution, the Federal Ministry of Health cannot act alone but must collaborate with other organizations. Examples of such collaboration include the following:

1. The energy companies must provide clean cooking, heating, and state-of-the-art lighting technologies in the homes and educate consumers about adopting clean fuels (liquid gas, ethanol), avoiding coal and kerosene use in the house, and cooking in areas with adequate ventilation.
2. The Department of Transportation must prioritize urban transit, walking, cycling networks in cities, so there is less reliance on vehicles. It works to shift technologies to heavy-duty cleaner vehicles and low-emissions vehicles and fuels, including fuels with reduced sulfur and particle content. Urban planning must make cities more compact and energy-efficient.
3. Homeowners and property owners must be encouraged to improve buildings' energy efficiency through healthy and affordable construction standards. Also, consumers must increase the use of low-emission fuels and renewable combustion.
4. The federal government must promote accessible power sources such as wind, hydropower and adopt cogeneration of power using mini-grids and rooftop solar power generation. It must reduce reliance on wood, diesel, and coal generators and protect against deforestation, occupational risks from coal mining, and fumes from the combustion of dirty fuels to protect the environment.
5. Waste Management Boards must invest in recycling, waste reprocessing, and improve biological waste management to produce biogas.
6. Industries must be encouraged to use clean technologies that reduce industrial smokestack emissions and improve urban and agricultural waste management, including capturing methane gas emitted from waste sites instead of incineration (for use as biogas).

7. The Federal Ministry of Health must collaborate with all sectors nationally, track data on air pollution-related diseases and health gains from critical interventions. It must also support the energy sector's needs based on assessments of disadvantaged groups' fuel and energy utilization. The industries should also support practices that introduce clean technologies, reduce fuel shortages, and promote renewable energy sources, particularly in rural communities that depend on diesel generators.
8. WHO must continue to provide the needed guidelines and build global databases to monitor health impact progress, determine which interventions have the most significant outcomes, and advocate for clean air.
9. Localities, regions, counties, and municipalities should develop policies to reduce tobacco smoking and second-hand smoking, set emission rate targets, and incentivize consumers to use energy-efficient appliances.
10. Non-governmental organizations and civil society must provide access to improve cooking utilities and support initiatives for clean home energy technologies and fuels.

Globally, the Ministry of Health in each country is the power player that keeps health on the national agenda. The inevitable question is why do governments and communities need the *Health in All Policies*? It is critically needed because the blueprint addresses the most significant health challenges, such as no infectious diseases, health inequities and inequalities, climate change, and spiraling healthcare costs. The circumstances under which an individual is born, grows up, lives, works and age, including the forces and systems affecting the broader society (economic and development policies, social norms, social policies, and political systems), are the social determinants of the health of an individual.

The framework for implementing the *Health in All Policies* has several vital components that the establishment must meet to put the approach into action. The organization or government must clearly articulate the structure of the planned activity, priorities, and plan for system monitoring, assessment, and dissemination. Furthermore, it must develop the support structures, evaluation and engagement processes, and human and resource capacity (WHO, 2017a). *The component strategies mentioned earlier are not in any fixed order of priority; instead, each country can adapt and adjust the elements in ways that are most relevant for its specific governance, economic, and sociocultural milieu.*

Is Health a "Consumption Good" or an "Investment Good"?

Health is a multidimensional construct with multiple aspects and different determinants that influence health outcomes. Factors influencing outcomes include the adequacy of health services, affordability, accessibility, appropriateness, and equitability in distributing services delivered from the multicenter system, private or public health facilities. There continues to be a concern about whether the health services offered from public or private health facilities can guarantee optimal patient and stakeholders' satisfaction with the services provided. The literature indicates that stakeholders are interested in ascertaining whether the care provided is appropriate and safe for the patients and the quality of care meets international best practices. A critical goal of healthcare delivery globally is achieving sustainable, high-quality care at a reasonable cost. This point of view is predicated on the assumption that quality of care can be measured, monitored, and improved. The demand for high-quality and affordable health care is elevated from the ever-evolving demographics, epidemiology, global political systems, and more significant complexities in diseases and the patients' preferences. The measurement of patient satisfaction is now widely accepted as a valid indicator of quality healthcare delivery. Other measures include the knowledge and competence of healthcare workers (HCWs), patient cooperation, health insurance, leadership, management styles in the health facilities, partnerships among referral systems, and HCW's job satisfaction.

In general, health care is generally not a refusable or elective service. It is a necessary service that substantially affects the costs. A workforce that is healthy and productive is essential for both industrial and economic growth. Poor health leads to absenteeism from work or reduced work capacity. Individuals with good health work more and earn more than those with poor health. Thus, the incentive is for government and employers to invest in health to increase productivity and income.

Without health, labor cannot produce goods and services. Therefore, the improvement of workers' health status is of interest to employers and stakeholders (Frimpong, 2014). The importance of health capital increases as production becomes increasingly health-intensive. The stock of health depreciates with aging, and occupation contributes to this depreciation because employees are often exposed to physical and chemical hazards. About two million people die annually worldwide because of work-related illnesses or injuries and occupational accidents, with 160 million new cases of work-related illness. Thus, a substantial part of the general morbidity of the population is related to work.

The existing literature is replete with various theories about health and development (Frimpong, 2014). The Grossman model of health demands that health is a durable capital good inherited but depreciated over time. Investment in health in equipment purchases and other inputs and depreciation is a natural deterioration of health over time. In Grossman's model, health enters the utility function directly as good people derive satisfaction from an investment, making more healthy time available for market and non-market activities. From practical perspectives, this model predicts that older people will be sick for longer time and have higher medical expenditures than younger people (Jones et al., 2012) have. The Grossman model has been studied extensively by introducing uncertainty in the model to assess the relationship between education and health, including whether the marginal efficiency of capital elasticity to education is less than or greater than one. Education will increase medical care demand if the curve is elastic (with elasticity more remarkable than one). Conversely, if the curve is inelastic, education will decrease medical care demand (Frimpong, 2014).

Grossman postulated that health is neither an investment good nor a consumption good, but a stock that benefits the individuals in two ways: first, by directly increasing utility and secondly by increasing healthy time available for other activities. However, this posit has been criticized for considering health as a dichotomous concept. A contrarian view is that health is both an investment and consumption good, and health provides both alternatives simultaneously (Muurinen, 1982).

Relationship Between Health and Development

Good health is central to happiness, overall well-being, and economic progress, as healthy populations live longer, are more productive, and have more money. Nevertheless, the relationship between health and the development of a society is complicated as it varies over time. Improved health has been one of the primary benefits of economic growth. This benefit occurs from the increase in income and from medical discoveries that contain diseases and disabilities. Health is part of a society's capital stock, and the differences between capital and physical capital must be recognized (Musgrove, 1993).

Many factors affect personal health status and a nation's ability to provide quality health services for its citizenry. For example, investments in roads can improve access to health services and safe life in emergencies. Inflation can impede health spending, and a public service budget freeze can limit hiring more health workers. The WHO has established a link between better health, development, and poverty and has advocated for higher government investment levels in health and prioritizing health within overall economic and action plans. Sadly, Nigeria has not taken this WHO's recommendation in its annual budgeting seriously. WHO's "health and development" efforts support health policies that respond to impoverished nations' needs. WHO also collaborates with donor organizations to ensure that aid for health care is adequate, effective, and targeted at priority needs (WHO, 2010a).

United Nations Development Goals

Between 2000 and 2015, the United Nations (UN) championed the implementation of eightmillennium development goals (MDGs) to combat poverty; HIV/AIDS, malaria and other diseases; hunger; illiteracy; environmental degradation; discrimination against women; achieve universal primary education; reduce child mortality; improve maternal health; and develop a global partnership for development (WHO, 2018, n.d.-b, n.d.-c). Unfortunately, Nigeria did not achieve the MDGs by the target date in 2015.

In September 2015, the UN adopted the sustainable developmental goals (SDGs) to replace the expired MDGs (UN, 2020). The SDGs build upon the MDGs' tenets to end global poverty, combat inequality and injustice, and address climate change to ensure that all people globally enjoy peace and prosperity by 2030. Nigeria embraced the 17 SDGs because they aligned with many of the federal government's long-term strategic plans. Specifically, the Nigerian federal government development priorities focus on poverty alleviation through job creation initiatives (SDG 1), health and well-being (SDG 3), education (SDG 4), gender equality (SDG 5), inclusive economy (SDG 8), peace and security (SDG 16), and partnerships (SDG 17).

SDG 1 (poverty) are consistent with the Nigerian federal government plan "to promote sustained, inclusive and sustainable economic growth, full and productive employment, and decent work for all" (United Nations Development Program – UNDP, 2020). With a population of 195.9 million and 60% less than 30 years of age, fulfilling this goal and taking advantage of the huge human capital resources will significantly transform the economy into a powerhouse. The unemployment rate in 2019 was 8.10%, a 0.15% decline from 2018 (8.24%) (Macrotrends, 2020). While the unemployment rate is down slightly, the informal sector that is largely unrecorded is booming (Jadesimi, 2015). Bringing most employed people into the formal (inclusive) economy as tax-payers and consumers would change the economic landscape and improve the nation's capacity to achieve UHC.

For SDG 3, Nigeria has one of the highest maternal mortality rates globally, but in recent years, the under-five mortality rates have declined from 157 to 132. Sadly, the coronavirus disease 2019 (COVID-19) pandemic has substantially stressed the already vulnerable health system. One of Nigeria's lessons from the crisis is prioritizing universal access to clean water and soap. Given that access to clean drinking water stands at 64%, there must be a more significant investment and commitment to UHC to ensure the most vulnerable are not left behind but rehabilitated to become valuable members of society (UN, 2020).

The out-of-school children are most impacted by poverty (SDG 1), low-quality education (SDG 4), unemployment (SDG 8), and limited access to the digital economy (SDG 17), which is a critical challenge confronting the country. With a booming population, regional disparities are significant. For example, about 78% of children in the Southwestern states of Nigeria can read full or part sentences, while only 17% of the Northeastern states can read. The disparity is due in part to the fact that education is allocated only 1.6% of GDP. More significant financial resources are needed to provide quality education to bridge the gap between the wealthy and the poor.

The country's informal sector economy (SDG 8) is one of the highest in Africa. About 75% of all new jobs are informal and account for 53% of the labor force and 65% of the GDP. Unfortunately, the youth have a combined unemployment and under-employment rate of 55.4%, or 24.5 million (UN, 2020). In a progressive and stable economic climate, educating the youth will transition them to productive employment and help reduce poverty (SDG 1) (UN, 2020).

To actualize the pledge to "leave no one behind," the federal government of Nigeria is collaborating with the private sector, civil society organizations, and UNDP to fast-track developmental programs for the poor to leave a better planet for future generations (UNDP, 2020). However, the SDGs' implementation faces enormous challenges as the health systems are overwhelmed by the COVID-19 pandemic and the economy that derives 86% of its revenue from oil and gas on a declining trajectory in the global economy.

Global Access to Health Care

About 50% of the global community cannot obtain essential health services. Consequently, annually, large numbers of households are pushed into poverty for paying out of pocket for their health care. Currently, 800 million people world-wide spend at least 10% of their household finances on healthcare expenses to take care of themselves, sick children, or other family members. These expenses are high enough to push about 100 million people into extreme poverty, which forced them to live on less than $2 a day. The number of people able to obtain essential health services, including immunization and family planning, insecti-cide-treated bed nets to prevent malaria, and antiretroviral treatment for HIV, has increased in the twenty-first century. Still, progress is highly uneven globally. For instance, there are wide gaps in healthcare services available in sub-Saharan Africa and Southern Asia. In other regions, primary healthcare services such as family planning and infant immunization are becoming more available. Lack of financial protection will increase financial distress for parents as they pay for these services out of their own pockets.

Only 17% of mothers and children in the poorest fifth of households in low- and lower-middle-income countries received at least six essential maternal and child health interventions, compared to 74% for the wealthiest fifth of households (WHO, 2017b).

In 2016, researchers from the Intelligence Unit of the Economist investigated how the healthcare systems in 60 countries worldwide are working to offer solutions to their populations' most pressing healthcare needs. The study developed a Global Access to Healthcare Index to examine access to health care in these 60 countries. The investigators used accessibility and healthcare-system indicators that evaluate the current record of accomplishment of each of the nations studied in meeting their country's healthcare needs. They also assessed the extent to which each country established the necessary health infrastructure needed to provide continued access. The study evaluated each nation on 23 sub-indicators within the two domains to determine whether citizens in each society have access to the appropriate health services. The Index examined access to care for patients with infectious diseases and non-communicable diseases, child and maternal health services, access to med-icines, and level of inequities in access (accessibility domain). The Index also mea-sured the conditions that allow for good access to adequate and relevant healthcare services, such as institutions, policy, and infrastructure (healthcare systems domain).

The findings revealed that accessibility performance is generally more robust than performance in the healthcare systems domain. Thus, suggesting that much more needs to be done to develop and extend coverage, the geographical reach of infrastructure, equity of access, and efficiency to improve health systems sustainability. Developed countries are among the top performers in the ranking system. The Index results revealed that political will and public faith in government institutions and other healthcare providers, even smaller, could perform well than in low-income countries (Chipman et al., 2017).

The top 20 high-performing countries in access to health care in ranking order are the Netherlands (first), followed by France, Germany, Australia, United Kingdom, Canada, Cuba, Italy, Japan, Spain, United States, Brazil, Israel, Taiwan, Thailand, Columbia, Kazakhstan, South Korea, Poland, Chile, Romania, and Turkey. However, the wealth of a nation is not the sole determinant to providing healthcare access, as several middle-income countries surpassed several high-income countries. For instance, Cuba ranked seventh, which is higher than Italy, rated eighth, Japan ninth, and Spain and the United States placed tenth. Other highly ranked middle-income countries are Brazil (joint 12th), Thailand 15th, Colombia (joint 16th), and Kazakhstan (joint 16th). The findings from this landmark study that are relevant to Nigeria are highlighted in Chap. 10.

Burden of Disease

The burden of disease (BOD) is the impact of a health condition measured by financial cost, mortality, morbidity, or other objective metrics. The BOD is a concept that describes death and loss of health due to diseases, injuries, and risk factors usually measured for all regions of the world. The health status is evaluated typically by measuring death rate, child mortality rate, or life expectancy. A focus on mortality provides little insight into the BOD, which affects the population's health but is not leading to death. However, assessing health outcomes by both mortality *and* morbidity (prevalence of disease) rates provide more comprehensive health outcomes information.

In mathematics terms, BOD = mortality *and* morbidity rates.

Alternatively,

$$BOD = \text{years of life lost}\left(YLL\right) + \text{years of a life lived with disability}\left(YLD\right)$$

where

YLL = Number of years of life a person loses as a consequence of dying early because of the disease
YLD = Number of years of life a person lives with a disability caused by the disease
BOD = Disability-adjusted life year (DALY).

Conceptually, one DALY is a loss of one year of healthy living because of either *premature mortality* or *disability*. The first data on *the Global Burden of Disease* (GBD) in the DALY unit was advocated in 1990 and published in the 1993 World Development Report by the World Bank. Presently, the Institute of Health Metrics and Evaluation (IHME) and the Disease Burden Unit of the WHO, created in 1998, publish the GBD. The GBD is categorized by age, types of disability and disease, by region and country.

On average, sub-Saharan Africa has the worst health in the world. With 11% of the global population, the region carries 24% of the worldwide disease burden. Africa has less than 1% of global health expenditure and only 3% of the global HCWs but accounts for almost 50% of the world's fatalities under 5 years. The region has the highest maternal mortality rate, bears a heavy toll from HIV/AIDS, tuberculosis, and malaria, and lacks the infrastructure to provide even primary health care to many citizens (World Bank Group, n.d.).

Overall, the global health burden rates vary from 40,000 to 70,000 DALYs per 100,000 individuals across high-burden countries such as sub-Saharan Africa. In North America, Europe, Middle East, North Africa, and Central Asia, the range is from 10,000 to 30,000 DALYs per 100,000. In 2016, the health burden was over 2.3 billion DALYs lost globally, with the most substantial burden in South Asia, with more than 25% of the total disease burden. The burden in sub-Saharan Africa is also high, with more than 20% of the global data. In 2004, the GBD in the DALY metric revealed that neuropsychiatric disorders are the most significant causes of disability, accounting for around 33% of all years lived with disability among adults 15 years and older, but account for only 2.2% of all deaths (World Bank, 2016).

Life Expectancy

Life expectancy measures the average number of years a person can expect to live based on the year of birth, his/her current age, and other demographic factors, including gender. In 2016, Nigeria's life expectancy ranked 178 globally, and the likelihood of a Nigerian dying between 15 and 60 years for men and women (per 1000 populations) was 372 and 333, respectively. In 2017, the probability of dying under 5 years (per 1000 live births) was 100 (WHO 2018; WHO 2019). In 2019, life expectancy for the year was 54.49 years, which is 0.58% higher than in 2018 when it was 54.18 years, 0.83% higher than in 2017 when it was 53.73 years. The life expectancy in the United States for 2019 was 78.87 years, representing a 0.08% increase from 2018 when it was 78.81 years – a 0.03% decline from 2017 when it was 78.84 years (World Health Ranking, 2016).

Comparatively, life expectancy in the United States increased for a decade from 1959 (69.9 years) to 2016 (78.9 years), but the pace slowed over time, and after 2014, decreased for three consecutive years. The decrease in life expectancy is due to the increase in deaths among working-age adults (25–64 years old) from the opioid epidemic, alcohol abuse, suicides, gun violence, and several organ systems-related diseases. The trend was more concentrated in the industrial Midwest and Northern New England regions. In 2019, life expectancy in the United States was substantially higher than in Nigeria by about 24.38 years. Between 1950 and 2019, Nigeria's life expectancy increased by 21.87 years from 32.62 to 54.49 years. In the

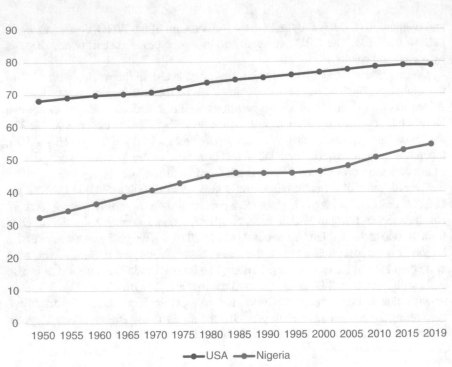

Fig. 2.2 Life expectancy in the United States and Nigeria from 1950 to 2019. (Sources: World Health Ranking, 2016, n.d.-b Countryeconomy.com n.d.)

same period, life expectancy in the United States increased from 68.14 to 78.87 years, an increase of 10.73 years (Fig. 2.2)

Hand Hygiene in Healthcare Settings

In the COVID-19 pandemic era, hand hygiene has taken center stage in the hospital environment. Clean hands are the most critical factor in preventing the spread of pathogens and antibiotic resistance in healthcare settings. In addition, hand hygiene reduces the incidence of healthcare-associated infections (HCAI). Each year, two million Americans get an infection in hospitals, and about 90,000 die because of HCAI. More widespread use of hand hygiene practices and antiseptic agents in the clinical setting is needed to promote patient safety and prevent infections. Plain soap can reduce bacterial counts, but antimicrobial soap is better, and alcohol-based hand rubs are the best. Comparatively, alcohol-based hand rubs are less damaging to the skin than soap and water. Alcohol-based hand rubs require less time, act faster, and a more efficient agent to reduce bacteria and even improve skin conditions. Hospital authorities should store alcohol-based hand rubs away from high temperatures or flames.

Wearing gloves reduces the risk of acquiring infections from patients, prevents transmission of flora from HCWs to patients, and reduces contamination from one patient to another (Fig. 2.3). Given the risks, HCWs must wear gloves when they contact blood or other body fluids before caring for patients. In addition, the same pair of gloves should be worn for only one patient and should not be washed or reused (Centers for Disease Control and Prevention – CDC, 2001; WHO, 2009).

Substantial evidence from the existing literature revealed that hand hygiene practices reduce the incidence of diseases. For instance, mothers who had their babies in the first obstetrics clinic at the General Hospital of Vienna had substantially lower mortality rates when HCWs used antiseptic agents to clean their hands than washing hands with plain soap and water (CDC, 2001). In addition, more recent studies found HCAI rates declined when HCWs performed antiseptic handwashing and adhere to recommended hand hygiene practices, which are generally poor, vary by occupation, but averaged around 40%.

When hands are visibly dirty, contaminated, or stained, HCWs must wash them with antiseptic agents or antimicrobial soap and water. When not visibly soiled, an alcohol-based hand rub must be used to decontaminate the hands routinely. Alcohol-based rub must be used when the hands are not visibly soiled to reduce bacterial counts.

Several factors identified in the literature that negatively affect adherence with recommended hand hygiene practices include irritation and dryness from antiseptic agents, the sinks not conveniently located, and lack of soap and paper towels. Other factors are not enough time, understaffing or overcrowding, the prioritization of patient needs, limited knowledge of institutional guidelines/protocols, forgetfulness, and disagreement with the recommendations. The perceived barriers to hand hygiene are the institution and HCWs peers. Thus, institutional and small-group dynamics must be initiated when implementing a system change to improve hand hygiene practice.

Organizational measures that can improve hand hygiene adherence include providing appropriate administrative support and financial resources, placing alcohol-based hand rubs at the entrance to patients' rooms or the bedside, and provide HCWs with pocket-sized sanitizers. Institutions must make available hand lotions or creams to minimize the occurrence of irritant contact dermatitis associated with hand washing. The time required for HCWs to leave what they are doing, go to a sink, and wash and dry their hands is a deterrent to frequent hand washing or hand antisepsis. Easier and rapid access to hand hygiene materials help improve adherence.

Another strategy to promote improved hand hygiene behavior is to monitor compliance to recommended hand hygiene practices and give feedback. Other techniques that can improve adherence to hand hygiene practices should be multimodal (i.e., use several different methods or procedures) and multidisciplinary (i.e., involve several other institutions and different HCWs). Patients and their families can be change agents in reminding HCWs to wash their hands. The following performance indicators and strategies can improve hand-hygiene compliance in health institutions:

1. Monitor the compliance to hand hygiene in each department or service unit
2. Monitor the volume of alcohol-based hand rub used each day
3. Monitor compliance with the establishment policies on wearing artificial nails
4. Provide ongoing feedback to HCWs about their compliance

Two issues remain unresolved. First, the effectiveness of the routine use of nonalcoholic-based hand rubs for hand hygiene in healthcare settings is unclear. Second, it is presently unknown whether the wearing of rings by HCWs affects the transmission of pathogens.

The Global Burden of Healthcare-Associated Infections

The criteria used by the U.S. Centers for Disease Control and Prevention (CDC) for nosocomial HCAI are challenging to meet in developing countries. The most frequently used measure is the surgical site infection, which is easier to define according to clinical criteria. In developed nations, HCAI diagnosis from surveillance studies relies mainly on microbiological and laboratory criteria. The pathogens detected most frequently in HCAI are from an infection site, both hospital-wide and in intensive care units (ICUs). In sophisticated and efficient health systems, the factors associated with the risk of acquiring an HCAI are virulence, capacity to survive in the environment, and antimicrobial resistance, the environment (ICU admission, prolonged hospitalization, invasive devices and procedures, antimicrobial therapy), and the host (low birth weight, underlying diseases, state of debilitation, immunosuppression, malnutrition).

HCAIs are a significant problem for patient safety; surveillance and prevention are of critical importance for hospitals and policymakers as they caused prolonged stay in the hospital, increased resistance of microorganisms to antibiotic therapy, massive long-term disability, the high financial burden for patients and their families, and excess deaths. The global dimension and scope of the HCAI burden are grossly underestimated (WHO, 2009).

The burden of HCAI is several-fold higher in developing countries than in industrialized nations. About 5–15% of patients hospitalized in developing countries are affected by HCAI, and HCAI impacts 9–37% of patients in the ICUs. In developing countries, neonatal infections are about 3–20 times higher among hospital-born babies than in industrialized nations. Studies from developing countries reported hospital-wide HCAI rates that are higher than in industrialized nations. However, most of the developing countries' investigations were in single hospitals, and the findings may not represent the problem across the entire country.

A one-day survey of the HCAI incidence in hospitals in Albania, Morocco, Tunisia, and Tanzania, found prevalence rates as high as 19.1%, 17.8%, 17.9%, and 14.8%, respectively. In developing countries, the risk of acquiring surgical site infection is substantially higher than in industrialized nations. For example, a pediatric hospital in Nigeria had a 30.9% HCAI prevalence rate; 23% was found in general surgery at a hospital in the United Republic of Tanzania and 19% in a maternity unit in Kenya. In these developing countries, the burden of HCAI in high-risk populations such as adults in ICUs and neonates is also several-fold higher in device-associated infection rates than reported in industrialized nations. Multivariate analysis studies of the HCAI risk factors from developing countries frequently identified prolonged hospital stay, surgery, intravascular and urinary catheters, and sedative medication (WHO, 2009).

In the United States, the HCAI incidence rate was 4.5% in 2002 and represents 9.3 infections/1000 patient-days, which correspond to 1.7 million patients affected – approximately, 99,000 deaths were due to HCAI. In 2004, the economic impact of HCAI was $6.5 billion. About 36% of hospital-wide infections in the United States are due to urinary tract infection, followed by surgical site infection (20%), bloodstream infection (BSI), and pneumonia (both 11%). Due to BSI and ventilator-associated pneumonia, the condition has a more harmful impact on mortality and extra costs than other causes. For example, the BSIs mortality rate in patients in the ICU is about 16–40%, and the extra length of hospital stay is about 7.5–25 days. Nosocomial BSI accounts for 250,000 deaths every year, with an increasing trend, particularly in cases due to antibiotic-resistant organisms. In the high-risk patients admitted to the ICUs, their HCAI burden increased substantially. The prevalence rates of infection acquired in ICUs vary from 9% to 37%, with crude mortality rates ranging from 12% to 80%. In the ICU, the infection rate was 13 per 1000 patient-days in 2002, and invasive devices such as a central venous catheter, mechanical ventilation, or urinary catheter are the most critical risk factors for acquiring HCAI.

In Europe, hospital-wide prevalence rates of patients affected by HCAI range from 4.6% to 9.3%. The prevalence rates of infection obtained in the ICUs range from 9.7% to 31.8%. Approximately five million HCAIs occur in acute care hospitals annually, which are 625 million extra days of hospital stay, representing a €13–24 billion economic burden. The mortality due to HCAI is about 1% (50,000 deaths/year) and contributes to death in roughly 2.7% of the cases (135,000 deaths/annual) (WHO, 2009).

Measuring Healthcare Outcomes

Health outcome is the change in the state of health of an individual, group, or population following an intervention, regardless of whether such action was intended to change health status (WHO, 1998). Outcome measures are the quality and cost targets that healthcare organizations work to improve. There are hundreds of outcome measures used in the clinical setting (Tinker, 2018). They range from changes in blood pressure in patients with hypertension to patient-reported satisfaction with care. However, it is crucial to measure health systems outcomes and use the results to improve the patient experience with healthcare delivery and improve population's health. Outcome measures can also reduce the per capita cost of health care and reduce burnout among HCWs. Although healthcare outcomes and goals are defined at the national level, each health system might set more aggressive goals that exceed the national targets.

Frequently, the government, accreditation agencies, insurance payers, and organizations that report on hospital quality of care and organizations that track national standards and financial incentives initiate healthcare outcome measures. It is critical for healthcare outcome measures to relate to patient safety or quality of care and positively influence healthcare delivery. It must also meet or exceed law and regulation and be accurately and readily measured.

In the United States, the Centers for Medicare and Medicaid Services (2021) uses outcome measures to calculate overall hospital quality by using seven indicators – mortality rate (22%), the safety of care (22%), patient experience (22%), hospitalization readmissions (22%), the effectiveness of care (4%), timeliness of care (4%), and efficient use of medical imaging (4%).

Mortality rate (aka death rate): The mortality rate is the number of deaths in a particular population, scaled to that population's size, per unit of time. The mortality rate is in units of deaths per 1000 people per year. For example, a mortality rate of 9.5 in a population of 1000 individuals means 9.5 deaths occurred annually in the entire population or 0.95% out of the total. Mortality is distinct from "morbidity," which is either the prevalence or incidence of disease and from the incidence rate, the number of new disease cases per unit of time.

The safety of care: Is used to track medical errors, skin breakdown, and HCAIs.

Readmission: Readmission is costly (and often preventable). In the United States, about $25 to $45 billion is spent annually on avoidable complications and unnecessary hospital readmissions. Readmission rates can be reduced to improve data collection's timeliness and accuracy, informing the decision-making process and monitoring performance.

Patient experience: It measures hospital stay experience and satisfaction with healthcare service delivery. It also includes real-time data on local service delivery improvement that will allow for a rapid response to problems identified.

The effectiveness of care: It measures the patients' compliance with the guidelines on best-practice care and the outcomes achieved. Examples include lower readmission rates for patients with kidney failure.

Timeliness of care: It measures patient access to healthcare services. Overcrowding in the emergency department is associated with increased inpatient mortality, increased length of hospital stays, and increased costs for patients admitted to the hospital.

Efficient use of medical imaging: Increasingly, it is becoming an essential indicator as it contributes to improved patient outcomes and more cost-efficient health care for all significant disease conditions. There is a need to prioritize three outcomes measurement essentials—data transparency, interoperability (sharing data between departments within an integrated system), and integrated care—to implement healthcare outcomes measurement successfully.

The following are examples of how healthcare systems can be designed to improve outcomes and processes:

1. By conducting a medication reconciliation system for patients with kidney failure at the time of discharge (process measure) can reduce rates of kidney failure readmission (outcome measure).
2. Implementing a fall risk assessment program for patients at the time of admission (process measure) can reduce rates of falls (outcome measure).
3. Using a skin assessment inventory (process measure) can prevent the breakdown of skin (outcome measure).

Assessment of Quality of Health Care

There are many models in the literature, including the WHO's "Recommended Quality of Care Framework," for measuring quality health care (WHO, 2006a, b), but the conceptual framework by Avedis Donabedian is the most widely recognized worldwide (Berwick and Fox, 2016). In 1966, Donabedian, a physician and health services scientist at the University of Michigan, proposed the quality of healthcare model for assessing the quality of health care (Donabedian, 2005). The model consists of three components: structure, process, and outcomes (Fig. 2.3).

The structure denotes the resources and environment in which health care is provided, such as hospital buildings, staff, financing, and equipment. The process entails the interaction between patients and HCWs within the health system. Finally, the outcomes are the effects of service delivery on the patients' health status and populations. Although there is no consensus agreement in the existing literature on the definition of "quality of health care," but there is a convergence of opinion that the definition should include healthcare characteristics, such as treatment effectiveness, acceptability, efficiency, the appropriateness of health interventions, and equity.

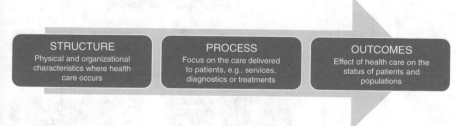

Fig. 2.3 Donabedian model for quality of health care. (Adapted from NHS England and NHS Improvement, n.d. Contains public sector information licensed under the Open Government License v3.0.)

Framework for Monitoring Performance of Health Systems

Over the years, several frameworks for measuring the performance of health systems have been proposed (Murray & Frenk, 2000). However, there is a vast difference in health outcomes for nations with similar income and education levels because of variations in health system performance. In response to this schism, the WHO, working with other global partners in 2000, reached a broad-based consensus on critical measures and effective methods and indicators of health systems performance capacity, such as "processes," "inputs," and "outputs" and to relate these with measures of "outcome." The framework for the evaluation of the health systems performance proposed by WHO in 2010 was based on six core pillars or "building blocks" such as governance and leadership, health service delivery, health workforce, health systems financing, access to essential medicines and vaccines, and health information system (WHO, 2010b; World Bank, 2006) (Fig. 2.4).

Governance, leadership, and health information systems reflect the basis for the overall policy and regulation of all the other health system components. The critical input component of the health system includes financing and the health workforce. The essential outputs for the availability and distribution of care within the health system are medical products, technologies, and service delivery. However, the WHO's framework does not include actions that influence people's behaviors in protecting and promoting health and healthcare services. Besides, the structure does not address the underlying social and economic determinants of health, such as gender inequities or education. Moreover, it does not deal with the firm and dynamic links and interactions across each component.

In evaluating global health system performance, the WHO recommended that an effective data generation system go beyond the health ministries and include other stakeholders and departments such as the national statistics offices, social services ministries, sports, and education. Therefore, a robust coordinating body that brings together the various stakeholders is warranted to establish a comprehensive and integrated plan to develop the health information and statistical system. Such a

Fig. 2.4 Six pillars of a healthcare system. (Source: WHO, 2010b)

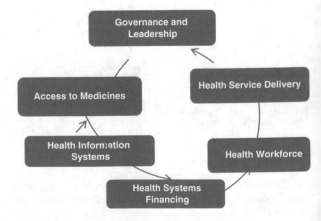

program should provide the basis for enhanced alignment and harmonization of technical and financial support from the collaborating partners. In addition, practical and affordable strategies must exist for generating timely and reliable data on health systems and appropriate investment available to develop the capacity to collect, manage, analyze, disseminate, and use the obtained information.

Health systems financing is a revenue collection method from primary and secondary sources (out-of-pocket payments), indirect and direct taxes, donor funding, and co-payment, voluntary and mandatory prepayments. The funds are accumulated in fund pools to share risk across large population groups, and the revenues are used to purchase goods and services from public and private providers for identified needs of the population, for example, the fee for service, capitation, budgeting, and salaries (Uzochukwu et al., 2015). A credible healthcare financing system must mobilize adequate resources to achieve efficiency and equity in spending. In addition, it must be affordable, of high quality, and goods and services adequately provided. Also, the money spent must be prudent to achieve the SDGs. Therefore, the mechanism for financing a healthcare system is a vital determinant for reaching UHC. In addition, the process determines whether health services are affordable and readily available to the citizen when needed.

Health information systems collect, process, analyze, and transmit the information required to organize and operate health services, research, and training. The importance of collecting and analyzing the system's data and using the results to improve service delivery cannot be overemphasized. Thus, policymakers in the health sector in small clinics, administrators of hospitals, directors of pharmaceutical companies, or ministers of health must always ask pertinent questions on their system's operations. Examples of relevant questions may include the recent increase in flu cases the beginning of a new epidemic? What will be the primary cause of death in the next 10–20 years? What treatment is more effective in the treatment of a particular disease? The information needed to answer these questions generally comes from various sources such as the *vital events registration data* on births, deaths, marriages, divorces, migrations, and *health facilities statistics* on patient diagnosis and services. It can also come from *public health surveillance* efforts to track and respond to disease trends, *census data, household surveys that* provide information on population sociodemographic characteristics, dynamic shifts, and *facilities monitoring and managing human* resources, assets, and finances.

Data collection on the workforce and financial expenditures must include information from both public and private practices. Health service data are critical to identify health trends and allocate resources effectively. Surveillance of outbreaks of infectious epidemics must be timely, rapid, and ongoing to provide early warning. Conversely, surveillance of changes in behavioral risk factors may take a longer time. Using preselected sites to have accurate and complete information will give reliable data than haphazardly selected sites when building health information systems.

Furthermore, the standardization of the data collection process will enhance the accuracy of the information. New technology is reshaping and expanding the methods used for collecting, storing, and processing information. The government must integrate health information systems into other centers to facilitate quicker responses and practical actions. For instance, the WHO's Regional Office is working with many African countries to use epidemiological and laboratory data in decision-making on population surveillance strategy to respond to the Ebola epidemic in the continent successfully.

The federal, state, and local government health departments and hospitals can use health information systems to improve the efficiency of health services. A study in rural Mali found the cost of childhood immunization programs in communities provided with health information systems was only US$1.47 per child, compared with US$2.79 per child in communities without health information systems (World Bank, 2006). Health information systems can help policymakers manage the health system and public policy development and influence clinical choices. However, health information systems also need to provide relevant data and generate new questions to better understand emerging diseases and healthcare delivery. Further work on the costs of developing data required for monitoring health systems strengthening is needed (WHO, 2010b).

Recent Advances and Innovations in Health Care

There are a plethora of recent advances and innovations in health care derived primarily from modern technology. The significant advancements and innovations include the following:

1. Several published case studies have used allogeneic human umbilical cord tissue-derived stem cells and autologous bone marrow-derived stem cells to treat patients with spinal cord injuries. In 2017, three patients at the California Institute for Regenerative Medicine with complete cervical spinal cord injuries received the oligodendrocyte progenitor cell transplant, a kind of cell found in the nervous system, with no adverse events. The researchers noted positive volitional controlled movement below the lesion. They planned to apply to the U.S. Food and Drug Administration for clinical trials to increase the sample size to 40 patients (Riordan, 2017).

   In 2019, a patient with quadriplegia had stem cells injected into his spinal cord and was above to walk only with minor gait abnormalities following intense physical therapy. Stem cell therapy is promising and will undoubtedly lessen the burden of care for patients with spinal cord injury.

2. Artificial intelligence applications help physicians make smarter diagnostic decisions during the evaluation, enhance the ease and accuracy of reading patient scans, and reduce physician burnout (Fig. 2.5). Machines assist physicians in learning algorithms, highlight problem areas on images, and quickly make sense of large amounts of data within a physician's Electronic Medical Records system. Thus, caring for patients has become working smarter, not harder (Ford, 2018).

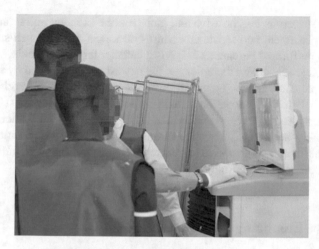

Fig. 2.5 A team of radiologists evaluating a patient imaging at UNIMED Teaching Hospital, Ondo City. (Photograph used with permission from UNIMED PRO)

3. Novel pharmacogenomics testing provided an alternative therapy for fighting the opioid crisis using the individual patient's genetic makeup to predict his/her metabolism of drugs, including opiate-based medicine. The testing is used to avoid adverse reactions and eliminate unnecessary and ineffective prescriptions, replacing them with more effective medications.

4. The use of *Visor®* for pre-hospital stroke diagnosis allows the timely response needed for stroke treatment. The new technology (hemorrhage scanning visor) detects bleeding in the brain and speeds up diagnosis and the ever-important time for stroke treatment. This advancement can lower the risk of disability and provide an opportunity for early recovery in patients with stroke.

5. Advances in immunotherapy now allow scientists to use the body's immune system to fight cancer through joint therapy concepts and engineered T-cells. With new immunotherapeutic targets and biomarkers, effective treatments are underway for all tumor profiles.

6. With the discover of 3D printing technology, medical devices are now effectively designed to match the patient's natural anatomy. The new technology shows greater acceptance by patients with increased comfort and improved clinical outcomes. Examples are its application in external prosthetics, cranial/orthopedic implants, and customized airway stents for diseases narrowing the airway, complicated heart surgeries, and total face transplants.

7. Computer technology is now used in healthcare education to create simulated and hybrid environments. The virtual/mixed reality medium provides simulation training that serves to enhance traditional instructional approaches. The new technology appeals to all types of learners: audio, visual, and kinesthetic.

8. Innovation in robotics provides surgeons better guidance that enhances extreme precision during spine, prostate, and endovascular surgeries. This minimally invasive robotic surgery has led to shortened recovery time and decreased pain.

9. Cardiac surgery is less invasive and more routine as many mitral and tricuspid valve replacement and repair procedures no longer require open surgery. The repair is performed percutaneously via a catheter through the skin.
10. Ribonucleic acid-based therapies are the newest technique used by scientists to modify patients' genetic composition at the ribonucleic acid level (Cleveland Clinic, 2019). The innovation is akin to deoxyribonucleic acid (DNA)-based gene therapies. It gives scientists the ability to detect the patient's genetic abnormality before it is translated into functioning (or nonfunctioning) proteins. This therapy is now used to treat rare genetic diseases such as Huntington's disease, cancer, and neurologic diseases.

Healthcare Financing Models

Universal health insurance coverage started in Germany in the 1880s when Chancellor Otto von Bismarck enacted a series of bills guaranteeing access to health care. Today, most high-income nations provide UHC for their citizens (Investopedia, 2020). In this book, UHC refers to a system where every citizen has access to the health services that they need—prevention, promotion, treatment, rehabilitation, and palliative care—without the risk of financial hardship when paying for them or go into bankruptcy. Implementation of UHC has a direct impact on the overall health and welfare of the population. Access to health services allows children to go to school and learn, makes citizens more productive, and actively contributes to their families and communities. It prevents being pushed into poverty when they have to pay for health services out of their own pockets (WHO, 2020). UHC is achievable under a government-run health system, a private health insurance system, or a combination of the two. A key element of financing UHC is sharing resources to spread health financial risks across the population. The system collects funds through taxation of workers who can afford to pay or compulsory earmarked contributions for health insurance.

In a *single-payer health system,* the government pays the healthcare claims, using money collected via the tax system. Hence, the government is the only (i.e., single) payer. At least 17 countries worldwide—Canada, Norway, Japan, Spain, the United Kingdom, Portugal, Sweden, Slovenia, Brunei, and Iceland—implement the single-payer system. Over 45.6 million Americans were uninsured in 2012, before President Barack Obama's Affordable Care Act (ACA). By 2019, about 8% of Americans had no health coverage; the ACA covered 26.1 million, but it is still not universal coverage. Medicare and the Veterans Health Administration in the United States are examples of single-payer systems. Medicare is a health insurance program launched in 1966 by the federal government. It provides health insurance coverage for Americans ages 65 years and older, individuals with end-stage renal disease and amyotrophic lateral sclerosis, and eligible younger people living with disabilities. Medicaid is a federal and state-funded insurance program that provides coverage for Americans with limited income and resources. It covers some services—nursing home care and personal care—not typically covered by Medicare.

The *multi-payer health system* allows several entities (e.g., insurance companies) to collect consumers' fees and pay for their healthcare services. In a *multi-payer health system*, as in the United States, citizens typically enroll in employer-sponsored health plans or individual market health plans that are not part of a single-payer system because their health insurance is not government-run. In these markets, several separate private insurance companies pay the enrollees' claims. The United States government invested heavily in health care with single-payer programs (Medicaid, Medicare, Veterans Health Administration, and *Children's Health Insurance* Program – CHIP) and has not achieved UHC and has the worse health outcome indices among the high-income countries. Surprisingly, the health system struggles under the double burden of the COVID-19 pandemic and the loss of income from elective surgery and routine medical care. The fallout from the COVID-19 crisis is the yearning for UHC to provide all Americans with health care (Investopedia, 2020).

Unlike the United States, other high-income countries such as Japan, Canada, the United Kingdom, Germany, Australia, Italy, Finland, and Switzerland provide UHC through government-run health systems (Montgomery, 2020). UHC is critical for sustainable development and poverty reduction and contributes to reducing social inequities. Achieving UHC is daunting, but all countries have a moral obligation to move more rapidly towards achieving it or maintain the gains already made. Several factors are needed to achieve UHC. They include adequate financing, a robust, efficient, well-run system that meets priority health needs through people-centered integrated care, affordability, so citizens do not suffer financial hardship while receiving services, sufficient essential medicines, technologies, and state-of-the-art equipment to diagnose and treat medical problems. Additional factors are an adequate number of well-trained, motivated health workers to deliver high-quality services based on the best available evidence, reducing out-of-pocket costs to patients, and progressive policies to address social determinants of health, such as education, living conditions, and household income, affecting people's health and services access. Canada operates a single-payer system and provides UHC; the hospitals are privately run, and they bill the government for services provided. The government does not employ health workers. The Canadian system is similar to the Medicare program in the United States (Investopedia, 2020).

In some countries, a *two-tier health insurance coverage system* is implemented. The government provides primary health insurance coverage, and those who can afford a higher standard of care obtain supplemental coverage. Nearly every citizen has supplemental insurance covering the deductibles and co-pays (out-of-pocket medical costs) not covered under the government plan in France. About 60% of Canadians purchase additional insurance coverage for dental, vision, and prescription drugs because the government-run plan does not pay for those services.

Globally, health systems are actively exploring new methods to control costs and use resources efficiently. In several countries, the critical decision to introduce a single-payer over a multi-payer healthcare system poses significant challenges. A systematic review by Petrou and associates in 2018 concluded that the single-payer system performs better in healthcare equity, risk pooling, and negotiation. In contrast, the multi-payer systems involve a higher administrative cost but provide additional options to patients and more challenging to be exploited by the government. The findings of the two systems' impact on efficiency and quality are somewhat tentative because of the available studies' methodological limitations.

Socialized medicine payer system—is a derogatory term coined in the United States—often used by the Republican Party to disparage the UHC in Cuba, Canada, and the United Kingdom. In reality, the socialized payer system takes the single-payer approach one step further as the government pays for health care and employs the healthcare workers that operate the hospitals. The socialized medicine system's primary criticisms are the lack of free-market competition among health providers, leading to lower costs. Critics of the system also assumed that government-run programs are poorly managed and unable to deliver high-quality service. The UK government runs the National Health Service (NHS), owns the hospitals, pays for services, and employs the healthcare workers.

In Nigeria, the tertiary hospitals and some highly resourced private hospitals in Lagos and Abuja can manage most diseases or ill-health conditions. However, the services of private hospitals are costly and usually out of reach for the poor. The federal and state governments own the secondary and tertiary hospitals and the primary employer of healthcare workers. The federal and state governments adopt a public-private partnership strategy to improve healthcare infrastructure. Many finance models are used, but the most common is the arrangement in which government provides infrastructure for the private entity to operate the health facility (UK Home Office, 2018). It is fair to infer that the financing models adopted in the country are ineffective, given that UHC is still a mirage even 60 years after independence. The healthcare funding mechanisms in Nigeria are described more comprehensively in Chap. 13.

Several developing countries around the world have moved closer to or already achieved UHC. Nepal, in 2008, introduced free UHC and is on track to achieve its health-related MDGs. Thailand, after 10 years of the UHC scheme, dramatically reduced impoverishment caused by out-of-pocket payments. El Salvador expanded health coverage by abolishing user fees and strengthening primary health care in rural areas. Africa, Liberia, Gabon, Ghana, Sierra Leone, and Rwanda have made substantial progress towards UHC (WHO, 2020).

Conclusion

A clear understanding of the information presented in this chapter is vital in consuming this book's contents. About 50% of the world's population cannot obtain essential health services, and large numbers of households are annually dragged into poverty for paying out of pocket for their health care. The sub-Saharan African region has the worst health globally and has the highest maternal mortality rate, and bears a heavy burden from the impact of HIV/AIDS, tuberculosis, and malaria. Sadly, the region lacks the infrastructures needed to provide primary health care to many of its citizens. The scope of the challenge calls for a reassessment of the traditional approaches to health care and the need for increased private sector participation in the region's overall health strategy. The Nigerian healthcare system is presently in a semi-comatose state, and the challenges in the health sector and recommendations on how to improve it are discussed more comprehensively in Chaps. 12 and 13.

Case Study: Practice Act and Ethical Code of Conduct

This case study will enable students to independently explore the ethical code of conduct and practice of their discipline. Students will access the website of their profession and answer the following questions:

1. What is the entry-level qualification needed to practice the profession?
2. Is a license required to practice the profession?
3. What are the requirements for the license?
4. Are assistants recognized in the profession, and what are their roles and responsibilities?
5. Who may supervise them?
6. What is the ratio for the supervision of the assistants?
7. Is there a provision for temporary licensure?
8. What would you consider an unethical behavior?
9. What are the sanctions for unethical practices?

References

Adeyanju, O., Tubeuf, S., & Ensor, T. (2017). Socioeconomic inequalities in access to maternal and child healthcare in Nigeria: Changes over time and decomposition analysis. *Health Policy and Planning, 32*(8):1111–1118. [online]. Available at: https://academic.oup.com/heapol/article/32/8/1111/3829669 Accessed 24 Oct 2020.

American Medical Association. (2015). *Healthy population equals healthy economy.* January 13. [online]. Available at: https://www.ama-assn.org/practice-management/economics/healthy-population-equals-healthy-economy. Accessed 16 Oct 2020.

Berwick, D., & Fox, D. M. (2016, Quarterly). Evaluating the quality of medical care: Donabedian's. *Milbank, 94*(2):237–241. [online]. Available at: https://www.ncbi.nlm.nih.gov/pmc/articles/PMC4911723/. Accessed 24 Oct 2020.

Centers for Disease Control and Prevention - CDC. (2001). *CDC nails nurses: U.S. Department of Health and Human Services.* [online]. Available at: https://www.infectioncontroltoday.com/hand-hygiene/cdc-nails-nurses; https://www.cdc.gov/healthywater/hygiene/hand/nail_hygiene.html. Accessed 24 Oct 2020.

Chinawa, J. M., Manyike, P. C., & Aniwada, E. C. (2016). Prevalence and socioeconomic correlates of autism among children attending primary and secondary schools in southeast Nigeria.

African Health Science, 16(4):936–942. [online]. Available at: https://www.ncbi.nlm.nih.gov/pmc/articles/PMC5398438/. Accessed 10 Jan 2021.

Chipman, A., Koehring, M., Boshnakova, A., Guerrero, C., Hurst, L., & Pannela, A. (2017). *Global access to healthcare: Building sustainable health systems.* [online]. Available at: https://perspectives.eiu.com/sites/default/files/Globalaccesstohealthcare-3.pdf. Accessed 24 Oct 2020.

Cleveland Clinic. (2019). *Cleveland clinic unveils top 10 medical innovations for 2019.* [online]. Available at: https://newsroom.clevelandclinic.org/2018/10/24/cleveland-clinic-unveils-top-10-medical-innovations-for-2019/. Accessed 24 Oct 2020.

Countryeconomy.com. (n.d.) *Country comparison Nigeria vs. the United States.* [online]. Available at: https://countryeconomy.com/countries/compare/nigeria/usa?sc=XE24. Accessed 22 July 2020.

Donabedian, A. (2005). Evaluating the quality of medical care. *The Milbank Quarterly, 83*(4):691–729. [online].

Ford, O. (2018). *Top 10 medical innovations for 2019.* [online]. Available at: https://www.mddionline.com/top-10-medical-innovations-2019. Accessed 24 Oct 2020.

Frimpong, A. O. (2014). Health as an investment commodity: A theoretical analysis. *Journal of Behavioural Economics, Finance, Entrepreneurship, Accounting and Transport, 2*(3):58–62. [online]. Available at: http://pubs.sciepub.com/jbe/2/3/1/. Accessed 24 Oct 2020.

Hooker, B. S. (2014) Measles-mumps-rubella vaccination timing and autism among young African American boys: A reanalysis of CDC data. *Translational Neurodegeneration, 3*:16. [online]. Available at: https://www.ncbi.nlm.nih.gov/pmc/articles/PMC4128611/. Accessed 10 Oct 2020.

Ichoku, H. E., Fonta, W. M., & Ataguba, J. E. (2013). Political economy and history: Making sense of health financing in sub-Saharan Africa. *Journal International Development, 25,* 297–309.

Investopedia. (2020). *Universal healthcare coverage.* [online]. Available at: https://www.investopedia.com/terms/u/universal-coverage.asp. Accessed 24 Oct 2020.

Jadesimi, A. (2015). *Nigeria and the sustainable development goals: Setting the course to 2030.* [online]. Available at: https://www.forbes.com/sites/amyjadesimi/2015/11/26/nigeria-and-the-sustainable-development-goals-setting-the-course-to-2030/?sh=45bcab744b78. Accessed 24 Oct 2020.

Jones, A. M., Rice, N., & Contoyannis, P. (2012). *The dynamics of health. The Elgar companion to health economics* (p. 15). Edward Elgar Publishing.

Macrotrends. (2020). *Nigeria unemployment rate 1991–2020.* [online]. Available at: https://www.macrotrends.net/countries/NGA/nigeria/unemployment-rate#:~:text=Nigeria%20unemployment%20rate%20for%202019,a%202.75%25%20increase%20from%202015. Accessed 24 Oct 2020.

Montgomery, K. (2020). *Differences between universal coverage and single-payer.* [online]. Available at: https://www.verywellhealth.com/difference-between-universal-coverage-and-single-payer-system-1738546. Accessed 24 Oct 2020.

Musgrove, P. (1993). Relations between health and development. Bol Oficina Sanit Panam, *114*(2):115–129. [online]. Available at: https://www.ncbi.nlm.nih.gov/pubmed/8466652. Accessed 24 Oct 2020.

Muurinen, J. M. (1982). Demand for health: A generalized Grossman model. *Journal of Health Economics, 1*(1), 5–28.

NHS England and NHS Improvement. (n.d.). *Online Library of Quality, Service Improvement and Redesign Tools: A model for measuring quality care.* https://www.england.nhs.uk/quality-service-improvement-and-redesign-qsir-tools/

Osypuk, T. L., Joshi, P., Geronimo, K., & Acevedo-Garcia, D. (2014). Do social and economic policies influence health? A review. *Current Epidemiological Report, 1*(3):149–164. [online]. Available at: https://www.ncbi.nlm.nih.gov/pmc/articles/PMC4429302/. Accessed 16 Oct 2020.

Oxfam International. (2020). *Nigeria: extreme inequality in numbers.* [online]. Available at: https://www.oxfam.org/en/nigeria-extreme-inequality-numbers. Accessed 24 Oct 2020.

Ranchod, S. (2016). A healthy society is a productive society. *City Press*. [online]. Available at: https://www.news24.com/citypress/voices/a-healthy-society-is-a-productive-society-20160603. Accessed 16 Oct 2020.

Riordan, N. H. (2017). *Stem Cell Institute: Stem cell therapy for spinal cord Injury*. [online]. Available at: https://www.cellmedicine.com/stem-cell-therapy-for-spinal-cord-injury/. Accessed 24 Oct 2020.

Sampson, S., & Felman, A. (2020). *What is good health?* Available at: https://www.medicalnews-today.com/articles/150999. Accessed 15 Mar 2021.

Tinker, A. (2018). *The top seven healthcare outcome measures and three measurement essentials*. [online]. Available at: https://www.healthcatalyst.com/insights/top-7-healthcare-outcome-measures. Accessed 24 Oct 2020.

U.S. Centers for Medicare and Medicaid Services. (2021). *Find and compare nursing homes, hospitals & other providers near you*. [online]. Available at: https://www.medicare.gov/care-compare/?providerType=Hospital&redirect=true. Accessed 15 Mar 2021.

UK Home Office. (2018). *Country policy and information note Nigeria: Medical and healthcare issues Version 2.0*. [online]. Available at: https://www.justice.gov/eoir/page/file/1094261/download. Accessed 20 May 2021.

UN - United Nations. (2020). *Nigeria: Sustainable development goals*. [online]. Available at: https://sustainabledevelopment.un.org/memberstates/nigeria. Accessed 24 Oct 2020.

UNDP. (2020). *Nigeria: Sustainable development goals*. [online]. Available at: https://www.ng.undp.org/content/nigeria/en/home/sustainable-development-goals.html. Accessed 24 Oct 2020.

Uzochukwu, B., Ughasoro, M. D., Etiaba, E., Okwuosa, C., Envuladu, E., & Onwujekwe, O. E. (2015). Healthcare financing in Nigeria: Implications for achieving universal health coverage. *Nigeria Journal of Clinical Practice*. [online]. Available at: http://www.njcponline.com/text.asp?2015/18/4/437/154196. Accessed 10 Oct 2020.

WHO. (1998). *Health promotion glossary*. [online]. Available at: https://www.who.int/healthpromotion/about/HPR%20Glossary%201998.pdf. Accessed 15 Mar 2021.

WHO. (2006a). *The world health report. Working Together for Health* (pp. 1–15). World Health Organization.

WHO. (2006b). *Quality of care: A process for making strategic choices in health systems*. Printed in France. [online]. Available at: https://www.who.int/management/quality/assurance/QualityCare_B.Def.pdf. Accessed 24 Oct 2020

WHO. (2007). The World Health Organization on health inequality, inequity, and social determinants of health. *Population Development Review, 33*, 839–843.

WHO. (2010a). *Health and development*. [online]. Available at: https://www.who.int/hdp/en/. Accessed 24 Oct 2020.

WHO. (2010b). *Monitoring the building blocks of health systems: A handbook of indicators and their measurement strategies*. Printed by the WHO Document Production Services, Geneva, Switzerland. [online]. Available at: https://www.who.int/healthinfo/systems/WHO_MBHSS_2010_full_web.pdf. Accessed 24 Oct 2020.

WHO. (2017a). *Health in All Policies: Framework for country action*. [online]. Available at: https://www.who.int/healthpromotion/hiapframework.pdf. Accessed 24 Oct 2020.

WHO. (2017b). *World Bank and WHO: Half the world lacks access to essential health services, 100 million still pushed into extreme poverty because of health expenses*. [online]. Available at: https://www.who.int/news-room/detail/13-12-2017-world-bank-and-who-half-the-world-lacks-access-to-essential-health-services-100-million-still-pushed-into-extreme-poverty-because-of-health-expenses. Accessed 24 Oct 2020.

WHO. (2020). *Health systems – Questions and answers on universal health coverage*. [online]. Available at: https://www.who.int/healthsystems/topics/financing/uhc_qa/en/. Accessed 24 Oct 2020.

WHO. (2018). *Millennium development goals (MDGs)*. [online]. Available at: https://www.who.int/topics/millennium_development_goals/about/en/#:~:text=The%20United%20Nations%20

Millennium%20Declaration,have%20specific%20targets%20and%20indicators. Accessed 10 Oct 2020.

WHO. (n.d.-b). *The burden of disease: What is it, and why is it important for safer food?* [online]. Available at: https://www.who.int/foodsafety/foodborne_disease/Q&A.pdf. Accessed 24 Oct 2020.

WHO. (n.d.-c). *Global Health Observatory data repository: Life expectancy by country: Nigeria and USA.* [online]. Available at: https://apps.who.int/gho/data/view.main.61200?lang=en. Accessed 22 July 2020.

World Bank. (2006). Chapter 7 – Pillars of the health system. In D. T. Jamison, J. C. Breman, A. R. Measham, G. Alleyne, M. Claeson, D. B. Evans, P. Jha, A. Mills, & P. Musgrove (Eds.), *Priorities in health: Disease control priorities project.* The International Bank for Reconstruction and Development. [online]. Available at: https://www.ncbi.nlm.nih.gov/books/NBK10265/. Accessed 24 Oct 2020.

World Bank Group. (n.d.). Health and education in Africa. *International Finance Corporation.* [online]. Available at: https://www.ifc.org/wps/wcm/connect/REGION__EXT_Content/Regions/Sub-Saharan+Africa/Investments/HealthEducation/#:~:text=People%20in%20Sub%2DSaharan%20Africa,of%20the%20global%20disease%20burden.&text=The%20region%20lacks%20the%20infrastructure,to%20many%20of%20its%20people. Accessed 24 Oct 2020.

World Health Ranking. (2016). *Nigerian life expectancy.* [online]. Available at: https://www.worldlifeexpectancy.com/nigeria-life-expectancy. Accessed 24 Oct 2020.

Zimmerman, E., & Woolf, S. H. (2014). Understanding the relationship between education and health. 50th year *National Academy of Medicine.* [online]. Available at: https://nam.edu/perspectives-2014-understanding-the-relationship-between-education-and-health/. Accessed 11 Jan 2021.

Chapter 3
The Evolutionary Developments, Threats and Opportunities Within the Nigerian Healthcare System

Learning Objectives

After reading this chapter, the learner should be able to:

1. Discuss the origin and developments of Western-style health care in Nigeria from 1472 to the contemporary era.
2. Discuss the current state of the Nigerian healthcare system.
3. Analyze why universal health care in Nigeria has been elusive for over 60 years.
4. Contextualize the present and future threats to the Nigerian healthcare system.
5. Describe opportunities within the Nigerian healthcare system.
6. Discuss the performance of the health system in Africa.

Introduction

Before 1472, traditional medicine was the only source of health care in Nigeria. Western-style health care was first imported into the country by the Portuguese navigators who arrived on the coast in 1472. Before contacting the early European explorers and missionaries, traditional medical practitioners (TMPs) such as herbalists, local midwives, bonesetters, and other esoteric practices were dominants. The strong influence of regional politics on socioeconomic development leads to policy inconsistency. Each successive administration is distinguished by its "interest" policies, which are often not aligned with the previous national health plans. Thus, although the Western-style health system in Nigeria continues to evolve, its origin and developments remain obscure to the rest of the world.

This chapter describes the evolutionary developments of Western-style health care in Nigeria from 1472 to the contemporary era, including why universal health care (UHC) has been elusive for over 60 years. The chapter also identifies the present and future threats and opportunities within the Nigerian health system.

Critical Milestones in the Development of Western-Style Healthcare System (1472–2019)

1472–1960: Traditional medicine was the healthcare delivery system in Africa before 1472. Western-style medical care was first imported into Nigeria by the Portuguese navigators who arrived on the coast. The establishment of the Roman Catholic Mission Hospital at St. Thomas Island off the Bight of Benin in 1504 marked the formal introduction of orthodox healthcare service in West Africa. However, the record of the Medical Examining Board in 1789 contained only the names of Europeans, mainly Dutch, Danish, and British nationals. In 1861, the British established the Colony and Protectorate of Nigeria, and by 1880, the first healthcare dispensary was opened at Obosi by the Church Missionary Society. Subsequently, the Roman Catholic Mission opened the Sacred Heart Hospital at Abeokuta in 1865. Later, they opened other dispensaries in Onitsha and Ibadan in 1886. By 1893, the Lagos Island General Hospital opened in Marina, Lagos, followed in 1898 by the St. Margaret's Hospital in Calabar (Nigerian Finder, 2020; Medical and Dental Council of Nigeria, 2018; Ogaji & Brisibe, 2015). The high mortality among Europeans who came to West Africa in the middle of the nineteenth century made the British Army train many West Africans as physicians and deployed them to serve in their native countries. Unfortunately, the details regarding the pioneer Nigerian physicians' contributions remained in obscurity (Balogun, 2020).

In the 1870s, the British colonial government provided medical services by constructing several clinics and hospitals in Lagos, Calabar, and other coastal trading centers. Unlike the missionary health establishments, the colonial government medical facilities were initially solely for Europeans' use. Later, they extended health services to African employees. As Europeans expanded their activities inland, government hospitals and clinics broadened to the other areas of the country. For example, the hospital in Jos was established in 1912 after the initiation thereof in tin mining.

World War I (1914–1918) had a substantially detrimental effect on the country's health services because many European and African medical personnel enlisted to serve in Europe. After the war, health facilities expanded considerably as the government established several medical assistants' schools. However, Nigerian physicians were prohibited from practicing in government hospitals during that era unless serving African patients. This practice led to protests and frequent involvement in the nationalist movement by physicians and other healthcare workers (Anonymous, n.d.-a).

After World War II (1939–1945), in response to nationalist agitation, the colonial government extended health and education facilities across the country. In 1946, the colonial masters announced a 10-year health development plan. Two years later, in 1948, the University of Ibadan opened, and it included a medical school and a University College Hospital. The Nigerian Medical Association (NMA), which represents physicians' interests, was established in 1951.

In 1952, Sudan Interior Mission (SIM) (later dubbed Serving in Mission) missionaries led by Dr. and Mrs. Campion opened a small maternity clinic, operating theater, outpatient department, and inpatient wards in Egbe, Kogi state. By 1955, a nursing school was established, and a midwifery school opened in 1977. By 1982, a Family Medicine Residency Program was established in the hospital with accreditation from the National Postgraduate Medical College of Physicians and later by the West African College of Physicians. In 1976, the medical complex was transferred to the Evangelical Church of West Africa (ECWA) (also known as Evangelical Church Winning All) and renamed Egbe Hospital to ECWA Hospital, Egbe. By 1986, Nigerians occupied all medical and administrative positions (ECWA Hospital, 2021).

Also, in 1952, the Gwandu native authority built a general hospital with a maternity and one male ward and two female wards in Birnin Kebbi. The Northern Nigerian government, Northwestern State government, Sokoto State government managed the hospital and were taken over by the Kebbi State government in August 1991. The government upgraded it to a specialist hospital. It was renamed the Sir Yahaya Memorial Hospital Birnin Kebbi to immortalize the 17th Emir of Gwandu, who had the vision to build a hospital at that time on his farmland without soliciting compensation. The hospital has over 290 capacity beds and is headed by a Chief Medical Director (WikiVisually, n.d.)

Coincidentally, again in 1952, the first medical school in Nigeria was established at the University College Hospital, Ibadan. Several nursing schools and two pharmacy schools were also founded, and by 1960, there were 65 government-owned nursing or midwifery training schools. In 1945, the National Orthopaedic Hospital was established in Shomolu, Lagos. The Ministry of Health developed the first colonial healthcare plan in 1946 to coordinate nationwide health services provided by the government, private companies, and missions. The health plan provided funding for hospitals and clinics concentrated in the urban centers but only allocated little funding for rural health centers. There were substantial disparities in the number of health facilities in the Southern region than in the North. Consequently, the government expanded health care to rural areas. The federal government developed the following national healthcare plans between 1945 and 2019 with the primary goal to provide UHC:

1. *1945–1955*: Queen Elizabeth's administration developed the First Colonial Healthcare Development Plan.

2. *1956–1962*: The Second Colonial Healthcare Development Plan was also developed by Queen Elizabeth's administration.
3. *1962–1968*: The First National Healthcare Development Plan was developed by President (Dr.) Nnamdi Azikiwe and Prime minister (Alhaji) Tafawa Balewa (1963–1966).
4. *1970–1975*: The Second National Healthcare Development Plan was developed by General Yakubu Gowon's administration.
5. *1975–1980*: The Third National Healthcare Plan was developed by General Olusegun Obasanjo.
6. *1981–1985:* President Shehu Shagari's administration developed the Fourth National Healthcare Plan.
7. *2004–2008:* President Olusegun Obasanjo's administration created the Healthcare Development Strategic Plan.
8. *2010–2015:* The Primary Healthcare Under One Roof Plan was developed by President Goodluck Jonathan administration.
9. *2016 –*: President Muhammadu Buhari's administration to date has developed three different health plans – The "Revitalization of Primary Health Care for Universal Health Coverage" plan, the "WHO Revised Third Generation Nigeria Country Cooperation Strategy" plan, and the "National Strategic Health Development Plan".

Queen Elizabeth's administration developed the First Colonial Healthcare Development Plan (1945–1955) to provide nationwide healthcare services for all. Queen Elizabeth's administration (1956–1962) also developed the Second Colonial Healthcare plan to provide national healthcare services for all. The colonial masters regionalized the Nigerian health system, and public hospitals provided free health care for civil servants and their family members. Hospitals owned by missionaries charged nominal fees and offered free services for the poor. In 1959, the second ECWA hospital was established in Jos, Plateau state.

By 1959, the Roman Catholics provided about 40% of the country's total mission-based hospital beds. There were 118 mission hospitals and 111 government hospitals. Roman Catholic hospitals were concentrated in the Southeastern and Midwestern regions, and by 1954, almost all the hospitals in the Midwest were owned by Roman Catholic missions.

1961–1990: The second-largest mission hospital owner was the Sudan United Mission in the Middle Belt region and the Sudan Interior Mission in the Northern states. By 1990, they both operated 25 hospitals and remained dominant components of the North's healthcare network. Christian missionaries also played an essential role in medical training and education. They provided training for nurses and other healthcare professionals (HCPs) and sponsored primary and advanced medical education in Europe. Many first-generation physicians were benefactors of this effort, which laid the groundwork for broader distribution and acceptance of orthodox medicine in the country (Anonymous, n.d.-a).

At independence in 1960, Nigeria's life expectancy was 37 years, higher than in several African and Asian countries. As life expectancy worldwide doubled, one would expect Nigeria to be between 70 and 74 years. Sadly, life expectancy is only 54.5 years and ranked the third lowest in the world. The lowest life expectancy rate is attributed to the fact that many Nigerians are superstitious and suspicious of orthodox medicine and promptly seek preventive and curative treatment. By 1960, the colonial masters had firmly established the allopathic health system in urban centers, and missionary activities had expanded to some rural communities.

President (Dr.) Nnamdi Azikiwe and Prime minister (Alhaji) Tafawa Balewa (1963–1966) developed the First National Healthcare Development Plan to expand rural health services. The administration builds upon the missionaries' skeletal framework by embracing their system and investing heavily in workforce development, awarding scholarships in many health fields—medicine, nursing, and physiotherapy—to study abroad. On return to the country, the pioneer Nigerian HCPs were accorded plum positions in the public sector – at the Federal Ministry of Health (FMH), medical schools, and University Teaching Hospitals (UTHs). The government also established modern hospitals in Ibadan, Lagos, Kano, and Enugu (Fig. 3.1). Recruitment of personnel and the purchase of state-of-the-art medical equipment became the government's priority.

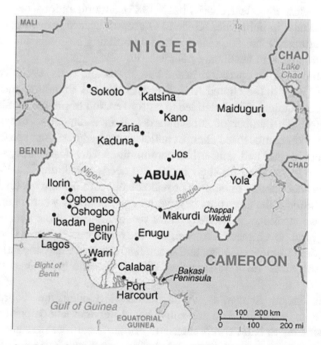

Fig. 3.1 The major cities in Nigeria. (Reproduced from: Nigeria map showing major cities as well as parts of surrounding countries and the Gulf of Guinea. *The World Factbook 2021*. Washington, DC: Central Intelligence Agency, 2021. https://www.cia.gov/the-world-factbook/)

The federal and state governments encouraged the public to use public hospitals, and allopathic drugs were provided free or heavily subsidized. The sudden interest in allopathic medications, over time, caused the shortage of highly skilled and knowledgeable TMPs. Most of the TMPs died without passing on their knowledge and skills to their sons. Unfortunately, most of the younger generation had embraced Western education and Christianity, which influenced their perception of traditional medicine as evil and inferior to allopathic drugs (Asakitikpi, 2019).

The Second National Healthcare Development Plan was developed by General Yakubu Gowon's (1979–1983) administration. The plan focused on providing primary health care to rural dwellers. However, despite the sudden national wealth from oil revenue, not much was done by General Gowon to achieve the 1946 National Healthcare Development Policy developed by the colonial masters. Corruption and waste depleted the national treasury, and suddenly austerity was declared by Gowon and the subsequent military and democratic administrations.

In the late 1970s and early 1980s, the global downturn in oil price and corruption in the public sector left the government treasury thin. Everyday consumables and drugs became scarce with irregular payment of public workers' salaries. It became clear that the government could no longer sustain the welfare model of healthcare financing and introduced fees for services provided in public health establishments. General Olusegun Obasanjo (1976–1979), President Shehu Shagari (1979–1983), and General Muhammadu Buhari (1983–1985) administrations began to preach austerity measures in public life. General Olusegun Obasanjo developed the Third National Healthcare Plan. The plan focused on building hospitals and health facilities but had no clear-cut healthcare policy.

The harsh economic condition in the late 1970s and early 1980s caused large migration of HCPs to the United Arab Emirates, United Kingdom, and the United States. The economic realities also led to a proliferation of private medical practice and a surge in the number of substandard and fake allopathic drugs, charlatan healthcare workers, unlicensed chemist outlets, drug peddlers, and spiritual healers. Health centers in rural and semi-urban communities were abandoned, and the rural dwellers were left to fend for their healthcare needs (Asakitikpi, 2019). Both the public and private sectors in tandem provide health care. Public health services are the responsibility of the three tiers of government, but primary care is the local government's responsibility. The states control secondary care at the general hospitals, while the federal government is in charge of the tertiary care provided at the UTHs, Federal Medical Centers (FMCs), and specialist hospitals. Also, the federal government is responsible for implementing disease-specific programs at all levels (WHO, 2018).

President Shehu Shagari's administration developed the Fourth National Healthcare Plan that focused on preventive health services and empowers states and local governments to build comprehensive/ primary health centers and health clinics. However, the government did not come close to achieving the aim of nationwide healthcare services for all. The coup that brought General Muhammadu Buhari to power in 1983 mentioned the poor service at the tertiary hospitals as one reason for government change. As a result, Buhari's Military administration revised the fourth national plan with emphasis on primary health care. It later adopted the World Health Organization's (WHO's) "health for all by 2000" goal, but Buhari's government and others that followed until today lacked the political will for its implementation.

By the mid-1980s, the economic conditions were further exacerbated by the local currency's devaluation due to the structural adjustment program implemented by General Ibrahim Babangida's military administration. Consequently, imported goods of all types doubled or tripled in price. The structural adjustment program initiated led to workers' mass retrenchment in public and private sectors, and access to healthcare services became difficult. As expected, private medical practitioners billed for their services, which led to a rise in healthcare costs.

In 1987, the federal government unveiled the primary healthcare plan to improve the collection and monitoring of health data to improve food supply and nutrition, maternal, childcare, family planning, and health education to prevent diseases and ensure the availability of essential drugs and vaccines in the country. The federal government also increased vaccination against primary childhood diseases and declared primary care as the cornerstone of national health policies; primary healthcare services are available mainly for rural dwellers. Still, primary healthcare coverage is not attained despite over 60 years of primary, secondary, and tertiary healthcare investments. The health care at the primary level is the least organized and least funded. The local government authorities have not been able to finance adequately and organize primary health care, creating a fragile base for the health system. Only 30% of the federal account is allocated based on population, and the least populous states often receive more revenues. At the state level, budget patterns between the North and the South have been systematically inequitable due to historical and political factors.

By the late 1980s, public healthcare establishments were severely impacted by rising costs, budget cuts, and materials shortages. Partly as a result of these problems, private health care facilities grew. The demand for orthodox health care far outstripped its availability. As government hospitals deteriorated, drugs and equipment were corruptly diverted to the private sector, and more physicians opened private practices. Free healthcare services became an issue of public policy contentions. The debate reached a crescendo in 1989 under General Ibrahim Babangida's military administration when the Constituent Assembly included a clause in the constitution specifying that free and adequate health care be available as a matter of right to all children younger than 18, people 65 and older, and individuals with disabilities. However, the provision was deleted from the draft constitution by Ibrahim Babangida and his governing council (Anonymous, n.d.-a). In retrospect, this decision was a missed opportunity to introduce UHC into the health system. Four decades later, UHC remains an illusion for the country.

1991–2018: In the late 1980s, shortage and fake drugs became a major national problem and led to the national drug policy enacted in 1990. Subsequently, the National Drug Law Enforcement Agency (NDLEA) was commissioned to address the challenges of inadequate drug availability, supply, and distribution. At the onset, the NDLEA recorded modest achievements in publishing an Essential Medicines List and a National Drug Formulary. Similarly, it introduced a drug registration procedure and established a statutory agency to administer and control drugs. As a result, the number of people in the country with access to essential medications required to treat chronic diseases, such as HIV and malaria, is estimated at 40%. However, over 60% of the population still lacks access to essential medicines. Accessibility to drugs is much better in urban areas, and many rural dwellers do not even have medical stores. In general, patients have access to generic drugs, which are cheaper and more affordable. Between 2002 and 2012, the availability of selected generic medicines in public health facilities was 26.2% compared to 36.4% in the private sector. Patients purchase drugs from both public and private pharmacy outlets. In rural areas, "patent medicine stores" are usually unregulated and unsupervised. As a result, between 15% and 75% of the country's total drugs were fake (MedCOI, 2018).

Realizing this major problem, the federal government took decisive action by stocking pharmaceutical products in the Central Medical Store in Lagos, where drugs are transported to different states. States also have their medical stores, where medical consumables are stored and transported to local government stores. From the local government stores, drugs are distributed to health facilities. Unfortunately, the bureaucrats later abused the drug distribution system due to corruption, and the process became chaotic and disorganized. Despite the modest progress made by the NDLEA, many areas of their operations still need to be reformed, including self-sufficiency in producing essential medicines, establishing an effective drug procurement and distribution system, harmonization, and updating the national drug policy.

President Olusegun Obasanjo's administration (2004–2008) developed the Healthcare Development Strategic Plan and launched the National Health Insurance Scheme (NHIS) and a national traditional medicine policy (Scott-Emuakpor, 2010). He was succeeded in 2009 by President Umaru Yar'Adua's administration, who inherited 33,303 general hospitals, 20,278 primary health centers and posts, 59 teaching hospitals, and federal medical centers in the country (Welcome, 2011). On November 23, 2009, President Umaru Yar'Adua abandoned the country's tertiary hospitals and traveled to Saudi Arabia to receive treatment for a heart condition. His departure from the country precipitated a constitutional crisis as many Nigerians made calls that Yar'Adua must step down as he was deemed unfit to continue in power. On May 5, 2010, he was pronounced dead, and Vice President Goodluck Ebele Jonathan succeeded him. The federal government declared 7 days of mourning in his memory.

In 2010, a major cholera epidemic broke out in the Northern states, extending to the Southern states with 3000 cases and 781 dead. The cholera outbreak in 2012 was estimated at three to five million cases annually and 100,000 to 150,000 deaths yearly. It was the worst outbreak in recent years. The number of cases was three times higher than that of 2009 and seven times higher than in 2008. Women and children accounted for four out of every five cases. In 2012, the FMH constituted the National Emergency Response and Preparedness Team to address disease prevention and control. Still, this has not helped matters, as every year the outbreak of different diseases that kill innocent people in their thousands is still prevalent. Despite this yearly outbreak, there has not been an effective and efficient emergency response and disease prevention system (Muhammad et al., 2017).

The "Primary Healthcare Under One Roof" plan was developed by President Goodluck Jonathan, but it is more rhetorical than a substantive action towards UHC (Aigbiremolen et al., 2014). By 2014, under Jonathan's administration, Nigeria had 134,000 hospital beds, which is 0.8 per thousand populations, below the other African region's rate. The number of hospital beds since 2009 grew at a compound annual growth rate (CAGR) of 3.8%, slightly higher than population growth, but at an insufficiently high quality to significantly impact the population bed ratio. There is an unequal distribution of personnel and infrastructures between the Southern and Northern states. There were 800 people per bed in the Southwest (Bendel, Lagos, Ogun, Ondo, and Oyo states), 1300 per bed in the Southeast (Anambra, Cross River, Imo, and Rivers states), 2200 per bed in the Middle belt (Bauchi, Benue, Gongola, Kwara, and Plateau states), and 3800 people per hospital bed in the North (Borno, Kaduna, Kano, Niger, and Sokoto states) (Anonymous, n.d.-a). The number of physicians grew at a CAGR of 2.7% since 2009, reaching 66,555 in 2014. The growth has been consistent with population growth – that is, the rate per thousand people has remained at 0.4, compared to 0.8 physicians per thousand people in South Africa. Nurses are in short supply in the country. There are about 268,000 nurses, which is equal to 1.5 nurses per thousand people. Dentists are also in short supply, with less than 3000 registered as of 2014 (MedCOI, 2018). Unfortunately, HCPs in public hospitals no longer have access to expensive medical therapeutic and diagnostic equipment because they are no longer functional. Still, the government does not have the resources to replace them.

The private health sector plays a dominant role in service delivery. They own 30% of the health establishments but provide over 60% of health service delivery (WHO, 2018). Private-sector healthcare services in Nigeria include hospitals, clinics and rehabilitation facilities, pharmaceutical stores, traditional medical practitioner centers, spiritual homes, and churches. Over the years, the major cities, such as Abuja, Enugu, Ibadan, Benin, Kano, Lagos, and Port Harcourt, have witnessed noticeable growth in the number of private facilities. The dominance of the private sector over public institutions betrays the Nigerian governments' relative inattention to healthcare delivery and conscious historical underfunding. Despite official promises to expand health care, a marked difference exists in the number and quality of health services provided in private and public facilities and between urban and rural areas.

Service delivery in the private sector is highly fragmented, consisting of small clinics and hospitals of less than ten beds with minimal facilities. However, there are a few reputable and medium-sized private hospitals across the country. The top five private hospitals in 2020 are Lagoon Hospital in Lagos, Primus Super Specialty Hospital in Abuja, Eko Hospital in Lagos, St. Nicholas Hospital in Lagos, and First Consultants Medical Center in Lagos. St. Nicholas Hospital is the foremost kidney transplant and dialysis center in the country.

Other highly regarded private hospitals are Reddington Hospital in Victoria Island, Lagos, and St. Edmund Eye Hospital in Surulere, Lagos, founded in 1965 by Dr. Edmund Abiola Akinocho. Reddington started in 2001 as a cardiac health center, became a full-fledged hospital in 2006, and pioneered the first digital cardiac catheterization and angiography in Nigeria. Reddington is now affiliated with Cromwell Hospital in London. St. Edmund Eye Hospital provides ambulatory eye surgeries with modern equipment in line with international standards. It has five beds for inpatient admission, with the capacity to handle over 4000 outpatients annually. Mission hospitals also deliver high-quality health care. For example, the Seventh-Day Adventist hospital in Ile-Ife, established in 1940, and Wesley Guild hospital in Ilesha became the nucleus of the University of Ife (now Obafemi Awolowo University) teaching hospital complex in 1975. Similarly, Baptist Medical Center in Ogbomosho, established in 1917, is a critical care institution serving the local communities and beyond. Many of the private health centers in the country are managed better than public health facilities. However, on average, healthcare cost is higher in private health establishments than in government hospitals (MedCOI, 2018).

President Muhammadu Buhari in 2017 launched the universal health coverage plan for primary health care aimed at delivering quality primary care services to all Nigerians – particularly the rural and vulnerable populations (United States Agency for International Development – USAID, 2017). In 2019, President Buhari again launched the Third Generation Cooperation Strategy based on WHO recommendation. The plan featured the country's long-term strategic plan towards attaining UHC and implementing the basic healthcare provision fund. Buhari's strategic goal was aligned with the Sustainable Development Goals (SDGs) and national health plan (WHO, 2019a). On January 9, 2019, President Buhari launched the second National Strategic Health Development Plan (2018–2022) to achieve UHC consistent with the 2014 National Health Act. The new plan focuses more on rural dwellers, children under 5 years, women, and the elderly. On the same occasion, President Buhari unveiled the first phase of the N55 billion primary healthcare funds to invest in human capacity-building and infrastructure (Onyedika-Ugoeze, 2020).

The Current State of the Nigerian Health System (2019–2021)

Alegbeleye (2019) aptly described the current state of the Nigerian health system as highly disorganized, unsanitary, unfriendly, and highly stressful to navigate. A visit to public hospitals in major cities highlights a depressing scene of too many patients and insufficient personnel to cater to them. Patients commonly sleep on the floor in hospital premises overnight or arrive hours before dawn to get a spot on the queue, with no guarantee of being attended before closure. Thousands of patients converge daily at the hospitals seeking treatment for various health problems but often leave in annoyance because of the quality of care (Ogundipe et al., 2015). Out of frustration, many patients turn to religion (traditional, Christianity, or Islamic) for a miracle cure instead of orthodox medicine that is expensive and arduous to navigate.

Nigeria's healthcare system is grossly underdeveloped and does not conform to many global best practices. The health system is organized into primary, secondary, and tertiary levels. However, the system is fragmented, with only a tiny fraction unified and organized into a functional unit. There is a referral process between these three levels. Unfortunately, the referral process is not always respected and is one of the system's central maladies. Diseases expected to be managed at the primary level often end up at the tertiary level because the primary level is fragile, with inadequate infrastructures and personnel (MedCOI, 2018). The healthcare system is divided into private and public health networks. Because of the low-quality services delivered in the public health facilities, most people relied on the private sector, where quality care is expensive and beyond most citizens' reach.

The health system's infrastructure remains low and insufficient to cater to the booming population. Much of the infrastructure is in the major cities, with urbanites getting four times as much access to health care as the rural dwellers. The federal and state governments have both adopted a public-private partnership strategy to improve healthcare infrastructure. Multiple models are utilized, but the most common is how the government solely finances the infrastructure and contracts it to a private franchise to operate the facility. In the tertiary health facilities in the Southern part of the country and the highly resourced private hospitals in Lagos, almost all diseases or ill-health conditions are managed. But the services are costly and usually out of the reach of the economically disadvantaged.

Typically, Nigerian public hospitals are divided into general wards, which provide outpatient and inpatient care for a nominal fee, and amenity wards charge higher prices but provide better care (Fig. 3.2). The general wards were usually overcrowded, with a long waiting period for registration and treatment. Patients frequently do not see a physician, but the nurse or other healthcare occupation workers treat them. Many drugs are often not available at the hospital pharmacy, and those available are usually dispensed without containers. Patients provide their

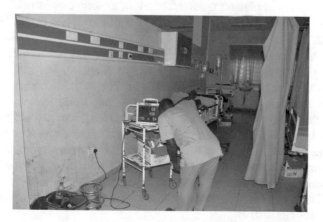

Fig. 3.2 A male medical ward at UNIMED, Ondo City. (Photograph used with permission from UNIMED PRO)

containers. The inpatient wards are often overcrowded; beds in corridors with mattresses on floors. Food is free for indigent patients. However, most patients have relatives or friends who prepare their food within the premises of the hospital. On the other hand, in the amenity wards, where the elites occupy, food, drugs, and better care are provided (Anonymous, n.d.-a).

Most countries worldwide are on the fast track of development, but Nigeria is on the decline. Like every aspect of Nigerian life, the health system is substantially better post-independence than today in 2021. For example, citizens of other nations, including the Saudi Arabia royal family, came to the University College Hospital, Ibadan, for treatment in the 1960s and 1970s (Mamora, 2020). Unfortunately, the current chaos and low quality of care provided in Nigeria's tertiary hospitals has made the health system a laughing stock worldwide. For over six decades, the politician and military rulers failed to provide UHC, a human rights issue of utmost importance.

Living in present-day Nigeria is exceptionally stressful because basic amenities are generally lacking – but citizens ingeniously improvise to obtain basic life necessities such as water and electricity. The power supply is lacking or epileptic in many cities, causing elite families to use solar devices or generators. Cases of carbon monoxide poisoning from generators are on the rise. Many families in urban centers lack access to clean water and have to use boreholes. The rural dwellers draw water from wells, open streams, or rivers. The country is practically a failed state as necessary social infrastructures (road, water, and electricity) are unreliable or nonexistent in the rural areas where 70% of the people live. Besides, health care is out of reach for over 95% of the population who are uninsured. On the other hand, the elites travel abroad to receive health care and send their children abroad for their education.

Aside from Abuja, the capital, many cities are poorly planned, usually overcrowded, with ineffective road networks and public transportation systems packed like sardines. Most cities lack waste management systems and other necessary structures for functionality and support for human habitation. One dangerous but conventional means of transportation is the use of motorcycles (*okada*) that are very prone to fatal accidents and a significant cause of injuries and deaths (Alegbeleye, 2019). In addition to unregulated food and poor nutrition, skin bleaching and fake drugs contribute to poor health. All of these factors and heavy traffic holdup in major cities present significant stressors to city dwellers.

Eke (2015) contends that South Africa's healthcare infrastructure is the most advanced on the African continent, while the Nigerian health system is still underdeveloped and lacks modern infrastructures. Due to the insecurity and poor working condition at home, Nigerian HCPs in large numbers have relocated to other African countries like Ghana, Zimbabwe, Namibia, Mozambique, and South Africa to work in their hospitals and universities. This setback is a reversal of fortune for Nigeria. President Shehu Shagari in 1983 expelled more than two million African workers, primarily Ghanaian, for outstaying their visas and taking jobs from Nigerians (Lawal, 1983; Legg, 2019).

Previous leaders build tertiary hospitals across the country to satisfy the "federal character" mandate but are unconcerned with their viability. What makes a health system reputable is not the aesthetics of the buildings but the commitment and competence of the HCPs and the facility's resources (Abubakar, 2019). Many health analysts and scholars have expressed concerns about the low quality of care provided in Nigeria's tertiary hospitals (Julius, 2015; Onwujekwe et al., 2018). As of January 2021, there are 57 tertiary hospitals in the country—21 UTHs, 23 FMCs, and 13 specialist hospitals—and they are listed in Chap. 4. Despite the many tertiary hospitals, the healthcare system is weak, as most hospitals are in name only, as little attention is invested in workforce development and infrastructures. Recommendations on tertiary hospital reforms are presented in Chap. 13.

More concerning about the current state of the tertiary hospitals is the widespread shortage of qualified HCPs. For example, the country has only 35,000 physicians, but by WHO's standard, it needs 237,000 physicians. The deficit is partially due to the massive migration of the HCPs abroad in search of greener pastures. The current stock of practicing physicians is about 35% less than the officially reported numbers because the data have never been updated since 1963. The physician's ratio is at 0.17 practitioners per 1000 population – among the lowest in Africa. The country has a shortage of all primary HCPs, and the density is estimated to be dismal to deliver essential health services effectively (MedCOI, 2018).

The geographic maldistribution of health establishments and human resources among the regions and the inadequacy of rural health centers persists. The shortage hardest hit is the Northeast region, followed by the Northwest. The Northeast region, where 14% of the population lives, has only 4% of the physicians, whereas the Southwest, with 20% of the population, has 43.9% of the physicians. With more people than the Southwest and a higher disease burden, the Northwest region has only 20% of the country's physicians. The low wages, underinvestment in healthcare infrastructure, and insecurity in the Northern states contribute to the inability to attract physicians to the health facilities. Most of the medical practitioners are concentrated in tertiary and secondary health facilities located in urban areas. This situation is due to the less attractive remuneration and the unattractive work conditions in rural areas (MedCOI, 2018).

Budget allocation to the health sector in the last two decades has not been up to 10% of the federal budget, even though African countries' leaders committed to allocating 15% in the Abuja declaration of 2001 (Abuja Declaration 2001). Since 1995, healthcare expenditure in Nigeria as a percentage of the GDP has never been up to 10%. It recorded the highest value of 9.2% in 2007 and the lowest at 3.7% in 2002 (Fig. 3.3). In the last decade, spending rose from 3.9% in 2010 to 6% by 2012. Unfortunately, the health budget decreased in 2013 to 4.0%, only 2.6% in 2014, 3.7% in 2016, 4.2% in 2017, and declined again to 3.9% in 2018 (World Bank, 2021). Nigeria's healthcare expenditure has been consistently lower than the average of 8.8% for the Organization for Economic Cooperation and Development (OECD) countries and 17.9% in the United States in 2017 (Martin et al., 2018).

Nigeria has one of the lowest ($217) healthcare expenditures per capita in the world; even Angola spends more per capita ($239) than Nigeria (Fig. 3.4). South Africa spends $1148, five times more per capita; Switzerland $6468, thirty times

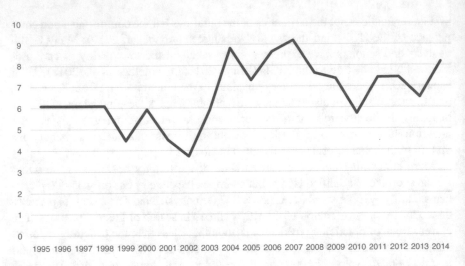

Fig. 3.3 Healthcare expenditure as a percentage of the GDP: 1995–2014. (Source: World Bank, 2021)

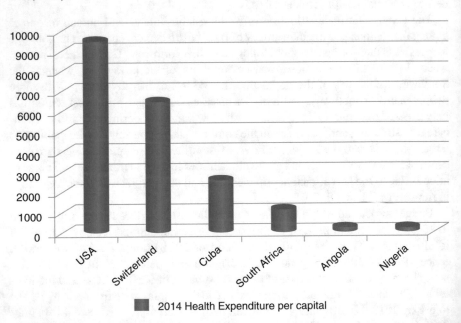

2014 Health Expenditure per capital

Fig. 3.4 Health expenditure per capita in Nigeria and in selected countries around the world. (Source: WHO, 2016a)

more per capita; Cuba spends $2475, eleven times per capital, while the United States spends $9403, 43 times per capita on health care than Nigeria (WHO, 2016a).

The federal government's inadequate funding of health care causes Nigerians to contribute substantially more toward their health than any country in Africa (Fig. 3.5). For example, in 2014, out-of-pocket expenses accounted for a whopping

Fig. 3.5 Out-of-pocket health expenditure (percentage of private spending on health) in selected countries around the world. (Sources: World Bank, 2017; WHO, 2016b)

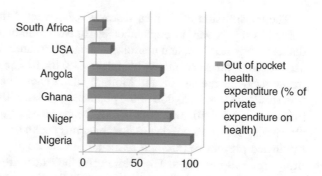

96% of the total healthcare expenses in Nigeria, compared to 67% in Ghana, 13% in South Africa, and 21% in the United States (World Bank, 2017).

The dismal health budget is reflective of the complacence of the Nigerian leaders towards the health sector. Similarly, the dingy health budget is the primary reason for the country's low-quality health care and why UHC has been a pie in the sky. Sadly, at the end of 2020, President Buhari's administration has failed to achieve the 30% health insurance coverage goal set in 2016. The current challenges facing the health system are discussed in greater detail in Chap. 5. The political and economic reforms needed to achieve universal and high-quality health care are discussed in Chapters 11 and 12. Chapter 14 discusses studies that explored consumers' and patients' levels of satisfaction with the Nigerian healthcare system.

Health Outcome Indicators

For decades, Nigeria's health system has one of the worst outcomes in the world. The infants, child, and maternal mortality indices and burden of communicable disease in the country are still unacceptably high, despite recent modest gains. Nigeria has one of the highest infant, child, and maternal mortality rates and ranked 153rd out of 187 countries on the United Nations' human development index. Nigeria is also ranked 187th out of 191countries. The health system is weak and the services delivered are of low quality with inequitable distribution and insufficient infrastructures (WHO, 2000, 2006, 2010a, 2010b, 2015, 2017b).

Nigeria's maternal mortality ratio is 814 per 100,000, and the mortality rate for children under five and infants is 104 and 70 per 1000 live births, respectively. A substantial disparity in health status exists across the different states and six geopolitical zones and rural/urban divide, education, and social class. Infectious diseases still constitute a significant public health problem: Malaria accounts for 27% of the global burden; tuberculosis (TB) prevalence is 323 per 100,000; HIV/AIDS prevalence is estimated at 3.2% – one of the highest burdens globally. Malnutrition is still prevalent, with a 43.6% stunting rate.

The transmission of Guinea worm was interrupted in 2013, and the last wild poliovirus report was in September 2016. Noncommunicable diseases, including diabetes, hypertension, and neurological disorders, are rising. Alcohol and tobacco use consumption is exceptionally high at 9.1% in 2015 and 17.4% in 2016, and road traffic accidents are significant. Mortality due to household and ambient air pollution stands at 99 per 100,000 of the population (WHO, 2018). The mortality rate for malaria is 146 per 100,000 populations (Muhammad et al., 2017). These unacceptable health outcomes are due to the penurious health service delivery compounded by limited preventive (pre and postnatal care, screening for specific diseases, and immunization) programs. The grim health indicators are attributed to the fact that over 95% of the population has no access to the aforementioned preventive healthcare services.

As of 2021, Nigeria has exceptionally high communicable and noncommunicable diseases and the world's highest disease-related morbidity and mortality. Infectious diseases, such as cholera, diphtheria, influenza, pneumonia, measles, mumps, tuberculosis, and nosocomial infections, are the primary causes of death. In addition to infectious diseases, diarrheal, malaria, diabetes mellitus, meningitis, prostate and breast cancer, liver disease, road traffic accidents, malnutrition, low birth weight, maternal conditions, tuberculosis, birth trauma, falls, violence, fires, drugs, and alcohol abuse also negatively contribute to the poor health outcomes. HIV/AIDS compound the disease burden and health challenges (World Health Ranking, 2016; Muhammad et al., 2017). Sadly, solutions to the disease burden are not in sight as the government has no coherent national health policy intensely focusing on UHC.

In the last decade, life-threatening contagious diseases have reduced substantially, and performance on key health indices slightly improved. Yet, Nigeria failed in 2015 to meet the United Nations' MDGs. In January 2016, after the MDGs' successes globally, the United Nations set in motion the 17 SDGs to end poverty by 2030 and ensure that the global community protects the planet and enjoys peace and prosperity. The 17 SDGs incorporated new interconnected ideas on economic inequality, innovation, climate change, peace, justice, and sustainable consumption; the first goal is eradicating extreme poverty in the world. Unfortunately, due to a lack of political will, Nigeria has made little or no progress on the 17 SDGs. Poverty in the country is at an all-time high. The challenge is complicated further by the fact that environmental pollution and climate challenges are on the ascendant. Given the above inadequacies, Nigeria is unlikely to meet the SDGs by 2030 unless some drastic interventions are taken to address these critical challenges.

The National Health Insurance Scheme Debacle

Before the Europeans arrived in Nigeria, the TMPs charged "fees" in barter and reciprocity. With the introduction of the Western-style health system, services were monetized and provided at a standard fee. The colonial masters did not directly extend services to rural dwellers but used medication as a platform for evangelism and associated traditional medicine with witchcraft, Satanism, and evil. The arrival of the missionaries led to the undermining and subsequent neglect of traditional medicine by the natives. With its humanistic and barter system, the TMPs expected some form of monetary reciprocity from patients and families. The missionary hospitals and maternities also charge some nominal fees for services. Thus, through the years, Nigerians became acquainted with paying for health services, and many were willing to pay when the federal and state governments could not sustain their welfare health scheme in the 1980s (Asakitikpi, 2019).

Asakitikpi (2019) proposed two models to explain the healthcare financing paradox in Nigeria. The first model supports the neoliberal health policy based on market forces and user fees for health services. The second (welfare model), which is in line with most government programs, advocates building more hospitals and health centers and expanding health insurance coverage. The two models have pros and cons, and both models have been implemented in the country with little success. In the past 60 years since independence, successive Nigerian governments have used a combination of the two models. However, none has achieved UCH – 95% of the uninsured population can still not access the health system because of the high cost (Awosusi et al., 2015; Ifijeh, 2015; NOIPolls, 2017; Amu et al., 2018; Aregbeshola & Khan, 2018).

The first Nigerian leader who introduced welfare model health and education systems was Chief Obafemi Awolowo – Nigeria's foremost federalist, a visionary and dynamic leader who advocated federalism as the sole basis for equitable national integration. As the premier of the Western region from 1954 to 1959, Chief Awolowo established the first television station in Africa in 1959. Additionally, he championed many progressive policies in education, social services, and agricultural practices. During his tenure, he provided free health care for children and free universal primary education (The Editors of Encyclopedia Britannica, 2020). He also increased health services delivery in the rural areas, diversified the economy, and democratized the local governments in the Western region (Your Dictionary, n.d.). He financed all the programs mentioned above from agricultural products (primarily cocoa), which was the regions' economy's mainstay. Having achieved so much with limited resources, many analysts wondered what would Chief Awolowo have done as Nigeria's President at the peak of the oil boom in the 1970s? That is a hypothetical question widely debated, but the public will never know the correct answer. Many of Chief Awolowo's critics believe he would have successfully implemented UHC.

Nigeria embraced the health insurance concept as far back as 1962, two years after independence, when the Lagos Social Health Insurance was enacted. Unfortunately, it was cut short for unknown reasons. The government provided free health care in public establishments. In the 1980s, the government disbanded the UHC policy due to the global slump in oil prices. In 1985, a committee set up by the FMH recommended launching a health insurance scheme by mid-1991. Unfortunately, their proposal did not see the light of the day until 8 years later, in 1999, when the National Health Insurance Scheme (NHIS) was established as a corporate body under Act 35 (Chukwudozie, 2015).

After independence in 1960, President (Dr.) Nnamdi Azikiwe/Prime Minister (Alhaji) Tafawa Balewa (1963–1966) implemented health care with little success. General Yakubu Gowon (1966–1975) had the best opportunity to provide UHC at the peak of the oil boom but lacked the political will, instead he wasted the nation's money on white elephant ventures. All the other Nigerian leaders after Gowon did not consider UHC number one in their budget priorities – General Murtala Mohammed (1975–1976), Major General Olusegun Obasanjo's (1976–1979), President Shehu Shagari's (1979–1983), Major General Muhammadu Buhari (1983–1985), General Ibrahim Babangida (1985–1993), interim President Ernest Shonekan (1993), General Sani Abacha (1993–1998), and General Abdulsalami Abubakar (1998–1999).

General Ibrahim Babangida's administration (1985–1993) introduced the health management organization (HMO) concept in the health system. Zenith Medicare Limited was registered in 1990 to offer health insurance policy for individuals, a small group of employers, and large corporate firms. Seven years later, in 1997, General Sani Abacha registered more HMOs to provide healthcare services to the public and corporate organizations – the Premium Health Limited in Ibadan, the MediPlan Healthcare Limited in Lagos, Prepaid Medical Services in Abuja, and the Healthcare International in Lagos. In 1998, the Total Health Trust opened in Lagos as a healthcare provider. Other HMO providers opened up in large cities around the country.

In 1999, the health system's chaos culminated in the flagship NHIS under Act 35 decree, which amended the Nigerian Health Insurance program incepted in 1962. The stated primary goal of NHIS is to provide quality health care to all Nigerians at an affordable cost for the poor. Although the NHIS was approved first in 1999, the government did not implement it for 6 years under two health ministers – Dr. Tim Menakaya (1999–2001) and Professor Alphonsus B. Nwosu (2001–2003). A national survey in 2004, before the formal launching of the NHIS, revealed that only 0.1% of Nigerians had health insurance coverage. Professor Eyitayo Lambo, as minister of health, launched the NHIS on June 6, 2005, and enrolled consumers in September of the same year. The NHIS was conceived as the critical pathway to improve the nation's dismal health outcomes.

The health insurance coverage is provided from the shared pool of funds contributed by the consumers who pay a fixed, regular amount that allows the Health Maintenance Organizations (HMOs) to fund the health system. It is primarily a risk-sharing arrangement program meant to improve resource mobilization and equity. The NHIS also regulates HMOs' private health insurance (NHIS, 2004). It covers inpatient hospital care for up to 15 days per year, outpatient care, maternal care for up to four live maternal births; preventative care including immunization; family planning and health education; consultation with specialists, and preventive dental care. Furthermore, the government provides free health care to children under the age of five and people with disabilities. It also provides a new bone marrow donor program for patients with leukemia, lymphoma, and sickle cell disease established in 2012 (Julius, 2015; Awosusi et al., 2015).

The administration of Olusegun Obasanjo in 2005 projected that Nigeria would achieve universal coverage within 10 years. By all indications, the NHIS was not pursued with vigor by the succeeding administrations. Sadly, the program fizzled out after Professor Lambo's tenure as health minister in May 2007. As of 2012, only four million Nigerians were enrolled, and 62 HMOs, 5949 healthcare providers, 24 banks, 5 insurance companies, and 3 insurance brokers were registered (Obalum & Fiberesima, 2012). Most enrollees as of 2015 are in the formal sector with abysmal coverage in the informal sector economy. Bauchi and Cross River have enrolled their employees around the same timeline, while eight other states—Lagos, Ondo, Oyo, Abia, Enugu, Gombe, Imo, and Jigawa Kaduna—have indicated interest. Four states—Lagos, Kwara, Ogun, and Akwa Ibom—are implementing state-led community-based health insurance programs to reach the economy's informal sector with varying coverage levels (Awosusi et al., 2015).

During the second term, Obasanjo's administration purchased significant state-of-the-art equipment, revamped the facilities in the tertiary hospitals, made drugs available in pharmacy outlets, and constant power supply in government hospitals became routine. However, Obasanjo's administration introduced fees for public hospitals' services due to the economy's downturn. Unfortunately, this decision led to a higher healthcare cost, which the lower class, made up over 75% of the population, cannot afford. Indeed, the neoliberal healthcare reforms benefitted only the upper and middle classes (Asakitikpi, 2019). The two administrations that succeeded Obasanjo—President Umaru Yar'Adua (2007–2010) and President Jonathan Goodluck (2010–2015)—did little to advance the implementation of the goals of the NHIS. By 2014, only five million people (3% of the population) had insurance coverage through the NHIS, and these are primarily workers in the formal sector, particularly federal civil servants. In the quest to accelerate progress towards UHC, the NHIS decentralized the implementation of the country's social health insurance program to the states (Okpani & Abimbola, 2015). Alhaji Umaru Yar'Adua, President Goodluck Jonathan, and the incumbent President Muhammadu Buhari (2015-) introduced some degree of user fees in public hospitals, which unexpectedly ushered in private health care. Private health centers have exponentially increased in the last three decades. With the expansion of private health care and the boom in the fake drug market, most Nigerians became suspicious of Western-style health care and resorted to traditional medicine (Asakitikpi, 2019).

The healthcare budget in 2014 at N262 billion ($1.6 billion) was the fourth largest allocation after defense, education, and finance (when including debt servicing). Advocacy groups and analysts believe that health allocation is grossly far less than what is needed to achieve UHC. In recent years, the per capita government expenditure on health has fluctuated between $21 and $29, which exceeds the $14 minimum benchmark recommended by the WHO for developing countries but far below the global average of around $615 (Oxford Business Group, 2015). Nigeria annually receives about $2 billion in health-related foreign aid and nongovernmental organizations, while other private groups account for some 3% of annual expenses. Individual out-of-pocket spending makes up the remainder (Oxford Business Group, 2015).

In 2016, President Buhari's administration amended the National Health Bill to make the NHIS affordable to consumers with equitable reimbursement for health-care providers. It expanded private sector participation to achieve 30% coverage by 2015. The new bill also proposed a new framework for drug distribution to reduce counterfeit and substandard medicine in the local market. Both goals were never achieved by the target date (Oxford Business Group, 2015).

In 2017, President Buhari's administration approved the second National Strategic Health Development Plan (NSHDP-II) that provides the path needed to support significant progress in improving the national health system's performance. It also emphasizes primary health care as the bedrock of the national health system and provides financial risk protection to all Nigerians, impoverished and vulnerable populations. In partnership with the FMH, the Nigerian Sovereign Investment Authority (NSIA) agreed to modernize and expand healthcare services through private sector participation. The cooperation will enhance the specialist hospitals and diagnostic centers' capacity to provide advanced healthcare services. So far, ten agreements have been signed between the NSIA, the FMH, and various healthcare facilities throughout the country, six of them already in advanced phases. In 2017, Lagos was the first state to pass the mandatory State-Based Health Insurance Scheme (SHIS) designed to reduce the financial burden of receiving health care and improving access to quality care (Olasunkanmi, 2017).

In 2019, President Muhammadu Buhari commissioned the Lagos University Teaching Hospital (LUTH) Cancer Centre. Varian Inc. USA supplied the equipment for the center. In addition to the partnership with the NSIA, the FMH has also set higher targets to increase healthcare access, aiming to increase the number of primary healthcare centers (PHCs) to ensure more accessible access to health care for 100 million Nigerians. To make this goal a reality, the FMH plans to build 10,000 PHCs with at least one PHC in each ward throughout the country (Eke, 2015).

As of 2020, there were about 40 accredited HMOs in the country, with each vying for more market share. In 2017, the former Minister of Health, Isaac Folorunso Adewole, confirmed that the federal government spent over N351billion on HMOs (Ovuakporie and Nwabughiogu, 2017). Unfortunately, the country has little to show for this massive expense as 120 million Nigerians still do not have health insurance coverage. For most people, payment for health care is primarily out of pocket. One significant barrier to increase NHIS participation rates is the nonmandatory nature of most health insurance in Nigeria. While most federal civil service employees are currently subscribed to the program, the NHIS is yet to capture most citizens, including those working in the large informal sector economy (Eke, 2015). Health insurance sector stakeholders, such as the NHIS and HMOs, call for legislation that makes health insurance mandatory. Because of the insurance market's competitive nature, the HMOs regularly cut prices to gain market share. The cuts often result in lower-quality services for patients (Eke, 2015). As of 2021, slightly over ten million Nigerians (4.8% of the population) have subscribed to the NHIS (Ezigbo, 2021).

Sadly, 16 years after President Obasanjo launched the NHIS, less than 5% of the population is insured (Awosusi et al., 2015; Ifijeh, 2015; NOIPolls, 2017; Amu et al., 2018; Aregbeshola & Khan, 2018). The insured are mostly government officials and private employees often forced to enroll in the program. Unfortunately, the exclusion of certain drugs and diseases—diabetes, sickle cell anemia, HIV, cancer—from most health insurance policies often leads many insured people to desperately seek treatment from the TMPs. A cornucopia of reasons has been offered for the lack of meaningful progress in universal coverage. Ifijeh (2015) avers that Nigerians are not seeking coverage due to a lack of awareness of the benefits they stand to gain from having better access to quality healthcare services. Other reasons adduced include the tepid support from the state governments, employers, and the high co-pay required from consumers. The delay in implementing the NHIS is unsettling when smaller and less economically endowed countries such as Rwanda boast of universal coverage. Substantial evidence revealed that public financing is critical to achieving UHC, but government expenditure on health in Nigeria has been dismal, and domestic resource mobilization is weak.

A study conducted by Odeyemi and Nixon in 2013, comparing the Nigeria's NHIS with that of Ghana that was launched simultaneously, reported that Ghana experienced a sharp decline in out-of-pocket expenditure in 2004 from 80% to 66%. In contrast, Nigeria saw high out-of-pocket expenditure levels, which persist at 93–95% from 2000 to 2010. Access to health services in Nigeria remains very low because NHIS has minimal impact on reducing finance-related health inequality. The private health insurance system operates based on flat-rate packages; how much each consumer pays as their annual insurance premium determines the coverage's extent. Macha et al. (2012) consider the private health insurance system regressive because it harmed equity and proposed a progressive healthcare financing system where the more affluent in the population pay more of their income for healthcare taxation than the needy.

Today, Nigeria's healthcare system is one of the most inefficient, with the worst health outcome indices globally (WHO, 2000, 2010a, 2010b). Healthcare spending has never risen to 10% of the gross domestic product (GDP), and over 95% of the population is uninsured. Recommendations on how Nigeria can achieve a universal and high-quality healthcare system are presented in Chapters 12 and 13.

Present and Future Threats to the Health System

Corruption: Several scholars and analysts contend that corruption is very pervasive in the health sector (Onwujekwe et al., 2018, 2019, 2020; Ogbaa, 2017; Ibenegbu, 2018; Tormusa & Idom, 2016). Allocated funds are usually diverted within the system, irrespective of the health budget percentage, due to corruption and public finance inefficiencies. Besides, corruption outside the health sector is more massive. Between 2006 and 2013, 55 Nigerians stole 1.35 trillion Naira ($6.8 billion; exchange rate of 150₦ to $1) meant, in part, to buy weapons to fight Boko Haram's six-year Islamist uprising. The stolen money can build 36 hospitals or provide education to the university level for 4000 children (Associated Press and Reuters, 2016).

In 2019, the federal government confirmed $400 billion was stolen through corrupt practices, and $40 million worth of jewelry was seized from former Minister of Petroleum Resources, Diezani Alison-Madueke (Nwezeh & Shittu, 2019). Some social critics linked the country's economic woes to continued spending spree culture, looting, lawlessness, and indiscipline, which are the modus operandi in national life (Suberu et al., 2015). Olamide opined that corruption poses a genuine threat to diversification because the assets that should be diverted to different economic sectors are upset by unlawful practices. The politicians and government establishments are against diversification but prefer to maintain the status quo. Indeed, corruption is a significant existential threat to the future of the country.

Socioeconomic Inequities: Beaumont and Abrak reported on a 2017 study by the Brookings Institute in the United States that found Nigeria, one of the two wealthiest economies in Africa, has overtaken India as the world's largest concentration of extreme poverty. Over 87 million Nigerians live in extreme poverty, compared to 73 million Indians. The study predicted that in the next 12 years, nine out of every ten most impoverished persons on the African continent would have nine out of every ten of the poorest people in the world (Beaumont & Abrak, 2018). Despite the austerity measures preached by the Nigerian leaders since the 1980s, Nigeria ranked second after Angola in Africa's top producers of sudden millionaires (Fig. 3.6).

Nigeria ranked highly in the number of millionaires in Africa, yet it ranked fifth globally in poverty after Chad, Madagascar, Zambia, and Haiti (Ferreira, 2019). About 40.1% of Nigerians live below the poverty line. Sokoto and Taraba states had the highest number of people living below the poverty line, while the lowest poverty rates are in the South-South and Southwestern states. Lagos state's poverty rate is

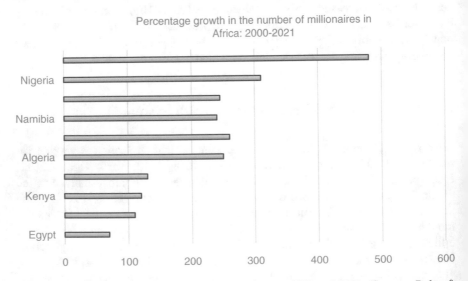

Fig. 3.6 Top producers of millionaires in Africa between 2000 and 2021. (Sources: Dolan & Yakowicz, 2020; Dawkins et al., 2021)

4.5% – the lowest rate in the country. In Nigeria, an individual is considered poor when they have less than 137,400₦ ($361) per year (Varrella, 2020). Nigeria is indeed a proverbial tale of two cities: the superrich in one lane and the destitute poor in the other lane. The vast socioeconomic inequities between the rich and the indigent are a threat to national stability and development as the poor may one day decide to revolt against the oppressive system.

Medical Tourism: Notwithstanding the enviable developments recorded in number of hospital buildings constructed across the country since independence, the human capital and physical infrastructure within the hospitals remain limited. Consequently, the services provided are substandard, low quality, and insufficient to cater to the fast-growing population. Annually, over 30,000 elite Nigerians and politicians travel to India, United Arab Emirates, South Africa, United States, and Europe to receive treatments for open-heart surgeries, brain surgeries, cancer, ophthalmology, and renal transplantation transplants (Fig. 3.7). On average, over 2500 Nigerians travel abroad monthly for health care, drawing between $ 1.5 billion from the country (NOIPolls, 2017, Eke, 2015, Huhuonline, 2021). By developing the nation's tertiary hospitals to a standard world level, the elites and politicians will spend their health care cost money at home instead of abroad.

In the middle of a global COVID 19 pandemic ravaging the country, President Muhammed Buhari traveled to the United Kingdom on March 31, 2021, to receive treatment for a chronic disease that Nigerian HCPs can effectively manage at home. Medical tourism is a threat to Nigeria's sovereignty as a nation and a drain on the economy. The funds spent on the medical jamboree can be used to develop the healthcare system.

Lack of Continuity of Policies and Ineffective Leadership: Some scholars and health analysts assert that the lack of meaningful progress in the health system and the health outcome indices is due to the lack of continuity in implementing the pro-

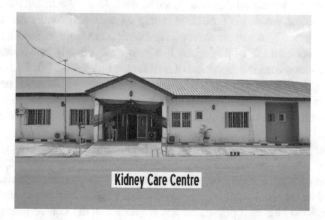

Fig. 3.7 UNIMED Kidney Care Center at Ondo City. (Photograph used with permission from UNIMED PRO)

posed health development plans since independence. Each administration often radically changes the national health plans implemented by the previous administration. In 2009, the Nigerian National Health Conference grandly described the health system as "weak as evidenced by lack of coordination, fragmentation of services, the dearth of resources, including inadequate and decaying infrastructure, drug and supplies, inequity in resource distribution, and access to care and very deplorable quality of care... the lack of clarity of roles and responsibilities among the different levels of government to have compounded the situation" (Nigeria National Health Conference, 2009). Indeed, the health system lacks good governance and needs effective leaders at all levels to turn things around for the better.

Nepotism and Tribalism: The current management of the universities and the UTHs reflects the decay and disorders in the larger society and a threat to the academy and health institutions' future. The system is mangled in corruption, tribalism, and mediocrity, as in every Nigeria's aspect of life. In the early years of university education in the country, Vice Chancellors' (VCs) appointment was based on merit without ethnic consideration. For example, the University of Ibadan routinely appointed non-Yoruba as the VC – Professor Kenneth Onwuka Dike (1960–1967), Professor Oritsejolomi Thomas (1972–1975), and Professor Tekena Tamuno (1975–1979). Today, the academy has become tribal enclaves where only "natives" are welcomed to apply for the VCs, even federal government-owned universities. The traditional rulers in the institution's jurisdiction are now the power brokers in selecting VCs (Varrella, 2020).

Population's Peculiar Demographics: Despite the various national health plans enacted since 1956, health access today is only 43.3%. The inadequacy of the healthcare delivery system is due to the population's peculiar demographics. About 55% of Nigerians are rural dwellers, and 45% are urbanites. Private practitioners provide about 70% of health care and only 30% by the government. Over 70% of drugs dispensed in the country are adulterated. Approximately 52–60% of the people work in the informal sector, where tax collection is only sporadic and "under the table." Thus, the NHIS is financially anemic because its revenue comes from only 40% of the entire population. About 40.1% of Nigerians live below the poverty line—less than $1 a day—and cannot afford the high cost of health care (Welcome, 2011). For the NHIS to be financially buoyant, the government must significantly reduce the percentage of the population in poverty and must reduce substantially those in the informal sector through job creation and opportunities that will promote self-actualization.

Brain Drain: Shortage of HCPs and insufficient funding are barriers to the implementation of UHC in the country. Nigerian HCPs are migrating abroad in enormous numbers because of poor working conditions. About 3936 Nigerian physicians, most of them trained in the local medical schools, currently practice in the United Kingdom, and another 4000 Nigerian physicians are employed in the United States healthcare system (Huhuonline, 2021). It is now evident that Nigeria has become a pipeline for the production of HCPs for developed countries. Although there are about 71,740 medical and dental practitioners listed on the Medical and Dental Council of Nigeria (MDCN), less than half of them (27,000) currently practice in the country. The problem of brain drain in the health sector has worsened the crisis. If the migration trend continues, the situation will pose an existential threat to the sustainability of the Nigerian healthcare system because the number of healthcare workers in the country is inadequate to serve the ever-growing population. It is conceivable that the continued deficit of HCPs will overwhelm the health system and eventually it will crash. A concerted effort is therefore needed to train more HCPs and retain those in the country by improving their service conditions.

Incessant Industrial Action: The Nigerian health system is notoriously known for regular industrial actions by HCPs. The strikes arise from disputes between physicians/dentists and the other HCPs over a range of issues relating to service conditions, the appointment of the minister of health, and the chief executive officer of the tertiary hospitals. The other HCPs allege that the government favors physicians/dentists in their conditions of service and appointments and have formed a union to counter the significant influence wielded by the Medical and Dental Council of Nigeria. Both feuding groups have frequently engaged in strikes, a situation that disrupts the nation's healthcare system. The constant labor strikes have caused untold hardship, suffering, and needless deaths across the country. It has also compelled many patients to seek care at private hospitals and clinics at a prohibitive cost, leaving those who cannot afford the cost of care at private hospitals at the doorstep of the TMPs with uncertain health outcomes. Besides the labor strikes, the country's HCPs are embroiled continuously in turf and territorial wars. Each health profession perceived the other as the enemy seeking to usurp their rights. The result is a lack of genuine collaboration in inpatient care and a threat to the health system's survival.

Weak Surveillance System Against Emerging Diseases: The health system lacks an effective medical surveillance system to track emerging diseases such as coronavirus disease 2019 (COVID-19) and bioterrorism. The health system had suffered several infectious disease outbreaks and mass chemical poisoning for several years. Besides efficient healthcare delivery, medical and epidemiological surveillance are critical functions of public health agencies charged with protecting the public from primary health threats – including emerging diseases and disaster outbreaks and bioterrorism. These deficiencies are threats to lives and national security. Consequently, it is desirable to build up the national capacity to prevent and track outbreaks of emerging pandemics and step up medical treatment and preventive measures to contain the disease spread over a large population (Welcome, 2011). Furthermore, a timely and accurate public health information system that can track disease outbreaks is needed to confront the multiple threats from emerging pandemics, bioterrorism, and climate changes impacts. At all levels, the government needs to strengthen workforce training capacity to address the challenges mentioned above.

Environmental Pollution: The WHO's particulate matter pollution benchmark is less than 10 µg/m^3, but the average in Nigeria is 26 µg/m^3 and only 8 µg/m^3 in the United States. Limited access to clean water constitutes a grave sanitation problem with debilitating life expectancy effects (Rine, 2019). The cases of unintentional carbon monoxide poisoning incidents are rising and are presently a public health problem. The familiar carbon monoxide exposure sources are from bush burning, fumes from the vehicle exhaust pipe, generator exhausts, outdoor cooking with firewood, barbecue, *Suya,* and indoor cooking stove.

Inhaling the air from the generator fume can cause headaches, dizziness, fatigue, vomiting, and nausea. Prolong exposure to moderate and high carbon monoxide levels increases heart disease risk and causes a shorter life span (Adekola, n.d.). At high doses, carbon monoxide causes unconsciousness and death in less than 3 min. In pregnant women, carbon monoxide poisoning can cause severe adverse fetal effects leading to hypoxia and damage to the nervous system. Other side effects include pneumonia, skin lesions, acute kidney failure, muscle necrosis, and visual problems. Specific preventive measures are needed to prevent the side effects of carbon monoxide on health. The government should launch a nationwide campaign directed at the youth to desist from setting bushes on fire. Additionally, the public health departments must educate generator owners not to place them in garages or near windows and stop self-repairing the device when they notice excess fume discharge. There is a dire need for active surveillance for proper generator use in the country (Heaalthfacts.ng, 2016).

Climate Change: Climate change is a real future threat to all nations, including Nigeria (Anonymous, n.d.-b). The United Nations Intergovernmental Panel on Climate Change recommends that carbon dioxide emission levels be cut to net zero by 2050 to prevent global warming of 1.5 °C above pre-industrial levels. Nigeria's climate has been changing with more frequent extreme temperatures, unpredictable rainfall patterns, a rise in coastal level and flooding, drought, desertification, land degradation, pollution of freshwater resources, and biodiversity loss. The direct effects of climate change generate heat waves, which causes unpredictable rainfall variation, heat stress, and drought are already adversely affecting agricultural production leading to food shortages. The condition is expected to get worse in the future if no mitigating intervention is implemented.

The Northern states' high vulnerability to climate change poses an imminent threat to national security through rising water in the coastal regions and food scarcity. Desert encroachment and steadily depleting vegetation and grazing resources in the Northern states have prompted massive emigration and resettlement to areas less threatened by desertification (Anonymous, n.d.-b). The emigration has exacerbated clashes among herders and farmers in different parts of the country and inter-ethnic conflicts that have produced fatalities (Haider, 2019). Eleven of the 36 states fall within the desert-prone zones affecting about 43 million people. Drought conditions in the North have also resulted in less drinking water. The menace of drought and desertification is an ecological disaster and future threat to sustainable development (The Federal Republic of Nigeria, 2018).

The indirect health impact of climate change in Nigeria produces malnutrition from food shortages, the spread of infectious disease, food and waterborne illness (e.g., typhoid fever, cholera). Adverse climate change is also associated with increased air pollution and higher temperatures with advanced meningitis cases (Haider, 2019).

Dismal Health Outcomes: Sub-Saharan Africa is notably lagging behind other regions of the world in meeting the MDGs – mainly, goals four to six focus on reducing child mortality, improving maternal health, malaria, HIV/AIDS, and other diseases by the year (United Nations Population Fund, n.d.). The high maternal mortality rate is among Nigeria's critical public health and developmental challenges. The high maternal fatalities are due to the delayed referral from unskilled providers, the lack of blood for transfusion during surgery, and the nonfunctional intensive care unit. Besides, the lifetime risk of dying from a pregnancy-related cause is 25 times higher in low-income countries than in high-income nation's hospitals (Aikpitanyi et al., 2019). Maternal death has a devastating impact on families and can cause long-term consequences for socioeconomic development.

One of the leading causes of child mortality globally is undernutrition and is estimated to cause at least half of all child deaths. Undernutrition is a critical determinant of maternal and child health and has significant adverse effects on children's brain and cognitive development. Undernutrition reduces the immunological capacity to defend against diseases and recurrent infections. This situation deprives the body of essential nutrients and leads to children's dismal growth, which adversely affects their future mental and physical development and learning capacity (De & Chattopadhyay, 2019).

Population Explosion: In 1960, Nigeria's population was 45.2 million, but it has dramatically surged to 201,062,775. Based on a growth rate of 3.2%, the country has witnessed over a 300% increase in 56 years. The population structure is predominantly young, with a median age of 18.2 years. The total dependency ratio is high at 89.2%, with a youth dependency of 84%. Put in the global context, Nigeria's population ranks number seven globally after China, India, United States, Indonesia, Brazil, and Pakistan. Nigeria's population surpasses Bangladesh, Russia, and Mexico (United Nations Population Fund, n.d.).

With 44% of the Nigerian population in extreme poverty, it drags down the financial resources needed to implement the UHC (Nigeria Demographic and Health Survey, 2013; The World Bank, 2020). Moreover, the population is growing more rapidly than available resources can sustain and quicker than the best attempt at any population control. Further population explosion will cause more severe competition for the health system's limited human and physical resources. The situation will worsen if urgent action is not taken to prevent further population growth.

Opportunities Within the Health System

Despite the multifaceted challenges discussed above, the federal government and entrepreneurs can resurrect the health system by exploiting the following ideas to invigorate the health system further.

Telehealth and Mobile Health Van for Health Services Delivery: Given decades of underfunding of health services, it is farsighted to explore cost control measures to make health more accessible, particularly in rural areas (WHO, 2010b). The HCPs can use telecommunications technology (telehealth) and mobile health clinics to replace the need to build expensive hospitals. The COVID-19 crisis unexpectedly caused a surge in new subscription levels for e-health service providers. Patients are now using telehealth platforms to consult HCPs to avoid visiting hospitals for fear of getting infected. The government has adopted the technology as part of its public health intervention programs, and clinicians foresee continuing growth in the demand for telehealth services in the future (Eke, 2015).

Partnership with Nigerian Healthcare Professionals in Diaspora: The earnings of Nigerians living abroad robustly impact their homeland economy. *Nigerian diaspora* accounts for over 33% of foreign migrant remittance flows to sub-Saharan Africa. Their remittance in 2018 was US$23.63 billion, which represented 6.1% of Nigeria's GDP – represents 83% of the federal budget and 11 times the foreign direct investment flows in the same year (Nevin & Omosomi, 2019). The economic power and expertise of the HCPs in the diaspora is a goldmine resource that the federal government can harness to develop the country.

Business Ventures: The health sector contributes 5% to GDP and remains a net importer of medical equipment and prescription drugs. The local production of medical products is limited to mundane items such as hospital beds and gurneys. Local pharmaceutical manufacturing companies can produce only over-the-counter medications, especially those for treating the common cold, malaria, headaches, and low-end prescription remedies. As the national disease pattern shifts from infectious diseases to lifestyle illnesses, pharmaceuticals sales are expected to reduce the dominance of anti-infection and anti-virus medications for new branded generic drugs (Oxford Business Group, 2015; Eke, 2015).

The primary driver of growth in healthcare demand in Africa is in the private sector. There are unique private sector business opportunities across the delivery chain in Nigeria. The United States is competitive in the sale of costly sophisticated diagnostic equipment to Nigeria. Test kits for malaria parasites, drug abuse, and infectious diseases such as HIV/AIDS and tuberculosis are also in high demand in Nigeria. The United States has a better opportunity than other countries to capture over-the-counter medications and supplements such as vitamins because of its high quality. China is a dominant offshore supplier of low-technology instruments that are cheap, and most private clinics can afford them. Vendors must register all medical devices and drugs imported into the country with the National Agency for Food

Drug Administration and Control (NAFDAC) and the Standards Organization of Nigeria (Eke, 2015). The registration process is painfully long as it requires several documents. Product counterfeiting is pervasive, and rights enforcement is weak.

Import tax in Nigeria is relatively low compared to other African countries. In 2013, the government stipulated a zero tariff on imported medical equipment, pharmaceutical manufacturing, and packaging materials to incentivize foreign investors. The zero tax rates are an incentive for entrepreneurs to do business in the country. But the duty rate of 20–25% on medical equipment is still being enforced. Imported drugs attract a 10% rate and 5% on pharmaceutical manufacturing equipment and packaging materials

In 2016, President Buhari's administration set a goal to achieve 30% health insurance coverage by 2015, but NHIS did not accomplish this goal till today. Consequently, prospective entrepreneurs have a unique opportunity to invest in insurance network ventures, increasing consumers' enrollment in the new health-care landscape. The expansion of the NHIS revenue will improve the quality of service provided within the health system. This development will give the HCPs better local career prospects and reduce the need for Nigerians to go abroad for treatment (Oxford Business Group, 2015).

New Health Facilities and Public-Private Partnerships: As part of the health sector intervention for the COVID-19 crisis, the Buhari administration plans to build 14 medical centers and expand two intensive care units in the six geopolitical zones. The project is expected to cost about $58 million. Federal and state governments are expected to use the public-private partnership model to attract private sector participation in health projects. For example, the Lagos State government is building 120–150 hospital beds (Medical Park facility) at US$247.3 million through a public-private partnership to provide a full spectrum of high-quality, cutting-edge facilities for medical and diagnostic services (Eke, 2015)

Electronic Medical Record Technology: Most Nigerian hospitals still store patient records manually using traditional paper methods. Affordable and straightforward Electronic Medical Record systems are now in great demand in the country. Also, medical consultants, personnel training, continuing education services, and hospital administration are badly needed in the health sector (Eke, 2015).

Performance of Health System in African Countries

Africans comprise 15% of the world's population, with a quarter of the global burden of disease and less than 3% of the worldwide healthcare professionals, but produce less than 1% of global research output. In 2020, African countries contributed only about 0.4% of their GDP towards research and development (Fig. 3.8). In contrast, Europe, Asia, and North America contributed 27%, 31%, and 37% of their GDP, respectively. Sadly, most West African countries spend less than 0.25% of their GDP on research and development, while most East and Southern African countries invest 1% or less (Olufadewa et al., 2020).

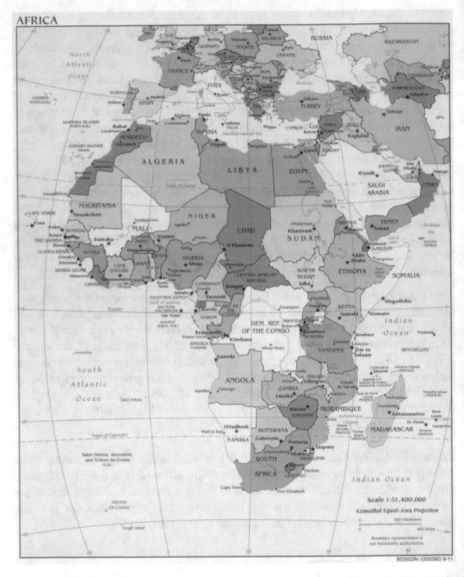

Fig. 3.8 Map of Africa. (Reproduced from: United States Central Intelligence Agency. (2011) Africa. [Washington, D.C.: Central Intelligence Agency] [Map] Retrieved from the Library of Congress, https://www.loc.gov/item/2012592672/)

Table 3.1 presents the health system performance indices for nine selected African countries – Ghana, Rwanda, Nigeria, South Africa, Kenya, Zimbabwe, Zambia, Tanzania, and Uganda (Fig. 3.8). Ghana and Rwanda have progressed the furthest toward achieving UHC. As of 2012, both countries provide UHC for the majority of their population. In the beginning, Rwanda provides its comprehensive health insurance mainly through foreign aid. In later years, the government made

Table 3.1 Comparison of the health system performance in Nigeria and selected African countries

	Country	2019 Population (million)	Health insurance coverage (% of the population insured)			Physician: people ratio	Health expenditure (% GDP)	WHO's (2000) overall health system performance ranking x/191
			Male	Both	Female			
1	Rwanda	12.6		91		1: 8919	6.6	172
2	Ghana	30.4	49.1		62.4	1:1000	3.6	135
3	Nigeria	201	3.1		1.1	1: 2000	3.7	187
4	South Africa	58.6		a		1:1000	9	175
5	Kenya	52.6	21.9		18.2	1:5000	5.7	140
6	Zimbabwe	14.7		9		1:10000	6.6	155
7	Zambia	17.9		a		1:6000	5	182
8	Tanzania	58.0	9.5		9.1	1:30000	5.6	152
9	Uganda	44.3		3		1:1000	7.2	149

Sources: (Worldometer, 2020; Aetna, 2021; WHO, 2000)
aNo national health insurance scheme

the system community-based and the ability to pay. The changes include a threefold increase in the minimum premium for the lowest tier of coverage, which some believe will be untenable for many of the country's poor.

Rwanda's health expenditure as a share of GDP was 6.6% in 2017. By 2019, Rwanda was close to attaining UHC because its President is committed to good health as a fundamental human right issue. Paul Kagame was elected in 2000 as the sixth and current President of Rwanda. The country has a 91% health insurance coverage and a 93% vaccination coverage rate. Over 90% of pregnant women give birth at a health center, and babies get vaccinated early in life, and there is a program designed specifically to remind mothers to come for a second dose. Children are immunized against 11 antigens, and the program embodies the UHC in the country (WHO, 2019b). In 2018, there were 1350 physicians in Rwanda, which translates to 1 physician per 8919 population (National Academy of Sciences, 2020).

Unlike Rwanda and Ghana, many African leaders lack the political will to implement NHIS or design innovative plans to fund UHC. In many countries that introduced NHIS, premiums and user fees were generally too high and challenging to collect. In Africa, premium-based models have not generated the robust financial revenue needed to initiate the UHC. Despite the financial constraints, many countries are slowly "moving in the direction" of implementing UHC by improving their NHIS plans (Appiah, 2012). Several countries like Nigeria, Tanzania, Kenya, Uganda, and Cameroon operate community-, private- or employer-based health insurance schemes, but their reach is minimal. Their plans offer protection for the poor and vulnerable populations but are unsustainable because they do not contribute adequate premiums to sustain the scheme.

Several countries continue to seek UHC funding through user fees while exempting vulnerable populations. For example, Mali and Burkina Faso have no user fees for children under five or pregnant women. In Nigeria, Tanzania, and Kenya, health insurance schemes have been introduced but only for public sector workers who pay monthly premiums. The majority of the workers are typically are not insured, or cannot afford, health insurance except, of course, for the very wealthy in the private sector (Appiah, 2012). In most West African countries, the formal sector (government) employees constitute only about 10–15% of the population, and their premiums are collected through payroll deductions. Unfortunately, most workers are in the informal sector, and managing their premiums is challenging because they do not earn fixed incomes.

Ghana has one of the highest health insurance coverage in Africa – 49.1% of males and 62.4% of the females are insured. The health system ranked 135th out of the 191 WHO's member states (Amu et al., 2018). In 2005, the Ghanaian government introduced the NHIS and financed it through monthly deductions of 2.5% of the formal economy worker's contribution to the social security fund, and a premium of between $4.80 and $32 per year for nongovernmental workers and a 2.5% national health insurance levy on goods and services. Children, pregnant women, the elderly, the impoverished, and the vulnerable have a premium exemption. In 2010, about 75% of the 24 million Ghanaians registered with the scheme, and 70% of enrollees were exempted from paying premiums (Appiah, 2012).

The public health service in Nigeria is financed through the NHIS, but only 1.1% of females and 3.1% of males are insured (Amu et al., 2018). Nigeria's health expenditure as a share of the GDP is a paltry 3.7%. Although Nigeria has a multidiscipline hospital network mainly in the urban areas, HCPs complain of low pay. In 2000, the WHO ranked Nigeria's health system's overall effectiveness at 187 among 191 member states. Since 2000, the government has implemented some initiatives, including family planning and immunization programs, to improve people's quality of life. Although the health system is improving, it faces many challenges, including a physician's low ratio at only 1 per 2000 people (low on a global scale), but better than Kenya, Zimbabwe, Zambia, Tanzania, and an inadequate infrastructure.

South Africa has a private health insurance plan covering about 16% of the population, but most people cannot afford the premium. South Africa has no NHIS system, but individuals can access the public health system regardless of nationality or immigration status. South Africa spends 9% of its GDP on health care, one of the highest in Africa. The health investment is on par with Spain and Malta, but the physician to population ratio is only 1–1000, well below the world average. The government supports low-income workers or people who cannot afford to serve private health insurance. South Africa's public health facilities are relatively well-equipped compared to other African nations, but the system is often overcrowded with long waiting times (Aetna, 2021).

In Zimbabwe, HCPs are in short supply, and necessary infrastructures such as beds, health information technology, and pharmaceuticals are limited and unreliable in several hospitals. The government in Zambia launched the NHIS in January 2020. Spending on health care in Kenya is only 5.7% of GDP – low by global standards but higher than that of its neighboring countries like Sudan and Ethiopia. Zimbabwe's health care system ranked 155th out of 191 in the WHO's, 2000 study. It has one physician per 10,000 people, and many private clinics in Zimbabwe will not treat patients until they have paid service fees upfront (Aetna, 2021).

As of 2019, Zambia has no NHIS, but the government plans to introduce UHC policy reforms to meet 2030 SDGs targets. In January 2020, the Zambian government announced a UHC benefits package covering contraceptive pills, implants, injectables, intrauterine devices, and emergency contraception. Zambia is the first country in the region to finance UHC for family planning and the first national-level advocacy for sexual and reproductive health and rights following the 2019 UN High-Level Meeting on UHC (Advance Family Planning, 2020).

Conclusion

Since independence in 1960, the various democratic and military governments of Nigeria have built hospitals and health centers but paid little attention to implementing UHC. Many vexing health disparities remained among the states, rural and urban areas, and across socioeconomic classes. The strong influence of politics on health and socioeconomic development leads to policy inconsistency. Each successive administration is distinguished by the "interest" policies they espoused, which are often not aligned with the initial national health plans. The future of the health system in Nigeria is at risk from a multitude of factors: medical tourism, ineffective leadership, nepotism and tribalism, brain drain, ongoing industrial action, weak surveillance system, air pollution and carbon monoxide poisoning, climate change,

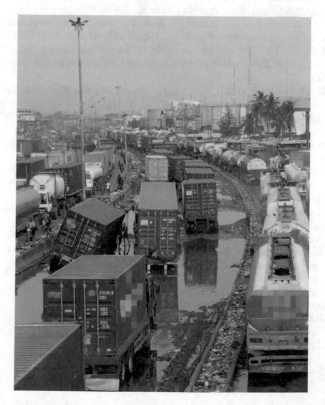

Fig. 3.9 Traffic situation in Lagos. (Photograph used with permission of Paschal Mogbo)

dismal health outcomes, and population explosion. However, corruption and inadequate funding are the primary reasons why over 95% of the population has access to health care – among the lowest in Africa. Pragmatic political and economic reforms are needed to make UHC a reality in the country

Case Study
Assume you live in a city infested with mosquitoes, and the condition of the roads that you travel to get to work daily is chaotic, as represented in Fig. 3.9. Discuss the implication of these environmental factors on the city dwellers' general health and quality of life.

References

Abubakar, S. A. (2019). *Unemployment among medical doctors*. [online]. Available at: http://www.gamji.com/article4000/NEWS4395.htm. Accessed 7 June 2021.

Adekola, A. (n.d.). *Carbon monoxide poisoning*. [online]. Available at: *https://adefolakeadekola. com/2018/12/30/carbon-monoxide-poisoning/#:~:text=CO%20poisoning%20in%20 Nigeria%20has%20some%20common%20sources%3A,the%20home%20and%2020%25%20 in%20the%20business%20environment*. Accessed 28 Dec 2020.

Advance Family Planning. (2020). *Zambia's national health insurance package covers range of family planning choices*. Bill & Melinda Gates Institute for Population and Reproductive Health. Department of Population, Family and Reproductive Health. Johns Hopkins Bloomberg School of Public Health. [online]. Available at: https://www.advancefamilyplanning.org/zambias-national-health-insurance-package-covers-range-family-planning-choices. Accessed 11 Apr 2021.

Aetna. (2021). *Health care quality in Africa: Uganda, Nigeria, Tanzania, Zambia, Kenya, Zimbabwe, and South Africa*. [online]. Available at: https://www.aetnainternational.com/en/about-us/explore/living-abroad/culture-lifestyle/health-care-quality-in-africa.html. Accessed 31 Jan 2021.

Alegbeleye, O. (2019). Access to healthcare is a right, not a privilege: The Nigerian state has to face up to this reality and revamp the healthcare system. *Global Hospital and Healthcare Management*. [online]. Available at: https://www.hhmglobal.com/knowledge-bank/articles/access-to-healthcare-is-a-right-not-a-privilege-the-nigerian-state-has-to-face-up-to-this-reality-and-revamp-the-healthcare-system. Accessed 24 Oct 2020.

Amu, H., Dickson, K. S., Kumi-Kyereme, A., & Darteh, E. K. M. (2018). Understanding variations in health insurance coverage in Ghana, Kenya, Nigeria, and Tanzania: Evidence from demographic and health surveys. *PLoS ONE, 13*(8): e0201833. [online]. Available at: https://journals.plos.org/plosone/article?id=10.1371/journal.pone.0201833. Accessed 10 Oct 2020.

Aregbeshola, B. S., & Khan, S. M. (2018) Predictors of enrolment in the national health insurance scheme among women of reproductive age in Nigeria. *International Journal of Health Policy Management, 7*(11):1015–1023. [online]. Available at: https://www.ncbi.nlm.nih.gov/pmc/articles/PMC6326643/. Accessed 10 Oct 2020.

Awosusi, A., Folaranmi, T., & Yates, R. (2015). *Nigeria's new government and public financing for universal health coverage*. [online]. Available at: https://www.thelancet.com/journals/langlo/article/PIIS2214-109X(15)00088-1/fulltext. Accessed 16 Oct 2020.

Anonymous. (n.d.-a). *Health: Nigeria*. [online]. Available at: http://countrystudies.us/nigeria/50.htm. Accessed 24 Oct 2020.

Anonymous. (n.d.-b). *Drought conditions and management strategies in Nigeria.* [online]. Available at: https://www.ais.unwater.org/ais/pluginfile.php/629/mod_page/content/6/ Nigeria_EN.pdf. Accessed 28 Dec 2020.

Appiah, B. (2012). Universal health coverage still rare in Africa. *CMAJ: Canadian Medical Association Journal, 184*(2), E125–E126. [online]. Available at https://www.ncbi.nlm.nih.gov/ pmc/articles/PMC3273529/. Accessed 31 Jan 2021.

Asakitikpi, A. E. (2019). *Healthcare coverage and affordability in Nigeria: An alternative model to equitable healthcare delivery.* [online]. https://doi.org/10.5772/intechopen.85978. https://www. intechopen.com/books/universal-health-coverage/healthcare-coverage-and-affordability-in-nigeria-an-alternative-model-to-equitable-healthcare-delive. Accessed 24 Oct 2020).

Associated Press and Reuters. (2016). Nigerian minister claims $6.8bn of public funds stolen in seven years. *Guardian.* [online]. Available at: https://www.theguardian.com/world/2016/ jan/19/nigerian-minister-claims-68bn-of-public-funds-stolen-in-seven-years. Accessed 28 Dec 2020.

AXA.com. (2019). Nigeria: Laying the groundwork for safe, quality healthcare. May 24. *AXA Magazine.* [online]. Available at: https://www.axa.com/en/magazine/nigeria-laying-the-groundwork-for-safe-quality-healthcare. Accessed 16 Oct 2020.

Balogun, J. A. (2020). Chapter 6: Pioneer Nigerian healthcare academicians. In *Healthcare education in Nigeria: Evolutions and emerging paradigms.* Routledge Publication. [online]. Available at: https://www.routledge.com/9780367482091. Accessed 23 Dec 2020.

Beaumont, P., & Abrak, I. (2018). Oil-rich Nigeria outstrips India as country with most people in poverty. *The Guardian*; 16 July. [online]. Available at: https://www.theguardian. com/global-development/2018/jul/16/oil-rich-nigeria-outstrips-india-most-people-in-poverty#:~:text=According%20to%20the%20authors%2C%20energy,with%20India's%20 73%20million%20people. Accessed 2 Jan 2021.

Chukwudozie, A. (2015). Inequalities in health: The role of health insurance in Nigeria. *Journal of Public Health in Africa, 6*(1):512[online]. Available at: https://www.ncbi.nlm.nih.gov/pmc/ articles/PMC5349265/. 23 Sept 2020.

Coutsoukis, P. (2020). *Nigeria history of modern medical services.* [online]. Available at: https:// photius.com/countries/nigeria/society/nigeria_society_history_of_modern_me~10005.html. Accessed 28 Dec 2020.

Dawkins, D., Shapiro, A., Khan, M., Wang, J., Peterson-Withorn, C., & Dolan, K. A. (2021). The Forbes billionaires' list: Africa's richest people 2021. *Forbes.* [online]. Available at: https:// www.forbes.com/sites/kerryadolan/2021/01/22/the-forbes-billionaires-list-africas-richest-peo ple-2021/?sh=4f8c738248f5. Accessed 27 July 2021.

De, P., & Chattopadhyay, N. (2019). Effects of malnutrition on child development: Evidence from a backward district of India. *Clinical Epidemiology and Global Health, 7*(3) 439–445. DOI: [online]. Available at: https://doi.org/10.1016/j.cegh.2019.01.014. Accessed 28 Dec 2020.

Dolan, K. A., & Yakowicz, W. (2020). Africa's richest people—And the tycoon who lost half his fortune. *Forbes.* [online]. Available at: https://www.forbes.com/sites/kerryadolan/2020/01/17/ africas-richest-peopleand-the%2D%2Dtycoon-who-lost-half-his-fortune/?sh=59f210642d85. Accessed Oct 2020.

ECWA Hospital. (2021). *Hospital history.* [online]. Available at: https://egbehospital. org/2013/03/12/egbe-nigeria-a-special-place/; https://egbehospital.org/egbe-hospital-history/. Accessed 15 Mar 2021.

WikiVisually. (n.d.). *Sir Yahaya Memorial Hospital.* [online]. Available at: https://wikivisually. com/wiki/Sir_Yahaya_Memorial_Hospital. Accessed 15 Mar 2021.

Eke, C. (2015). Healthcare Resource Guide: Nigeria. *Export.gov.* [online]. Available at: https://2016.export.gov/industry/health/healthcareresourceguide/eg_main_092285.asp. Accessed 28 Dec 2020.

Ferreira, F. H. G. (2019). *Measuring and monitoring global poverty at the World Bank: A brief overview.* [online]. Available at: http://pubdocs.worldbank.org/en/537241551878505289/ PovertySmackdown-FranciscoFerreira.pdf. Accessed 10 Oct 2020.

Haider, H. (2019). *Climate change in Nigeria: Impacts and responses*. K4D Helpdesk Report 675. Brighton, UK: Institute of Development Studies. . [online]. Available at: https://assets.publishing.service.gov.uk/media/5dcd7a1aed915d0719bf4542/675_Climate_Change_in_Nigeria.pdf. Accessed 28 Dec 2020.

Heaalthfacts.ng. (2016). *Generator fumes and the danger on our health*. [online]. Available at https://healthfacts.ng/effects-of-generator-fume-on-health/;   https://www.ais.unwater.org/ais/pluginfile.php/629/mod_page/content/6/Nigeria_EN.pdf. Accessed 28 Dec 2020.

Huhuonline. (2021). *Editorial: Buhari's medical tourism in London*. [online]. Available at: https://huhuonline.com/index.php/home-4/opinions/14460-editorial-buhari-s-medical-tourism-in-london. Accessed 31 Mar 2021.

Ibenegbu, G. (2018). *What are the problems facing healthcare management in Nigeria?* [online]. Available at: https://www.legit.ng/1104912-what-the-problems-facing-healthcare-management-nigeria.html. Accessed 10 Oct 2020.

Ifijeh, M. (2015). Only five percent of Nigerians are covered by health insurance. *This Day Newspaper*. November 12. [online]. Available at: http://allafrica.com/stories/201511121412.html9. Accessed 16 Oct 2020.

Julius. (2015). Nigerian healthcare system. The good and the bad. *VisitNigeria.com.ng*. [online]. Available   at: http://www.visitnigeria.com.ng/nigeria-healthcare-system-the-good-and-the-bad/. Accessed 16 Oct 2020.

Lawal, S. (1983). *Ghana must go: The ugly history of Africa's most famous bag*. [online]. Available at: http://atavist.mg.co.za/ghana-must-go-the-ugly-history-of-africas-most-famous-bag. Accessed 24 Jan 2021.

Legg, P. (2019). Shehu Shagari obituary. *The Guardian,* US Edition. [online]. Available at:https://www.theguardian.com/world/2019/jan/09/shehu-shagari-obituary. Accessed 24 Jan 2021.

Mamora, O. (2020). Saudi Arabian royal family used to visit Nigeria for treatment – Health minister. *Punch*. March 3. [online]. Available at: https://punchng.com/saudi-arabian-royal-family-used-to-come-to-nigeria-for-treatment-health-minister/. Accessed 24 Oct 2020.

Martin, A. B., Hartman, M., Washington, B., & Catlin, A. (2018). National health care spending in 2017: Growth slows to post–great recession rates; share Of GDP stabilizes. *Health Affairs, 38*(1). [online]. Available at: https://www.healthaffairs.org/doi/full/10.1377/hlthaff.2018.0508. Accessed 4 Jan 2021.

Macha, J., Harris, B., Garshong, B., et al. (2012). Factors influencing the burden of health care financing and the distribution of health care benefits in Ghana, Tanzania and South Africa. *Health Policy Planning, 27*, i46–i54.

MedCOI. (2018). *Country policy and information note Nigeria: Medical and healthcare issues*. [online]. Available at: https://www.justice.gov/eoir/page/file/1094261/downloadMedCOI2018

Muhammad, F., Abdulkareem, J. H., & Chowdhury, A. B. M. (2017). Major public health problems in Nigeria: A review. *South East Asia Journal of Public Health, 7*(1):6–11. [online]. Available at: https://www.banglajol.info/index.php/SEAJPH/article/view/34672. Accessed 18 Jan 2021.

NationalAcademyofSciences.(2020).*EvaluationofPEPFAR's(President'sEmergencyPlanforAIDS Relief) contribution (2012–2017) to Rwanda's Human Resources for Health Program*. [online]. Available at: https://www.ncbi.nlm.nih.gov/books/NBK558442/#:~:text=Including%20physician%20specialists%20and%20general,MOH%2C%202018a%2Cb. Accessed 1 Feb 2021.

Nations Population Fund. (n.d.). *Sexual and reproductive health*. [online]. Available at: https://www.unfpa.org/sexual-reproductive-health. Accessed 16 Oct 2020.

Nevin, A. S., & Omosomi, O. (2019). Strength from abroad: The economic power of Nigeria's diaspora. *PricewaterhouseCoopers Limited*. [online]. Available at: https://www.pwc.com/ng/en/pdf/the-economic-power-of-nigerias-diaspora.pdf. Accessed 16 Oct 2020.

Nigeria Demographic and Health Survey. (2013). *National Population Commission*. Republic of Nigeria Abuja, Nigeria ICF International Rockville, Maryland, UK June 2014. [online]. Available at: https://dhsprogram.com/pubs/pdf/FR293/FR293.pdf. Accessed 16 Oct 2020.

Nigeria National Health Conference. (2009). *Communique*. Abuja, Nigeria. [online]. Available at: http://www.ngnhc.org. Accessed 28 Dec 2020.

Nigerian Finder. (2020). *Brief history of health care in Nigeria*. https://nigerianfinder.com/history-of-health-care-in-nigeria/

NOIPolls. (2017). *Emigration of Nigerian medical doctors: Survey report.* [online]. Available at: https://noi-polls.com/2018/wp-content/uploads/2019/06/Emigration-of-Doctors-Press-Release-July-2018-Survey-Report.pdf. Accessed 10 Oct 2020.

Nwezeh, K., & Shittu, H. (2019). *Nigeria: U.S.$400 billion looted from treasury – Govt.* [online]. Available at: https://allafrica.com/stories/201909130041.html. Accessed 28 Dec 2020.

Obalum, D. C., & Fiberesima, F. (2012). Nigerian National Health Insurance Scheme (NHIS): An overview. *The Nigerian Postgraduate Medical Journal, 19*(3):167–174. [online]. Available at: https://www.researchgate.net/publication/232246860_Nigerian_National_Health_Insurance_Scheme_NHIS_an_overview#:~:text=History%20of%20NHIS%20The%20Scheme,have%20been%20accredited%20and%20registered. Accessed 10 Oct 2020.

Odeyemi, I. A. O., & Nixon, J. (2013). Assessing equity in health care through the national health insurance schemes of Nigeria and Ghana: A review-based comparative analysis. *International Journal for Equity in Health, 12,* 9–26.

OECD. (2002). *Nigeria.* [online]. Available at: https://www.oecd.org/countries/nigeria/1826208.pdf. Accessed 16 Oct 2020.

Ogaji, D., & Brisibe, S. F. (2015). The Nigerian health care system: Evolution, contradictions and proposal for future debates. *Port Harcourt Medical Journal, 9*:S79–S88. [online]. Available at: https://www.researchgate.net/publication/306315335

Ogbaa, M. (2017). *A Nigerian story: How healthcare is the offspring of imperialism and corruption.* [online]. Available at: https://www.theelephant.info/features/2017/11/16/a-nigerian-story-how-healthcare-is-the-offspring-of-imperialism-and-corruption/. Accessed 10 Oct 2020.

Ogundipe, S., Obinna, C., & Olawale, G. (2015). Shortage of medical personnel: Tougher times ahead for Nigerians. 27 January. *Vanguard.* [online]. Available at: https://www.vanguardngr.com/2015/01/shortage-medical-personnel-tougher-times-ahead-nigerians-1/. Accessed 16 Oct 2020.

Olufadewa, I. I., Adesina, M. A., & Ayorinde, T. (2020). From Africa to the World: Reimagining Africa's research capacity and culture in the global knowledge economy. *Journal of Global Health, 10*(1):010321. [online]. Available at: https://www.ncbi.nlm.nih.gov/pmc/articles/PMC7101491/. Accessed 1 Feb 2021.

Onwujekwe, O., Odii, A., Mbachu, C., Hutchinson, E., Ichoku, H., Ogbozorf, P. A., Agwu, P., Obi, U. S., & Balabanova, D. (2018). *Corruption in the Nigerian health sector has many faces: How to fix it.* University of London. [online]. Available at: https://ace.soas.ac.uk/wp-content/uploads/2018/09/Corruption-in-the-health-sector-in-Anglophone-W-Africa_ACE-Working-Paper-005.pdf. Accessed 10 Oct 2020.

Onwujekwe, O., Agwu, P., Orjiakor, C., McKee, M., Hutchinson, E., Mbachu, C., Odii, A., Ogbozor, P., Obi, U., Ichoku, H., & Balabanova, D. (2019). Corruption in Anglophone West Africa health systems: A systematic review of its different variants and the factors that sustain them. *Health Policy and Planning, 34*(7):529–543. [online]. Available at: https://academic.oup.com/heapol/article/34/7/529/5543565. Accessed 10 Oct 2020.

Onwujekwe, O., Orjiakor, C. T., Hutchinson, E., McKee, M., Agwu, P., Mbachu, C., Ogbozor, P., Obi, U., Odii, A., Ichoku, H., & Balabanova, D. (2020). Where do we start? Building consensus on drivers of health sector corruption in Nigeria and ways to address It. *International Journal of Health Policy Management, 9*(7):286–296. [online]. Available at: https://pubmed.ncbi.nlm.nih.gov/32613800/. Accessed 26 Dec 2020.

Onyedika-Ugoeze, N. (2020). President launches 2018–2022 National strategic health development plan. [online]. *The Guardian.* Available at: https://guardian.ng/news/president-launches-2018-2022-national-strategic-health-development-plan/. Accessed 30 Dec 2020.

Oxford Business Group. (2015). *Opportunities for private companies in Nigeria's health care sector, and efforts to improve provision.* [online]. Available at: https://oxfordbusinessgroup.com/overview/opportunities-private-companies-nigerias-health-care-sector-and-efforts-improve-provision. Accessed 30 Dec 2020.

Rine, R. (2019). Nigeria's life expectancy in 2019: Matters arising. *TNV. The Nigerian Voice.* [online]. Available at: https://www.thenigerianvoice.com/news/277752/nigerias-life-expectancy-in-2019-matters-arising.html. Accessed 16 Oct 2020.

Scott-Emuakpor, A. (2010). The evolution of health care systems in Nigeria: Which way forward in the twenty-first century. *Nigerian Medical Journal, 51*:53–65. [online]. Available at: http://www.nigeriamedj.com/text.asp?2010/51/2/53/70997. Accessed 23 Jan 2020.

The Federal Republic of Nigeria. (2018). *Federal Ministry of Environment National Drought Plan.* Available at: https://knowledge.unccd.int/sites/default/files/country_profile_documents/1%2520FINAL_NDP_Nigeria.pdf. Accessed 28 Dec 2020.

Tormusa, D. O., & Idom, A. M. (2016). The impediments of corruption on the efficiency of health-care service delivery in Nigeria. *Online Journal of Health Ethics, 12*(1). [online]. Available at: https://aquila.usm.edu/ojhe/vol12/iss1/3/. Accessed 10 Oct 2020.

USAID. (2017). *Nigeria's President commits to revitalizing 10,000 primary health care centers.* [online]. Available at: https://www.hfgproject.org/nigeria-commits-revitalizing-10000-primary-health-care-centers/. Accessed 30 Dec 2020.

Varrella, S. (2020). Poverty headcount rate in Nigeria as of 2019, by state. *Statistica.* [online]. Available at: https://www.statista.com/statistics/1121438/poverty-headcount-rate-in-nigeria-by-state/#:~:text=An%20individual%20is%20considered%20poor,in%20Nigeria%20lived%20in%20poverty. Accessed 28 Dec 2020.

Welcome, M. O. (2011). The Nigerian health care system: Need for integrating adequate medical intelligence and surveillance systems. *Journal of Pharmacy Bioallied Science, 3*(4), 470–478. https://doi.org/10.4103/0975-7406.90100. Accessed 28 Dec 2020.

WHO. (2020). *Health and development.* [online]. Available at: https://www.who.int/hdp/en/. Accessed 16 Oct 2020.

WHO. (2019a). *Rwanda: The beacon of Universal Health Coverage in Africa.* [online]. Available at: https://www.afro.who.int/news/rwanda-beacon-universal-health-coverage-africa. Accessed 15 Mar 2021.

WHO. (2019b). *President Buhari launches WHO's revised third generation country cooperation strategy.* [online]. Available at: https://www.afro.who.int/news/president-buhari-launches-whos-revised-third-generation-country-cooperation-strategy. Accessed 30 Dec 2020.

WHO. (2018). *Nigeria.* [online]. Available at: https://apps.who.int/iris/bitstream/handle/10665/136785/ccsbrief_nga_en.pdf;jsessionid=3FA2142ADB26766C98CB2FD927F164A0?sequence=1. Accessed 16 Jan 2021.

WHO. (2017a). *Joint External Evaluation of IHR Core Capacities of the Federal Republic of Nigeria.* Geneva: World Health Organization. Licence: CC BY-NC-SA 3.0 IGO. [online]. Available at: https://apps.who.int/iris/bitstream/handle/10665/259382/WHO-WHE-CPI-REP-2017.46-eng.pdf?sequence=1. Accessed 28 Dec 2020.

WHO. (2017b). *Health is a fundamental human right.* [online]. Available at: https://www.who.int/mediacentre/news/statements/fundamental-human-right/en/#:~:text=The%20right%20to%20health%20for,them%2C%20without%20suffering%20financial%20hardship.&text=That's%20why%20WHO%20promotes%20the,in%20the%20practice%20of%20care. Accessed 16 Oct 2020.

WHO. (2016a). *Global health observatory (GHO) data: World health statistics 2016: Monitoring health for the SDGs.* [online]. Available at: https://www.who.int/gho/publications/world_health_statistics/2016/en/. Accessed 10 Oct 2020.

WHO. (2016b). *Global health observatory (GHO) data: World health statistics: Out-of-pocket expenditure (OOP) per capita in PPP Int$.* [online]. Available at: https://www.who.int/data/gho/data/indicators/indicator-details/GHO/out-of-pocket-expenditure-(oop)-per-capita-in-ppp-int. Accessed 27 July 2021.

WHO. (2015). *World health statistics Part I: Global health indicators.* [online]. Available at: https://www.who.int/gho/publications/world_health_statistics/EN_WHS2015_Part2.pdf. Accessed 10 Oct 2020.

WHO. (2011). *The Abuja declaration: Ten years on.* [online]. Available at: https://www.who.int/healthsystems/publications/abuja_declaration/en/; https://www.who.int/healthsystems/publications/abuja_report_aug_2011.pdf?ua=1. Accessed 16 Oct 2020.

WHO. (2010a). *Health and development.* [online]. Available at: https://www.who.int/hdp/en/. Accessed 24 Oct 2020.

WHO. (2010b). Telemedicine in the member states: Opportunities and developments. Report on the second global survey on eHealth. *Global Observatory for eHealth series* – Volume 2. [online]. Available at: http://www.who.int/goe/publications/goe_telemedicine_2010.pdf. Accessed 16 Oct 2020.

WHO. (2008). *Health systems financing: Toolkit on monitoring health systems strengthening.* [online]. Available at: http://www.who.int/health-info/statistics/toolkit_hss/EN_PDF_Toolkit_HSS_Financing.pdf. Accessed 10 Oct 2020.

WHO. (2006). *Quality of care: A process for making strategic choices in health systems.* Printed in France. [online]. Available at: https://www.who.int/management/quality/assurance/QualityCare_B.Def.pdf. Accessed 24 Oct 2020.

WHO. (2000). *The world health organization's ranking of the world's health systems, by rank.* [online]. Available at: https://photius.com/rankings/healthranks.html. Accessed 10 Oct 2020.

World Bank Data. (2010). *Current health expenditure per capita (current US$).* [online]. Available at: https://data.worldbank.org/indicator/SH.XPD.CHEX.PC.CD. Accessed 10 Oct 2020.

World Bank. (2017). *Out-of-pocket expenditure (% of current health expenditure).* [online]. Available at: https://data.worldbank.org/indicator/SH.XPD.OOPC.CH.ZS. Accessed 27 July 2021.

World Bank. (2021). *Current health expenditure (% of GDP).* [online]. Available at: https://data.worldbank.org/indicator/SH.XPD.CHEX.GD.ZS?locations=NG. Accessed 4 Jan 2021.

Worldometer. (2020). *Countries in the world by population.* [online]. Available at: https://www.worldometers.info/world-population/population-by-country/. Accessed 10 Oct 2020.

Your Dictionary. (n.d.). [online]. Available at: https://biography.yourdictionary.com/chief-obafemi-awolowo. Accessed 28 Dec 2020.

Chapter 4
The Organizational Structure and Leadership of the Nigerian Healthcare System

Learning Objectives

After reading this chapter, the learner should be able to:

1. Compare the management of health services in Nigeria with the United States and United Kingdom
2. Describe the differences in the roles of the university teaching hospitals, federal medical centers, and specialty hospitals
3. Describe the Nigerian healthcare structure
4. Enunciate the three levels of government and their responsibilities in providing health services
5. Discuss the impacts of the private sector in the delivery of health care in the country.
6. Compare the management and leadership of health departments in Nigeria with the norms in developed countries
7. Discuss the debate on the disharmony and unhealthy rivalry among healthcare professionals in Nigeria
8. Describe the roles of the Minister of Health and the appropriate skills needed to be successful in the position
9. Discuss the controversy on the surgeon general position in Nigeria

Introduction

Indigenous medical practice in Nigeria is much older than modern health services, introduced about 500 years ago into what is now known as Nigeria through the trans-Sahara trade routes and by the European traders, explorers, colonial military,

© The Author(s), under exclusive license to Springer Nature Switzerland AG 2021
J. A. Balogun, *The Nigerian Healthcare System*,
https://doi.org/10.1007/978-3-030-88863-3_4

and civilian administrators, and the missionaries (Osuhor, 1978). Over the years, the Nigerian healthcare system and clinical practice have evolved in response to changes in disease patterns, patients' needs, and societal expectations. A social commentator described the health system as fraught with several challenges due to lack of planning, policy mismatch, underfunding, poor condition of service, archaic infrastructure, uneven distribution of hospitals in the six geopolitical zones, low technology, including political instability and decline in the economy in the last decade (Omojuwa, 2015; Nasir El-Rufai, 2015).

All over the world, including Nigeria, the Federal Ministry of Health (FMH) is the health sector's primary power player. The Ministry bears the responsibility for providing safe, quality, affordable, adequate, equitable, and accessible health services. Hence, it is critical to understand the Ministry's administrative structure and functions as a predicate to understanding the country's healthcare system's performance. In Nigeria, the Minister of Health is the Chief Executive Officer (CEO) in charge of the FMH and assisted by the commissioner of health in the 36 states.

In the United States, health services are managed by the Department of Health and Human Services, also known as the Health Department, and is organized into 11 divisions: Administration for Children and Families, Administration for Community Living, Agency for Healthcare Research and Quality, Agency for Toxic Substances and Disease Registry, Centers for Disease Control and Prevention, Centers for Medicare and Medicaid Services, Food and Drug Administration, Health Resources and Services Administration, Indian Health Service, National Institutes of Health, and Substance Abuse and Mental Health Services Administration.

The United Kingdom's publicly funded health system is managed by the National Health Service (NHS), the second-largest single-payer healthcare delivery system in the world after Brazil. The NHS provides health care to all legal United Kingdom residents, with most services free at the point of use. Emergency care and treatment of infectious diseases are free for most people, including visitors (Brown, 2003).

This chapter analyzes the organizational structure of the FMH, the healthcare system, the impacts of the private sector on healthcare delivery. The chapter investigates the widely held perception that physicians and men dominate the health system's leadership worldwide, including Nigeria. It also discusses the causes of *disharmony and unhealthy rivalry among healthcare professionals, the roles of the minister of health, and* the debate surrounding the surgeon general's position.

Operational Definitions

To fully understand the issues discussed in this chapter, it is pertinent to operationalize the following basic terms:

1. An *organization* is a group of people hired and assembled to accomplish well-defined goals.
2. A *healthcare organization* is an institution, hospital, or clinic that provides services to meet the target population or community's health needs. It may be pri-

vately (for-profit) funded or owned by the government or nongovernment establishments. Examples are the state general hospitals, university teaching hospitals (UTHs), specialist hospitals, proprietary religious hospitals, or non-governmental organizations.

3. An *organizational structure* outlines how certain activities are directed to achieve the organization's mission and determines how information flows between the various levels. The activities include rules, roles, and responsibilities. In a centralized organizational scheme, decisions flow from the top down. On the other hand, in a decentralized system, decision-making power is distributed at the organization's different levels (Kenton, 2021).

4. *Leadership*, also known as headship, is the CEO or an individual in authority who exerts power and influence on the followers.

5. *Leadership style* is the CEO or leader's behavior responsible for coordinating and administering teams, organizations, or systems.

Organization Structure of the Federal Ministry of Health

The organizational structure for the FMH is a moving target because every minister of health tends to restructure the organization's operations instead of building upon the accomplishments of their predecessors. The lack of consistency makes it difficult to measure progress. The following organizational structure is President Buhari's second-term structure, which is different from his first term and those of the previous governments.

The organizational structure of the FMH between 2015 and 2019 consisted of six divisions: Hospital Services, Nursing, Regulatory and Professional Schools, Dentistry, National Blood Transfusion Services/Laboratory, and Trauma/Medical Emergency Response and Disaster Management, and two program units (e-Health, Telemedicine and Continuing Professional Discipline, and the National Cancer Control Program and Nuclear Medicine) (FMH, 2020). The FMH was reorganized, in early 2020, into the following eight departments and five units:

1. Food and Drug Services Department: Six divisions – Pharmaceutical Services, Drug Vaccine Development, National Product Supply Chain Management Program, Food, Chemical, Water and Cosmetic, Planning, Monitoring, Evaluation, and Information/Special Duties Unit, and Traditional Medicine Development

2. Hospital Services Department: Six divisions – Hospital Service, Nursing, Regulatory and Professional Schools, Dentistry, National Blood Transfusion Services/Laboratory, Trauma/Medical Emergency Response, and Disaster Management and two programs (e-Health, Telemedicine, and Continuing Professional Discipline and National Cancer Control Program and Nuclear Medicine)

3. Information and Communication Technology (ICT): Three divisions – Service Delivery and Support, Data Center Management, and e-Health Strategy and Solution

4. Family Health: Five divisions – Child Health, Gender, Adolescent School Health and Elderly Care, Reproductive Health, Health Promotion, and Saving One Million Lives Program
5. Public Health: Nine divisions – Climate Change/Environmental Health, Noncommunicable Diseases Control Program, Neglected Tropical Diseases, Occupational Health and Safety, Port Health Services, National Tuberculosis, and Leprosy Control Program, National Malaria Elimination Program, HIV/AIDS and Viral Hepatitis Program, and Epidemiology Services
6. Health, Planning, Research, and Statistics: Five divisions – Policy and Planning, International Cooperation, Monitoring and Evaluation, Research Knowledge and Management, and Health System Strengthening
7. Procurement
8. Reform Coordination and Service Improvement (FMH, 2020).

The five new units are Legal Services, Traditional, Complementary and Alternative Medicine, Public-Private Partnership/Diaspora Unit, Port Health Division, and Servicom (FMH, 2020). Unlike other countries (U.S. Department of Health & Human Services, 2020; Ministry of Health and Welfare, 2017; Tikkanen et al., 2020; Wu et al., 2010), the website of the Nigerian FMH did not publish an organogram that will help delineate the lines of communication within the organization. Sadly, conspicuously missing at the federal level is the lack of a unit to plan for medical rehabilitation, hospice and palliative care, and people living with disabilities.

The federal government established at least one tertiary health institution in each state. There are currently 21 UTHs (Table 4.1) and 23 Federal Medical Centers (FMCs) evenly distributed across the country (Table 4.2). Lagos state is the only exception with both an FMC and a UTH. Most of the FMCs are located in the state capital, especially in situations where the highest secondary health institution provided by the state government does not adequately meet the demands for specialist healthcare delivery for the citizens.

In addition to the UTHs and FMCs, 13 specialty hospitals are distributed more or less evenly across the country (Table 4.3). The chief medical director (CMD) is the CEO of the UTH, FMCs, and specialist hospitals. The CMD reports to the Board of Management appointed by the federal government and accountable to the minister of health. The CMD implements the policies and the day-to-day operations of the hospital. Candidates for the position are legislatively mandated to be medical or dental practitioners registered with the Medical and Dental Council of Nigeria (MDCN) with more than 12 years of postgraduate experience. Also, the candidate must be a Fellow of the National Postgraduate Medical College of Nigeria (NPGMCN) or the West African College of Physicians/Surgeons and must be a consultant for a minimum of 5 years.

The hospital services division is responsible for supervising the three major federal tertiary hospitals: UTHs, FMC, and specialty hospitals. The CMD, a physician, is appointed by the FMH at the hospital management board's recommendation to administer the hospitals' daily operations and chairs the

Table 4.1 University Teaching Hospitals in Nigeria

1. Abubakar Tafawa Balewa University Teaching Hospital, Bauchi
2. Ahmadu Bello University Teaching Hospital, Zaria
3. Aminu Kano University Teaching Hospital, Kano
4. Federal Teaching Hospital, Abakaliki
5. Federal Teaching Hospital, Gombe
6. Irrua Specialist Teaching Hospital, Irrua
7. Jos University Teaching Hospital, Jos
8. Lagos University Teaching Hospital, Lagos
9. Nnamdi Azikiwe University Teaching Hospital, Nnewi
10. Obafemi Awolowo University Teaching Hospital Complex, Ile-Ife
11. University of Abuja Teaching Hospital, Gwagwalada
12. University of Benin Teaching Hospital, Benin City
13. University College Hospital, Ibadan
14. University of Calabar Teaching Hospital, Calabar
15. Usmanu Danfodiyo University Teaching Hospital, Sokoto
16. University of Ilorin Teaching Hospital, Ilorin
17. University of Maiduguri Teaching Hospital, Maiduguri
18. University of Nigeria Teaching Hospital, Enugu
19 University of Port Harcourt Teaching Hospital, Port Harcourt
20. University of Uyo Teaching Hospital, Uyo
21. National Hospital, Abuja

management board that provides the oversight for each hospital. The director of administration for the hospital reports to the CMD for the day-to-day general administration of the hospital and the chief administrative adviser and secretary to the management board. Candidates for the director of administration position must minimally have a first degree in health services management, humanities, or social sciences from an accredited university and at least 20 years of post-qualification experience.

A postgraduate degree in a relevant field is an added advantage. The appointment of the leadership of the FMH, UTHs, and specialist hospitals is a controversial issue.

The nursing division maintains oversight of the nursing profession's activities, working in conjunction with the Nursing and Midwifery Council of Nigeria as its subordinate regulatory agency. The dentistry division advises the federal government on all oral health matters, policy formulation, resource mobilization, monitoring and evaluation of such policies, supervising oral health in schools and research institutions, and delivering affordable and effective oral healthcare services.

The national blood transfusion services' core function is to provide a centrally coordinated blood transfusion service within the national health plan. It also offers safe, adequate, and quality blood in an equitable and accessible manner. The national blood transfusion service centers are located in Abeokuta, Abuja, Ado-Ekiti, Benin, Calabar, Enugu, Ibadan, Jalingo, Jos, Kaduna, Katsina, Lokoja, Maiduguri, Nangere, Owerri, Port Harcourt, and Sokoto.

Table 4.2 Federal Medical Centers in Nigeria

1. Federal Medical Center, Abakaliki, Ebonyi State
2. Federal Medical Center, Abeokuta, Ogun State
3. Federal Medical Center, Asaba, Delta State
4. Federal Medical Center, Abuja, Federal Capital Territory
5. Federal Medical Center, Azare, Bauchi State
6. Federal Medical Center, Bida, Niger State
7. Federal Medical Center, Birnin-Kebbi, Kebbi State
8. Federal Medical Center, Birnin Kudu, Jigawa State
9. Federal Medical Center, Ebute-Meta, Lagos State
10. Federal Medical Center, Gombe, Gombe State
11. Federal Medical Center, Gusau, Zamfara State
12. Federal Medical Center, Ido Ekiti, Ekiti State
13. Federal Medical Center, Jalingo, Taraba State
14. Federal Medical Center, Katsina, Katsina State
15. Federal Medical Center, Keffi, Nasarawa State
16. Federal Medical Center, Lokoja, Kogi State
17. Federal Medical Center, Makurdi, Benue State
18. Federal Medical Center, Nguru, Yobe State
19. Federal Medical Center, Owerri, Imo State
20. Federal Medical Center, Owo Ondo State
21. Federal Medical Center, Umuahia, Abia State
22. Federal Medical Center, Yenagoa, Bayelsa State
23. Federal Medical Center, Yola, Adamawa State

Table 4.3 Federal Specialty Hospitals in Nigeria

1. Federal Neuro-Psychiatric Hospital, Abeokuta, Ogun State
2. Federal Neuro-Psychiatric Hospital, Uselu, Edo State
3. Federal Neuro-Psychiatric Hospital, Calabar
4. Federal Neuro-Psychiatric Hospital, Enugu
5. Federal Neuro-Psychiatric Hospital, Kaduna
6. Federal Neuro-Psychiatric Hospital, Kware, Sokoto State
7. Federal Neuro-Psychiatric Hospital, Maiduguri
8. Federal Neuro-Psychiatric Hospital, Yaba, Lagos State
9. National Orthopaedic Hospital, Dala, Kano State
10. National Orthopaedic Hospital, Enugu
11. National Orthopaedic Hospital, Igbobi, Lagos State
12. National Eye Centre, Kaduna
13. National Ear Centre, Kaduna

The trauma/medical emergency response and disaster management division advise the federal government on health emergencies and disaster management. The division also formulates policies, monitors, and evaluates the implementation of health emergencies and disasters. The e-health/telemedicine program includes services on health-related Internet information sites, automated online therapy, online consultations (real time), online pharmacies, telehealth, home monitoring systems, and virtual clinics. The national cancer control program and nuclear medicine advises the federal government on cancer diseases, maintains a national Cancer Registry, develops policies, monitors and evaluates cancer treatment outcomes (FMH, 2020). The health professional regulatory boards and non-degree awarding health professional schools report to the FMH (2020).

Healthcare System Structure

One in every four sub-Saharan people resides in Nigeria, making it Africa's most populous country and the seventh in the world. With 42.5 million people at the time of independence in 1960, Nigeria's population has quadrupled to 205.9 million as of June 13, 2020. It will become the third-largest nation globally, with 399 million people by the year 2050 (World Education WES, 2017). Many health analysts aver that Nigeria has one of the most complicated health systems in Africa. The health system has a three-tier structure, with primary care, including Africa traditional medicine as the foundation, secondary care as the supporting pillars, and tertiary care at the apex (Fig. 4.1).

Nationwide, the three government levels (federal, state, and local) share responsibilities for providing health services and programs. The burden of implementing primary health care (PHC) lies within the purview of the local governments; secondary health care belongs to state governments, while the federal government is

Fig. 4.1 Organogram on the Nigerian healthcare system

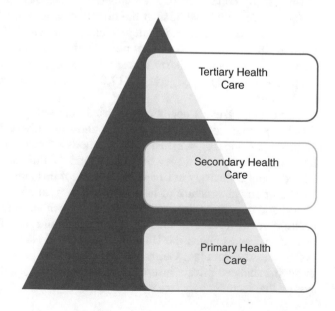

responsible for tertiary health care. Nationally, the private sector also plays a critical role in the provision of medical services. In addition to providing technical assistance to local government health programs and facilities, the state ministry of health is responsible for the training of nurses, midwives, medical laboratory technicians, and sanitarians at the state general hospitals.

The federal government is responsible for providing policy guidance, planning and technical assistance, and coordinating the national health policy's implementation. Although there is input at the state level, the federal government is primarily responsible for disease surveillance, drug regulation, vaccine management, and healthcare professional (HCP) education. While the federal government oversees the UTHs, specialist (psychiatric and orthopedic) hospitals, and the FMCs, the 774 local government authorities manage the PHC facilities' operations within their domains. The oversight includes the provision of primary health services, community health hygiene, and sanitation. The government-run healthcare system's apparent limitations and challenges have increased prominence and relevance to the private sector (profit and nonprofit) and traditional medicine practitioners (TMPs), bonesetters, and spiritual healers.

The 774 local government authorities in the country have 7580 hospitals, representing 44.4% of the total. Next, the private sector had 7373 hospitals, which is 43.2% of the total. The state government had 1385 hospitals (8.1%), religious institutions had 330 hospitals (1.93%), communities had 249 (1.5%), and the federal government had 151 hospitals (0.9%) of the total (Nwakeze & Kandala, 2011). However, the country's number of health facilities is speculative because many private hospitals are not duly registered (Bello, 2018). The PharmAccess Foundation, in 2015, indicated that Nigeria has five hospital beds per 10,000 population and 23,640 public and private hospitals in 2005. In April 2014, a study conducted in six states (Abia, Benue, Edo, Kaduna, Lagos, and Nasarawa) revealed that 32% of the private health facilities were not registered, and the government cannot independently validate 53% of those listed. The findings suggest that government records are incomplete and inaccurate due to employee misconduct (PharmAccess Foundation, 2015). Nwakeze and Kandala, in 2011, estimated that Nigeria has 17,038 hospitals unevenly distributed among the 36 states.

The health system's operation is a triad delivery system consisting of conventional western medicine, complementary and alternative medicine (CAM), and traditional medicine (Fig. 4.2). The three methods are recognized and regulated by the federal government, and they operate in tandem with each other. CAMs are discussed comprehensively in Chaps. 6, 7, and 8 of this publication.

The principal structure of healthcare delivery in Nigeria is through the public sector, and the mechanism has not changed much since independence. Generally, health care worldwide is funded through taxation, out-of-pocket payments, and insurance. For example, the United Kingdom and New Zealand fund their health system mostly from tax; Germany, France, and Switzerland support their system through mandated private insurance. In Nigeria, the health sector is a tax-funded system that includes user fees with very little regulation or quality assurance across

Fig. 4.2 Healthcare
delivery systems in Nigeria

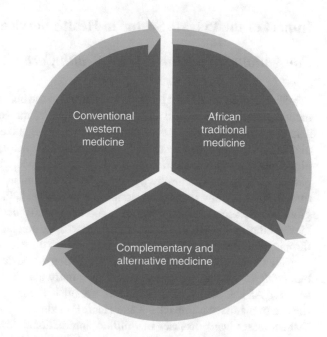

the various government tiers. Tax-funded models for funding services have failed in the other sectors of the Nigerian economy, and there is no reason to expect it to work in the health sector (Ventures, 2015).

The government encourages employers to provide generous health benefits to their workers and dependents, but there is no monitoring mechanism to track conformance. As a result, in most cases, workers pay healthcare costs out of pocket. In a 1993 survey, about 85% of the study respondents reported paying out of pocket for services; 10% of the urbanites incurred out-of-pocket expenses than 4% by rural dwellers who indicated their employers paid for their health expenses. An earlier survey of 2751 employers conducted in 1988 by Ogunbekun and associates (1999) revealed that employee health benefits accounted for 6.5% of the payroll. For the most part, they pay for their service on a fee-for-service arrangement.

Due to historical and political factors at the state level, budget patterns have been systematically inequitable between the North and the Southern states. About 60% of the public primary healthcare facilities (health posts and dispensaries that provide essential curative services) are in the Northern states. Only 30% of the federal account is distributed based on population, and often the least populous states receive more revenues. More hospitals are in the Southwest region than in the Southeast and fewer hospitals in the Northern region. Much of the healthcare infrastructure is in the urban centers, providing four times as much access to health care as those living elsewhere. Because of the deteriorating condition of government hospitals and health centers, most Nigerians rely on the private sector, where good treatment is expensive and beyond the reach of the poor. On average, private healthcare costs are higher than the public (UK Home Office, 2018).

Impact of the Private Sector in Health Service Delivery

Conventional Medicine Private Health Care

In addition to the FMH, the other power players in the health system are the government departments at federal and state levels, donors, and community organizations. The nonprofit sector consists of nongovernmental organizations, civil society organizations, the legal, organizational forum such as the incorporated trustees, companies limited by guarantee, unincorporated associations, charitable trusts, political parties, cooperatives, friendly societies, and trade unions. In Nigeria, the philanthropic statutory law recognizes nonprofits in various fields such as education, religion, health, social services (sports), and community development. However, the lack of empirical research makes it difficult to draw any factual inference on philanthropic or subsector activities.

Nigeria has the largest Christian population in Africa, with over 85 million belonging to various denominations. The country also has the largest Muslim faith in West Africa. Many church leaders establish foundations through which they make a humanitarian impact – Kanu Heart Foundation is an indigenous foundation that addresses heart diseases in children. International donor agencies usually support the nonprofit sector. The primary church-related foundations in Nigeria include Chris Oyakhilome Foundation, David Oyedepo Foundation, David Ibiyeomie Foundation, and the OPM Foundation. They support social initiatives, including taking care of the poor, orphans, widows, and victims of natural disasters, renovating schools, and providing free schools and scholarships. The private foundations also support health programs such as eradicating polio, HIV/AIDS prevention, and maternal and child health care. They also engage in health research and education on birth control and teenage pregnancies (Okaomee, n.d.).

In many developing countries, the private sector's share of total health spending is three or four times the amount of public health expenditure. The ratio of private to public facilities is between 5:95 and 30:70. In post-apartheid South Africa, half of the healthcare expenditure is from the private sector; only 16% of the population has health insurance coverage, while the remaining 84% depending on the public health system or payout of their own pockets for private care. Without any doubt, many South Africans do not have their needs met by the current healthcare system (Ranchod, 2016).

In Nigeria, due to the stronghold of governmental presence in the healthcare sector, after 1960 and in 1980, the tendency for policymakers to view the industry as a competitor rather than a partner, the size and composition of private sectors are even scantier compared to many other African countries (Ogunbekun et al., 1999). By the mid-1980s, the private healthcare market snowballed, which witnessed a deep economic recession with falling social expenditures and household incomes in real terms. Private establishments now account for over 60% of healthcare services in the country. The low quality and shortage of health services in public facilities have made the private sector an attractive choice for consumers. However, in recent years, private practitioners' cost of medical services has grown faster than the average rate of inflation. The government's ineffective regulation and surveillance have led to weak control over the clinical activities of private industry HCWs (Asakitikpi, 2019).

Many private health facilities in Nigeria operate without an appropriate license by the State Ministry of Health. Many often do not annually report caseloads, number, and classification of employees and technologies. Data on private sector personnel resources is compromised because many HCPs employed in the private sector are employed full time in the public sector. In 1991, about 30% of all health institutions and 43% of beds in Ogun state were private hospitals, and 50% of physicians and 33% of nurses and midwives worked in the private setting. In 1999, for-profit healthcare providers were responsible for 31% of the 11,757, primarily small-sized clinics/hospitals (less than 15 beds) that provided surgical, medical, and maternity care (Ogunbekun et al., 1999).

Group medical practice is uncommon, and investor-owned (for profit) hospitals are exceedingly rare. Private clinical practice is essentially a solo enterprise and primarily concentrated in six states (Lagos, Oyo, Imo, Anambra, Bendel, and Kaduna), representing about 80% of the total number of registered facilities and beds in the country. A similar pattern exists in the distribution of retail pharmacies, marked by imbalances in favor of the urban centers.

In Lagos, about 75% of the retailers are in urban areas and more than 80% in Ogun state. In Oyo State, 83% of the physicians and 93% of the private practice specialists were in Ibadan, representing 41% of the state population. Sadly, due to the high investment cost required to develop a practice, only a few privately owned dental clinics exist, even in urban centers. In 1991, less than 2% of Lagos's health facilities were dental clinics (Ogunbekun et al., 1999).

The health sector's contribution to the Nigerian economy is minuscule – approximately 2–5% of the gross domestic product. Before the 1980s, the government financed the bulk of health expenditure, but the economic recession and structural adjustment program shifted the burden to employers and households. By 1990, private sources invested 60% of total health expenditure, in contrast to 35% by the government. In recent years, the share of health expenditure from the private sector further increased. In 1994, only 20% of the total health spending came from public sources, at a time when international assistance declined. The relative growth in private health expenditure is due to several factors, including the decline in health budgets, the initiation of the cost-recovery process in government hospitals, and inconsistent public policy (Ogunbekun et al., 1999).

The rapid increase in the private healthcare sector buffered the inadequacies in the government provision of services to patients at all levels. For instance, in 1985, only 40% of the population had access to modern health services; by 1995, it increased to 65% due to the expanded PHC program and continued service expansion from the private sector.

In 1992, 50% of all family planning consumers received their products from private clinics. Between 1980 and 1991, the private sector also doubled the immunization coverage for children in less than one year. In the 1990s, private hospitals served as the General Practice Residency site for physicians/dentists and surpassed the government hospitals' investment in medical equipment and technology. The unplanned and uncontrolled expansion of the private market proved very difficult to monitor effectively by the government, causing increased malpractice reports. At the same time, intra-sector competition compromised the efficiency in the delivery of services (Ogunbekun et al., 1999).

Before the 1990s, the price for medical care was set independently by owners of clinics and hospitals and guided by the local market forces. Expectedly, the cost of services varied widely across the country. In that environment, some providers charged low fees to remain competitive. Still, clinicians could not provide high-quality service under a situation that promotes unethical practices among solo practitioners. The government stepped in to harmonize payments initiated in the 1990s to reduce price levels to conform with the amount charged in 1992 by ethical physicians/dentists. The immediate effect alone caused a steep (53%) rise in the consumer price – the singular highest increase for any one year up to that date.

The harmonization fees further increased in 1995. The growth is attributed to the high cost of drugs and medical equipment and the high price of funds in a deregulated economic environment. The 1991 pay rise for HCPs employed in government hospitals also led to substantial pay in the private sector. The situation produced a considerable increase in healthcare costs up to 200% between 1992 and 1995 (Ogunbekun et al., 1999). Over 60% of the population still lack access to medicines. The proportion of people with access to essential medications required to treat chronic diseases, such as malaria and HIV, is estimated at 40% (UK Home Office, 2018).

Traditional Medicine Private Health Care

The bureaucratic structure and high cost of accessing government-owned general and specialist hospitals and tertiary teaching hospitals have increased the demand for private health establishments, predominantly catering to middle-class cadres. The cost of unadulterated drugs and private healthcare delivery services are generally high and not easily accessible to the poor. Consequently, the lower and middle socioeconomic classes typically consult complementary and alternative medicine practitioners, unqualified and unlicensed chemist shop owners, traditional drug hawkers, TMPs, faith healers in spiritual homes and churches. The roles of complementary and alternative medicine practitioners, TMPs, and faith healers are discussed more comprehensively in Chaps. 6, 7, and 8.

The Nigerian health system is flush with the massive circulation of fake, substandard, and adulterated pharmaceutical products estimated to be between 15% and 75% of total drugs in the country (UK Home Office, 2018). The ubiquitous drug peddlers play a unique role in the health system by targeting unskilled, low-income, and manual workers. They typically sell substandard energy-boosting medications, aphrodisiacs, multivitamins, blood tonic, analgesics in bus stops, marketplaces, and commercial busses (Asakitikpi, 2019). Many of the drugs are sourced from Asian countries – China, Thailand, and India.

Like the drug peddlers, traditional drug hawkers are found at bus stops and marketplaces. They also meet specific consumers' needs, although sometimes the clientele spectrum cuts across socioeconomic classes. Their remedies are packaged in bottles, wrapped in paper and nylon sachet, and sold to the public. They market them to their clientele to treat infections, diarrhea, skin rash, pile, eczema, dysmenorrhea, ringworm, low sexual drive, and low sperm count (Asakitikpi, 2019).

Traditional drug hawkers enjoy extensive patronage primarily because of the low cost of their products and cultural engagement with their clients. The price of their products is relatively low because they are locally sourced. They display a high level of familiarity with the remedies they sell and the ailments they claim to cure. To demonstrate the efficacy of their products, they advertise using the bull horns, public address systems, and patients suffering from the condition they claim their drugs can cure. They market their products by displaying them in commercial busses and engaging commuters. First, they pray in the local language. Then they wish their listeners "Alafia" or good health, discuss the symptoms associated with various diseases, and then present their listeners with the remedies that will cure the conditions. They also discuss the Western allopathic medicines' equivalent of their product and their efficacy. However, they are quick to pinpoint the high cost of purchasing allopathic drugs and their side effects. The discussion of the Western allopathic medicines' side effects usually convinces their audience to patronize their products. Interestingly, both the educated and the uneducated public and some middle-income socioeconomic class patronize the traditional hawkers and drug peddlers (Asakitikpi, 2019).

Traditional drug hawkers and peddlers of Asian drugs complement each other. They are the most common healthcare providers among the vast majority of low-income socioeconomic classes in urban centers, and they play a significant role in the healthcare system. Although TMPs are found in urban centers, they are the predominant primary healthcare provider in rural areas. They still retain the traditional informal structure of health care, but they have now introduced service fees (Asakitikpi, 2019).

Management and Leadership of the Health Departments

In the United States and the United Kingdom, the health departments' leader is called the "secretary of health." In both countries, the appointment of the secretaries of health and the major hospitals' CEOs are based on merit and qualifications that include administrative experience, mellowed temperament, and excellent human relations skills. In Nigeria, the health system's leadership is the minister of health at the federal level and the commissioner of health at the state level. The Chief Medical Director (CMD) oversees the daily operations of the UTHs, FMCs, and specialist hospitals. The CMD position is statutorily allocated to physicians/dentists.

In most cases, physicians/dentists are appointed by the minister of health. The other HCPs assert that this arrangement is inconsistent with the democratic ideals of governance and transparency. They affirm that the present situation is absurd and inconsistent with the practice in other parts of the world. To test this claim, eighty randomly selected countries from the WHO member states were surveyed to evaluate the widely held perception that physicians and men dominate the health system's leadership around the world, including Nigeria (Table 4.4).

Data collected in October 2019

The data presented in Table 4.4 revealed that 37 (46%) of the current ministers of health in WHO member nations are physicians. The remaining 43 (54%) are from other professions such as law, theology, public health, engineering, accountancy, pharmacy, toxicology, social work, academy, politics, library science, health economy, and journalism. Women are highly underrepresented in the sample. Only 24 (30%) of the health ministers are women.

It is pertinent to put the earlier findings into a global context by comparing them with the United States (HHS.gov, 2021). Of the 13 Senate-confirmed secretaries of health in the United States from 1980 to 2021, only three (23%) were physicians and five (38%) lawyers (Table 4.5). The incumbent and previous secretaries of health are lawyers. About 67% of the secretaries of health are men and 33% women. Compared to the WHO member nations, where 46% of health secretaries are physicians (Table 4.4), in the United States, physicians are less appointed as secretary of health. Like Nigeria, men are appointed more often as secretary of health in the United States.

Leadership of the Federal Ministry of Health

With the disharmony and unhealthy rivalry among HCPs in Nigeria, many technocrats and health analysts attributed it to ineffective leadership at all health sector levels (Lambo, 2019; Oleribe et al., 2016, 2018). Nigerians are among the best brains globally, and the country is endowed with capable administrators and technocrats at home and in the diaspora. Still, successive governments have not been able to put honest and visionary leaders at the FMH consistently. Since the first republic, the healthcare system has been in travail and riddled with various crises. The multifaceted challenges have inhibited the implementation of consistent policies and raised questions, doubts, and fears, all of which suggest ineffective leadership at all health system levels. It is relevant to identify the professions of the individuals who have been at the reins of affairs in the health sector.

The names and professions of the ministers of health in Nigeria from 1952 to 2020 are presented in Table 4.6. Within the 68 years from 1952 to 2020, physicians served for 34 years, and all the other professionals combined served for 34 years. The data revealed that within the 68 years, the government appointed 27 ministers of health. Of the 27 ministers, 48% (13) were physicians compared to 46% by WHO member nations (Table 4.4). The remaining 52% (14) were politicians, lawyers,

Table 4.4 Profile of the ministers of health for 80 randomly selected WHO member nations

Serial #	Country	Name of Minister	Gender	Profession	Tenure
1	Zimbabwe	Pagwesese David Parirenyatwa	Male	Physician	2013–2018
2	Congo Brazzaville	Jacqueline Lydia Mikolo	Female	Politician	2016 to date
3	Democratic Republic of Congo	Victor Makwenge Kaput	Male	Physician	2007–2018
4	Rwanda	Diane Gashumba	Female	Physician	2016 to date
5	Cameroon	Andre' Mama Fouda	Male	Engineer	2007 to date
6	Bangladesh	Zahid Maleque	Male	Politician	2019 to date
7	Switzerland	Susanna Huovinen	Female	Politician	2014 to date
8	The Gambia	Isatou Touray	Female	Politician	2018 to date
9	China	Ma Xiaowei	Male	Physician	2018 to date
10	Morocco	Prkhalid AIT Taleb	Male	Physician	2019 to date
11	Swaziland	Sibongile Ndiela-Simelane	Female	Accountant	2019 to date
12	Lesotho	Nkaku Kabi	Male	Lecturer	2017 to date
13	Finland	Aino-Kaisa Pekonen	Female	Nursing	2019 to date
14	Italy	Roberto Speranza	Male	Politician	2019 to date
15	Israel	Benjamin Netanyahu	Male	Diplomat	2017 to date
16	Ireland	Simon Harris	Male	Politician	2016 to date
17	Croatia	Milan Kujundzic	Male	Physician	2016 to date
18	Japan	Katsunobu Kato	Male	Economics	2019 to date
19	Vietnam	Thi Kim Tien	Female	Physician	2011 to date
20	Myanmar	Myint Htwe	Male	Physician	2016 to date
21	Ukraine	Zoriana Skaletska	Female	Lawyer	2019 to date
22	Poland	Lukasz Szumowski	Male	Physician	2018 to date

(continued)

Table 4.4 (continued)

Serial #	Country	Name of Minister	Gender	Profession	Tenure
23	Saudi Arabia	Tawfiq Al Rabiah	Male	Lecturer	2016 to date
24	Peru	Zulema Thomas	Female	Health administrator	2019 to date
25	South Korea	Park Neugh-hu	Male	Social worker	2017 to date
26	Sri Lanka	Rajitha Senaratne	Male	Dentist	2015 to date
27	Romania	Victor Costache	Male	Physician	2019 to date
28	Mali	Samba Sow	Male	Physician	2017 to date
29	Tunisia	Sonia Ben Cheikh	Female	Physician	2019 to date
30	Netherlands	Hugo de Jonge	Male	Teacher	2017 to date
31	Burundi	Thaddee Ndikumana	Male	Physician	2019 to date
32	Singapore	Gan Kim Yong	Male	Engineer	2011 to date
33	Malaysia	Dzulkefly Bin Ahmed	Male	Toxicologist	2018 to date
34	Greece	Vassilias Kikilias	Male	Physician	2019 to date
35	Thailand	Piyasakol Sakolsatayadron	Male	Physician	2016 to date
36	Indonesia	Terawan Agus Putranto	Male	Physician	2019 to date
37	New Zealand	David Clark	Male	Theology/ Philosophy	2017 to date
38	Bahrain	Faea Bint Saeed Al Saleh	Female	Librarian	2015 to date
39	Iran	Saeed Namaki	Male	Pharmacist	2019 to date
40	Malawi	Peter Kumpalume	Male	Physician	2014 to date
41	Kenya	Cleopa Kilonzo Mailu	Male	Geneticist	2015 to date
42	Uganda	Jane Aceng	Female	Pediatrician	2016 to date
43	Tanzania	Ummy Ally Mwalimu	Female	Lawyer	2015 to date
44	Botswana	Alfred Madigele	Male	Physician	2018 to date

Table 4.4 (continued)

Serial #	Country	Name of Minister	Gender	Profession	Tenure
45	Namibia	Kalumbi Shangula	Male	Physician	2018 to date
46	Angola	Silvia Lutucuta	Female	Physician	2019 to date
47	Brazil	Ricardo Barros	Male	Engineer	2016 to date
48	Barbados	Jeffery D. Bostic	Male	Politician	2018 to date
49	Guyana	Volda Ann Lawrence	Female	Accountant	2018 to date
50	Trinida Tobago	Terrence Deyalsingh	Male	Pharmacist	2015 to date
51	Nepal	Bhanu Bhakta Dhakal	Male	Politician	2019 to date
52	Hungary	Gabor Zombor	Male	Physician	2014 to date
53	Allgeria	Mokhtar Hasbellaoui	Male	Physician	2017 to date
54	Philipines	Francisco Duque	Male	Physician	2017 to date
55	Ghana	Kwaku Agyaman Manu	Male	Accountant	2017 to date
56	Libreria	Bernice Dahn	Female	Physician	2015 to date
57	Mozambique	Nazira Karimo Vali Abdula	Female	Physician	2015 to date
58	France	Agnes Buzyn	Female	Physician	2017 to date
59	Bolivia	Ariana Campero Nava	Female	Physician	2015 to date
60	Sychelles	Jean Paul Adam	Male	Political economist	2016 to date
61	Sweden	Annika Strandhall	Female	Politician	2017 to date
62	Portugal	Marta Temido	Female	Health economist	2018 to date
63	Armenia	Arsen Torosyan	Male	Public Health	2018 to date
64	Argentina	Adolfo Rubinstein	Male	Physician	2017 to date
65	South Africa	Zweli Mkhize	Male	Physician	2019 to date
66	Sierra Leone	Abu Bakarr Fofanah	Male	Physician	2014 to date

(continued)

Table 4.4 (continued)

Serial #	Country	Name of Minister	Gender	Profession	Tenure
67	Venezuela	Carlos Alvarado	Male	Physician	2018 to date
68	Spain	Maria Luisa Carcedo	Female	Physician	2018 to date
69	Russia	Veronica Skvortsova	Female	Physician	2012 to date
70	India	Harsh Vardhan	Male	Physician	2019 to date
71	Nigeria	Osagie Emmanuel Ehanire	Male	Physician	2019 to date
72	United Kingdom	Matt Hancock	Male	Economist	2018 to date
73	United States	Alex Azar	Male	Lawyer	2018 to date
74	Germany	Jens Spahn	Male	Politician	2018 to date
75	Canada	Patricia Hajdu	Female	Social work	2019 to date
76	Denmark	Magnus Heunicke	Male	Journalist	2019 to date
77	Norway	Bent Hoie	Male	Lawyer	2013 to date
78	Australia	Greg Hunt	Male	Lawyer	2017 to date
79	Cuba	Roberto Morales Ojeda	Male	Physician	2018 to date
80	Mexico	Jorge Alcocer Varela	Male	Researcher	2018 to date

military officers, journalists, academics, pharmacists, parasitologists, and nurses. Coincidentally, the pharmacist, parasitologists, and nurse served as health minister for a brief period. The pharmacist served for only four months, the nurse for three months, and the parasitologists for less than two years. Of the 27 ministers of health, only 4% (one) is a woman. Compared to other WHO member countries, where 30% of the health ministers are women, Nigerian women are disproportionately under-represented as ministers of health. The findings in this chapter debunked the widely held perception that physicians are appointed ministers of health in higher numbers in Nigeria than in the other parts of the world. Nigeria's health system is in turmoil and inefficient, not because of the higher number of physicians who served as ministers of health, but because of their ineffectiveness in managing the FMH and the hospitals.

In 2015, Alalade provided relevant biographical information about the *ministers of health in Nigeria from 1950 to 2015*. Drawing on the data from that article and

Table 4.5 The Secretaries of the United States Department of Health and Human Services from 1980 to 2021

Serial #	Name – Gender	Profession	State	Tenure in office	Appointing president
1	Patricia Roberts Harris - Female	Lawyer	District of Columbia	May 4, 1980–January 20, 1981	Jimmy Carter
	William Mckiee[a]		New Mexico	January 20, 1981–January 22, 1981	Ronald Reagan
2	Richard S. Schweiker - Male	Businessman and politician	Pennsylvania	January 22, 1981–February 3, 1983	Ronald Reagan
	Speedy Long[a]		Louisiana	February 3, 1983– March 9, 1983	Ronald Reagan
3	Margaret M. Heckler - Female	Politician and Lawyer	Massachusetts	March 9, 1983– December 13, 1985	Ronald Reagan
4	Otis R. Bowen - Male	Politician and Physician	Indiana	December 13, 1985–March 1, 1989	Ronald Reagan
5	Louis Wade Sullivan - Male	Physician	Georgia	March 1, 1989–January 20, 1993	George H. W. Bush
6	Donna Shalala - Female	Politician and academic	Wisconsin	January 22, 1993– January 20, 2001	Bill Clinton
7	Tommy G. Thompson - Male	Lawyer and politician	Wisconsin	February 2, 2001– January 26, 2005	George W. Bush
8	Michael O. Leavitt - Male	Politician	Utah	January 26, 2005– January 20, 2009	George W. Bush
	Charles E. Johnson[a]		Utah	January 20, 2009– April 28, 2009	Barack Obama
9	Kathleen Sebelius - Female	Businesswoman and politician	Kansas	April 28, 2009– June 9, 2014	Barack Obama
10	Sylvia Mathews Burwell - Female	Politician and economist	West Virginia	June 9, 2014–January 20, 2017	Barack Obama
	Norris Cochran[a]		Florida	January 20, 2017–February 10, 2017	Donald Trump

(continued)

Table 4.5 (continued)

Serial #	Name – Gender	Profession	State	Tenure in office	Appointing president
11	Tom Price - Male	Physician	Georgia	February 10, 2017– September 29, 2017	Donald Trump
	Don J. Wright[a]		Virginia	September 29, 2017–October 10, 2017	Donald Trump
	Eric Hargan[a]		Illinois	October 10, 2017–January 29, 2018	Donald Trump
12	Alex Azar Male	Lawyer	Indiana	January 29, 2018– January 19, 2021	Donald Trump
13	Xavier Becerra – Incumbent - Male	Lawyer	California	January 27, 2021	Joseph Biden

Source: HHS.gov, 2021
[a]Temporary appointment; not confirmed by the US Senate

other published sources, an analysis of the job performance of the long-serving and consequential health ministers is presented next.

The late Professor Olikoye Ransome-Kuti, a pediatrician, was appointed by General Ibrahim Babangida as minister of health and served in the 1980s until 1992. As the longest-serving minister of health, he was a man of honor and integrity who introduced the concept of PHC to the nation. Professor Kuti succeeded in implementing the PHC policy. The WHO analytical expert review team commended his efforts and recommended the institutionalization of PHC through establishing the National Primary Healthcare Development Agency (Lambo, 2015, 2019). In 1976, Professor Kuti developed the Basic Health Services Scheme (BHSS), which many experts posited failed because of the astronomical cost needed for its implementation, which the national government could not afford. The implementation of the BHSS would have required the nation to devote most of its resources to health care for five years. The BHSS required too many health facilities in each local government area: one comprehensive health center, four primary health centers, five health clinics for each health center, some mobile clinics, and colossal health personnel. In 1988, Professor Kuti again proposed a "health policy" that never took off the ground during his eight-year tenure. A key achievement during his tenure was the attainment of 80% immunization coverage for fully immunized children. This achievement was short-lived because of the withdrawal of foreign donors' financial support in opposition to the unpopular Abacha regime (Ihekweazu, 2015).

Professor Olikoye Ransome-Kuti, during his seven-year tenure as health minister (1985–1992), tried unsuccessfully to fully achieve the Alma Ata Declaration goal, which declared that health is a fundamental human right. After he left office in

Table 4.6 Ministers of Health in Nigeria: 1952–2020

	Names	Tenure date	Gender	Number of years	Profession/ occupation
1	Chief S.L. Akintola	1952–1956	Male	4	Politician
2	Chief Ayo Rosiji	1957–1959	Male	2	Lawyer
3	Alhaji Waziri Ibrahim	1959–1961	Male	2	Politician
4	Senator Dr. Majekodunmi	1961–1965	Male	4	Physician
5	Mallam Aminu Kano	1972–1974	Male	2	Politician
6	Group Capt. Dan Suleiman	1975–1977	Male	2	Military officer
7	Dr. Peter Ogbang	1977–1979	Male	2	Academic
8	Dr. D.C. Ugwu	1979–1983	Male	4	Physician
9	Sam Paul Wampama	October–December, 1983	Male	0.25	Politician
10	Commondore Patrick Koshoni	January–October, 1984	Male	0.66	Military officer
11	Emmanuel Nsan	1984–1985	Male	1	Physician
12	Olikoye Ransome-Kuti	1985–1992	Male	7	Physician
13	Christopher Okoji (interim)	1993	Male	1	Physician
14	Julius Adelusi Adeluyi	August–November, 1993	Male	0.33	Pharmacist
15	Sarki Tafida	1993–1995	Male	2	Physician
16	I.C. Mabuleke	1995–1997	Male	2	Journalist
17	Jubril Ayinla	1997–1998	Male	1	Military officer
18	Debo Adeyemi	May 1998–1999	Male	0.5	Physician
19	Dr. Tim Menakaya	1999–2001	Male	2	Physician
20	Alphonsus B. Nwosu	2001–2003	Male	2	Parasitologist
21	Eyitayo Lambo	2003–2007	Male	4	Health economist
22	Adenike Garage	2007–2008	Female	1	Physician
23	Oshotimehin Babatunde	2008–2010	Male	2	Physician
24	Onyebuchi Chukwu	2010–March, 2015	Male	5	Physician
25	Khaliru Hassan	March–May, 2015	Male	0.25	Nursing
26	Isaac Folorunsho Adewole/ Osagie Emmanuel Ehanire	2015–2019	Male	4	Physicians
27	Osagie Emmanuel Ehanire/ Adeleke Olorunnimbe Mamora	August 2019 to date	Male	1	Physicians

1992, the PHC system collapsed (Lambo, 2010). Successive military and democratic governments failed to allocate enough funds to provide PHC consistent with the Alma Ata Declaration goal. Professor Ransome-Kuti's vision of shifting the responsibility for PHC to the local governments turned out, after all, not to be such a good idea. Because the general misconception is that PHC is for the rural people, the city dwellers think it is inferior to receive service from a PHC facility (Falae, 2018).

Professor ABC Nwosu, a parasitologist at the University of Nigeria Nsukka, was appointed by President Olusegun Obasanjo as a special adviser on political matters on May 29, 1999, and later served as minister of health from 2001 until 2003. Professor Nwosu had no significant policy changes or paradigm shifts introduced during his term as minister of health. Professor Eyitayo Lambo succeeded him.

Professor Eyitayo Lambo, a health economist, and seasoned technocrat, was appointed minister of health during President Olusegun Obasanjo's second term. He served from July 2003 until May 2007 without any scandal and no single industrial strike in the health sector. Professor Lambo shepherded a health sector reform after the system was ranked low in the WHO's assessment of its member nations in 2000. He oversaw the national program's merging on immunization with the National Primary Healthcare Development Agency and launched the National Health Insurance Scheme on June 6, 2005 (Alalade, 2015). Professor Lambo upgraded most tertiary hospitals and instituted the National Health Insurance Scheme and the national blood transfusion service. Many analysts credit him with revising and retooling the health policy plan that Professor Kuti proposed in 1988. A social critic described Professor Lambo's plan as a model blueprint for providing high-quality health care in developing nations (Nasir El-Rufai, 2015). One commentator opined that Professor Lambo is the best minister of health the country has ever had. He outperformed the surgeons and other medical professionals who held the office without tangible achievement (Tam, 2015).

Professor Adenike Grange, a pediatrician, was appointed the first Nigerian woman minister of health on July 25, 2007, by President Umaru Yar'Adua. However, she was arrested in February 2008 on the instigation of President Yar'Adua, for the handling of contract awards and the N300 million unspent funds in the 2007 budget. The money was meant to be returned to the treasury but was allegedly shared by FMH officers as bonuses (Nkwazema & Nwezeh, 2008). Professor Grange asserted that her director misadvised her (Agande & Shuaibu, 2008). In March 2008, President Yar'Adua accepted her resignation (Idonor & Akor, 2008). A court of appeal in Abuja, in December 2009, released Professor Grange from facing prosecution, and all charges were dropped (TsaAbuja, 2008; Ise-Oluwa Ige, 2009).

The late Professor Babatunde Osotimehin was appointed minister of health by President Goodluck E. Jonathan to replace Dr. Grange, and he left office in March 2010 when Jonathan dissolved his cabinet. Professor Osotimehin showed interest in reproductive health and human rights issues but did not record any significant legislative or policy achievement, nor did he strategically position the FMH during his tenure.

Professor Onyebuchi Chukwu, an orthopedic surgeon, served as minister of health in President Jonathan's administration beginning in April 2010 and was re-appointed in June 2011. Although Professor Chukwu was dismissed in 2008 as the chief medical officer of Ebonyi UTH due to an unsolved allegation of fraud (The Nation Archive, 2014), President Jonathan still appointed him minister for health. Professor Chukwu's tenure was marred by the most frequent and worst industrial strikes that led to the sacking of 16,000 resident physicians protesting for 8 weeks against poor conditions of service (Alalade, 2015; Adeloye et al., 2017). The President of The Nigeria Labor Congress chastised Professor Chukwu for dishonoring the National Industrial Court's verdict and repudiated an earlier agreement with the unions (Vanguard, 2013). To his credit, Professor Chukwu eradicated the guinea worm in Nigeria during his tenure, and he successfully led the fight against the Ebola virus outbreak in 2014. He resigned as minister for health in October 2014 to run unsuccessfully for governor in Ebonyi State.

Professor Isaac Folorunso Adewole was appointed minister for health on October 12, 2015, by President Muhammadu Buhari. Dr. Osagie Emmanuel Ehanire was appointed minister of state. Professor Adewole was replaced in June 2019 after Buhari's re-election for the second term, and Dr. Osagie Emmanuel Ehanire became the minister of health. He is credited with implementing the Basic Healthcare Provision Fund and executing the world's largest population-based HIV/AIDS survey. He obtained the bill's presidential assent that created the Nigerian Center for Disease Control and launched Nigeria's first electronic health registry (Ihekweazu, 2015). There were six industrial strikes in the health sector (between April 2016 and April 2017) during Professor Adewole's tenure (Oleribe et al., 2018; Adeloye et al., 2017; Campus Times, 2013). The HCPs put the PHC system on life support as the tertiary hospitals could not serve their designated top tier role as the nation's specialist referral centers. As a result of the chaos in the health system, minor conditions typically seen in the primary health centers, clinics, or general hospitals, without a referral, are now managed at the tertiary hospitals.

During the second term of President Muhammadu Buhari's administration, he appointed two ministers to run the health ministry on August 21, 2019 – Dr. Osagie Emmanuel Ehanire as the senior minister and Dr. Adeleke Olorunnimbe Mamora, the minister of state. But less than a year in their tenure as health minister, resident physicians went on strike during the coronavirus disease 2019 (COVID-19) pandemic over complaints of inadequate personal protective equipment, welfare, and better benefits concerns (Aljazeera.com, 2020; Sotunde et al., 2020).

Overall, 48% of the ministers of health that served for 34 years (for 50% of the time from 1952 to 2020) were physicians. They all had distinguished professional careers, yet the health system that they managed is one of the most inefficient in the world with poor health outcome indicators (WHO, 2000, 2006, 2015, 2016) and perpetually marred by industrial strikes (Oleribe et al., 2016, 2018; Adeloye et al., 2017). Only Professor Ransome Kuti and Professor Eyitayo Lambo had a widely acclaimed performance as health ministers (Tam, 2015; Nasir El-Rufai., 2015). Many physicians were catapulted into the leadership position because their political connection had no tangible achievement during their tenure in office. It is fair to conclude that a good knowledge of medicine and a successful medical career do not often translate into effective leadership in steering the nation's healthcare system's ship. The country desperately needs uncompromised visionary leaders, irrespective of the profession, with good management and strategic planning experiences to address the healthcare system's multifactorial challenges. One critic opined that it is shortsighted and uninformed to think that the best physicians must always be the health minister, overlooking other healthcare team members' competence (Tam, 2015).

The Functions of the Health Minister and Skills Needed to Be Successful

The health sector's continuous industrial strike has been attributed to poor management by several ministers of health and the CMDs of the tertiary hospitals. It is, therefore, pertinent to highlight the personal qualities and roles, and responsibilities of the minister of health. An in-depth review of the literature on organizational behavior revealed that a medical qualification is not a prerequisite criterion to be successful as a health minister. Instead, the following requirements and skills are needed to be successful:

1. The individual should be a visionary and a strategic thinker, an outsider, a skillful communicator who knows political realities and can collaborate with other power players to achieve the strategic plan. Must have the right political attitude to issues and balance various health-related interests, including physicians/dentists and other health professionals.
2. The health minister position requires the officeholder to scan the environment, develop and effectively manage a strategic action plan with timelines, evaluate results, collect feedback for performance improvement, inspire all stakeholders to achieve the vision, and cultivate meaningful relationships with political leaders, other ministers, and leaders from different health organizations and international partners.
3. The minister of health must provide effective leadership and governance by engaging the private sector, NGOs, and donors with vested interests in health using political, communication, and advocacy skills to make economic and political arguments with the Minister of Finance, the President, and the legislative leadership. In addition, the minister must be a good steward accountable for results and transparency in using available resources, strengthening consumer demand for better health services, promoting health, and providing essential public health functions directly or through private-sector agencies (Omaswa and Boufford, 2014).
4. The minister of health must have the organization and management skills needed to build coalitions toward a coherent policy agenda with an in-depth understanding of how the government at large and the health department are working. Furthermore, the minister must effectively communicate the value and importance of health-related issues and delineate priorities in health. He must be able to identify and select competent collaborators to organize multidisciplinary working groups. Some technocrats opined that the health minister must have no present or past conflicts of interest, including ties with the pharmaceutical industry, private hospitals, or other health-related economic activities (Lambo, 2019).

The Controversy Over the Surgeon General Position

The surgeon general title originated in the seventeenth century and is today used in several of the 53 commonwealth nations and most of the 29 North Atlantic Treaty Organization (NATO) countries for a senior military medical officer or a senior uniformed physician commissioned by the government and entrusted with public health responsibilities. In the United Kingdom, the head of the military medical services is the surgeon general. The three senior service medical directors hold the position with vice admiral, lieutenant general, or air marshal ranks. In the United States, the chief public health officer is the surgeon general. Also, the three military services appoint a surgeon general for the army, navy, and air force. A few states elect a surgeon general as well.

In the past decade, Nigeria has considered creating a surgeon general position as part of its colonial health administration lineage as a member of the commonwealth. The proposal generated intense controversy in the health sector. Some critics wondered why carry on with the colonial experience and the surgeon general's value-added function to solving Nigerian demonstrable health challenges? Some argued that the surgeon general must be a physician or dentist. This proposal assumed that such a model would end the health sector disputes by opening up the health minister position to other HCPs. Others argued that this proposal could be counterproductive since it would be construed (and rightly so) that other HCPs should have a legal hold on the health minister's position, provided the surgeon general is the exclusive right of the physicians and dentists (Lambo, 2019). If Nigeria must have a surgeon general, why should the person not be a commissioned medical professional? The national assembly considered a bill to create the general surgeon position but did not receive enough votes to pass. It faced stiff opposition from other HCPs and even politicians, and it is unclear if and when the bill will be brought up for reconsideration. Many critics affirm that the functions spelled out in the proposed law undermine the minister of health position. If the bill "as is" becomes law, it will undoubtedly become another source of friction among the HCPs.

It is relevant to discuss here the lessons that Nigeria can learn from other countries. A few countries worldwide (United States, United Kingdom, Canada, and South Africa) have commission-designated physicians for the surgeon general position. In the United States, the surgeon general is generally considered the megaphone on health matters during the typical political climate, but the post may be on its way to oblivion. In the current era of budget austerity, many technocrats in Washington, DC, have demanded eliminating the position to save money because the Department of Health and Human Services can absorb the surgeon general's role. Over the years, the post has generated undeserved controversies that put some presidents in a political crossfire from the opposing party. Dr. Everett Koop, a pediatric surgeon who served as the 13th surgeon general during President Ronald Reagan's administration from 1982 to 1989, is the only surgeon general to become a household name in the United States (The Washington Post, 2013). Dr. Koop was known for his advocacy against tobacco use, prevention of AIDS, abortion, and his support for disabled children's rights.

Dr. Joycelyn Elders, a pediatrician who served as surgeon general from 1993 to 1994 during President Bill Clinton's administration, was the second woman, the second person of color, and the first African American to serve in that role. Dr. Elders is best remembered for her frank discussion on controversial issues such as drug legalization, masturbation, and distributing contraception in schools. However, because of her many controversial views among conservatives, she was forced to resign in December 1994 (Unbound Magazine. (n.d.)).

Dr. Jerome Adams, an anesthesiologist, was the surgeon general during the COVID-19 crisis. However, because of the political quadriremes in Washington, DC, Dr. Adams was relegated into the background. Dr. Anthony Fauci, Director of the National Institute of Allergy and Infectious Diseases since 1984, is the point man and respected spokesperson of the Trump Administration's White House Coronavirus Task Force addressing the COVID-19 pandemic. Dr. Fauci and not Dr. Adams, the surgeon general, is considered the most trusted medical figure in the country. At 80 years of age, Dr. Fauci is an American hero who is still working hard to keep America safe from pandemics.

A 2019 published book by Mike Stobbe detailed how politics crippled the effectiveness of previous surgeons generals in the United States. The position of surgeon general competes for funding and attention with the secretary of the Department of Human and Health Services and the director of the Centers for Disease Control and Prevention (CDC). Many health experts argued that in an era of declining budgets, a low profile and ineffective surgeon general is a waste of resources and should be disbanded (Stobbe, 2019). The proposed surgeon general position has already generated hatred among HCPs, and many well-meaning Nigerians have recommended that the idea be scrapped. Instead, they suggested that a committee within the Department of Health be constituted and charged with determining whether the nation's President or Governor be relieved of his/her position if found to be in poor health and cannot discharge the roles and responsibilities of the office. In the era of austerity and declining revenue in Washington, DC, the surgeon general's image and reputation are on the decline. Thus, it may be unnecessary to have a surgeon general in Nigeria amid the disharmony and tension among the HCPs. Such an appointment will add fuel to an already toxic relationship in the health sector.

Conclusion

The appointment of the leadership (health minister, CMDs of the UTHs, FMCs and specialist hospitals, and surgeon general) within the hierarchy of the FMH is a contentious issue and a primary cause of hatred and disharmony within the healthcare system. *Compared to the WHO member nations, physicians are less often appointed as secretary of health in the United States, and there is no significant gender difference in such appointments. The findings in this chapter debunked the general perception of inequity across professions in the selection of minister of health in Nigeria compared to WHO member countries. But Nigerian women are disproportionately underrepresented as ministers of health.* The country is endowed with capable administrators and technocrats at home and in the diaspora; unfortunately, successive governments have not been able to consistently appoint honest and visionary leaders to deliver on universal health care.

Case Study

Review the organizational structure of the Department or Ministry of Health in the United States, Singapore, Taiwan and South Korea from the following links:

1. USA:
   https://www.hhs.gov/about/agencies/orgchart/index.html
2. Singapore:
   https://www.commonwealthfund.org/international-health-policy-center/countries/singapore
3. Taiwan:
   https://www.mohw.gov.tw/cp-114-246-2.html
   https://www.ncbi.nlm.nih.gov/pmc/articles/PMC3960712/
4. South Korea:
   https://www.mohw.go.kr/eng/am/am0102.jsp?PAR_MENU_ID=1001&MENU_ID=100115

Using the information presented in this chapter, construct an organogram for the Federal Ministry of Health in Nigeria.

References

Adeloye, D., David, R. A., Olaogun, A. A., Auta, A., Adesokan, A., Gadanya, M., Opele, J. K., Owagbemi, O., & Iseolorunkanmi, A. (2017). Health workforce and governance: The crisis in Nigeria. *Human Resources for Health, 15*:32. [online]. Available at: https://human-resources-health.biomedcentral.com/articles/10.1186/s12960-017-0205-4#citeas. Accessed 16 Oct 2020.

Agande, B., & Shuaibu, I. (2008). Health ministers quit. *The Vanguard.* [online]. Available at: http://allafrica.com/stories/200803260005.html. Accessed 16 Oct 2020.

Alalade, A. F. (2015). Adewole stands "on the shoulders of giants": The 18 torchbearers of the Nigerian health sector. *Nigeria Health Watch.* [online]. Available at: https://nigeriahealthwatch.com/adewole-stands-on-the-shoulders-of-giants-the-18-torchbearers-of-the-nigerian-health-sector/#.XvKKgChKg2w. Accessed 16 Oct 2020.

Aljazeera.com. (2020). *Nigerian doctors strike over lack of PPE, welfare concerns.* [online]. Available at: https://www.aljazeera.com/news/2020/06/nigerian-doctors-strike-lack-ppe-welfare-concerns-200615084342885.html. Accessed 16 Oct 2020.

Asakitikpi, A. E. (2019). *Healthcare coverage and affordability in Nigeria: An alternative model to equitable healthcare delivery.* [online]. Available at: https://www.intechopen.com/books/universal-health-coverage/healthcare-coverage-and-affordability-in-nigeria-an-alternative-model-to-equitable-healthcare-delive. Accessed 19 May 2021.

Bello, O. (2018). What is the number of hospitals in Nigeria? May 13. *Quora.* [online]. Available at: https://www.quora.com/What-is-the-number-of-hospitals-in-Nigeria. 23 Sept 2020.

Brown, L. D. (2003). Comparing health systems in four countries: lessons for the United States. *American Journal of Public Health, 93*(1):52–6. [online]. Available at: https://www.ncbi.nlm.nih.gov/pmc/articles/PMC1447691/. 16 Mar 2021.

Campus Times. (2013). Professor Adewole's transformation by hype. *Campus Times, 5.* [online]. Available at: https://campustimesui.wordpress.com/2013/12/05/professor-adewoles-transformation-by-hype/. 23 Sept 2020.

Falae, V. (2018). *Trace the history of primary health care in Nigeria*. [online]. Available at: https://naijaquest.com/history-primary-health-care-nigeria/. Accessed 16 Oct 2020.

FMH. (2020) [online]. Available at: http://www.health.gov.ng/index.php/department/hospital-services; https://www.health.gov.ng/. Accessed 16 Oct 2020.

HHS.gov. (2021) [online]. Available at: HHS Historical highlights: Secretaries of HHS and HEW. https://www.hhs.gov/about/historical-highlights/index.html. Accessed 26 Mar 2021.

Idonor, D., & Akor, S. (2008) Fired! Yar'Adua sacks health minister over N300m scam. *Daily Champion*. [online]. Available at: https://allafrica.com/stories/200803260402.html. Accessed 16 Oct 2020.

Ihekweazu, C. (2015). Professor Eyitayo Lambo's "tour de force" and call to action. *Nigeria Health Watch*. [online]. Available at: https://nigeriahealthwatch.com/professor-eyitayo-lambos-tour-de-force-and-call-to-action/#.XvKEqihKg2w. Accessed 16 Oct 2020.

Ise-Oluwa, Ige. (2009). N300m scam: Appeal court acquits ex-health minister, Grange. *The Daily Vanguard*. [online]. Available at: http://www.vanguardngr.com/2009/12/n300m-scam-appeal-court-acquits-ex-health-minister-grange/. Accessed 16 Oct 2020.

Kenton, W. (2021). Organizational structure. *Investopedia*. [online]. Available at: https://www.investopedia.com/terms/o/organizational-structure.asp. Accessed 17 Nov 2021.

Lambo, E. (2019). *Managing inter professional disharmony in Nigeria's health sector for health security*. A presentation at the 55th annual scientific conference and workshop of the Association of Medical Laboratory Scientists of Nigeria, Abuja, 5 Sept 2019.

Lambo, E. (2015). *Primary healthcare: Realities, challenges, and the way forward*. Paper presented at the first Annual Primary Healthcare Lecture organized by the National Primary Healthcare Development Agency (NPHCDA) at Shehu Musa Yar'Adua Center, Wuse Zone 4, Abuja, 8th December 2015.

Lambo, E. (2010). *Healthcare services in Nigeria at 50*. Paper presented at the 27th Annual Health Week Organized by the University of Ilorin Medical Students Association at the Africa Hall, University of Ilorin Mini Campus Ilorin, Nigeria. 25th May 2010.

Ministry of Health and Welfare. (2017). Address: No.488, Sec. 6, Zhongxiao E. Rd., Nangang Dist., Taipei City 11558, Taiwan (R.O.C.) [online]. Available at: https://www.mohw.gov.tw/cp-114-246-2.html. Accessed 16 Oct 2020.

Nasir El-Rufai. (2015). Nigeria's health sector: Challenge and solutions that work. *Omojuwa.com*. [online]. Available at: http://omojuwa.com/2015/02/nigerias-health-sector-challenge-and-solutions-that-work-nasir-el-rufai/. Accessed 16 Oct 2020.

Nkwazema, S., & Nwezeh, K. (2008). Yar'Adua moves against health minister. *This Day*. Archived from the original on 27 August 2008. [online]. Available at: https://web.archive.org/web/20080827203433/http://odili.net/news/source/2008/mar/3/299.html. Accessed 16 Oct 2020.

Nwakeze, N. M., & Kandala, N. B. (2011). The spatial distribution of health establishments in Nigeria. *African Population Studies, 25*(2) [online]. Available at: https://www.researchgate.net/publication/274945986_The_spatial_distribution_of_health_establishmentsin_Nigeria. Accessed 23 Sept 2020.

Ogunbekun, I., Ogunbekun, A., & Orobaton, N. (1999). Private health care in Nigeria: Walking the tightrope. *Health Policy and Planning, 14*(2), 174–181.

Okaomee, A. (n.d.). The nonprofit sector and philanthropy in Nigeria. *Learning to Give*. [online]. Available at: https://www.learningtogive.org/resources/nonprofit-sector-and-philanthropy-nigeria. Accessed 16 Oct 2020.

Oleribe, O. O., Ezieme, P. I., Oladipo, O., Akinola, E. P., Udofia, D., & Taylor-Robinson, S. D. (2016). Industrial action by healthcare workers in Nigeria in 2013–2015: An inquiry into causes, consequences, and control-A cross-sectional descriptive study. *Human Resource Health, 27*;14(1):46. [online]. Available at: https://pubmed.ncbi.nlm.nih.gov/27465121/. Accessed 16 Oct 2020.

Oleribe, O. O., Udofia, D., Oladipo, O., Ishola, T. A., & Taylor-Robinson, S. D. (2018). Healthcare workers' industrial action in Nigeria: a cross-sectional survey of Nigerian physicians. *Human Resource Health, 16*: 54. [online]. Available at: https://www.ncbi.nlm.nih.gov/pmc/articles/PMC6192190/. Accessed 16 Oct 2020.

Omaswa, F., & Boufford. (2014). *Strong ministries for strong health systems: Handbook for ministers of health*. With contributions from Peter Eriki and Patrick Kadama.

Omojuwa. (2015). *Nigeria's health sector: Challenge and solutions that work – Nasir El-Rufai*. [online]. Available at: https://facesinternationalmagazine.org.ng/?p=2648. Accessed 16 Oct 2020.

Osuhor, P. C. (1978). Organisation of health services in Nigeria. *Health Popul Perspect Issues, 1*(1):1–11. [online]. Available at:https://pubmed.ncbi.nlm.nih.gov/10297868/. Accessed 16 Oct 2020.

PharmAccess Foundation. (2015). *Nigerian health sector market study report.* [online]. Available at: https://www.rvo.nl/sites/default/files/Market_Study_Health_Nigeria.pdf. 23 Sept 2020.

Ranchod, S. (2016). A healthy society is a productive society. *City Press.* [online]. Available at: https://www.news24.com/citypress/voices/a-healthy-society-is-a-productive-society-20160603. Accessed 16 Oct 2020.

Sotunde, A., Ukomadu, A., Ohuocha, C., Heinrich, M., & Merriman, J. (2020). Nigerian doctors strike for better benefits during coronavirus crisis. *Reuters.* [online]. Available at: https://www.reuters.com/article/us-health-coronavirus-nigeria-healthcare/nigerian-doctors-strike-for-better-benefits-during-coronavirus-crisis-idUSKBN23M1BZ. Accessed 16 Oct 2020.

Stobbe M. (2019). Surgeon general's warning: *How politics crippled the nation's doctor.* 1st Edition. [online]. Available at: https://www.amazon.com/Surgeon-Generals-Warning-Politics-Crippled/dp/0520272293 (Accessed: 16 October 2020).

Tam, A. A. (2015). Healing the ills in the ailing Nigerian health system. *The Guardian.* [online]. Available at: https://guardian.ng/features/healing-the-ills-in-the-ailing-nigerian-health-system/. Accessed 16 Oct 2020.

The Nation Archive. (2014). *Did Prof. Chukwu, current health minister, defraud Ebonyi State of N36 Million?* http://saharareporters.com/2014/08/21/did-prof-chukwu-current-health-minister-defraud-ebonyi-state-n36-million

The Washington Post. (2013). *Highlights of the career of C. Everett Koop, only surgeon general to become a household name.* February 25.

Tikkanen, R., Osborn, R., Mossialos, E., Djordjevic, A., & Wharton, G. A. (2020). International healthcare profiles: Singapore. *The Commonwealth Fund.* [online]. Available at: https://www.commonwealthfund.org/international-health-policy-center/countries/singapore. Accessed 16 Oct 2020.

TsaAbuja, G. (2008). N300m scam: Grange, Aduku, Ogandi, others docked, remanded in EFCC custody. The Daily. Sun. 9 April 2008. [online]. Available at: http://www.vanguardngr.com/2009/12/n300m-scam-appeal-court-acquits-ex-health-minister-grange/. Accessed 16 Oct 2020.

UK Home Office. (2018). *Country policy and information note Nigeria: Medical and healthcare issues Version 2.0.* [online]. Available at: https://www.justice.gov/eoir/page/file/1094261/download. Accessed 20 May 2021.

Unbound Magazine. (n.d.) *The legend who put her career on the line for sexual health.* [online]. Available at: https://unboundbabes.com/blogs/magazine/legend-career-on-line-sexual-health. (Accessed: 16 October 2020).

U.S. Department of Health & Human Services. (2020). *HHS organizational chart.* [online]. Available at: https://www.hhs.gov/about/agencies/orgchart/index.html. Accessed 16 Oct 2020.

Vanguard. (2013). *NLC blames health workers' strike on Chukwu.* August 27. [online]. Available at: https://www.vanguardngr.com/2013/08/nlc-blames-health-workers-strike-on-chukwu/. Accessed 16 Oct 2020.

Ventures. (2015). How strikes are killing Nigeria's public health system. *Ventures.* January 17. [online]. Available at: http://venturesafrica.com/how-strikes-are-killing-nigerias-public-healthcare/. Accessed 10 Oct 2020.

WES -. (2017) Education in Nigeria. [online]. Available at: https://wenr.wes.org/2017/03/education-in-nigeria (Accessed: 23 January 2020).

WHO. (2000). *The world health organization's ranking of the world's health systems, by rank.* [online]. Available at: https://photius.com/rankings/healthranks.html. Accessed 10 Oct 2020. https://photius.com/rankings/world_health_systems.html. Accessed 10 Oct 2020.

WHO. (2006). The world health report. In *Working Together for Health* (pp. 1–15). World Health Organization.

WHO. (2015). *World health statistics.* Part I: Global health indicators. [online]. Available at: https://www.who.int/gho/publications/world_health_statistics/EN_WHS2015_Part2.pdf. Accessed 10 Oct 2020.

WHO. (2016). *Global health observatory (GHO) data: World health statistics 2016: Monitoring health for the SDGs.* [online]. Available at: https://www.who.int/gho/publications/world_health_statistics/2016/en/. Accessed 10 Oct 2020.

Wu, T. Y., Majeed, A., & Kuo, K. N. (2010). An overview of the healthcare system in Taiwan. *London Journal of Primary Care* (Abingdon), *3*(2):115–119. [online]. Available at: https://www.ncbi.nlm.nih.gov/pmc/articles/PMC3960712/. Accessed 10 Oct 2020.

Chapter 5
The Vulnerabilities of the Nigerian Healthcare System

Learning Objectives

After reading this chapter, the learner should be able to:

1. Identify the challenges facing the implementation of universal health care in Nigeria
2. Analyze the factors impacting effective delivery of high-quality health care in Nigeria
3. Apply the WHO's framework to discuss the challenges within the Nigerian healthcare system
4. Describe the significant achievements and contributions of Nigeria to global health

Introduction

The Nigerian health system is one of the most inefficient globally (WHO, 2000). The first national health plan in Nigeria was developed in 1946 by the colonial masters with the primary goal to provide universal health care (UHC) to the citizen. Successive governments have put forth policy development plans to reform the health system, but UHC remains a pie in the sky. The first casualty of a decline in oil revenue has always been the defunding of primary health care, followed by education (Scott-Emuakpor, 2010).

The maternal and infant mortality rate in Nigeria is worse than the sub-Saharan African average. Thousands of children still die annually from vaccine-preventable diseases because the primary healthcare system is highly ineffective and has deteriorated substantially in the last two decades. Furthermore, Nigeria did not achieve most of the United Nations' eight health-related Millennium Development Goals (MDGs) by the 2015 target date (PharmAccess Foundation, 2015). This failure necessitates President Muhammadu Buhari's administration to consider creative ways of responding to the 2030 sustainable development goal 3 (SDG 3) on UHC and poverty. Sadly, at the end of 2020, Buhari's administration failed to achieve the 30% health insurance coverage goal set in 2016. The pertinent question that concerned technocrats and policymakers repeatedly ask is: Why is the Nigerian health system unable to perform to its full potential? This chapter's dual objectives are to identify the factors that make UHC unattainable and determine the challenges facing the effective delivery of high-quality health care in the country.

Methodology

This chapter's objectives were implemented by conducting an exhaustive search of the literature on the PubMed database using the following combinations of keywords: Nigeria, health system, challenges, UHC, and high-quality care. No date, gender, or geographical limitations were stipulated during the searches. The number of "hits" generated at each stage is presented in Table 5.1. The fourth stage of the literature search produced 34 "hits," but only 11 are relevant to the objectives of the study identified. The fifth stage search had seven "hits," but only one of the "hits" is relevant to the study's objectives. Only articles published in the English language were reviewed.

Only one quantitative study addressed the challenges facing the implementation of UHC in Nigeria (Umeh, 2018), while 11 other quantitative studies focused on the barriers against affordable and high-quality health care (Ejughemre, 2013; Odeyemi & Nixon, 2013; Gadzama et al., 2014; Uzochukwu et al., 2015; Okebukola & Brieger, 2016; Aregbeshola, 2018; Ozawa et al., 2019; Kiri and Ojule, 2020; Ozumba et al., 2019; Akinleye et al., 2020; Uguru et al., 2020). Additionally, 17 reviews and critique articles on the Nigerian healthcare system were identified (WHO, 2000, 2006, 2015, 2016; Fajola et al., 2007; Scott-Emuakpor, 2010; Welcome, 2011; Ogbebo, 2015; Orekunrin, 2015; Federal Ministry of Health (FMH), 2016; Ojo and Akinwumi, 2015; Julius, 2017; Ogbaa, 2017; Fosco, 2018;

Table 5.1 Output of literature search on the PubMed database on December 18, 2020

Stage of Search	Keywords	Outputs
1	Nigeria	56,068
2	Nigeria, health system	6776
3	Nigeria, health system, challenges	632
4	Nigeria, health system, challenges, universal healthcare	34
5	Nigeria, health system, challenges, universal healthcare, high quality care	7

Muhammad et al., 2017; Lopez, 2019; Asakitikpi, 2019). Other relevant publica-tions were obtained from the Google search engine database and references in the articles/reports cited above. The articles/reports on the vulnerabilities of the health-care system were categorized into six building blocks using the WHO's framework for gauging the performance of health systems (WHO, 2010).

Health System Vulnerabilities

Vulnerability #1: Poor Governance and Ineffective Leadership

For decades, the health sector leadership has poorly managed the three-tier health structures at all levels. A myriad of governance-related challenges that bedevil the health system includes a lack of political will and poor planning, ineffective leader-ship, corruption, wrong policy priorities, and severe political and economic stresses. Because the leaders misappropriated funds at the federal and state levels, the local governments rarely get their budget allocations, affecting primary healthcare ser-vices. The local level considerably lost its autonomy as successive state govern-ments' grabbed control of administrative functions and finances. The state power grab renders the local government primary care implementation ineffective (Ogbaa, 2017; Ojo and Akinwumi, 2015; Ohansa and Orimisan, 2012; Uzochukwu et al., 2015).

Corruption is endemic in many aspects of Nigerian life, and health care is not an exemption. In 2018, the health sector was deemed the third most corrupt govern-ment branch (Ibenegbu, 2018). But due to cultural reasons, it is a challenge to deci-pher what constitutes corruption and the different ways it manifests itself because what would be considered corrupt in many countries is deemed reasonable in Nigeria – like accepting bribes and diverting patients to private practices. Many leaders, including healthcare chief executive officers (CEOs), do not believe accept-ing a bribe is good but deem it reasonable if they are involved but unreasonable if an imaginary person commits the act. For example, the health sector was rocked in 2015 by a scandal of an impersonator, Martins Ugwu, employed in the FMH as a physician for 9 years before being uncovered (Ogbebo, 2015).

Amid all the scandals, President Goodluck Jonathan declared stealing by his ministers is not corruption and ignored allegations of fraud involving his cabinet members. However, his Minister for Petroleum, Ms. Diezani Allison-Madueke, was charged for money laundering and made to refund $90 billion of stolen money to the Economic and Financial Crimes Commission (Kazeem, 2015; Tnv Nigerian Voice, 2016). Critics bemoaned the lackluster performance of President Muhammadu Buhari's inability to deliver on its signature campaign promise to fight corruption. Nigeria dropped four spots to 146 out of 180 countries on the 2019 Transparency International's corruption index, marking its lowest ranking. The performance brought added scrutiny, with many Nigerians wondering about Buhari's commit-ment to his anti-graft campaign promise (Munshi, 2020). Another survey study conducted by the *US News and World Report* of 80 countries worldwide revealed that Nigeria is the most corrupt nation. The top ten countries after Nigeria were Colombia, Pakistan, Iran, Mexico, Ghana, Angola, Russia, Kenya, and Guatemala (World Population Review, 2020).

Vulnerability #2: Low-Quality Health Service Delivery

Nigeria has one of the most obstinate healthcare delivery systems globally, and achieving UHC remains a dream. Despite the various reforms geared towards UHC, less than 5% of the population is insured. One empirical research study investigated UHC implementation barriers in Nigeria and three other African countries – Ghana, Kenya, and Tanzania (Umeh, 2018). The findings of the study revealed the following five factors that obviate UHC:

1. Extreme poverty and the inability of the needy to pay health insurance premiums.
2. Corruption.
3. High informal sector economy, and most workers are mostly uninsured.
4. High NHIS dropout rate.
5. Underfunded health system.

About 44% of Nigerians live below the poverty line—on less than $1 a day—and cannot afford health insurance premiums. Moreover, the weak referral practice between the three tiers of the health system, caused by poor managerial functions and untapped health information systems, is responsible for its ineffectiveness. Another major shortcoming of healthcare delivery is the absence of adequate medical intelligence and surveillance systems to track disease outbreaks and environmental biohazards that are the first line of approach to an effective healthcare system (Welcome, 2011).

From 1970 to 2018, the informal sector economy's size in Nigeria ranges between 47% and 67%, accounting for 56% of the gross domestic product (GDP). On average, annually, the country loses about 56% of potential tax revenue to informality. In 2018 alone, the estimated tax revenue loss was about ₦3.5 trillion. The key drivers of informality in the economy are the regulatory burden, unemployment, and unregulated institutions (Tonuchi et al., 2020). The informality also precludes collecting any substantial revenue for the National Health Insurance Scheme (NHIS). It will be a hard sell to convince the poor to invest in government programs in a country that payment is made for electricity, but the power supply is epileptic or not delivered at all in several states. The distrust in government-run services (electricity and health) among the poor and the vulnerable population has to be broken for any significant uptake in the NHIS.

Abdulraheem and associates (2012) contend that primary health care, which is the bedrock of the healthcare system, caters to less than 20% of potential patients because the rural dwellers constitute 48% of the population, lack the necessary infrastructures, and their health centers are poorly equipped. The rural dwellers rely mainly on ambulatory care services that are often poorly organized and leave them at the mercy of quacks and faith healers. Social amenities, such as clean pipe-borne water, access to passable roads, electricity, suitable accommodation, reputable schools, Internet connectivity, and transportation, are lacking in the rural areas. Consequently, most healthcare professionals (HCPs) are not willing to live under such horrific conditions.

In a cross-sectional survey of 1600 women from Enugu State, Ozumba, and associates found inequities in access to quality health service. The statistically significant primary driver for the disparities is where the mothers live. Mothers who are urban dwellers and educated, with the elderly and affluent, had better healthcare access than their counterparts. Living in the urban center, distance to the health facilities, and being rich determine access to health service when needed (Ozumba et al., 2019).

A mixed-method cross-sectional descriptive study by Uguru and associates investigated the determinants and challenges of providing access to oral health care in Enugu state. Their findings revealed that the cost of raw materials (100%), personnel (98%), infection control resources (98%), geographical location (98%), government policies (88%), and the price of other goods (81%) influenced the provision of dental caries treatment services. Adequate access to dental services is a significant concern that affects all aspects of health care and a critical factor to achieving UHC (Uguru et al., 2020).

Nigeria has the second-largest number of people living with HIV and accounts for 9% of the global HIV burden. Similarly, Nigeria has the highest malaria burden globally, which remains the top cause of morbidity and mortality among children. In the last decade, the child and maternal mortality rates in the country have slightly decreased (Federal Ministry of Health, 2016) (Table 5.2).

Table 5.2 Child and maternal mortality rates in Nigeria in the global context

Serial #	Indicator	2003	2008	2013	Cuba[a] 2015	United States[b] (2015)	United Kingdom[b] (2015)
	Child mortality per 1000 live births						
1	Neonatal mortality	48	40	37	3	3.6	2.4
2	Infant mortality	100	75	69	4	6.5	4.2
3	Post neonatal mortality	52	35	31			
4	Child mortality	112	88	64			
5	Under-five mortality	201	157	128	6	6.5	4.2
6	Maternal mortality per 100,000 births (WHO/ UNICEF)	1000	545	576	38	14	9

Source: Federal Ministry of Health, 2016
[a]https://www.unicef.org/infobycountry/cuba_statistics.html#0
[b]http://data.unicef.org/topic/child-survival/neonatal-mortality/

Despite the improvement in the last decade, Nigeria still has one of the highest (worst) child and maternal mortality rates in the world; ranks tenth after Chad, Somalia, Central Africa, Sierra Leone, Burundi, Guinea-Bissau, Liberia, Sudan, and Cameroon (United Nations Children's Fund – UNICEF, n.d.; World Bank Data, 2010). The high child and maternal mortality rates are primarily due to inadequate access to quality health care in rural and remote areas and the shortage of physicians and midwives. Despite the horrendous child and maternal mortality rates, less than 10% of the health budget is for primary care. More concerning is that over 80% of the budget is for curative care offered in the tertiary (teaching/specialist) institutions (FMH, 2016)

The top ten causes of death in Nigeria are malaria, lower respiratory infections, HIV/AIDS, diarrhea, road traffic injuries, protein-energy malnutrition, cancer, meningitis, stroke, and tuberculosis. Malaria alone accounts for over a quarter of the death among children under 5 years of age, 30% of childhood death, and 11% of maternal fatalities. Nigeria has the second-highest HIV burden globally – 3.4 million Nigerians live with HIV (Muhammad et al., 2017). Malaria is a significant health and developmental problem, with a prevalence rate of 919 per 100,000 populations. It is the primary cause of morbidity and mortality in infants and young children in the country (Table 5.3). About 75% of malaria deaths occur in children under five, and malaria causes one in every ten maternal deaths (Labiran et al., 2008).

Nigeria has the second-largest HIV epidemic in the world, with 1.9 million people living with the infection and 180,000 AIDS-related deaths. HIV prevalence among adults aged 15–49 years is only 1.4%, compared to 19.2% in South Africa and 12.9% in Zambia. In 2015, Nigeria reported 227,000 new HIV infection cases, but unfortunately, only 51% of adults with HIV receive antiretroviral treatment. The South-South region of Nigeria has the highest HIV prevalence rate at 3.1% among adults aged 15–49 years. HIV prevalence is also high in the North-Central (2.0%) and South-East (1.9%) and lower in the South-West (1.1%), the North-East (1.1%), and the North-West (0.6%) zones (UNAIDS, 2019). The above unacceptable health indices emanate from abysmal health service delivery compounded by limited

Table 5.3 The top ten disease morbidity and mortality rates in Nigeria

Rank	Morbidity	Rate (%)	Rank	Mortality	Rate (%)
1	Malaria	70.5	1	Malaria	53.9
2	Diarrhea	14.2	2	Diarrhea	17.1
3	Dysentery	5.5	3	Pneumonia	7.4
4	Pneumonia	4.8	4	Dysentery	4.9
5	Sexually transmitted diseases	2.0	5	AIDS	3.3
6	Tuberculosis	0.6	6	Cerebrospinal meningitis	3.3
7	Measles	0.4	7	Cholera	3.2
8	AIDS	0.4	8	Measles	1.8
9	Cholera	0.4	9	Neo-natal tetanus	1.4
10	Pertussis	0.3	10	Tuberculosis	1.3

Sources: UNICEF, n.d.; World Bank Data, 2010

preventive programs for pre- and postnatal care, screening for specific diseases, and immunization. Over 95% of the population has no access to preventive healthcare services.

Researchers from the Intelligence Unit of the Economist in 2016 examined the healthcare systems in 60 countries worldwide to determine their most pressing healthcare needs. They found the lowest-performing countries (in ranking order) in the equity of healthcare access were India, Kenya, Ukraine, Nepal, Afghanistan, Nigeria, Democratic Republic of Congo, Cambodia, Afghanistan, Ethiopia, and Bangladesh came last. Five countries (Bangladesh, Cambodia, the Democratic Republic of Congo, the Dominican Republic, and Ukraine) have no specific policies (or not yet implemented) to guarantee access to health care for children. Moreover, 16 countries have no particular policies (or not yet implemented) to ensure access to health care for the unemployed. The top ten performing countries in access to child and maternal health services in ranking order were China (#1), followed by Thailand, Cuba, Taiwan, Brazil, United Kingdom, Canada, South Korea, Netherlands, and Uzbekistan. Most countries have or near achieving high coverage rates in essential child and maternal health services, including immunization, birth facilities, and family planning. Across all countries by income level the trend reflects a higher priority given to health care for women and girls. Unfortunately, Nigeria still lags in measles immunization coverage (Koehring, 2018).

Notwithstanding the scourge of the diseases and abhorrent health outcomes, successive governments in Nigeria only pay lip service to UHC. The exact number of healthcare facilities in Nigeria is open to debate because many private health institutions are not registered with the government (Bello, 2018). The data from the FMH in 2016 indicated there were 34,173 healthcare establishments/facilities in the country as of December 2011. Of the figure, 30,098 (88%) are primary care centers (dispensaries, maternities and clinics), 3992 (12%) are secondary (general/private hospitals) level facilities, while 83 (1%) are tertiary (teaching/specialist) facilities. More than 66% of these facilities are government-owned (Federal Ministry of Health, 2016) (Table 5.4).

When put in a global context, the number of healthcare facilities in Nigeria is grossly inadequate. For example, Cuba, a developing country like Nigeria, with a population of only 11.3 million in 2007, has 248 hospitals, 470 polyclinics, 289 maternity homes, and 54,857 medical care beds, 14,650 social service beds. The number of medical care beds and social service beds (per 1000 population) was 4.9 and 1.3, respectively (Cuba Health Profile, 2007).

Table 5.4 Types and number of healthcare facilities in Nigeria

Serial #	Funder	Primary level (dispensaries/ maternities/clinics)	Secondary level (general/private hospitals)	Tertiary level (teaching/specialist hospitals	Total
1	Public	21,808	969	73	22,850
2	Private	8290	3023	10	11,323
3	Total	30,098	3992	83	34,173

Source: Federal Ministry of Health, 2016

Nigerian tertiary hospitals have limited state-of-the-art diagnostic and therapeutic equipment to provide high-quality health care because 78% of the budget is from personnel salary and welfare. In 2018, 93% of allocations to federal government-owned hospitals was expended on recurrent expenditure items – primarily personnel costs, and to a lesser degree, overhead expenses. In 2016, the recurrent expenditure made up approximately 97% of total allocations to federal government-owned hospitals (Onigbinde et al., 2018). Consequently, the tertiary hospitals have no funds left to invest in capital projects – buildings, major diagnostic and therapeutic equipment, power generating plants, and consumables. Most of the tertiary hospitals lacked well-trained healthcare specialists. The infrastructure deficit in hospitals and the poor working conditions of the HCPs have been part of the bane of the country's healthcare system.

The electricity supply in Nigeria is erratic and a significant drag on the delivery of an efficient healthcare system. Only about 40% of the households are connected to the electricity grid, and those with electricity supply, including health facilities, experience power outages around 60% of the time (Parmar, 2015). Healthcare services are interrupted with each power failure, thereby putting laboratory reagents and vaccines that have to be stored at optimum temperatures at risk. More importantly, the human suffering associated with the interruption in healthcare services due to equipment malfunction and power outages cannot be quantified in pecuniary terms.

Vulnerability #3: Shortage of Healthcare Workforce

In 1962, there were only 1354 physicians and 58 dentists in Nigeria. A decade later, in 1972, the number of physicians and dentists increased to 3112 (56%) and 124 (53%), respectively. However, the Nigerian population grew by 21% from 54,000,000 in 1962 to 68,000,000 in 1972, making the numerical improvement in physicians and dentists less impactful (Scott-Emuakpor, 2010).

By 2005, the number of HCPs also increased to 39,210 physicians (30 per 100,000 people), 2773 dentists (2 per 100,000 people), 1224,626 nurses (100 per 100,000 people) 769 physiotherapists (0.62 per 100,000 people), and only 519 radiographers (0.42 per 100,000 people) (Federal Ministry of Health, 2016).

In 2013, a total of 71,740 physicians and dentists were registered with the Medical and Dental Council of Nigeria (MDCN), but only 27,000 practices in the country. At the same time, about 7000 Nigerian physicians and dentists' practice in the United Kingdom and the United States (Obinna, 2019). Five years later, in 2018, 72,000 physicians and dentists were registered with the MDCN, but only 35,000 practices in the country.

In addition to the scarcity of physicians, dentists, and nurses, other HCPs are in short supply in Nigeria. For instance, the physiotherapists per population ratio (density) in 2015 stands at one physiotherapist to 63,349 Nigerians, and it is one of the highest (i.e., worst) in the world. When compared to other countries around the

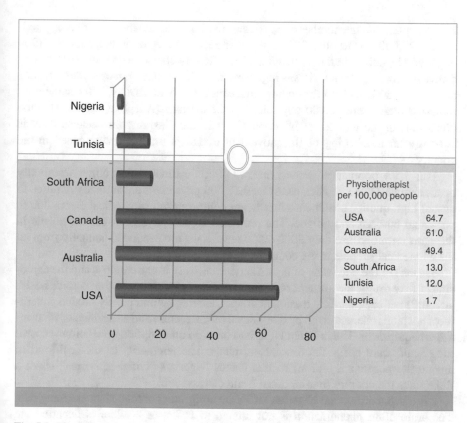

Fig. 5.1 Physiotherapist workforce (per 100,000 people) in selected countries around the world. (Reprinted from Balogun, J. A. (2020b). The path to our destiny: The transitioning of physiotherapy in Nigeria from occupation to a true profession. *Journal of the Nigeria Society of Physiotherapy*, 19(1), 19-35. Figure 1. https://doi.org/10.5897/JNSP2020.0004, licensed under the terms of the Creative Commons Attribution License (https://creativecommons.org/licenses/by/4.0/))

world, the shortage is more dramatic (Fig. 5.1). Nigeria has only 1.7 physiotherapists per 100,000 people, while Tunisia has 12, South Africa has 13, Canada has 49.4, Australia has 61.4, and the United States has 64.7 (Balogun, 2020b).

The exact number of Nigerian HCPs in the diaspora is unknown and open to wide speculation based on the source of information. Okoro and associates (2014) claimed there were 4500 Nigerian physicians in the United States. Three years later, in 2017, the Nigerian Medical Association's former president, Dr. Osahon Enabulele, stated that there were 8000 Nigerian physicians employed in the United States (Ighobor, 2017). On the other hand, Mitchell (2018) indicated that over 4700 physicians trained in Nigeria worked for the United Kingdom NHS and provided a substantial subsidy. The Association of Nigerian Physicians in the Americas in 2020 stated there were 4000 Nigerian-born or trained physicians in North America.

In 2017, NOIPolls indicated that the difference between physicians registered with the MDCN and those practicing in Nigeria is about 37,000. The registrar of the

MDCN noted that the number of physicians working outside the country is approximately 20,000 (NOIPolls, 2017). Another report in 2018 indicated only 1903 Nigerian physicians in the United Kingdom (Reality check, 2018). In 2019, Abang estimated over 72,000 physicians registered with the MDCN, but over 50% practice abroad, and 2000 had left the country in recent years. The MDCN, in the same year, indicated there were 40,000 physicians in the country (Adegoke, 2019). The discrepancies in the number of Nigerian HCPs in the diaspora are because there is currently no monitoring of the movement of HCPs trained and licensed in the country.

At a 3.5% population growth rate, NOIPolls estimated that Nigeria currently needs about 303,333 physicians. At least 10,605 physicians are annually required to ensure high-quality health care that is not compromised by medical errors due to personnel burnout and fatigue. The projected 10,605 physicians are unrealistic in the short term because only 3000–3500 physicians are produced annually from all the 44 medical schools in the country (NOIPolls, 2017).

Because of the poor state of health service delivery in the country, and the explosion of fake drugs, the affluent Nigerians have lost confidence in the nation's health system. They seek medical treatment abroad, leaving behind poorly funded government hospitals characterized by dilapidated infrastructure and a shortage of state-of-the-art equipment. The indigent Nigerians have no other option on where to receive their health care but at the decrepit hospitals. The popularity of medical tourism among the politicians and aristocrats makes Nigeria's "Giant of Africa" claim a fluke since the country runs an elitist healthcare system.

It is disconcerting that Nigerian HCPs are emigrating abroad at an alarming rate. The brain drain phenomenon is not limited to HCPs as academics departed the country in large numbers in the late 1970s. However, the current pace of HCPs' emigration abroad for greener pasture, seven during the COVID-19 pandemic, has reached a new height (Business Hallmark, 2021). Many health analysts described the situation as a "ticking time bomb" for the country. The top preference destination countries that Nigerian physicians emigrate to, in ranking order, are the United Kingdom, United States, Canada, Saudi Arabia, Australia, UAE, Caribbean Island, Ireland, and South Africa (NOIPolls, 2017; Fosco, 2018; Abang, 2019). About 90% of the physicians surveyed indicated they have plans to seek job opportunities abroad, while the nation's worsening health sector grapples with industrial strikes (NOIPolls, 2017).

Nigeria spends between $1 and $1.5 billion annually on medical tourism to India, Egypt, Dubai, and the United Kingdom for cardiology, orthopedics, neurology, cosmetic and renal transplant surgeries, including cancer and renal dialysis care (Ajimotokan, 2019; Onyenucheya, 2018; Basiru et al., 2018; NOIPolls, 2017; Okafor, 2017; Makinde, 2016; VOA, 2019; Punch, 2016; International Medical Travel Journal, 2014; Ajobe et al., 2013). In 2005, the wife of a Nigerian president died in Spain after undergoing cosmetic surgery. President Buhari traveled to the United Kingdom in June 2016 to treat "a persistent ear infection." This situation is an embarrassment for a country with a national ear hospital and over 250 otolaryngologists (Makinde, 2016). The exorbitant cost associated with medical tourism is another waste that could be better harnessed to develop the health-care system.

The House of Representatives failed in 2019 to approve a bill seeking to restrict public officials from taking foreign medical trips at public expense. They shame-lessly argued the proposed law discriminated against their human rights and pun-ished them for the government's failure to develop the healthcare system (Adelakun, 2020). Sadly, nothing has changed; the elites still have their focus on foreign medi-cal trips. The broken political system will require more than the clarity and sensibil-ity that the coronavirus disease 2019 (COVID-19) pandemic revealed to the Nigerian leaders that the healthcare system is long overdue for an overhaul. There is a press-ing need to institute a different set of morality and ethics that will promote good governance, clamp down on corruption, and discourage citizens' penchant taste for foreign goods.

Vulnerability #4: Paltry Health Systems Financing

As discussed in Chap. 2 of this publication, the mechanism for funding health care is a critical determinant for reaching UHC. Only through robust funding of the health sector by the national government will UHC be a reality. Health care in Nigeria is financed through different sources, including but not limited to tax reve-nue, self-out-of-pocket payments (OOPs), donor funding, and social and commu-nity health insurance programs (Uzochukwu and associates (2015). The NHIS officially launched in 2005 by President Olusegun Obasanjo's administration was designed to provide financial risk protection and reduce the high burden of OOP expenditure by individuals and households. The program created social health insurance for public sector employees, including careers of community-based health insurance, private health insurance, and voluntary health insurance. The overarch-ing goal of NHIS is to provide access to quality health care for all Nigerians and achieve UHC. Sadly, 15 years later, these goals remain a pipe dream. OOP spending constitutes nearly 90% of the total private health spending, placing a significant burden on households. About 60% of all health spending is financed directly by families without insurance. The uneven distribution of resources has affected health-care financing, particularly OOP expenditure Daily Trust (2017).

Despite the launching of the NHIS, over 95% of Nigerians currently have no insurance needed to provide access to health care (Awosusi et al., 2015; Ifijeh, 2015; NOIPolls, 2017; Amu et al., 2018; Aregbeshola and Khan, 2018). The low enroll-ment in the NHIS is due to the population's peculiar demographics. About 48% of Nigerians live in rural areas and 52% in urban areas (Worldometer, 2020). Private vendors provide about 70% of health care, and the government offers only 30%, and over 70% of the drugs dispensed are substandard (Welcome, 2011).

The revenue for financing health care is collected from pooled (budget alloca-tion, direct and indirect taxation, and donor funding) and unpooled sources; both contribute over 70% of total health expenditure. The unpooled sources include OOP payments (informal or formal direct payments to HCPs following service provision) and payments for goods (medical products such as bednets or condoms). Despite these health-financing options, spending is still disproportionately distributed across the health system, with regional inequity in healthcare expenditure (Uzochukwu et al., 2015). The persistent and significant weakness of the Nigerian health financ-ing system's functioning is due to the low public spending, very high levels in out-of-pocket expenditures (one of the highest in the world), and impoverishment due to healthcare costs and increased incidence of catastrophic health spending. Different efforts are explored to increase public funding of health alongside other options such as public-private partnerships and international development assis-tance at all levels of government.

Empirical evidence from other nations worldwide suggests that it is challenging to achieve UHC from contributory insurance schemes, particularly with a large informal sector economy like Nigeria (Aregbeshola, 2018). The challenges to expanding health insurance coverage in Nigeria include convincing state govern-ments to buy into the national health insurance scheme and the shortage of HCPs to meet the anticipated increased demand. Private voluntary health insurance has shown a low potential to expand coverage, decentralizing health insurance to the states, and community-based health insurance has limited potential to extend access to the impoverished, vulnerable, and informal sector populations (Okebukola & Brieger, 2016).

To accelerate progress towards achieving UHC in Nigeria, Aregbeshola (2018) recommended a tax-based, noncontributory, universal health-financing system as the primary funding mechanism supplemented by social health insurance and its decentralization to states for formal sector employees and private voluntary health insurance should cover wealthy individuals. On the other hand, Ejughcmre (2013) proposed that the Nigerian government must bolster NHIS revenue by leveraging private resources and promoting innovations and expertise.

Odeyemi and Nixon (2013) compared Nigeria and Ghana's health and economic indicators after a decade (2000–2010) of initiation of the NHIS program. In 2010, healthcare expenditure in both countries was about 5% of the GDP, but public spending was 38% of Nigeria's total expenditure and 60% in Ghana. Over the 10 years, the private OOP expense in Ghana fell from 80% to 66% of total expendi-ture but remained at over 90% in Nigeria. The NHIS coverage in Nigeria was a dismal 3.5% in Nigeria and over 65% in Ghana. Nigeria's health insurance package has variable benefits options depending on the membership category, while Ghana has the same benefits across all beneficiaries.

A constant feature of Nigeria's budget is the inadequate funding of health care by successive governments since independence. Since 1995, healthcare expenditure in Nigeria recorded the highest value of 9.2% in 2007 and the lowest at 3.7% in 2002.

In the last decade, spending rose from 3.9% in 2010 to 6% by 2012. Unfortunately, the health budget decreased in 2013 to 4.0%, only 2.6% in 2014, 3.7% in 2016, 4.2% in 2017, and declined again to 3.9% in 2018 (The World Bank, 2021).

On April 27, 2001, African leaders held a meeting at Abuja, where they pledged to devote at least 15% of their annual budget to health care (The Abuja declaration, 2011). For 19 consecutive years after the pledge, Nigeria is yet to allocate 15% of its budget to health. As of 2011, only four African countries (Zambia, Malawi, Liberia, and Rwanda) met the pledge, but in 2017, only Sierra Leone (15.10) and Liberia (15.50) met the benchmark (Fig. 5.2).

The health expenditure (as a share of GDP) in Nigeria is only 3.9% in 2018 and when compared to the United States (17.90%), Netherlands (12.40%), Lesotho (11.60%), Germany (11.30%), United Kingdom (9.40%), and Cuba (11.70%) is insignificant (Central Intelligence Agency World Fact Book, 2021). Compared to

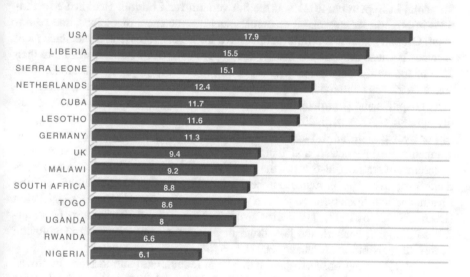

Fig. 5.2 Health expenditure (as a share of GDP in 2017) of selected countries around the world. (Source: CIA, 2021)

Table 5.5 Nigeria's healthcare expenditure in 2016 (as a percentage of GDP), vis-à-vis selected African countries

Country	Health expenditure (% of GDP)	Ranking (53/55 African States)
Angola	3.3	51
Ethiopia	4.9	36
Nigeria	3.7	45
South Sudan	2.7	53

Source: USAID, 2017

other African countries (Table 5.5), the 2016 health spending for Nigeria (3.7%) lagged behind Ethiopia at 4.9% and barely higher than Angola at 3.3%, and South Sudan at 2.7% (United States Agency for International Development – USAID, 2017).

Vulnerability #5: Limited Access to Essential Medicines and Vaccines

The WHO every two years publishes a model list of essential medicines as a guide for countries to adopt or adapt following local priorities and treatment guidelines (WHO (2021). The first list for adults was released in 1977, and the first list for children was published in 2007. WHO updated the 22nd Essential Medicines List for adults in September 2021 and the 8th version for Children Healthcare institutions in Nigeria lack essential resources, such as vaccines, medicines, and equipment. Globally, about 2 billion people have no access to essential medicines and vaccines because they are too costly, unacceptable, or of low quality for more than 25% of the world population (Ozawa et al., 2019). One in every ten medications sold in Africa is adulterated. The problem is particularly rife in Nigeria, where primary hospitals and pharmacy outlets purchase their medicines at unsafe open-chain drug markets (AXA.com, 2019).

For over two decades, Nigeria has struggled without adequate infrastructure to eliminate the production and distribution of counterfeit drugs. The successive Nigerian government also lacks the political will to enforce legislation and standards properly. The growing numbers of deaths prompted the public and the Pharmaceutical Society of Nigeria to pressure the government to enact legislation (Decree No. 21 of 1998). The decree prohibited the sale and distribution of counterfeit, adulterated, banned, and fake drugs or poisons in open markets and without a license of registration (Adebayo, 2017).

Counterfeit drugs pose substantial threats to reducing infant mortality, improved maternal health, and combating HIV/AIDS, malaria, and other diseases. Adulterated drug proliferation causes treatment failures, organ dysfunction or damage, worsening chronic disease conditions, and many deaths (Adebayo, 2017). Fake drugs are the most lucrative counterfeit business, with a global market worth roughly $200bn. Africa accounts for around 42% of the world's cases. In Nigeria, fake malaria medication accounts for 12,300 deaths annually and $893 m in costs (Millar, 2020).

To address the counterfeit menace, Medsafe, a Nigerian health tech company, developed a platform that allows pharmacies to manage their medication needs by linking manufacturers directly to hospitals and pharmacies. The platform ensures that any drugs procured are safe and cost-effective. Additionally, RxAll and TrueSpec Africa developed AI-powered scanners to determine the legitimacy of drugs. The scanned information is linked to a database that quickly determines whether or not it is genuine. Another mobile scanner (FD Detector) was developed by an entrepreneurial team of Nigerian teenage girls to uncover fake drugs at the point of purchase (Millar, 2020). Technological innovations from private enterprises will continue to make a real difference in the fight against counterfeit drugs.

Globally, over 10 million children under 5 years die – 24% of the fatalities are due to vaccine-preventable diseases. Nigeria is one of the low-income nations faced with the "double burden" of the high prevalence of infectious diseases and the rising prevalence of noncommunicable diseases. Immunization rates in Nigeria are among the lowest in the world. In Northern Nigeria, barely 10% of children receive all of their routine vaccines. Similarly, the vaccine uptake against tetanus is equally low among women (Ophori et al., 2014).

Vaccination or immunization, the administration of antigenic materials to produce immunity to a disease, is arguably the essential public health strategy against the six killer diseases of childhood – measles, pertussis, diphtheria, tetanus, tuberculosis, and poliomyelitis.

Vaccination is used for a clearly defined target group and does not require any significant lifestyle change. It relieves the healthcare system's strain and the money saved for other critical healthcare services (WHO, 2019). Immunization, the process by which a person becomes protected against disease, is one of the most cost-effective health investment strategies accessible to control and eliminate life-threatening infectious diseases, a primary cause of suffering, disability, and death in hard-to-reach and vulnerable populations. The immunization schedule in Nigeria is as follows:

- At birth: OPV0, HBV1, BCG
- 6 weeks postpartum: OPV1, DPT1, HBV2
- 10 weeks old: OPV2, DPT2
- 14 weeks old: OPV3, DPT3, HBV3
- 9 months old: Measles, Yellow fever, Vitamin A1
- 15 months old: Vitamin A2

- In pregnant women, the immunization schedule is:
- TT1 at first contact, no protection
- TT2 4 weeks later; 80% protection for 3 years
- TT3 6 months later; 95% protection for 5 years
- TT4 one year later or in the subsequent pregnancy 99% protection for 10 years
- TT5 one year later or in subsequent pregnancy 99% protection for life.

Globally, about 2 billion people have no access to essential medicines and vaccines because they are too costly, unacceptable, or of low quality for more than 25% of the world population (Ozawa et al., 2019). The poor health outcome indices in the country are attributed, in part, to the low immunization rate against the six killer diseases and the limited annual screening for the major diseases. Healthcare institutions in Nigeria lack essential resources, such as a vaccine, medicine, and equipment. A nationwide program on immunization introduced from 1979 to 1997, called Expanded Program on Immunization, was created to control the occurrence of all vaccine-preventable diseases by vaccination of children below 11 months, pregnant women, and women of reproducing age. The immunization prevents and eradicates measles, diphtheria, pertussis, neonatal tetanus, yellow fever, cerebrospinal meningitis, poliomyelitis, and tuberculosis.

In the last two decades, effective vaccines against pneumonia, another childhood killer, have become available. The benefits of pneumococcal and *Haemophilus influenzae* type b vaccines have been demonstrated in studies from different parts of the world, including Nigeria. Unfortunately, an effective vaccine for malaria and HIV infection is still elusive. Fortunately, several effective COVID-19 vaccines are now widely available in high-income countries, but it will take some time for them to be widely available in Nigeria.

It is now known that some vaccines are less effective in developing countries than in the industrialized world. When clinical trials are undertaken, such efforts come years after the vaccine is licensed in the industrialized world. Thus, clinical trials of vaccines in Nigeria are inescapably needed because it is not a priority of the pharmaceutical companies in high-income nations (Abdulkarim et al., 2011).

After three consecutive years without a poliovirus case, Nigeria was declared free of the disease by the WHO in 2019. This development was a heartening milestone watched with cautious optimism. Some northern states banned vaccination in 2003. In 2012, the country accounted for more than 50% of all polio cases worldwide and nearly derailed the global drive to eradicate the disease in the country. The WHO monitors the situation to ensure a robust surveillance system to track the wild poliovirus (Mackenzie, 2019). As of May 2021, Nigerian response to the COVID-19 pandemic has been lackluster, with a poorly coordinated national strategy to curtail the virus's spread.

In 2020, the Nigerian government committed more resources to prevent vaccine-preventable diseases through immunization efforts. Of the nearly N91 billion capital budget, the FMH allocated N44.5 billion for the Basic Health Care Provision Fund, and the remaining N46.5 billion was allocated for other activities. Specifically, N22.73 billion was budgeted for the Global Alliance for Vaccines and Immunizations, N4.8 billion for polio eradication initiatives, and N815 million for procurement of non-polio supplementary immunization activities vaccine, and N4 billion for procurement of vaccines and devices (Adepoju, 2020).

Within the ambit of the COVID-19 preparedness and response project, the Nigerian government, on September 30, 2021, received a $400 million loan to provide financing for safe and effective COVID-19 vaccine acquisition and deployment within the country, with the primary goals to break the chain of local transmission and limit the spread of the virus. The loan will enable President Buhari's government to meet the pronouncement to vaccinate 51% of the population in two years (The World Bank. (2021). As of November 22, 2021, seven different types of COVID-19 vaccines from various countries around the world are available in Nigeria - Moderna (mRNA-1273), Pfizer/BioNTech (BNT162b2), Gamaleya (Sputnik V), Janssen (Johnson & Johnson - Ad26.COV2.S), Oxford/AstraZeneca (AZD1222), Serum Institute of India (Covishield (Oxford/AstraZeneca formulation), Sinopharm (Beijing - BBIBP-CorV (Vero Cells). None of the vaccines is undergoing clinical trials in the country (McGill COVID19 Vaccine Tracker Team (2021).

The percentage of the total population that has been fully vaccinated against COVID-19 varies widely around the world. As of November 20, 2021, 53.5% of the world population has received at least one dose of a COVID-19 vaccine, with 28.26 million doses administered daily. About 7.78 billion doses of the vaccine have been given globally. Unfortunately, only 5.2% of people in low-income countries have received at least one dose.

In Nigeria, 9.48 million doses of COVID-19 vaccine have been administered, and only 3.4 million Nigerians (representing 1.7% of the population) are fully vaccinated as of November 22, 2021 (Google, 2021). At the same time frame, a more significant share of the population is fully vaccinated in Singapore (91.9%), United Arab Emirates (88.4%), Portugal (87.8%), Brazil (60%), United States (57.8%), Mexico (49.4%), Russia (37.1%), Indonesia (32.8%), India (29.6%), Pakistan (22%), and 20.4% in Bangladesh (Global Change Data Lab., 2021).

Vulnerability #6: Weak Health Information Systems

The health information system consists of six parts – human resources (workforce), indicators, data sources, data management, information products, and information use. The FMH launched the National Health Management Information System (NHMIS) in the 1960s to coordinate the nation's medical statistics information for human resources, hospital activities, mortality, morbidity, birth, and death data in hospitals. National policy was introduced in 2006 and revised in 2014, but the health information system remains weak and unable to fulfill its mandate because of underinvestment in health. The health information system evolved in a haphazard and fragmented fashion due to organizational weaknesses. The unplanned reporting demands resulted in the distortion of the nation's health information system, with many programs and institutions operating multiple parallel systems (FMH, 2014).

Today, the nation's NHMIS focuses more on routine health data at the expense of other essential components and faces a myriad of challenges, including lack of funding, staff shortage, limited resources, inadequate coordination of data flow, complexity, and overlap of data collection instruments, lack of feedback to peripheral levels, and a massive backlog of unprocessed data (Abubakar, n.d.). The data collection process is fragmented, inconsistent, and the medical record in most Nigerian hospitals are still manually processed and not computerized (Fig. 5.3). The health information system in the country is disease-focused because of the requirements of foreign donor organizations and their specific reporting obligations towards diseases such as HIV/AIDS, malaria, and TB.

Evaluations of the Nigerian health information system by Meribole and associates in 2018 identified weak governance and ineffective leadership, turf wars, ambiguities of roles and responsibilities, limited financial incentives, and poor technical skills as the major challenges facing the system. The absence of interagency coordination and collaboration produced silos and inefficiency with the NHMIS. The system has not effectively leveraged the growing information and communications

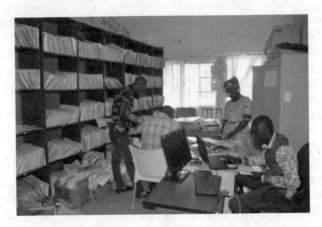

Fig. 5.3 Patients' medical records in most Nigerian hospitals are still not computerized. (Photograph used with permission from UNIMED PRO)

technology penetration in the country and explores opportunities for standardization and intersystem operation planning.

Kiri and Ojule (2020) analyzed 76 available publications from sub-Saharan African countries that implemented NHIS to identify the program's challenges. Only a few of the studies addressed the critical obstacles to effective implementation, management, and sustenance in the various countries where acts of forgery, counterfeiting, and other forms of fraud are rampant. The authors described the potential role of using electronic medical record systems (EMRS) in low technology-resourced countries. They discussed how EMRS could mitigate the challenges posed by most of the peculiar problems associated with poor infrastructure.

Like their counterparts in the developing world, clinicians in Nigeria are now using telehealth to deliver healthcare services and medical education with positive outcomes (Akinleye et al., 2020). This practice is particularly beneficial in the COVID-19 era, where social distancing is a critical element of preventative measures to lower infection risk.

Research productivity and timely dissemination are yardsticks for measuring the level of innovation within a health system. Health research is a global endeavor, and investigators increasingly recognize that their research efforts are enhanced by collaborating with colleagues in other multiple centers and countries and engaging in joint training of HCPs. Unfortunately, the research outputs from sub-Saharan Africa have not matched those from different parts of the world. A study by the World Bank in 2014 revealed that although Africa constitutes 16% of the world's population, it produces only 1% of the global research outputs, with only 198 researchers/1 million people in Africa, compared to 455 in Chile and 4500 in the United States and the United Kingdom (World Bank, 2014)

It is estimated that sub-Saharan Africa will require an additional 1 million PhDs, especially those qualified to conduct cutting-edge research if the continent is to meet up to half of the research momentum currently going on in the Western countries. The study also found that all African countries produce about 27,000 research publications annually, equivalent to the total number of papers generated in a small country such as the Netherlands. Three nations (Egypt, Nigeria, and South Africa) account for these publications in Africa. Most research publications in Africa now emanate from South Africa, Egypt, Nigeria, Algeria, Kenya, Morocco, and Tunisia, with South Africa as the most research productive country on the continent (World Bank, 2014)

As the most populous country on the Africa continent, with the highest number of universities, Nigeria's research productivity is below par and unacceptable. In the 1970s, Nigerian universities and teaching hospitals surpassed other African nations in terms of quality, human and fiscal resources, and research productivity. With the increased number of universities, specialist hospitals, and medical research centers, this is no longer the case. The universities can turn around the declining academic standards by focusing on research activities that address local developmental challenges that improve citizens' quality of life. Unfortunately, in some universities, many senior academics are promoted to professorial rank with low research output. Such professors are not able to train graduates who can conduct meaningful and impactful research in their discipline. University administrators should prod the government to fund ongoing capacity-building workshops and seminars in research methodology and biostatistics to address the problem.

Major Achievements and Contributions of Nigeria to Global Health

Despite the multitudes of challenges within the Nigerian health system, it is not all doom and gloom. There are several areas that the system has contributed meaningfully to global health. One of the best-kept secrets is the contribution of Nigeria to the evolution of primary care education. Before they became a common practice in other parts of the world, the Faculty of Health Sciences at Obafemi Awolowo University, Ile-Ife, in 1972, pioneered medical curriculum with an emphasis on primary health care.

The faculty adopted a Bachelor of Science degree as the entry requirement for the clinical year of its medical and dentistry curricula. Further, Ife jettisoned the artificial division created between preventive and curative medicine and questioned the rationale for laying undue emphasis on hospital development at the expense of rural health services, dispensaries, and maternity centers. This curricula innovation and other evolutionary and emerging developments in healthcare education in the country were the centerpieces of a recent book published by this author (Balogun, 2020a). The remaining section of this chapter presents Nigeria's shinning contributions to primary health care, itinerant/community-based physiotherapy services, effective containment of the spread of the Ebola virus, and the primary medical and surgical discoveries in the country.

Genesis of Primary Health Care and Itinerant/ Community-Based Physiotherapy Systems

Post-independence, in 1960, Nigeria's healthcare services focused primarily on curative care at the expense of preventing illnesses. However, 15 years later, the National Basic Health Services Scheme was developed to provide primary health care, offer medical training, and build health facilities, but neglected investment in new technology and community participation (Alenoghena et al., 2014). Unfortunately, the scheme remained a brilliant idea that never took off the ground until 1985 when Olikoye Ransome-Kuti, professor of pediatrics at the College of Medicine, University of Lagos, was appointed the health minister. During his seven years' tenure, from 1985 to 1992, he developed a national health policy that emphasized primary health care and the importance of disease prevention. He relocated the responsibility for primary health care to the local governments by encouraging vaccination and free immunization for children, among other things, launched a nationwide campaign against HIV/AIDS. In 1993, following a military coup, Professor Ransome-Kuti was removed as Minister of Health. His tenure is often described as the era of effective and innovative primary health care in Nigeria.

The emergence and global interest in primary health care occurred during the late 1970s and early 1980s (Marcos Cueto, 2004). The primary healthcare concept was globally adopted in the declaration at the International Conference on Primary Health Care held in Alma Ata, Kazakhstan, in 1978 (known as the "Alma Ata Declaration"). The Alma-Ata Conference declaration became a core concept of the WHO's Health For All (WHO, 2016). The statement triggered global interest in primary health care among HCPs and institutions, governments, civil society organizations, researchers, and grassroots organizations dedicated to solving the inequalities in health worldwide. China, barefoot doctors inspired the Alma-Ata Conference declaration (Marcos, Cueto, 2004; Bulletin of the WHO, 2008).

During the early 1970s, physiotherapy services were confined to the four walls of the hospitals, and physiotherapists were not considered to have a stake in disease prevention. In 1973, Chief Christopher Ajao conceived itinerant and community-based physiotherapy practice to bring physiotherapy services to rural areas. This development was before WHO initiated the concept of community-based rehabilitation in 1978. Chief Ajao collaborated with the Canadian University Services Overseas (CUSO), through the Canadian Embassy in Lagos, to recruit physiotherapists to bring into friction his idea. The international nongovernment development organization (CUSO) recruits qualified Canadians to work for two years as volunteers in developing countries (Benning, 1969; Stuart, 2012). Under this partnership, with CUSO, several Canadian physiotherapists were deployed annually to Oyo state to serve in the rural areas. Before his political appointment, in 1974, Chief Ajao introduced the concept of itinerant and community physiotherapy programs-that he conceived in 1973. He implemented it throughout the entire Oyo state by bringing physiotherapy services to the doorstep of the disenfranchised and those with disabilities. To implement the plan, he deployed the Canadian-and Nigerian-trained physiotherapists to work in rural communities. This move was a departure from having physiotherapists work only at Adeoyo Hospital in Ibadan, the state capital. In addition to working in their primary domicile community, the physiotherapists assigned to the program drove government vehicles from their domicile station to the rural areas to provide physiotherapy services and return to their base at the end of the workday. Chief Ajao's ingenuity displayed to the world Nigeria's contribution to innovative thinking in healthcare delivery. The itinerant and community physiotherapy programs that he conceptualized are now standard practice across the globe.

A retrospective study conducted in 1988 by Abereoje evaluated the impact of the itinerant and community-based physiotherapy programs implemented in the rural communities of Oyo state. The finding revealed that both itinerant and community physiotherapy schemes made physiotherapy services accessible to rural dwellers. The community physiotherapy scheme served more patients and effectively met the rural population's healthcare needs than the itinerant physiotherapy scheme. However, the study found no statistically significant difference (p > 0.05) in the treatment duration for both systems (Abereoje, 1988).

Community Health Workers

The advent of community health workers in Nigeria became imperative in the 1970s because all attempts to persuade physicians/dentists to work in the rural areas failed. It failed because the medical education offered in the Nigerian pioneer universities (Ibadan and Lagos), except for the University of Ife (now Obafemi Awolowo University), did not equip the physicians/dentists with the skills needed to work in the community setting. Secondly, the lack of basic amenities, such as water, electricity, and schools in the rural areas made working there unattractive to many physicians/dentists. The curriculum of nurses/midwives, like physicians/dentists, did not also adequately prepare them to deliver primary health services. Thus, most Nigerian nurses/midwives during that era prefer to work in a hospital setting.

Because of the challenges mentioned above, the Minister of Health, Professor Ransome-Kuti, introduced a new cadre of primary HCPs in 1978 to serve rural areas. Community health practitioners comprise of Community Health Officers, Community Health Supervisors (which training was stopped in 1990), and Community Health Assistants (now Community Health Extension Workers (CHEWs), and Community Health Aides (now Junior Community Health Extension Workers (JCHEWs). The CHEWs remained the core occupation in the Nigerian primary healthcare system (Ibama et al., 2015).

A quasi-experimental study by Uzondu and associates in 2011 evaluated the benefits of the CHEWs in the provision of essential maternal, newborn, and child health services in Jigawa state. The CHEWs are explicitly trained to provide health care for mothers and their babies. They educate women on the tenets of safe pregnancies, the importance of prenatal and postnatal care, how to access healthcare resources, and how to deliver healthy babies. They live in the same neighborhoods as their patients and connect them with HCPs. The study's findings revealed the training of CHEWs in Jigawa state improved access to health care, and the number of women who received prenatal care doubled. With transportation problems resolved, visits to health clinics increased dramatically to 500% through an organized taxi driver's network. Clinic attendance also surged from 1.5 visits to 8 for each month per 100 people.

Furthermore, in just one year, women giving birth in health centers doubled, and those receiving prenatal care increased from 6% to 21%. More importantly, the health outcomes were sustained during the two subsequent years. This unique healthcare delivery by CHEWs is Nigeria's innovative contribution to the world healthcare system (Uzondu et al., 2015). The following factors possess significant challenges for Nigerian CHEWs in meeting their critical roles in the health system:

1. The CHEWs are in short supply, and the available workforce is distributed unevenly across the country. Although the rural communities where CHEWs serve constitute about 70% of the Nigerian population, the primary healthcare facilities' distribution is predominately in the urban areas. Thus, coverage and the attainment of the Sustainable National Development goal are unrealistic.
2. Most primary healthcare facilities are in a state of disrepair. With equipment and infrastructure either absent or obsolete, the referral system is almost nonexistent, nonfunctional, or facing severe criticism and rejection by the higher-level care providers.
3. Successive governments in the country showed weak political will to provide human capacity building, physical resources, and infrastructure.
4. Reaching rural communities poses a major logistical challenge due to poor roads. Thus, it is challenging to provide functional health facilities to all communities.
5. Most CHEWs and policymakers have limited knowledge of disease prevention and primary care, resulting in poor quality healthcare services.
6. Inadequate education with a limited retraining program commensurate with the roles and responsibilities of the CHEWs. Limited sponsorship for in-service training and continuing professional education is needed for proficiency and enhancement of clinical skills.
7. The poor condition of service and remuneration dampens the zeal to render critical roles towards National Development: Payment of salary and promotion are not regular.

All of these factors affect CHEW morale and engendered care and national development (Solomon-Ibama & Dennis, 2016).

A significant health systems reform introduced in 2007 by President Obasanjo's administration is the community-based health insurance scheme. The program profoundly changed the processes of healthcare delivery at several hospitals and clinics around the country. A case in point is the development of the "Green Hospital Energy" at Obio Cottage Hospital, owned by the Shell Petroleum Development Company of Nigeria. The community-based project reduced the cost of power utilization in the hospital from $300–$1500/month to $180–$500/month and increased facility utilization to 340 patients/day. Other positive outcomes were a 51% decrease in patient transit time from 3.8 h to 1.7 h, a 53% decline in the process steps from 72 to 35, and a reduction in specimen processing from 2 h 25 min to 13 min for the introduction of the aired oven.

Furthermore, the program reduced the registration time and manual handling of client records with an electronic and authentication system for tracking enrolment and financial resources, thus leading to improved quality of care. Remote healthcare delivery using modern technology saved lives and decreased care costs for patients diagnosed through video and audio reports. The transformative program improved the patients' satisfaction and increased the demand for healthcare services in the facility (Fajola et al., 2007).

Another health systems restructuring introduced in 2015 is mobile technology in preventing chronic diseases, maternal care, and the management of Ebola and malaria epidemics. The innovative program improved medical systems' efficacy through improved patient tracking and reporting, including critically needed health services to underserved communities. The increased use of mobile technology strengthened clinicians' capacity and improved the delivery of maternal and child health services. The program brought the much-needed medical expertise to front-line HCPs by systematizing the collection of patient information, tracking the spread of epidemics, and enhanced the diagnosis and treatment provided (Rosenberg et al., 2015).

A significant contemporary development in the healthcare system was removing the bottlenecks associated with access to quality health care. Patients in Asaba can now call their physician and get consultations online through video or audio systems. The new technology called "complete care" allows patients to consult with their physicians/dentists, make payments, and book appointments for follow-up visits. The technology has a unique capability that enables patients to schedule home visit appointment with their healthcare providers (Oladapo, 2018).

Medical and Surgical Discoveries

In 1972, Professor Fabian Udekwu and Professor Yakoub (an Egyptian and British citizen) at the University of Nigeria Teaching Hospital (UNTH) Enugu scheduled a patient for the cardiopulmonary bypass pump surgery, thinking he had an aortic, pulmonary window – a pathology that rightly deserved open-heart surgery. However, they later found out that the patient had ductus arteriosus, which they repaired, but the patient does not require open-heart surgery (Grillo and Adeloye, 2009). The first open-heart surgery in the country, performed with foreign partners' assistance, took place at UNTH on February 1, 1974. In recognition of this feat and other cardiac surgical operations that followed, the federal government in 1984 designated UNTH the National Cardiothoracic Center of Excellence (Nwafor et al., 2017).

The University of Ibadan College of Medicine and its affiliated University College Hospital (UCH) is Nigeria's oldest university and center of excellence for training HCPs, and medical research in West Africa. By 1976, Professor Samuel Adetola Adebonojo and Professor Ayodele Falase at UCH successfully performed the first implantation of a permanent transvenous cardiac pacemaker in Nigeria. The procedure is now performed routinely at UCH Ibadan and other university teaching hospitals. Both Professors Fabian Udekwu and Isaac Grillo pioneered open-heart surgery in the country. Professor Udekwu and his surgical team, assisted by the International College of Surgeons, were the first to insert a cardiopulmonary bypass pump in Nigeria (Grillo and Adeloye, 2009).

In 1978, the first indigenous team of surgeons at UCH performed open-heart surgery without a foreign professional's assistance or presence. The surgical team led by Isaac Adetayo Grillo, and Samuel Adetola Adebonojo, Olu Osinowo, and 'Wole Adebo was assisted by two anesthesiologists, Dr. O. Akinyemi and Dr. C.E. Famewo; a cardiologist, Dr. O. Falase; a cardiopulmonary pump technician, Mr. S.O. Osanyintuyi and an operating room (theatre) scrub nurse, Mrs. Omotosho. In preparing for the surgery, the surgical team collaborated with veterinary surgeons in the Faculty of Veterinary Medicine and Surgery at Ibadan (Professor Adelola Adeloye and Dr. Layo Idowu) to perfect their surgical techniques by operating on six dogs. Subsequently, Professor Grillo and his team performed five more open-heart surgeries. Three of the six patients had long-term survivals. One of the patients died on the table due to disseminated intravascular clotting. Another patient died on the ward when walking a month post-surgery. The autopsy showed ventricular septal defect Dacron patch blowout due to infection. The sixth patient died on the table due to the low left ventricular muscle wall remnant to support circulation. Unfortunately, there was no intra-aortic balloon available to use for temporary support of circulation. The UCH program died a natural death due to exhaustion and dwindling support from the hospital workforce and concerns relating to the high cost of the operation and the prolonged time spent on postoperative care (Grillo and Adeloye, 2009).

Subsequently, the fortunes of the UCH workforce plummeted after the nation's oil boom was mismanaged, leading to economic doom. Many surgeons and academicians faced hardship in paying their real estate loans due to bank interest rates, which skyrocketed from 6% to 23%. This development caused Isaac Grillo, Samuel Adebonojo, Olu Osinowo, and many other academicians and professionals to migrate to Saudi Arabia, Kuwait, and the other Gulf States for employment, leaving the nation's hospitals and universities in shambles.

Between 1974 and 1981, the National Cardiothoracic Center of Excellence at UNTH completed 46 cardiac operations cases in children ranging from 6 months to 16 years. Twenty-five of the 46 patients were operated on for congenital heart defects, and 21 were operated on for acquired heart disease. During the same period from 1978 to 1983, the UCH performed six open-heart surgeries. By the year 2000, UNTH and UCH performed 102 cases of open-heart and 48 cases of closed-heart surgeries (Nwafor et al., 2017). As of December 2011, the direct cost of open-heart surgery in Nigeria ranges from $6230 to $11,200. This price remains competitive with other developing countries such as India, Egypt, and South Africa (Falase et al., 2013).

Despite the limited resources and the multiple challenges in the health sector, several significant accomplishments occurred in the university teaching hospitals across the country. For instance, in 2016, surgeons at Lagos State University Teaching Hospital successfully performed their first bone bridge surgery and cochlear implant surgery without any foreign expatriate's inputs. A team of urologists and nephrologists at the hospital also completed its first kidney transplant, and the patient was discharged from the hospital in good condition. Similarly, surgeons at Obafemi Awolowo University Teaching Hospital Complex, Ile-Ife, successfully performed open-heart surgery on six children, aged 1–5 years, in collaboration with foreign professionals (Alao and Omofoye, 2016).

In the same year, in 2016, surgeons at the Abubakar Tafawa Balewa Teaching Hospital in Bauchi led by Professor Haruna Liman successfully performed an innovative bladder surgery (neobladder reconstruction) for an 18-year-old cancer patient with a 5-year history of passing blood in his urine and later diagnosed with malignant cells in his bladder tissues. The surgical procedure controlled the tumor from spreading and increasing the patient's chance of survival and quality of life (Oputah, 2016).

In 2017, surgeons at the University of Benin Teaching Hospital, through a partnership with the University of Basel, Switzerland, treated patients with sickle cell anemia. They completely removing the sickled red blood cells through one arm and replace them with un-sickled healthy blood cells through the other limb at the same time. Following the treatment, the pain and crisis associated with the disease decreased substantially, and the procedure was repeated twice a year with minimal cost. With enough donors, the patients only pay for the blood used. This development is significant since Nigeria has the highest number of sickle cell carriers globally, with about 3% of the population suffering from the disease (Bazuaye, 2017).

In the same year, cardiovascular education recorded a significant feat as two female consultant cardiologists—Dr. Ifeoluwa Adewoye and Dr. Mirabel Nwosu—made history on March 21, 2017, solely performed cardiac catheterization, under the mentorship of Professor Kamar Adeleke at Babcock University Teaching Hospital. The 1-year intensive training is considered "remarkable" because it takes cardiologist trainees in developed countries at least 3 years of experience in the catheterization laboratory and 300 assisted procedures before they are allowed to perform it independently. It costs over $100,000 for a resident to receive cardiac catheterization training in the United States. The training of the two women cardiologists is significant because only four male cardiovascular interventionists were practicing in the country at the time, all of whom trained in the United States and Canada (Adeleke, 2017).

How Nigeria Effectively Contained the Spread of Ebola

In 2012, swine flu (H1N1) spread to Lagos, and Dr. Ameyo Stella Adadevoh was the first physician to diagnose and alert the Ministry of Health. Less than 2 years later, she was again the primary physician to identify another contagious virus – Ebola. On July 20, 2014, Nigeria experienced an outbreak of Ebola virus disease (EVD) with the arrival of an infected airline traveler exposed to EVD in Liberia before he flew to Lagos to participate in the Economic Community of West African States conference. On arrival at the Murtala Mohammed International Airport, he collapsed and was taken to a private hospital—First Consultants Medical Centre—because the physicians/dentists employed at all government hospitals in the country were on an indefinite strike. Dr. Adadevoh was the physician on duty at the private hospital when the patient arrived on July 20, 2014. He was treated by the medical staff and nurses at the hospital but died 5 days later, on July 25, 2014.

Dr. Adadevoh worked for 21 years at the private hospital as a consultant physician and endocrinologist but had never seen a patient with EVD before. Still, she correctly diagnosed her first patient when she was threatened by Liberian officials who wanted the patient to be discharged to attend the Economic Countries of West African States conference. Dr. Adadevoh stood her ground and insisted that she would not release him for the greater public good. Her keen perception, courage, and steadfastness prevented a significant outbreak of EVD in Nigeria.

At the time, the health system was ill-prepared for an Ebola outbreak, and three of her colleagues who treated the indexed patient contracted the disease and died. Although the FMH responded to the Ebola outbreak rapidly, 19 additional EVD cases were reported in Lagos and Port Harcourt. The rapid response instituted by the FMH curtailed the epidemic within 3 months. The WHO declared Nigeria EVD-free on October 20, 2014, after no new cases were observed for 42 days (WHO, 2014). The FMH traced all the 20 EVD patients in Nigeria to the first indexed patient treated by Dr. Adadevoh and her colleagues. Their heroic efforts and bravery differentiated the Ebola outbreak in Nigeria from Sierra Leone, Guinea, and Liberia, where the indexed patients were not initially promptly diagnosed. Dr. Adadevoh's sacrifice prevented a national and possibly global catastrophe (Althausa et al., 2015; Otu et al., 2017).

For over two decades, Nigeria's healthcare network rates among the worst globally. A 2018 study in the *Lancet* ranked Nigeria 142nd out of 195 countries in healthcare access and quality. However, a recent improvement in the health system is the human and physical infrastructures developed to end polio – decentralizing disease control networks. Improved vaccine storage means the health system is better equipped to fight other emerging diseases such as measles and Ebola. Among the methods developed across the country are a series of Emergency Operation Centers (EOCs) – centralized offices staffed by HCPs from different aid agencies and government health workers supervised by a national EOC in Abuja. The offices in each state are responsible for coordinating immunization programs. A group of trained health workers collects data at a local level and quickly responds to disease outbreaks without a federal response. The bureaucratic process of letter writing and visits to Abuja are no longer needed (Lopez, 2019).

The Bill and Melinda Gates Foundation, in 2012, funded the first EOCs established. Two years later, the EOC system faced its biggest test in July 2014, with the Ebola outbreak in Lagos. No doubt the systems put in place by the polio eradication program, particularly its decentralized, rapid-response structure, were responsible for this effective national response. Similarly, the polio program helped improve vaccine storage across the country. With the funding for polio eradication, there are now cold storage spots around the country that enable vaccines to be stored at an average temperature of 40F (5C), which is necessary for them to be effective (Lopez, 2019).

Recent Improvements in Health Outcomes

Infant and maternal mortality rates are improving, polio is now partially eradicated, and measles outbreaks and the prevalence of malaria, HIV, and TB are all down through nationwide immunization programs and more effective means to distribute vaccines (Oxford Business Group, 2015). Additionally, new HIV infections in Nigeria have decreased by 35% over the past 3 years due to an increased number of treatment centers offering free antiretroviral therapy from just 25 in 2001 to more than 800 by 2015. Malaria cases are also down due to the new strategies of subsidized antimalarial distribution and the provision of insecticide-treated mosquito nets to the vulnerable population (Oxford Business Group, 2015).

Professor Friday Okonofua and his research team at the Women's Health and Action Research Centre at Benin City demonstrated through an intervention study that the active involvement of hospital managers and policymakers in the implementation of the FMH Maternal and Perinatal Death Surveillance and Response project led to a seven-fold reduction in maternal mortality ratio and significant improvement in quality of care and decline in maternal mortality ratio in referral hospitals (Aikpitanyi et al., 2019).

Conclusion

The five corrupt practices affecting the standard of patient care in Nigeria include procurement-related fraud, under-the-counter payments, health financing-related crime, employment-related bribery, and unreported absenteeism from work. Despite the various reforms geared to increase health service delivery, less than 5% of Nigerians currently have health insurance coverage. Nigeria ranks seventh among other countries worldwide with a shortage of HCPs because those locally produced emigrate abroad at an alarming rate; 90% of physicians have plans to seek job opportunities outside the country, as the nation's worsening health sector grapples with HCP strikes. For 19 consecutive years after the Abuja declaration pledge, Nigeria has yet to allocate 15% of its budget to health. Thus, the country has one of the lowest ($217) health care expenditures per capita globally.

The literature review identified multiple factors responsible for the low-quality health care delivery. They include ineffective leadership, antiquated infrastructure, epileptic power supply, interprofessional conflicts, brain drain effect, absence of a centralized planning system, lack of investment in facilities and prescription drugs, and waste. Five key elements that forestall the implementation of UHC were identified. They are lack of political will and commitment by successive governments that ruled the country and poor governance, corruption, underfunded health system, high informal sector economy, extreme poverty, and the poor's inability to pay health insurance premiums.

Case Study

Watch the video, *History Brief: Daily Life in the 1930s in the United States* by typing the following web address into your browser https://www.youtube.com/watch?v=gkAfjRolNCI

After watching the video, answer the following questions:

1. How does living in the United States in the 1930s compare to daily life in Nigeria today?
2. List the top ten diseases that you think will be prevalent in the United States in the early twentieth century.
3. Compare these top ten conditions with the leading ten causes of death in the United States in 2017; see Table 5.6.
4. Discuss the reasons for the shift in the disease pattern.

Table 5.6 Leading ten causes of death in the United States in 2017

Serial #	Cause of death	Number of deaths*	Percentage of total deaths (%)
1	Heart disease	647,457	23.5
2	Cancer	599,108	21.3
3	Accidents/unintentional injuries	169,936	6
4	Chronic lower respiratory disease	160,201	5.7
5	Stroke and cerebrovascular diseases	146,383	5.2
6	Alzheimer's disease – Dementia	121,404	4.3
7	Diabetes	83,564	3
8	Influenza and pneumonia	55,672	2
9	Kidney disease	50,633	1.8
10	Suicide	47,173	

Source: * Tavella and Nichols, 2019

References

Abang, M. (2019). Nigeria's medical brain drain: Healthcare woes as doctors flee. *Al Jazeera News*. [online]. Available at: https://www.aljazeera.com/indepth/features/nigeria-medical-brain-drain-healthcare-woes-doctors-flee-190407210251424.html. Accessed 10 Feb 2020.

Abereoje, O. (1988) An evaluation of the effectiveness of itinerant and community phys-iotherapy schemes in meeting the primary health care needs in Oyo State, Nigeria. *Physiotherapy Practice* (4): 194–200. [online]. Available at: https://www.tandfonline.com/doi/abs/10.3109/09593988809160149. (Accessed: 10 October 2020).

Abubakar, A. A. (n.d.). Health management information system in Nigeria. [online]. Available at: http://www.pitt.edu/~super7/43011-44001/43561.ppt. Accessed 10 Oct 2020. The Abuja declaration. (2011) Ten years on. WHO. [online]. Available at: https://www.who.int/health-systems/publications/abuja_declaration/en/ https://www.who.int/healthsystems/publications/abuja_report_aug_2011.pdf?ua=1" (Accessed:16 October 2020).

Adebayo, A. (2017). Fake medicine in Nigeria – When the drugs don't work. *Inventa International*. [online]. Available at: https://www.lexology.com/library/detail.aspx?g=6b2f05d6-1ecd-4e72-aba7-2c86ef70a8f9. Accessed 27 May 2021.

Adegoke, Y. (2019). Does Nigeria have too many doctors to worry about a 'brain drain'? *BBC* Africa, Lagos. [online]. Available at: https://www.bbc.com/news/world-africa-45473036. Accessed 10 Feb 2020.

Abdulkarim AA, Ibrahim RM, Fawi AO, Adebayo OA, Johnson AWBR. (2011) Vaccines and immunization: *The past, present and future in Nigeria*. [online]. Available at: https://www.ajol.info/index.php/njp/article/view/72382 (Accessed: 17 November 2021).

Abdulraheem, I. S., Olapipo, A. R., & Amodu, M. O. (2012). Primary healthcare services in Nigeria: Critical issues and strategies for enhancing the use by the rural communities. *Journal of Public Health and Epidemiology, 4*(1), 5C13.

Abereoje, O. (1988). An evaluation of the effectiveness of itinerant and community phys-iotherapy schemes in meeting the primary health care needs in Oyo State, Nigeria. *Physiotherapy Practice, 4*, 194–200. [online]. Available at: https://www.tandfonline.com/doi/abs/10.3109/09593988809160149. Accessed 10 Oct 2020.

Abubakar, A. A. (n.d.). Health management information system in Nigeria. [online]. Available at: http://www.pitt.edu/~super7/43011-44001/43561.ppt. Accessed 10 Oct 2020.

Adegoke, Y. (2019, April 25). Does Nigeria have too many doctors to worry about a 'brain drain'? *BBC* Africa, Lagos. [online]. Available at: https://www.bbc.com/news/world-africa-45473036. Accessed 10 Feb 2020.

Adelakun, A. (2020, June 18). Nigerian leaders have still not learned. *Punch Newspaper*. [online]. Available at: https://groups.google.com/forum/?utm_medium=email&utm_source=footer#!msg/usaafricadialogue/2YRl2gKUQGk/yM28m4VfAAAJ. Accessed 10 Oct 2020.

Adeleke, K. (2017). *Nigerian cardiologists record breakthrough in heart surgery*. [online]. Available at:https://www.vanguardngr.com/2017/03/nigerian-cardiologists-record-breakthrough-heart-surgery/. Accessed 10 Oct 2020.

Aikpitanyi, J, Ohenhen, V, Ugbodaga, P, Ojemhen, B, Omo-Omorodion, BI, Ntoimo, LFC, Imongan, W, Balogun JA, Okonofua, FE. (2019). *Maternal death review and surveillance: The case of Central Hospital, Benin City, Nigeria. Plos One* 19; 14 (12). [online]. Available at: https://www.ncbi.nlm.nih.gov/pmc/articles/PMC6922332/. (Accessed: 16 October 2020).

Ajimotokan, O. (2019, March 21). Korea jostles for slice of Nigeria's $1B medical tourism spend-ing. *This Day*. [online]. Available at: https://www.thisdaylive.com/index.php/2019/03/21/korea-jostles-for-slice-of-nigerias-1b-medical-tourism-spending/. Accessed 10 Oct 2020.

Ajobe, A. T., Alhassan, A., Chung, S., Leonard, J., & Ahmad, R. (2013). Nigeria: How Nigerians spend billions on medical tourism. *Daily Trust*. [online]. Available at: https://allafrica.com/stories/201301071129.html. Accessed 10 Oct 2020.

Akinleye, F. E., Akinbolaji, G. R., & Olasupo, J. O. (2020). Towards universal health coverage: Lessons learnt from the COVID-19 pandemic in Africa. *The Pan African Medical Journal, 35*(Suppl 2), 128. https://doi.org/10.11604/pamj.supp.2020.35.2.24769

Alao, T., & Omofoye, T. (2016). *Lagos, Ife teaching hospitals record surgical feats*. [online]. Available at: https://guardian.ng/news/lagos-ife-teaching-hospitals-record-surgical-feats/. Accessed 10 Oct 2020.

Alenoghena, I., Aigbiremolen, A. O., Abejegah, C., & Eboreime, E. (2014). *Primary health care in Nigeria: Strategies and constraints in implementation.* [online]. Available at: https://www.ajol.info/index.php/ijcr/article/view/107665. Accessed 10 Oct 2020.

Althausa, C. L., Lowa, N., Musa, E. O., Shuaib, F., & Gsteigera, S. (2015). Ebola virus disease outbreak in Nigeria: Transmission dynamics and rapid control panel. *Epidemics, 11*, 80–84.

Amu, H., Dickson, K. S., Kumi-Kyereme, A., & Darteh, E. K. M. (2018). Understanding variations in health insurance coverage in Ghana, Kenya, Nigeria, and Tanzania: Evidence from demographic and health surveys. *PLoS One, 13*(8), e0201833. [online]. Available at: https://journals.plos.org/plosone/article?id=10.1371/journal.pone.0201833. Accessed 10 Oct 2020.

Aregbeshola, B. S. (2018). A tax-based, noncontributory, health-financing system can accelerate progress toward universal health coverage in Nigeria. *MEDICC Review, 20*(4):40–45. [online]. Available at: en (scielosp.org). Accessed 23 Dec 2020.

Aregbeshola, B. S., & Khan, S. M. (2018). Predictors of enrolment in the national health insurance scheme among women of reproductive age in Nigeria. *International Journal of Health Policy Management, 7*(11), 1015–1023. [online]. Available at: https://www.ncbi.nlm.nih.gov/pmc/articles/PMC6326643/. Accessed 10 Oct 2020.

Asakitikpi, A. E. (2019). *Healthcare coverage and affordability in Nigeria: An alternative model to equitable healthcare delivery.* [online]. Available at: https://www.intechopen.com/books/universal-health-coverage/healthcare-coverage-and-affordability-in-nigeria-an-alternative-model-to-equitable-healthcare-delive. Accessed 23 Dec 2020.

Awosusi, A., Folaranmi T., & Yates, R. (2015). *Nigeria's new government and public financing for universal health coverage.* [online]. Available at: https://www.thelancet.com/journals/langlo/article/PIIS2214-109X(15)00088-1/fulltext. Accessed 16 Oct 2020.

AXA.com. (2019, May 24). Nigeria: Laying the groundwork for safe, quality healthcare. *AXA Magazine.* [online]. Available at:https://www.axa.com/en/magazine/nigeria-laying-the-groundwork-for-safe-quality-healthcare. Accessed 16 Oct 2020.

Balogun, J. A. (2020a). *Chapter 5: The evolution of healthcare education in Nigeria. Chapter 7: Emerging paradigms in healthcare education in Nigeria in: Healthcare education in Nigeria: Evolutions and emerging paradigms.* Routledge Publication. [online]. Available at: https://www.routledge.com/9780367482091. Accessed 23 Dec 2020.

Balogun, J. A. (2020b). The path to our destiny: The transitioning of physiotherapy in Nigeria from occupation to a true profession. *Journal of the Nigeria Society of Physiotherapy, 19*(1), 19–35. [online]. Available at: https://www.researchgate.net/publication/346679736_The_path_to_our_destiny_The_transitioning_of_physiotherapy_in_Nigeria_from_occupation_to_a_true_profession. Accessed 18 Dec 2020.

Basiru, S., Oluyemi, J., Abdulateef, J., & Atolagbe, E. (2018). Medical tourism in Nigeria: Challenges and remedies to healthcare system development. *International Journal of Development and Management Review, 13*(1), 223–238.

Bazuaye, A. (2017). Nigeria records breakthrough in sickle cell treatment. [online]. Available at: https://www.cvcnigeria.org/view.php?id=7. Accessed 10 Oct 2020.

Bello, O. (2018, May 13). What is the number of hospitals in Nigeria? *Quora.* [online]. Available at: https://www.quora.com/What-is-the-number-of-hospitals-in-Nigeria. Accessed 10 Octo 2020.

Benning, J. A.. (1969). *Canadian university service overseas and administrative decentralization.* [online]. Available at: https://onlinelibrary.wiley.com/doi/pdf/10.1111/j.1754-7121.1969.tb00276.x. Accessed 10 Oct 2020.

Business Hallmark. (2021) Hundreds of Nigerian doctors set to emigrate to Saudi Arabia as country's health sector worsens. [online]. Available at: https://hallmarknews.com/hundreds-of-nigerian-doctors-set-toemigrate-to-saudi-arabia-as-countrys-health-sector-worsens/ (Accessed: 23 November 2021).

Bulletin of the World Health Organization. (2008). Consensus during the cold war: Back to Alma-Ata. *World Health Organization.* [online]. Available at: http://www.who.int/bulletin/volumes/86/10/08-031008/en/. Accessed 10 Oct 2020.

Central Intelligence Agency (CIA). (2021). *The world factbook.* [online]. Available at: https://www.cia.gov/the-world-factbook/countries/nigeria/. Accessed 20 Apr 2021.

Cuba Health Profile. (2007). [online]. Available at: https://www.medicc.org/publications/cuba_health_reports/cuba-health-data.php. Accessed 10 Oct 2020.

Cueto, M. (2004). The origins of primary health care and selective primary health care. *America Journal Public Health, 22*(94), 1864–1874. [online]. Available at: http://ajph.aphapublications.org/doi/10.2105/AJPH.94.11.1864. Accessed 10 Oct 2020.

Daily Trust. (2017, April 25). FG, states spend 4% of budgets on health. *Daily Trust.* [online]. Available at: https://www.dailytrust.com.ng/fg-states-spend-4-3-of-n13-5tr-budgets-on-health.html. Accessed 10 Oct 2020.

Ejughemre, U. J.. (2013). Accelerated reforms in healthcare financing: The need to scale up private sector participation in Nigeria. *International Journal of Health Policy Management, 9* 2(1), 13–19. https://doi.org/10.15171/ijhpm.2014.04.

Fajola, A. O., Ogbimi, R. N., Oyo-Ita, A., Mosuro, O., Mustapha, A., Umejiego, C., Fakunle, B., & Uduma, C. (2007). *Innovative approaches to healthcare delivery in resource-limited settings: Lessons from Nigeria.* [online]. Available at: https://www.onepetro.org/conference-paper/SPE-183622-MS. Acessed 10 Oct 2020.

Falase, B., Sanusi, M., Majekodunmi, A., Ajose, I., Idowu, A., & Oke, D. (2013). The cost of open-heart surgery in Nigeria. *The Pan African Medical Journal, 14*, 61.

Federal Ministry of Health. (2016). *National health policy 2016: Promoting the health of Nigerians to accelerate socio-economic development.* [online]. Available at: https://extranet.who.int/countryplanningcycles/sites/default/files/planning_cycle_repository/nigeria/draft_nigeria_national_health_policy_final_december_fmoh_edited.pdf. Accessed Oct 2020.

FMH. (2014). *Nigeria health information system policy.* [online]. Available at: https://ehealth4everyone.com/wp-content/uploads/2015/09/Nig-Health-Info.pdf. Accessed 10 Oct 2020.

Fosco, M. (2018). Doctor drain: An exodus from Nigeria threatens its healthcare system. *Ozy.* [online]. Available at: https://www.ozy.com/around-the-world/doctor-drain-an-exodus-from-nigeria-threatens-its-health-care-system/87072/. Accessed 23Dec 2020

Gadzama, G. B., Bawa, S. B., Ajinoma, Z., Saidu, M. M., & Umar, A. S. (2014). Injection safety practices in a main referral hospital in Northeastern Nigeria. *Nigeria Journal of Clinical Practice, 17*(2), 134–139. [online]. Available at: https://doi.org/10.4103/1119-3077.127420 (Accessed: November 23 2021).

Global Change Data Lab. (2021) Coronavirus (COVID-19) vaccinations. Our World In Data. [online]. Available at: https://ourworldindata.org/covid-vaccinations (Accessed: November 24, 2021).

Google. (2021) COVID-19 vaccine: *Nigeria.* [online]. Available at: https://www.google.com/search?q=How+many+Nigerians+vaccinated+for+covid-19&rlz=1C1CHZN_enUS938US938&oq=How+many+Nigerians+vaccinated+for+covid-19&aqs=chrome..69i57.18456j1j7&sourceid=chrome&ie=UTF-8 (Accessed: November 23 2021).

Gadzama, G. B., Bawa, S. B., Ajinoma, Z., Saidu, M. M., & Umar, A. S. (2014). Injection safety practices in a main referral hospital in Northeastern Nigeria. *Nigeria Journal of Clinical Practice, 17*(2), 134–139. https://doi.org/10.4103/1119-3077.127420

Grillo, I. A., & Adeloye, A. (2009). Open heart surgery in Nigeria from beginning to date. *Annals of Ibadan Postgraduate Medicine, 7*(2), 17. [online]. Available at: https://www.ncbi.nlm.nih.gov/pmc/articles/PMC4111008/. Accessed 10 Oct 2020.

Ibama, A. S., Atibinye, D., & Obele, R. (2015). Community health practice in Nigeria – Prospects and challenges. *International Journal of Current Research, 7*(01), 11989–11992. [online]. Available at: https://journalcra.com/sites/default/files/issue-pdf/7095.pdf. Accessed 10 Oct 2020.

Ibenegbu, G. (2018). What are the problems facing healthcare management in Nigeria? [online]. Available at: https://www.legit.ng/1104912-what-the-problems-facing-healthcare-management-nigeria.html. Accessed 10 Oct 2020.

Ifijeh, M. (2015, November 12). Only five percent of Nigerians are covered by health insurance. *This Day.* November 12. [online]. Available at: http://allafrica.com/stories/201511121412.html. Accessed 10 Oct 2020.

Ighobor, K. (2017). Diagnosing Africa's medical brain drain: Higher wages and modern facilities are magnets for Africa's health workers. *Africa Renewal.* [online]. Available at: https://www.

un.org/africarenewal/magazine/december-2016-march-2017/diagnosing-africa%E2%80%99s-medical-brain-drain. Accessed 10 Feb 2020.

International Medical Travel Journal – IMTJ. (2014). *Nigeria spends $1 billion on outbound medical tourism.* [online]. Available at: https://www.imtj.com/news/nigeria-spends-1-billion-outbound-medical-tourism/. Accessed 10 Oct 2020.

Julius. (2017). *Nigeria healthcare system: The good and the bad.* [online]. Available at: http://www.visitnigeria.com.ng/nigeria-healthcare-system-the-good-and-the-bad/. Accessed 23 Dec 2020.

Kazeem, Y. (2015, October 2). Nigeria's ex-petroleum minister has been arrested in London for money laundering. *Quartz Africa.* [online]. Available at: https://qz.com/africa/516617/nigerias-ex-petroleum-minister-has-been-arrested-in-london-for-money-laundering/. Accessed 10 Oct 2020.

Kiri, V. A., & Ojule, A. C. (2020). Electronic medical record systems: A pathway to sustainable public health insurance schemes in sub-Saharan Africa. *Nigeria Postgraduate Medical Journal, 27*(1), 1–7. https://doi.org/10.4103/npmj.npmj_141_19

Koehring, M. (2018). Global access to healthcare. *The economist intelligence unit.* [online]. Available at: https://eiuperspectives.economist.com/healthcare/global-access-healthcare. Accessed 10 Oct 2020.

Labiran, A, Mafe, M, Onajole, B, Lambo, E. (2008). Health workforce country profile for Nigeria. *Africa Health Workforce Observatory,* 8.

Lopez, O. (2019, September 19) Nigeria's health care system on the mend: Reducing bureaucracy and improving vaccine storage have helped health experts better respond to disease outbreaks. *US News and Report.* [online]. Available at: https://www.usnews.com/news/best-countries/articles/2019-09-19/nigeria-slowly-improving-its-health-care-system. Accessed 10 Oct 2020.

Mackenzie, D. (2019, August 23). Wild polio has been eradicated in Nigeria but infections will continue. *Health Analysis.* [online]. Available at: https://www.newscientist.com/article/2214302-wild-polio-has-been-eradicated-in-nigeria-but-infections-will-continue/. Accessed 10 Oct 2020.

Makinde, O. A. (2016). Physicians as medical tourism facilitators in Nigeria: Ethical issues of the practice. *Croatian Medical Journal, 57*(6), 601–604. [online]. Available at: http://www.cmj.hr/2016/57/6/28051285.htm. Accessed 21 Feb 2021.

Meribole, E. C., Makinde, O. A., Oyemakinde, A., Oyediran, K. A., Atobatele, A., Fadeyibi, F. A., Azeez, A., & Ogbokor, D. (2018). The Nigerian health information system policy review of 2014: The need, content, expectations and progress. *Health Information and Libraries Journal.* [online]. Available at: https://onlinelibrary.wiley.com/doi/full/10.1111/hir.12240. Accessed 10 Oct 2020.

Millar, A. (2020). *The rise of fake medicines in Africa.* [online]. Available at: https://www.pharmaceutical-technology.com/features/counterfeit-drugs-africa/. Accessed 27 May 2021.

Mitchell, P. (2018) Poor countries subsidise the NHS by training doctors – Compensate them. *The Guardian.* [online]. Available at: https://www.theguardian.com/education/2018/jun/18/poor-countries-subsidise-the-nhs-by-training-doctors-compensate-them. Accessed 10 Feb 2020.

Muhammad, F., Abdulkareem, J. H., & Chowdhury, A. B. M.. (2017). *Major public health problems in Nigeria: A review.* [online]. Available at: 10.3329/seajph.v7i1.34672 https://www.researchgate.net/publication/322158989_Major_Public_Health_Problems_in_Nigeria_A_review. Acessed 10 Oct 2020.

Munshi, N. (2020, January 28). Nigeria makes anti-corruption moves amid criticism over progress. *Financial Times.* [online]. Available at: https://www.ft.com/content/42ae53b2-411d-11ea-a047-eae9bd51ceba. Accessed 10 Oct 2020.

Nichols, H. (2019). What are the leading causes of death in the US? *Medical News Today.* [online]. Available at: https://www.medicalnewstoday.com/articles/282929. Accessed 10 Oct 2020.

NOIPolls. (2017). *Emigration of Nigerian medical doctors: Survey report.* [online]. Available at: https://noi-polls.com/2018/wp-content/uploads/2019/06/Emigration-of-Doctors-Press-Release-July-2018-Survey-Report.pdf https://noi-polls.com/new-survey-reveals-8-in-10-nigerian-doctors-are-seeking-work-opportunities-abroad/. Accessed 10 Oct 2020.

Nwafor IA, Eze JC, Ezemba N, Chinawa JM, Onyekwulu FA, Nwafor MN. (2017) Changes in the open heart surgery protocol and outcomes in a Nigerian national cardiothoracic center of excellence over 42 Years. *Therapeutic Advances in Cardiology* 1.2; 97-104. [online]. Available at: https://www.scientiaricerca.com/srtaca/pdf/SRTACA-01-00017.pdf (Accessed: 17 November 2021.

Obansa, S. A. J., & Orimisan, A. (2012). *Healthcare financing in Nigeria: Prospects and challenges.* [online]. Available at: https://www.researchgate.net/publication/283609489_Health_care_financing_in_Nigeria_Prospects_and_challenges. Accessed10 Oct 2020.

Obinna C. (2019) Why Nigerian doctors are rushing abroad – NMA, others. Vanguard https://www.vanguardngr.com/2019/04/why-nigerian-doctors-are-rushing-abroad-nma-others/.

Odeyemi, I. A., & Nixon, J. (2013). Assessing equity in health care through the national health insurance schemes of Nigeria and Ghana: A review-based comparative analysis. *International Journal of Equity Health, 22*(12), 9. https://doi.org/10.1186/1475-9276-12-9.

Ogbaa, M. (2017) *A Nigerian story: How healthcare is the offspring of imperialism and corruption.* [online]. Available at: https://www.theelephant.info/features/2017/11/16/a-nigerian-story-how-healthcare-is-the-offspring-of-imperialism-and-corruption/. Accessed 10 Oct 2020.

Ogbebo, W. (2015). *The many problems of Nigeria's health sector.* [online]. Available at: https://infoguidenigeria.com/problems-of-nigeria-health-sector-and-possible-solutions/. Accessed 10 Oct 2020.

Ojo, T. O., & Akinwumi, A. F. (2015). Doctors as managers of healthcare resources in Nigeria: Evolving roles and current challenges. *Nigerian Medical Journal, 56*(6), 375–380.

Okafor, P. (2017, August 23). Nigeria loses $1bn annually to medical tourism. *Omatseye Vanguard*, [online]. Available at: https://www.vanguardngr.com/2017/08/nigeria-loses-1bn-annually-medical-tourism-omatseye/. Accessed 10 Oct 2020.

Okebukola PO, Brieger WR. (2016) Providing universal health insurance coverage in Nigeria. *Int Q Community Health Educ*;36(4):241–46. [online]. Available at: https://pubmed.ncbi.nlm.nih.gov/27389041/ (Accessed: 23 September 2021).

Okoro, C. C., Omeluzor, S. U., Itunu, A., & Bamidele, I. A.. (2014). Effect of brain drain (human capital flight) of librarians on service delivery in some selected Nigerian universities. *SAGE Open,* July–September 1–11[online]. Available at: https://journals.sagepub.com/doi/pdf/10.1177/2158244014541131. Accessed 10 Oct 2020.

Oladapo, M. (2018). *Nigerian doctors record breakthrough with patient's online video/audio call consultations.* [online]. Available at: https://www.independent.ng/nigerian-doctors-record-breakthrough-with-patients-online-video-audio-call-consultations/amp/. Accessed 10 Oct 2020.

Onigbinde, O., Samuel, A., Faleye, A., Olaleye, O., Jolayemi, T., Fauziyyah, A., Yusuf, R., & Omokhaye, H. (2018). *Policy brief first quarter.* [online]. Available at: https://yourbudgit.com/wp-content/uploads/2018/04/Nigeria-Health-Budget-Analysis.pdf. Accessed 24 May 2021.

Onyenucheya, A. (2018) Reversing medical tourism in Nigeria. *The Guardian*. October 25. [online]. Available at: https://guardian.ng/features/reversing-medical-tourism-in-nigeria/. Accessed: 10 Oct 2020.

Ophori, E. A., Tula, M. Y., Azih, A. V., Okojie, R., & Ikpo, P. E. (2014). Current trends of immunization in Nigeria: Prospect and challenges. *Tropical Medicine and Health, 42*(2), 67–75. [online]. Available at: https://www.ncbi.nlm.nih.gov/pmc/articles/PMC4139536/. Accessed 18 May 2021.

Oputah, D. (2016) Medical breakthrough as Nigerian surgeons construct bladder for cancer patient. *The Will.* [online]. Available at: https://thewillnigeria.com/news/medical-breakthrough-as-nigerian-surgeons-construct-bladder-for-cancer-patient/. Accessed 10 Oct 2020.

Orekunrin, O. (2015). Nigeria's healthcare problems: A three-pronged solution. [online]. Available at: [online]. Available at: https://politicalmatter.org/2015/07/11/10769/. Accessed 10 Oct 2020.

Otu, A., Ameh, S., Osifo-Dawodu, E., Alade, E., Ekuri, S., & Idris, J. (2017). An account of the Ebola virus disease outbreak in Nigeria: Implications and lessons learned. *BMC Public Health, 18*, 3. [online]. Available at: https://www.ncbi.nlm.nih.gov/pmc/articles/PMC5504668/. Accessed 10 Oct 2020.

Oxford Business Group. (2015). *Opportunities for private companies in Nigeria's health care sector, and efforts to improve provision*. [online]. Available at: https://oxfordbusinessgroup.com/overview/opportunities-private-companies-nigerias-health-care-sector-and-efforts-improve-provision. Accessed 30 Dec 2020.

Ozawa S, Shankar R, Leopold C, Orubu S. (2019) Access to medicines through health systems in low- and middle-income countries. *Health Policy Plan*;34(Supplement_3):iii1–iii3. [online]. Available at: https://pubmed.ncbi.nlm.nih.gov/31816069/ (Accessed: 23 September 2021).

Ozumba, B. C., Onyeneho, N. G., Chalupowski, M., & Subramanian, S. V. (2019). Inequities in access to maternal healthcare in Enugu State: Implications for universal health coverage to meet vision 2030 in Nigeria, *International Quarterly Community Health Education, 39*(3), 163–173. [online]. Available at: https://journals.sagepub.com/doi/10.1177/0272684X18819977?icid=int.sj-full-text.similar-articles.2. Accessed 23 Jan 2020.

Parmar, H. (2015, September 8). *Healthcare business challenges in Nigeria*. [online]. Available at: https://www.linkedin.com/pulse/healthcare-business-challenges-nigeria-hemraj-parmar-mba/. Accessed 10 Oct 2020.

PharmAccess Foundation. (2015). *Nigerian health sector market study report*. [online]. Available at: https://www.rvo.nl/sites/default/files/Market_Study_Health_Nigeria.pdf. Accessed 23 Jan 2020.

Punch. (2016, October 14). Nigeria spends $1bn annually on medical tourism. *Punch*. [online]. Available at: https://punchng.com/nigeria-spends-1bn-annually-medical-tourism/. Accessed 10 Oct 2020.

Reality Check. (2019, May 13). NHS staff shortage: How many doctors and nurses come from abroad? *BBC News*. [online]. Available at: https://www.bbc.com/news/world-48205445. Accessed 10 Oct 2020.

Rosenberg, D. J., West, D. M., Okuzu, O. N., Oshin, A., & Theobald, D. (2015). *Mobile technology and health: The newest front line in healthcare innovation in Africa*. [online]. Available at: https://www.brookings.edu/events/mobile-technology-and-mhealth-the-newest-frontline-in-health-care-innovation-in-africa/. Accessed 10 Oct 2020.

Scott-Emuakpor, A. (2010). The evolution of health care systems in Nigeria: Which way forward in the twenty-first century. *Nigerian Medical Journal, 51*, 53–65. [online]. Available at: http://www.nigeriamedj.com/text.asp?2010/51/2/53/70997. Accessed 23 Jan 2020.

Solomon-Ibama, A., & Dennis, P. (2016). Role of community health practitioners in national development: The Nigeria situation. *International Journal of Clinical Medicine, 7*, 511–518. [online]. Available at: https://www.scirp.org/journal/paperinformation.aspx?paperid=68938. Accessed 10 Oct 2020.

Stuart, R. (2012). *CUSO International*. [online]. Available at: https://www.thecanadianencyclopedia.ca/en/article/cuso-international. Accessed 10 Oct 2020. Tavella, VJ, Nichols, H. (2019) What are the leading causes of death in the US? Medical News Today. [online]. Available at: https://www.medicalnewstoday.com/articles/282929 (Accessed: 10 October 2020).

Tavella, VJ, Nichols, H. (2019) What are the leading causes of death in the US? Medical News Today. [online]. Available at: https://www.medicalnewstoday.com/articles/282929 (Accessed: 10 October 2020).

The Association of Nigerian Physicians in the Americas – ANPA. (2020). *Vision and mission in action*. [online]. Available at: https://anpa.org/mission-vision/. Accessed 10 Feb 2020.

Tnv Nigerian Voice. (2016). #Diezani refunds 90 billion dollars – *CNN*. [online]. Available at: https://www.thenigerianvoice.com/thread/51654/221309/1https://www.facebook.com/RetiredMembersOfNigerianArmedForcesRemenaf/posts/diezani-refunds-90-billion-dollar-cnn-confirmedi-start-to-imagine-what-a-normal-/1293893257328938/. Accessed 10 Oct 2020.

Tonuchi, E. J., Idowu, P., & Mimiko, D. O. (2020). How large is the size of Nigeria's informal economy? A MIMIC approach. *International Journal of Economics, Commerce and Management, 8*(7), 204–228. [online]. Available at: https://www.researchgate.net/publication/343345347_How_large_is_the_size_of_Nigeria's_informal_economy_A_

MIMIC_Approach#:~:text=Findings%20from%20the%20MIMIC%20model,to%20 informality%2C%20with%20the%20estimated. Accessed 21 Dec 2020.

Uguru, N., Onwujekwe, O., Ogu, U. U., & Uguru, C. (2020). Access to oral health care: A focus on dental caries treatment provision in Enugu Nigeria. *BMC Oral Health, 19*(1), 145. https:// doi.org/10.1186/s12903-020-01135-1

Umeh, C. A. (2018). Challenges toward achieving universal health coverage in Ghana, Kenya, Nigeria, and Tanzania. https://doi.org/10.1002/hpm.2610 [online]. Available at: Challenges toward achieving universal health coverage in Ghana, Kenya, Nigeria, and Tanzania – Umeh – 2018 – The International Journal of Health Planning and Management – Wiley Online Library. Accessed 24 Dec 2020.

UNICEF. (n.d.) *Nigeria: Key demographic indicators.* [online]. Available at: https://data.unicef. org/country/nga/. Accessed 23 July 2021.

UNAIDS. (2019). New survey results indicate that Nigeria has an HIV prevalence of 1.4% [online]. Available at: https://www.unaids.org/en/resources/presscentre/pressreleaseandstate-mentarchive/2019/march/20190314_nigeria (Accessed: 10 October 2021).

USAID. (2017, January 26). *Global health.* [online]. Available at: https://www.usaid.gov/nigeria/ global-health. Accessed 10 Oct 2020.

Uzochukwu, B., Ughasoro, M. D., Etiaba, Okwuosa, C., Envuladu, E., & Onwujekwe, O. E. (2015). Healthcare financing in Nigeria: Implications for achieving universal health coverage. *Nigeria Journal of Clinical Practice.* [online]. Available at:http://www.njcponline.com/ text.asp?2015/18/4/437/154196. Accessed 10 Oct 2020.

Uzondu, C. A., Doctor, H. V., Findley, S. E., Afenyadu, G. Y., & Ager, A. (2015). Female health workers at the doorstep: A pilot of community-based maternal, newborn, and child health service delivery in Northern Nigeria. *Global Health Science Practice, 3*(1), 97–108. [online]. Available at: https://www.ncbi.nlm.nih.gov/pmc/articles/PMC4356278/. Accessed 10 Oct 2020.

VOA. (2019) Nigeria losing $1B annually to medical tourism, Authorities say. May 10. *VOA.* [online]. Available at: https://www.voanews.com/africa/nigeria-losing-1b-annually-medical-tourism-authorities-say. Accessed 10 Oct 2020.

Welcome, M. O. (2011). The Nigerian health care system: Need for integrating adequate medical intelligence and surveillance systems. *Journal of Pharmacy and Bioallied Sciences, 3*(4), 470–478. [online]. Available at: https://www.ncbi.nlm.nih.gov/pmc/articles/PMC3249694/. Accessed 10 Oct 2020.

WHO. (2000). *The world health organization's ranking of the world's health systems, by rank.* [online]. Available at: https://photius.com/rankings/healthranks.html. Accessed 10 Oct 2020.

WHO. (2006). *The world health report. Working Together for Health* (pp. 1–15). World Health Organization.

WHO. (2010). *Monitoring the building blocks of health systems: A handbook of indicators and their measurement strategies.* [online]. Available at: https://www.who.int/healthinfo/systems/ monitoring/en/. Accessed 10 Oct 2020.

WHO. (2014). *Are the Ebola outbreaks in Nigeria and Senegal over?* [online]. Available at: https:// www.who.int/mediacentre/news/ebola/14-october-2014/en/. Accessed 15 Mar 2021.

WHO. (2015). *World health statistics. Part I: Global health indicators.* [online]. Available at:https://www.who.int/gho/publications/world_health_statistics/EN_WHS2015_Part2.pdf. Accessed 10 Oct 2020.

WHO. (2016). *Global health observatory (GHO) data: World health statistics 2016: Monitoring health for the SDGs.* [online]. Available at: https://www.who.int/gho/publications/world_ health_statistics/2016/en/. Accessed 10 Oct 2020.

WHO. (2019). *Access to medicines and vaccines: Report by the director-general.* [online]. Available at: https://apps.who.int/gb/ebwha/pdf_files/WHA72/A72_17-en.pdf. Accessed 10 Oct 2020.

The World Bank. (2021) Current health expenditure (% of GDP). [online]. Available at: https:// data.worldbank.org/indicator/SH.XPD.CHEX.GD.ZS (Accessed: 18 November 2021).

World Bank. (2014). *A decade of development in sub-Saharan African science, technology, engineering, and mathematics research.* A report by the World Bank and *Elsevier.* [online]. Available at: http://documents.worldbank.org/curated/en/237371468204551128/pdf/910160 WP0P126900disclose09026020140.pdf. Accessed 10 Oct 2020.

World Bank Data. (2010). *Current health expenditure per capita (current US$).* [online]. Available at: https://data.worldbank.org/indicator/SH.XPD.CHEX.PC.CD. Accessed 10 Oct 2020.

World Population Review. (2020). *Most corrupt countries 2020.* [online]. Available at: http:// worldpopulationreview.com/countries/most-corrupt-countries. Accessed 10 Oct 2020.

Worldometer. (2020). *Countries in the world by population: Coronavirus report.* [online]. Available at: https://www.worldometers.info/world-population/population-by-country/ https:// www.worldometers.info/coronavirus/#countries. Accessed 10 Oct 2020.

Chapter 6
The Spectrum of Complementary and Alternative Medicine

Learning Objectives

After reading this Chapter, the learner should be able to:

1. Identify and discuss the different types of complementary and alternative medicine (CAM)
2. Distinguish between complementary, alternative, and integrative medicine
3. Articulate the philosophies of mainstream orthodox medicine and CAM
4. Deconstruct the similarities and differences between mainstream conventional medicine and CAM
5. Describe the treatment principles for each CAM method
6. Discuss the global demand for the use of CAM
7. Analyze the need for and utilization of CAM in the United States
8. Objectively evaluate CAM treatments and products

Introduction

During the past decade, interest in complementary and alternative medicine (CAM) has surged because the global public attitude about the remedies has been positive. The CAM spectrum is herbal medicine, massage, homeopathy, mud bath, acupuncture, Chinese herbs, Tuina massage, Tai Chi, Qigong, music therapy, wax bath, reflexology, and dance therapy. It also includes hydrotherapy, mind and spirit therapies, self-exercise therapies, radiation and vibration, osteopathy, chiropractic, aromatherapy, moxibustion, and therapeutic fasting and dieting, to mention a few. However, these therapies' clinical effectiveness and safety remain controversial as advocates often make outlandish and unsubstantiated claims.

© The Author(s), under exclusive license to Springer Nature Switzerland AG 2021
J. A. Balogun, *The Nigerian Healthcare System*,
https://doi.org/10.1007/978-3-030-88863-3_6

Globally, scientists currently do not fully understand the mechanisms of action and safety of most CAM practices and products. Studies from the United States found integrative medical treatments safe and effective in many conditions but interact with prescribed medications with severe adverse side effects (Lucas, 2006; Taylor et al., 2006; Elmer et al., 2007; University of California, San Francisco, 2020). There is currently little empirical evidence on the chemical composition, therapeutic effectiveness, and safety of most CAM remedies worldwide. The majority of CAM enthusiasts perceive their treatments to be "natural" and safe. This perception is misplaced without the knowledge of the chemical composition and toxicity of the products. The interactions between CAM remedies and Western medications are not well documented. The side effects reported mainly by CAM users include chemical burns following the application of herbal products on the skin, anorexia, nausea and vomiting, general malaise, diarrhea, and undesired weight loss. Unfortunately, most HCPs are not familiar with these adverse effects and the alternative medical systems, biological-based therapies, energy therapies, manipulative and body-based therapies, and mind-body therapies (Frass et al., 2012; Fan, 2005).

This chapter introduces the primary CAM systems currently gaining popularity worldwide. It presents the classification and differences between orthodox medicine, CAM, and integrative medicine. The chapter also discusses the origin, treatment philosophy, therapeutic efficacy, and safety of acupuncture, chiropractic, osteopathy, traditional Chinese medicine, Ayurveda, naturopathy, homeopathy, aromatherapy, and spirituality.

Classification of Complementary and Alternative Medicine Systems

CAM is an amalgam of different therapies from various medical and healthcare practices and systems that are not considered conventional Western medicine. There are more than 100 systems of alternative medicine used all over the world. The classification of CAM systems routinely changes continually, as the therapies found to be safe and effective are embraced by conventional health care, and new treatment approaches emerge. The primary CAM treatments are classified into five broad categories: Alternative medical systems, biological-based therapies, energy therapies, manipulative and body-based therapies, and mind-body therapies (Frass et al., 2012; Fan, 2005). Some of the medical systems belong to more than one category. For example, traditional Chinese medicine is under the alternative medical methods, but some of its therapies also belong to the mind-body interventions (e.g., Tai Chi and Qi gong), and some belong to the biologically based treatments such as herbs, foods, and vitamins (Fig. 6.1).

Alternative health systems are traditional practices independently similar to allopathic (orthodox) medicine utilized by individual cultures worldwide. Examples

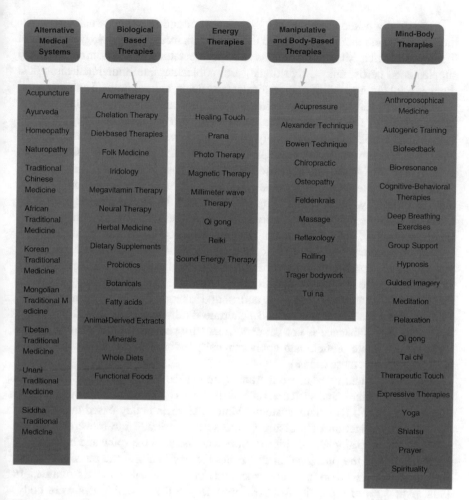

Fig. 6.1 Classification of CAM systems. (Sources: Frass et al., 2012; National Cancer Institute, 2021. Adapted from Table 1 in: ©2012 Frass, et al. Originally published in *Ochsner Journal*, 12(1), 45–56. Use and Acceptance of Complementary and Alternative Medicine Among the General Population and Medical Personnel: A Systematic Review. http://www.ochsnerjournal.org/content/12/1/45, released under the terms of the Creative Commons Attribution License (https://creativecommons.org/licenses/by/4.0/))

include indigenous healing systems such as African, Chinese, Korean, Mongolian, Tibetan, Unani, Siddha, Ayurveda traditional medicine, and homeopathy. The diagnostic and treatment philosophy of alternative health systems practitioners is patient-centered rather than disease-centered (Koithan, 2009). They share a perspective to the effect that imbalances, whether inherited or acquired, in the patient's overall constitution, are the primary manifestation of disease or dysfunction and not disease localized in a specific organ isolated from the rest of the body.

Biologically based therapies use "substances found in nature" such as aromatherapy, chelation therapy, diet-based therapies, folk medicine, iridology, and neural therapy. Biologically based treatments also include natural products, such as dietary supplements, herbs, unique nutritional, orthomolecular, and individual biological therapies, including probiotics, botanicals, fatty acids, animal-derived extracts, vitamins, minerals, proteins, amino acids, whole diets, and functional foods. Several investigations of the efficacy of the dietary supplements have been reported, but none of the studies has compellingly proven effectiveness. Nevertheless, biologically based therapies are increasingly popular. The CAM literature estimates that more than 95% of Americans have used biologically based treatments (Tabish, 2008).

Energy therapies use energy fields to promote health and healing. Biofield therapies affect energy fields surrounding and penetrate the human body by applying direct or indirect pressure on these fields. Examples are Qigong, Reiki, Prana, Healing Touch®, and Therapeutic Touch. Bioelectromagnetic-based therapies employ an unconventional use of electromagnetic fields, such as pulsed, magnetic, and alternating current or direct current fields, to treat asthma or cancer or manage pain and migraine headaches (Tabish, 2008). Examples are phototherapy, magnetic therapy, millimeter wave therapy, and sound energy therapy (Koithan, 2009). Biofield therapies that surround and penetrate the human body affect the energy fields, but their existence is not yet experimentally proven. Some forms of energy therapy manipulate biofield and apply manual pressure and use the hand to move the joints through these fields.

Manipulative and body-based therapies are the movement of one or more parts of the body structures and systems, such as the bones and joints, the soft tissues, and the circulatory and lymphatic systems. Manipulative and body-based therapies are the manual application of pressure to the soft tissues and the movement of the patient's joints. Examples are chiropractors who focus on the spine and how manipulating it affects the preservation and restoration of health – the physiotherapists apply manual pressure to the muscles and tendons to normalize those structures. In 1998, over 50% of the visits to CAM providers in the United States were body-based therapies, such as acupressure, Alexander technique, Bowen technique, Feldenkrais, Rolfing, Trager bodywork, Tui na, osteopathic manipulation, chiropractic, massage, and reflexology.

Mind-body therapies focus on the intrinsic link between human thoughts and physiological functioning to positively influence health and well-being. Examples of mind-body therapies are anthroposophical medicine, autogenic training, bioresonance, deep breathing exercises, meditation, prayer, biofeedback, guided imagery, relaxation, hypnosis, and expressive therapies such as dance, art, and music. As research uncovers the efficacy of mind-body therapies, such as cognitive-behavioral therapies and patient support groups, previously considered CAMs are now viewed as mainstream conventional treatments (Koithan, 2009). Biofeedback is a mind-body therapy that uses the responses from a variety of monitoring procedures and equipment to teach patients to control specific involuntary body functions, such as heart rate, blood pressure, and muscle.

Distinction Between Complementary and Alternative Medicine and Integrative Medicine

The term "complementary medicine" refers to medical practices used together with conventional medicine. For example, the use of acupuncture to treat the side effects of cancer treatment and hypnotherapy in conjunction with pain medications to reduce anxiety and enhance relaxation in people recovering from severe burns is considered complementary medicine.

The term "alternative medicine" is the treatment and healthcare practices outside of standard medical care. For example, traditional African medicine and treatment of heart disease with chelation therapy – a method of removing excessive metals from the blood instead of using the standard approach – are considered alternative medicine. Alternative medicine has been in existence for hundreds and, in some cases, thousands of years. The holistic approach to health care is labeled "alternative" for various scientific, cultural, and political reasons in the West. It is challenging to evaluate the efficacy of alternative practices (e.g., acupuncture) scientifically in the same way that medications are tested. The medical establishment relies on scientific evidence (rather than clinical experience) when evaluating alternative medicine's safety and effectiveness. Many alternative treatments that have not been thoroughly tested (or cannot be thoroughly tested) are considered "unscientific" by Western standards – for example, using alternative medicine such as a special diet rather than taking medications to treat attention-deficit/hyperactivity disorder.

The term "integrative medicine" is often interchangeably used with complementary and alternative medicine, but there is a subtle difference between the two terms. Integrative medicine practitioners typically blend appropriate CAM with mainstream medicine rather than add one CAM (e.g., herbs) treatment to standard medical treatment. Integrative medicine treatment for Alzheimer's disease may include a combination of: (1) drugs that increase certain brain chemicals, (2) exercise therapies, such as walking programs and relaxation training to reduce anxiety and improve behavior, (3) antioxidants (such as vitamin E and ginkgo biloba) that scavenge free radicals, and (4) music therapy to boost the immune system.

Differences in Treatment Philosophy Between Mainstream Medicine (Standard Care) and Complementary and Alternative Medicine

The goal of conventional (orthodox) medicine is to locate (diagnose) the real source of a particular disease and then remove it surgically or treat it with medication (Fig. 6.2). For example, if a patient has an infection, mainstream physicians will prescribe an antibiotic to kill the invading bacteria. Conversely, CAM practitioners

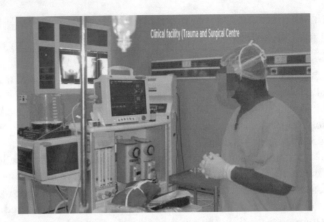

Fig. 6.2 A surgeon at UNIMED Teaching Hospital preparing for surgery. (Photograph used with permission from UNIMED PRO)

take a more "holistic" approach to health care. They consider health and disease a complex interaction of several factors involving the physical, spiritual, mental, emotional, genetic, environmental, and social systems.

CAM practitioners will focus on the whole body to promote good health or treat a disease and consider all of these factors.

Although CAM treatments vary widely, they share several commonalities. The focus is on treating the whole person's physical, emotional, social, and spiritual imbalance. Prevention of illness is a primary concern, and treatments are individualized. Treatments administered by CAM practitioners focus on the causes of disease rather than the symptoms, and the procedures support the natural healing processes of the body.

Complementary Medical Systems

Acupuncture Acupuncture is the most popular component of traditional Chinese medicine (TCM) – a system used for healing purposes as far back as 200 BC. Then, knowledge of acupuncture slowly spread from China along the Arabian trade routes toward the West. Around 1680, the first medical description of acupuncture by a European physician was by Willem ten Rhijne, who was employed at an East India Company and observed acupuncture in Japan. Subsequently, there was a flurry of interest in the United States and the United Kingdom by the first half of the nineteenth century, leading to some publications in the peer-reviewed scientific journals, including a *Lancet* editorial article entitled "Acupuncturation." However, by mid-century, acupuncture fell into disrepute, and interest in it lay dormant, though acupuncturists briefly resurrected. In the United States, academic programs in acupuncture include a Doctorate of Acupuncture and Oriental Medicine, Master of

Science (Traditional Oriental Medicine), Master of Science in Acupuncture, and Certificate in Chinese Herbology Licensed Acupuncturists.

Acupuncture is an innovative and holistic, drug-free treatment that addresses the patient's well-being, including a health maintenance treatment program. During the treatment procedure, an acupuncturist inserts needles and gently jiggles it as it goes in at specific micro-pressure points where the energy pathway is close to the skin's surface along the meridians intending to change the natural balance of energies. The patients do not feel pain, but they may feel a twitch or a quick twinge sensation as the needle is initially inserted but disappears as the needle is inserted completely. After a few minutes, the patient will relax and may even doze off. The acupuncturist quickly removes the needles without pain at the end of the treatment session.

The Chinese claim that acupuncture stimulates the body's natural healing mechanisms and restores balance to the Qi. There are presently no empirical data in support of the Qi and meridian pathway theory. Acupuncturists claim dry needling increased blood flow, body temperature, white blood cell activity (responsible for the immune system's functioning), reduced cholesterol and triglyceride levels, and regulated blood sugar levels.

For decades, the Chinese have used acupuncture for pain modulation and treatment of many varieties of diseases. Similarly, neuromuscular electrical stimulation is commonly employed in Western medicine to modulate pain, augment muscle strength, and enhance blood flow in peripheral vascular disease patients. The traditional Chinese theories of how acupuncture works are still being challenged fiercely in the West, most notably in the United Kingdom and the United States. Many rehabilitation specialists believe that electrical stimulation of acupuncture points with surface electrodes can elicit similar physiological and therapeutic effects as those produced by acupuncture techniques (Balogun et al., 1998). However, much remains unknown by clinicians and scientists in the West about the basic tenets of Eastern medicine. Moreover, many of the acupuncture concepts are at odds with the "germ theory" of disease subscribed to in the West. Given the schism, full integration of acupuncture into Western medical practice is not going to be easy. However, indications are that scientists and clinicians in the West and East are currently engaged in collaborative research. Ongoing investigations are steps in the right direction toward fostering East/West treatment philosophies (Balogun, 1999).

Physiotherapists in the West now use electroacupuncture to stimulate the points linked to the patient's symptoms to facilitate the flow of *Qi* (Sinay, 2019). Two needles are placed around the point, and an electrotherapy machine delivers an electrical impulse to the needles. Thus, electroacupuncture increases the potential healing effects of standard acupuncture (Fig. 6.3).

There are many theories on the mechanisms of action of acupuncture, but evidence on the clinical effectiveness of acupuncture therapy is still elusive for many conditions, such as chronic pain. The ancient meridian theory has been debunked in the West and replaced by a neurological model that acupuncture needles stimulate nerve endings and alter brain function, particularly the central pain inhibitory mechanisms.

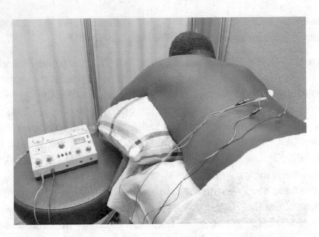

Fig. 6.3 Application of electroacupuncture to modulate pain. (Photograph used with permission of Paschal Mogbo)

In the past two decades, research into acupuncture therapy has grown exponentially, increasing at twice the rate of the investigation into conventional biomedicine. Findings from systematic reviews and meta-analyses have provided a more reliable indication of acupuncture's value in treating nausea (from various causes), dental pain, back pain, and headache. There have been over 13,000 studies, including hundreds of meta-analyses, 1000 systematic reviews summarizing the results of thousands of human and animal studies from 60 countries. The studies covered various clinical topics such as chronic pain, cancer, pregnancy, stroke, mood disorders, sleep disorders, and inflammation, to name a few. Several studies in the West have documented the effectiveness of acupuncture in acute pain management. However, the mechanisms of action of this therapy are still not fully understood within the Western system of health care (Koppelman, 2018).

The pertinent literature was summarized, in 2010, by the Australian Department of Veteran Affairs, and the review was updated in 2014 by the United States Department of Veteran Affairs and then again in 2017 by John McDonald and Stephen Janz. They concluded by saying, "our study found evidence for the effectiveness of acupuncture for 117 conditions, with stronger evidence for acupuncture's effectiveness for some conditions than others. Acupuncture is considered safe in the hands of a well-trained practitioner and is cost-effective for some conditions. The quality and quantity of research into acupuncture's effectiveness are increasing" (Koppelman, 2018).

In a randomized controlled trial (RCT), Schroeder and associates (2017) investigated the effectiveness of acupuncture on stress perception among patients at a large, urban college campus. The patients ($N = 62$) were randomly assigned into experimental acupuncture or sham acupuncture groups and received treatment once a week for 12 weeks. Each patient completed Cohen's global measure of perceived stress scale (PSS-14) at five periods – before treatment, at 6 weeks, 12 weeks, and 6 weeks and 12 weeks post-treatment. The patients in both groups showed a significant initial decrease in perceived stress scores. However, at 3 months post-treatment, the experimental acupuncture group showed a significantly more substantial treatment effect than the sham acupuncture group.

A meta-analysis in the *Journal of Pain* in 2018 revealed that acupuncture is beneficial in managing several chronic pain disorders. In addition, the pain relief is persistent for at least 12 months following treatment. The authors inter-alia concludes that "the effects of acupuncture are not completely explicable in terms of placebo effects," but cautioned that "factors other than the specific effects of needling at correct acupuncture point locations" contribute to the benefits derived from receiving acupuncture (Devitt, 2018).

Zhang and associates' meta-analysis study provides evidence that acupuncture is an effective and safe treatment in stroke rehabilitation – for post-stroke depression. Furthermore, ex post facto analyses of their data revealed that acupuncture alone improved depressive symptoms better than drug therapy (Zhang et al., 2019). The World Health Organization (WHO) and the National Institutes of Health in the United States believe that acupuncture is practical and effective in treating infertility, back pain, headache, insomnia, sciatica, sports injuries, heart problems, and stress. The WHO has concluded that acupuncture effectively evokes analgesia, protects the body against infections, and regulates various physiological functions. Although acupuncture is most often used to reduce pain, it can also change the disease's pathogenesis. Research studies suggest that needling and other acupuncture techniques elicit various effects in the peripheral (body) and the central (brain) systems. One theory about its mechanism of action is that the stimulated nerve fibers convey signals first to the spinal cord by activating the body's central nervous system and the brain. The spinal cord and brain then release hormones (endorphins) responsible for making us feel less pain while improving overall health. Using brain images, scientists have confirmed that acupuncture increases the patients' pain threshold, explaining why it produces long-term pain relief (Mandal & Cashin-Garbutt, 2019).

Studies funded by the National Institutes of Health in the United States revealed that acupuncture therapy is an effective treatment when used alone or in combination with conventional therapies to treat several chronic disorders such as headaches, menstrual cramps, tennis elbow, fibromyalgia, myofascial pain, osteoarthritis, low back pain, carpal tunnel syndrome, asthma, dental pain after surgery, addiction, nausea caused by surgical anesthesia and cancer chemotherapy and in stroke rehabilitation (Johns Hopkins Medicine, 2020). Although relatively few complications are associated with acupuncture therapy, adverse effects resulting from the use of non-sterile needles and improper delivery of treatments can cause infections, punctured organs, collapsed lungs, and injury to the central nervous system (National Center for Complementary and Integrative Health – NCCIH, 2019).

Chiropractic Chiropractic is a complementary treatment concerned with diagnosing, treating, and preventing neuro-musculoskeletal disorders and their general health effects. The profession espouses the theory that the improper alignment of the 21 vertebrae ("vertebral subluxation") is the cause of diseases and disorders. The roots of chiropractic care date back to the beginning of recorded time.

Publications from China and Greece in 2700 BC and 1500 BC mentioned manipulating the spine and maneuvering the lower extremities to ease the lower back pain. Also, Hippocrates, the Greek physician who lived from 460 to 357 BC in his writings, spoke to the relevance of chiropractic treatment when he declared, "Get knowledge of the spine, for this is the requisite for many diseases."

Spinal manipulation gained momentum in the late nineteenth century in the United States, when Daniel David Palmer, in 1895, founded the Chiropractic profession in Davenport, Iowa. Palmer was a self-taught healer who studied the spinal structure and manipulative techniques that cured a man of deafness and acute back pain by realigning a displaced vertebra in his back. In 1897, Daniel David Palmer opened the Palmer School of Chiropractic; it is still one of the 17 chiropractic institutions in the United States. The Chiropractic profession exists in over 100 countries, mainly in North America, Europe, and Australia. Throughout the twentieth century, chiropractors in the United States gained legal recognition in all 50 states, and the profession is the third-largest independent health profession in the Western world. In the United States, 52,000 licensed chiropractors treat over 20 million patients a year. A chiropractic degree requires the same duration of training as a medical degree. Chiropractic education includes clinical experience, basic sciences, structural (spinal), and functional (nervous system) diagnoses.

The putative role of chiropractic in non-musculoskeletal disease has been a source of controversy since its inception. The medical establishment does not fully embrace chiropractic in part because of their ritualistic and metaphysical origins, claims of innate intelligence, chiropractic subluxation, including the lack of scientific evidence supporting spinal dysfunction or subluxation as the sole cause of the disease and broad spectrum of visceral disorders that are unrelated to the neuro-musculoskeletal system (Heid, 2017).

A 2006 Gallup Poll in the United States rated chiropractic last among health professions about ethics and honesty because many physicians believe the concepts of chiropractic "are not based on solid science and its therapeutic value has not been demonstrated beyond a reasonable doubt" (Ingraham, 2020). Chiropractors have many disagreements about their profession. There is an ideological chasm between the two schools of thought within the chiropractic professions – "mixers" who want to modernize the profession, and the "straights," traditional chiropractors who believe the old ways and take the founding concepts literally as health care (Ingraham, 2020).

Straight chiropractors are a minority group considered as purists who adhere to the philosophical principles set forth by Palmer. Straights retain metaphysical and ritualistic beliefs and practices. Straights believe that vertebral subluxation leads to interference with an "innate intelligence" exerted via the nervous system and is the primary underlying risk factor for many disorders and diseases. They consider the medical diagnosis of patient complaints (which they rate as the "secondary effects" of subluxations) unnecessary for chiropractic treatment. They also focus exclusively on the detection and correction of vertebral subluxation via spinal adjustment. Straights do not "mix" other types of therapies in their practice but instead prefer to remain a separate profession distinct from mainstream health care (Ingraham, 2020).

On the contrary, mixers, representing the majority group, are open to mainstream medicine but retain some belief in vertebral subluxation. They incorporate and "co-join" diagnostic and treatment techniques from osteopathic, orthodox medicine, acupuncture, homeopathy, along with nutritional supplements, herbal remedies, and physical therapy modalities such as exercise, massage, ice packs, moist heat, and biofeedback.

Several systematic studies have evaluated the effectiveness of chiropractic spinal manipulation in treating back pain and disability. The studies found a low to moderate treatment effect. The studies' evidence was rated down because of the small sample size (Goertz et al., 2018). In 2019, Goertz and Coulter implemented a multi-site, comparative effectiveness study among 750 US active-duty military personnel with low back pain. The sample, aged 18–50 years, were assigned to receive either usual medical care (UMC) alone ($n = 375$) or standard medical care plus chiropractic care (UMC + CC; $n = 375$). The UMC consists of treatments recommended by the patient physicians for low back pain, including prescription medications, physical therapy, or specialist referral. Chiropractic care included a combination of spinal manipulation, physical therapy modalities, and self-care recommendations. The patients rated their low back pain (LBP) intensity on a 10-point numerical rating scale and with an LBP-related functional disability obtained from the Roland Morris Disability Questionnaire administered online. Other outcome measures included a responder analysis, pain medication use, global LBP improvement, and patient satisfaction. The investigators measured the outcomes at baseline (during the prior week), two, four, six (primary endpoint), and 12 weeks' periods. Overall, the patients assigned to the UMC + CC group reported statistically significant mild to a moderate short-term reduction in LBP intensity (mean difference: -1.1; 95% CI, -1.4 to -0.7), physical disability (mean difference: 2.2; 95% CI, -3.1 to -1.2) and in the secondary outcome measures than the UMC group. The findings met established thresholds for moderate clinical effects – no related severe adverse events in either group. The side effects reported by the UMC + CC group consisted of transient muscle and joint stiffness (Goertz and Coulter, 2019).

In mainstream orthodox medicine, chiropractic is a controversial treatment. This is because, in part, some people experience stiffness, tiredness, and minor aches for a few days post-manipulation while their body adjusts to the new alignment. Besides, few cases of severe adverse effects resulting from damage to blood vessels (cervical vertebra artery) and stroke have been reported in the literature. During cervical manipulation, chiropractors often apply sudden rotation and force that can cause a small tear in the artery walls in the neck and form a blood clot at the site, which may later break free to block a blood vessel in the brain and cause a stroke (Ingraham, 2020). The incidence of stroke following cervical manipulation is rare: only about 1 out of 3 million manipulations, which are a small risk when compared to between 210,000 and 440,000 patients each year admitted to the hospital, suffer some preventable injuries that contributes to their death (Ernst, 2007; Turner et al., 2018; Vickers & Zollman, 1999).

Vertigo or unilateral facial paresthesia is a warning sign that may precede stroke onset by several days. Increased stroke risks associated with chiropractic visits are likely due to patients with headaches and neck pain from dissection (already in progress) seeking care before their (eventual) stroke. That data make medical errors the third-leading cause of death in America, behind heart disease, which is the first, and cancer, second. The consensus scientific evidence is that chiropractic effectiveness in treating lower back pain is at par with other manual therapies. There is no credible evidence on the efficacy of chiropractic in the treatment of visceral conditions (Painter, 2020).

Osteopathy The genesis of osteopathy dates back to the nineteenth century, but the profession has philosophical roots way back to the Hippocratic teaching in the fourth century BC. The osteopathy philosophy was developed in 1874 by Andrew Taylor Still, a Missouri physician and surgeon who recognized the importance of treating illness within the whole body's context. Still, the son of an itinerant Methodist preacher, was born in Virginia in 1828 and practiced medicine and farming. At the age of six, Still's father moved the family to Tennessee to accept a circuit preacher's position.

Globally, the scope of practice of osteopathy varies by country. In the United States, osteopathy is an alternative therapy, and osteopathic medicine is mainstream healthcare practice. Osteopathic physicians trained in the United States practice the entire scope of modern medicine and are called doctors of osteopathy (DOs). Osteopaths trained outside the United States are not physicians and are limited in practice to non-invasive manual therapies, nutritional, postural, and health education. In Canada, Europe, and Australia, osteopathy is considered an alternative treatment.

The American Osteopathic Association uses the terms "osteopathic physician" and "osteopathic medicine" to distinguish individuals trained in osteopathic medicine in the United States from osteopaths trained in osteopathy, the restricted-scope form of practice outside of North America. Osteopathic manipulative treatment (OMT in the United States or only "osteopathic treatment" in other countries) is the application of manually guided thrusts to improve physiologic function and support homeostasis that has been altered by somatic dysfunction: an impaired function of the skeletal, arthrodial, myofascial structures and their related vascular, lymphatic and neural elements.

Still's early education was a typical rural schooling experience with a hefty dose of discipline, a little bit of reading, writing, and arithmetic. He was frustrated with what he viewed as the ineffective and hazardous nature of remedies at that time. In the late 1800s, none of today's miracle drugs, including antibiotics, was available.

Dr. Still believed that the physician's role in treating disease was to restore proper musculoskeletal function to the body. At the age of 10, Dr. Still suffered from frequent headaches and nausea. Consequently, he built a rope swing, 8–10 inches off the ground between two trees, and lay down on it swinging back and forth. He wrote, "I lay stretched on my back, with my neck across the rope. Soon I became easy and went to sleep, got up in a little while with a headache all gone" (The Osteopathic Cranial Academy, 2018). Following this experience, he continued to use the swing as a "treatment" device every time he had a headache. Thus, he conceptualized osteopathy on the philosophy that all body systems are interrelated and dependent on good health.

Dr. Still theorized that dysfunction in the musculoskeletal system causes most diseases and that the body's structure and function are inseparable. He argued that the human body could stimulate its healing mechanisms, having the inherent capacity to defend, repair, and remodel itself. He wrote, "the body is an integrated unit of mind, body, and spirit ... Man is Triune" (Osteopathic Medical Foundation, n.d.). Out of necessity, Dr. Still looked first to nature's own ability to heal and found a way to access this ability within the body.

As a surgeon, Dr. Still observed that diseased organs were substantially congested during surgery, and he sought a non-surgical means of alleviating this congestion. He eventually developed a method of improving restricted tissues, using his hands to relieve the congestion. He used this body self-correcting capacity as the cornerstone of the osteopathic philosophy that he developed. The ailments his patients suffered include acute dysentery and sciatica. While many of his patients improved dramatically, others improved a little bit. Considering the other therapeutic tools available at the time, he was more effective than many other allopathic physicians during his era.

Dr. Still became a Kansas state and territorial legislator and a free-state leader. During the American Civil War, he lived near Baldwin City, Kansas, developed the practice of osteopathy, and coined the term "osteopathy." He established the American School of Osteopathy (now called AT Still University of the Health Sciences) in 1892 at Kirksville, Missouri. The school taught mobilization, manipulation, nutrition, and lifestyle modifications, rather than surgery and drug therapies. The State of Missouri granted the school the right to award the doctor of medicine (MD) degree, but Dr. Sill was dissatisfied with conventional medicine's limitations and instead chose to retain the doctor of osteopathy (DO) degree distinction. Vermont became the first state in 1896 to license DOs. In 1898, the American Institute of Osteopathy launched the Journal of Osteopathy, and by that time, four other States recognized the profession. In 1901, the American Osteopathic Association was formed to regulate the occupation.

Even during Still's lifetime, the early osteopathic colleges began teaching drug therapy. Orthodox medicine continued to oppose osteopathy until 1962, when DOs had full practice rights in all 50 states. By 1973, the California Medical Association recognized the DOs as voting members. The International Osteopathic Association in 2012 approved June 22 every year as the "World Osteopathy Day" to mark the day osteopathy was founded by Still. At various times Still called himself a "magnetic healer" and a "lightning bonesetter." Some of his maneuvers resembled those used by British bonesetters and magnetic physicians of his time. On December 12, 1917, Andrew Taylor Still died from the complications of the stroke he had sustained 3 years earlier. His influence gradually weakened as drugs became more clinically practical and introduced into the curriculum. As modern medicine emerged, the practice of osteopathy became less frequent. Nevertheless, many osteopathic physicians continue to value the wisdom of the original teachings and seek a deeper understanding of osteopathy.

Osteopathic training has become identical to conventional allopathic medical schools. They still grant the DO degree, and they always teach osteopathy. Most DOs are primary care practitioners specializing in family medicine, internal medicine, obstetrics, gynecology, or pediatrics. A few DOs are employed in other medical specialties. Although osteopathic manipulations were initially intended and used to treat all forms of diseases, they are mainly used to treat musculoskeletal disorders. The DOs learn manipulation therapies (hands-on adjustments of muscles, bones, and ligaments) and use these in conjunction with the more conventional medical treatments.

Although Dr. Still was opposed by conventional physicians, his osteopathic concept is robust and made a lasting impression on medicine throughout the world. Osteopathic and conventional basic science research has validated many of Still's original ideas. Today, even the conventional medical establishment globally has formed many manual medicine societies, and the specialties of Physical Medicine and Rehabilitation benefitted tremendously from much of Still's pioneering work. Still and his followers linked every disease or illness to structural dysfunction in the spine. They posited that when problems arise in the spine, the nerves send signals of that abnormality to the body's organs. He called these spinal problems "osteopathic lesions" ("osteo" for bone and "pathic" for diseased) and devised osteopathic manipulation techniques to treat them. The following is a sample of the numerous osteopaths Still mentored over the long period of his impressive career:

1. Daniel David Palmer, a magnetic healer from Davenport, Iowa, came to Kirksville in 1893 to be treated by Still.
2. John Martin Littlejohn, in 1900, established the Littlejohn College of Osteopathy and Hospital in Chicago, Illinois, where he taught and practiced until 1913 when he returned to London and founded the British School of Osteopathy in 1917. Littlejohn taught without a break at the British school until the outbreak of World War II in 1939.
3. William Garner Sutherland, DO, extended osteopathic principles to the study of the cranium and developed a diagnostic and therapeutic modality involving the motion of the bones of the cranium and manipulation of the subtle flow of energy in the body. This osteopathic concept has spread worldwide. There are colleges in England, Canada, and other parts of Europe whose activities and operations are informed by these principles.
4. J. M. Littlejohn invited John Wernham to study osteopathy in 1928. After that, Wernham studied, lectured, and practiced for over 70 years, guided by the teachings of Dr. Littlejohn. Taking advantage of his longevity, Wernham produced an extensive library of osteopathic texts. The Maidstone College of Osteopathy was founded in 1984 by John Wernham and devoted to Dr. J. M. Littlejohn's teaching philosophy. The institution was renamed John Wernham College of Classical Osteopathy in 1996 in honor of the founder. The College honors Wernham's legacy by offering postgraduate courses on classical osteopathy and publishing books. Born in 1907, Wernham practiced, taught, wrote, and published in various osteopathy areas until his death in February of 2007 at 99.

5. A small subdivision of UK osteopathic practitioners is known as "classical osteopaths." They followed John Martin Littlejohn and John Wernham's teaching and referred to their practice as a "total" body adjustment style.

Three primary philosophical schools of thought in osteopathy are classical, cranial, and cranial sacral therapy. Classical osteopaths claim that "total" body adjustment treatment leads to successful patient outcomes in many "functional and pathological disorders" such as infections and degenerative conditions. This school of thought places great emphasis on the clearance of the products of metabolism. However, their approach is contentious even within their school, which takes us next to cranial osteopathy. Like classical brethren, cranial osteopaths are a controversial specialty of osteopathy that seeks to revitalize the small rhythms ordinarily present at the skull's sutures. Cranial osteopaths feel the rhythm at the lines between the skull bones, evaluate the quality of that rhythm, and apply subtle, indirect force to enhance its movement and pulsation. This treatment assists the cerebrospinal fluid in flowing and circulating, offering the central nervous system nutrition, detoxification, and protection from trauma. Cranial osteopathy is the precursor to cranial sacral therapy developed by John Upledger.

Osteopathy is generally regarded as a safe treatment and only associated with minor side effects, such as mild to moderate soreness or pain in the treatment area, headache, and fatigue. These untoward side effects typically develop within a few hours of a treatment session and usually get better on their own within 2 days. In rare cases, severe complications are linked to OMT involving the neck performed by osteopaths. These include tearing an artery wall leading to a stroke, resulting in permanent disability or even death.

Certain health conditions (osteoporosis, fractures, acute inflammatory conditions, and infections, blood-clotting disorders, such as hemophilia, cancer, and multiple sclerosis) are contraindicated to osteopathy treatment. Osteopathy is also not recommended for patients taking blood-thinning medicines, such as warfarin and those having a course of radiotherapy.

Several prospective studies have demonstrated the effectiveness and safety of osteopathic manipulative treatment (OMT) as an adjunct to standard medical care (Licciardone et al., 2013a, 2013b; Hensel et al., 2016; Noll et al., 2016). A review of OMT articles over six decades by Vick and associates (1996) did not find any serious adverse event. They speculated that using the RCT method to evaluate the efficacy and safety of OMT would be cost-prohibitive, requiring thousands of patient encounters. Consequently, Seffinger (2018) recommended gathering efficacy and safety data on serious adverse events more pragmatically through a practice-based research network instead of using the RCT strategy.

The *Journal of the American Osteopathic Association,* in 2018, published a practice-based research network study by Degenhardt and associates. They interviewed 880 patients treated with OMT procedures involving more than 1800 office encounters. All the clinicians but two (one was an MD and the other a foreign-trained osteopath) were US-trained osteopathic physicians. To limit reporting bias, the patients reported to the researchers any adverse events immediately after

OMT. The study revealed that OMT's adverse events were generally mild (e.g., pain/discomfort), and no serious adverse event was reported (Degenhardt et al., 2018).

Adverse events from manual therapy procedures similar to high-velocity, low-amplitude OMT performed by non-osteopathic physicians have been documented (Carnes et al., 2010; Nielsen et al., 2017). But Degenhardt and associates (2018) observed far fewer adverse event cases from high-velocity, low-amplitude OMT techniques than reported in previous retrospective studies (Licciardone et al., 2013a, 2013b; Hensel et al., 2016; Noll et al., 2016).

Considerable evidence from RCTs exist on the beneficial effects of spinal manipulation for treating back and neck pain. The existing studies are often criticized for failing to exclude non-specific effects of treatment. A well-known example is the United Kingdom's clinical trial involving 741 patients with low back pain randomized to chiropractic or hospital outpatient care. The treating clinicians in both groups were free to treat patients as they saw fit. The study concluded that "chiropractic almost certainly confers worthwhile, long-term benefit." However, a recent systematic review of this and similar trials highlights methodological weaknesses, such as the fact that commonly used outcome measures such as pain and disability scores are assessed by patients and therefore unblinded (Vickers & Zollman, 1999).

In one clinical trial that used blinded assessment of outcome, patients with back or neck pain were randomized to routine general practitioner care, placebo (deactivated thermotherapy), physiotherapy, or manipulation. The study found physiotherapy and manipulation superior to placebo and general practitioner care after 6 weeks, and after one year of follow-up, manipulation was superior to physiotherapy.

In addition to back and neck pain, other RCTs have also indicated that manipulative treatment effectively treats headaches, including migraines. The number of such studies is small to confirm credible external validity. Moreover, there is no valid evidence of the benefit of spinal manipulation in many of the other musculoskeletal conditions that are commonly treated by osteopathy and chiropractic. Aside from dysmenorrhea, a small number of studies have shown a positive effect of manipulative therapy. But current evidence did not benefit other disorders related to smooth muscles or viscera, such as asthma and hypertension.

There has been little research on cranial osteopathy (Vickers & Zollman, 1999). Several critics contend that the knowledge base of osteopathy is not anchored in science. Limited empirical data exist that demonstrated osteopathy's effectiveness in treating medical conditions other than low back pain. Currently, no convincing empirical data show osteopathy effective in treating asthma, dysmenorrheal, shoulder pain, migraines, sinusitis, stress, or depression.

There are currently 26 Osteopathic Medical Schools in the United States that have produced over 70,000 osteopathic physicians (ValueMD, 2005). Only about 2000 osteopaths practice the original healing art, with some osteopaths using manipulation as an adjunct to their conventional practices. Over 100 million people annually visit DOs in the United States, and the American Osteopathic Association approves over 200 teaching hospitals.

Alternative Medical Systems

Traditional Chinese Medicine Traditional Chinese Medicine (TCM) practice dates back to 200 B.C. Other Eastern countries, such as Korea, Japan, India, and Vietnam, have all developed their unique TCM versions. The Native American, Aboriginal, African, Middle Eastern, Tibetan, Central, and South American cultures have developed their traditional medical systems. Ancient medicines include Chinese, Asian, Pacific Islander, American Indian, and Tibetan practices. Conventional oriental medicine emphasizes Qi's proper balance or disturbances (pronounced as "chee"), or vital energy, in health and disease. TCM is an alternative medical system used to diagnose, treat, and prevent illnesses for more than 2000 years (Tabish, 2008).

The early writings about TCM date back to 200 B.C, and classical Chinese texts recorded herbal medicine and acupuncture, including the theory, practice, diagnosis, and treatment of various diseases – over many centuries, it has been refined. The method of TCM stayed in Asia for centuries. Chinese immigrants have been practicing TCM in the United States since the mid-nineteenth century. Still, it remained unknown to most Americans before 1971 when James Reston, a *New York Times* reporter covering former President Richard Nixon's trip to China, had an emergency appendectomy. Post-surgery, he was treated with acupuncture to relieve pain, and his stories about this experience fascinated the American public. Over the years, TCM has become a mainstream alternative medicine practiced in the United States.

Traditional Eastern medicine consists of techniques and methods that include oriental Shiatsu massage, acupuncture, acupressure, Moxibustion (burning an herb near the skin), Cupping, and herbal supplements Qigong (a form of energy therapy). Chinese medical orthodoxy believes that disease is the alterations in the normal flow of Qi (pronounced as "chee") via meridians such that "Yin" and "Yang" are imbalanced. It theorizes that diseases are a function of three primary "causes": (1) external or environmental factors, (2) internal emotions, and (3) lifestyle factors such as diet. In the Asian/Chinese culture, Yin (the black) contains a seed of Yang (in the form of a white dot).

Each limb has six channels, three Yin channels on the inside and three Yang channels outside. The specific meridian is the "channels" or "vessels" for transporting blood and body fluids and Qi around the body. Each of the 12 regular channels corresponds to the five Yin organs, the five Yang organs, Pericardium, and San Jiao. The arm Yin meridians are Lung, Heart, and Pericardium, while the arm Yang meridians are the Large Intestine, Small Intestine, and Triple Warmer. The leg Yin meridians are Spleen, Kidney, and Liver. The leg Yang meridians are the Stomach, Bladder, and Gall Bladder. The five Yin and the five Yang organs have no anatomical equivalent in Western medicine, though they relate to processes in the body (Kootenaycolumbiacollege, 2018).

Like the Yin and Yang approach, the five-element philosophical theory is ancient and universal in what it embodies. The method is embedded intricately into Chinese culture's fabric and the foundation of Chinese disciplines, such as Feng Shui, the

Martial Arts, and the Ching. The theory posits that there are five "organ" systems in the body: Kidney, Heart, Spleen, Liver, and Lung. The five-organ system corresponds to more than individual body parts; it is a healing system. For example, the kidney represents the urinary system in its entirety, along with the adrenal glands that sit on top of the kidneys. The heart represents both the brain and the heart. The Chinese description of "organs" is not identical to the body's physical and anatomical organs in Western medicine.

The five-element philosophical theory provides a framework to diagnose and treat all health issues: body, mind, emotions, and spirit. The five elements include the internal organs, and the interconnected and interacting relationships between them repeatedly fall out of balance, creating health issues. With their treatment interventions, TCM practitioners seek to rebalance these organ relationships.

Lee and associates claimed that "throughout the 5000-year history of China, more than 300 epidemics were recorded, and TCM were used effectively to combat each of these epidemics' infections and saved many lives." Following the outbreak of coronavirus disease 2019 (COVID-19) in the Wuhan district, Lee and his associates conducted a retrospective analysis of the herbal preparations used in China to treat COVID-19. The authors claimed they found TCM is beneficial in the treatment of virus infection. When they compared their result with Western medicine, they argued, "TCM is superior in preventing infected patients escalated to severe cases and reduced the number of patients admitted to the intensive care unit (ICU)." One of the hospitals surveyed reported the "efficacy rate" of TCM treatment was 99.2%. The TCM was used in conjunction with the treatment provided to patients in the ICU receiving Western medicine. The investigators found TCM was effective in the recovery phase of the infection for patients released from the ICU. The meridian system, which guides all TCM treatments of human diseases, was provided as the scientific evidence for treating COVID-19 infection, particularly for treating acute lung injuries, which is the common symptom of the disease (Lee et al., 2021). The external validity of this study is minimal. The design did not meet the rigorous clinical trial scientific inquiry methods in the West. For example, there was no randomization in the study design. The dependent variables monitored were very subjective, and the researchers tested no hypothesis and, therefore, did not use any inferential statistics to compare the two groups.

A national survey in the United States showed that one in five Americans use TCM and Tai chi practices to treat medical conditions such as stroke, heart disease, mental disorders, respiratory diseases (bronchitis and the common cold), and mixed results. The studies were of low quality in experimental design, and the researcher can draw no valid conclusions about their effectiveness. More concerning is that herbal products are often contaminated with undeclared plant or animal material, drugs (such as the blood-thinner warfarin and the non-steroidal anti-inflammatory agent diclofenac), and heavy metals (such as arsenic, lead, and cadmium). Contamination with pesticides or compounds called sulfites could cause asthma or severe allergic reactions; or incorrect herbs, some of which have caused organ damage. Also, manufacturing errors resulting from one herb being mistakenly replaced with another can cause serious complications (NCCIH, 2019).

Tai chi combines specific postures with mental focus, breathing, relaxation, and gentle movements. Research findings revealed that tai chi treatment might improve balance and stability in older people and those with Parkinson's disease, reduce knee osteoarthritis pain, fibromyalgia, and back pain, and improve mood. Tai chi and a similar qi gong technique are relatively safe and unlikely to cause any severe injury, but they are associated with minor aches and pains. Therefore, pregnant women should consult with their healthcare providers before beginning tai chi, qi gong, or any high-intensity exercise program (NCCIH, 2019).

In the United States, the Food and Drug Administration (FDA) classifies TCM herbal medicine as "dietary supplements," and manufacturers do not need to get pre-market approval but are responsible for ensuring that the products are safe and claims of effectiveness are supported by scientific evidence (University of Minnesota, 2016).

There are currently 35 oriental medicine training programs in the United States. Recently, nine Chinese medical institutions and Ohio University College of Osteopathic Medicine joined forces to study TCM's mechanism and its application in Western medicine. Similarly, the University of Pittsburgh created an International TCM Center to coordinate research efforts with similar institutions in China. Australia introduced TCM in its national medical system in 2012, and both Portugal and Hungary formally approved it in their healthcare system in 2013.

Ayurveda Ayurveda, also called Ayurvedic medicine, is an alternative medicine healing system developed in India more than 3000 years ago in Sanskrit. Ayurveda, derived from Atharvaveda, is from the Sanskrit words Ayur (life) and Veda (science or knowledge), whose translation means life science or knowledge of life (Johns Hopkins University, 2021). Dhanvantari, the physician to the gods in Hindu mythology, is the progenitor of Ayurveda (Augustyn, 2021). It has grown into a well-established medical system due to the untiring efforts of the icons of "gurukulas" and the herbal industries of India, especially the Patanjali, Dabur, Zandu, Baidyanath, and Himalaya. The influence of Ayurveda is so profound that the Middle East and Europe's impact could not deter its popularity among the citizens of India (Balkrishna & Misra, 2017).

Ayurvedic medicine has both preventive and curative components. The preventive aspect emphasizes a strict code of personal and social hygiene, depending on individual, climatic, and environmental needs, Yoga, and exercises. The curative part involves the use of herbal medicines, external preparations, physiotherapy, and diet. The preventive and therapeutic measures are adapted to meet the personal requirements of each patient (Augustyn, 2021). Today, Ayurveda is a comprehensive natural healing system that focuses equally on the body, mind, and spirit and strives to restore the individual's innate harmony. The primary Ayurvedic treatments are diet, exercise, meditation, herbs, massage, exposure to sunlight, and controlled breathing. In addition, Ayurveda follows a traditional diet and engages in regular detoxes believed to rid toxins' body and mind and ultimately prevent illnesses. However, many health experts are skeptical of detoxification's purported benefits (Davidson and Tinsley, 2020).

Ayurvedic preparations are used commonly in Asian countries, including India, Bangladesh, Pakistan, Afghanistan, Nepal, Sri Lanka, and Myanmar. In addition, they are gaining popularity in the United States, Canada, United Kingdom, and Australia, where they are used as dietary supplements. Ayurvedic preparations are made from leaves, roots, barks, or whole plants with/without the addition of metallic and non-metallic substances called 'Bhasma' (Sarker, 2014). The knowledge of traditional medicinal plants is passed on through generations right from India's Vedic period.

Ayurvedic products are potentially toxic, and the formulations may cause arsenic poisoning. A study published in the *Journal of the American Medical Association* in 2008 revealed that 20% of Ayurvedic products made in the United States and India contained detectable lead, mercury, or arsenic. The researchers identified 25 websites selling Ayurvedic products and found 673 Ayurvedic products. They subsequently randomly selected 230 out of the 673 produced and purchased them. They received 193 of the 230 products purchased online, and when analyzed, 21% contained detectable levels of lead, mercury, or arsenic (Food and Drug Administration, 2008).

A 2015 study from the United States found 40% of patients using Ayurvedic preparations had elevated lead blood levels, and some had elevated blood levels of mercury. About 25% of the supplements tested had high levels of lead, and 50% had high levels of mercury – another 2015 case study linked elevated blood lead levels in a 64-year-old woman with Ayurvedic products purchased online. The latter study was published in the US Centers for Disease Control and Prevention's (CDC) *Morbidity and Mortality Weekly Report* (NCCIH, 2020). Most Ayurvedic remedies consist of combinations of herbs and other medicines, an occurrence that makes it challenging to delineate which ones are safe and effective. The following four studies from the US National Center for Complementary and Integrative Health (NCCIH) found Ayurveda to be effective.

1. A 2013 clinical trial conducted among 440 patients with knee osteoarthritis compared two Ayurvedic formulations of plant extracts against the natural product glucosamine sulfate and the drug celecoxib. All the treatment types produced similar pain reduction and improvements in function.
2. An exploratory study on rheumatoid arthritis funded by NCCIH in 2011 among 43 patients found conventional treatment with methotrexate and Ayurvedic treatments (which included 40 herbal compounds) produced similar effective outcomes.
3. Another small short-term clinical trial that evaluated five Ayurvedic herbs among 89 men and women with type 2 diabetes produced some benefits. However, weak study designs prevent any externally valid conclusion on the effectiveness of Ayurveda in the treatment of diabetes.
4. Two studies evaluated the benefits of turmeric – an herb used in Ayurvedic preparations – to treat ulcerative colitis and found it to be beneficial. The sample size of the two studies was small. One of the studies published in 2005 included only ten patients, while the other research published in 2006 had 89 patients (NCCIH, 2020).

The long history of Ayurveda notwithstanding, its scientific pedestal is lacking because no randomized, double-blind, placebo-controlled studies have been published on its efficacy. Recent debates on the toxicity of heavy metals (lead, mercury, and arsenic) in Ayurvedic preparations have brought attention to their safety. In addition, there is the possibility of bacterial contamination in the preparation of *Asava* and *Arista* – the two popular ingredients used in the preparation of Ayurvedic formulation. The fermentation technique is applied to polyherbal materials.

In an editorial published in 2014 by Sarker in the *Journal of Homeopathic Ayurvedic Medicine*, inter-alia contends that Ayurvedic medicines "can be a potential and effective alternative for the treatment of diseases like cancer, diabetes, renal impairment, immunoimpotency or sexual weakness, weight loss or to reduce obesity, AIDS, immunosuppression or autoimmunity, heart diseases, neurological disorders, in which modern medicines have limited, or no success rate or have serious adverse effects." However, these claims should be taken with a dose of caution because they have not been bolstered by rigorous scientific evidence.

Guha and Cameron (2016) argued that Ayurveda defies the double-blind placebo-controlled strategy of experimentation because individual treatment is the fundamental tenet of Ayurveda. Each session is highly customized according to each patient's needs since no two persons are alike. For example, individuals are treated with a different formulation or diet for the same disease. Thus, Guha and Cameron posited those studies measuring outcomes "of a single treatment on large numbers of people are impossible within the Ayurvedic system."

In 1971, the government of India commissioned the Indian Medical Council to integrate indigenous practices with orthodox Western medicine. Most Ayurvedic medicine practitioners work in rural areas, providing primary health care to at least 500 million people (Augustyn, 2021). Despite the lack of rigorous double-blind placebo-controlled evidence, the Indian government currently licenses Ayurveda, Siddha, Unani, and Homeopathy practitioners. Ayurveda is offered at several universities at the bachelor's degree level, making it qualify for licensure status (Tabish, 2008). The Indian government also authorizes other therapies, such as Panchakarma and massage, related to Ayurveda.

The practice of Ayurveda and practitioners' training in the United States is not regulated – no state currently requires a license to practice (NCCIH, 2020). In contrast, the WHO presently recognizes Ayurveda as a traditional system of medicine. The formal definition of health by the WHO was adapted from the teaching of Ayurveda (Guha & Cameron, 2016).

Naturopathy Naturopathy is an alternative therapy that focuses on natural remedies to stimulate and support the body's healing ability. It is a holistic system of treating disease without pharmaceuticals or surgery but using special diets, herbs, vitamins, and massage to assist natural healing processes. Naturopathic practitioners strive to find the cause of disease by understanding the patient's body, mind, and spirit. The standard treatments include nutritional counseling, herbal medicine, homeopathic medicine, acupuncture, hydrotherapy, massage, hot and cold packs, electric currents, and sound waves to manipulate the muscles, bones, and spine.

Hippocrates, a Greek physician who lived 2400 years ago, is often considered the progenitor of naturopathy. In Europe, traditional and indigenous medicines combined with Traditional Chinese Medicine came together uniquely in Germany to form a distinct profession termed naturopathy. However, as we know today, naturopathy was founded and named by German physician Benedict Lust in 1892. Lust immigrated to the United States in 1896, wherein, in 1902, he established the Unborn Health Institute in New Jersey. Lust sought a holistic system of treating disease without pharmaceuticals or surgery and strived to find the cause of illness by understanding the patient's body, mind, and spirit – Man is Triune: three in one – like Dr. Still's teaching. He emphasized natural cures, proper bowel habits, and good hygiene as the primary tools for health. Basic dietary principles, such as increasing fiber intake and minimizing saturated fats, were his teaching and treatment tenets.

Naturopathy became popular in the United States between 1920 and 1930, and medical practitioners from various specialties came together to form the Naturopathic Medical Society. By 1920, over 10,000 practitioners joined the Society. Between 1920 and 1930, twenty Naturopathic Colleges existed in the United States. However, only five Naturopathic Colleges are in the United States and two in Canada. Between 1940 and 1950, naturopathy fell out of favor because of the discovery of antibiotics to treat many diseases. As a result, people abandoned the natural way of treating conditions. Following the discovery of antibiotics in 1948, conventional medicine came into prominence, and naturopathy faded in America. In the 1970s, naturopathy regained some popularity as Americans developed a new appreciation for alternative and "holistic" approaches to medicine, leading to a renaissance and acceptance of alternative health care.

Today, naturopathy is practiced in the United States, Australia, Canada, New Zealand, and the United Kingdom. Like medical school, neuropathic education is 4 years in duration, and students take the same basic sciences as medical students. Naturopathic practitioners' study holistic and non-toxic approaches to treatment with an emphasis on wellness and disease prevention. Naturopathic physicians receive training in diet and clinical nutrition, acupuncture, hydrotherapy, homeopathic medicine, botanical medicine, psychology (behavioral change), counseling, physical medicine, pharmaceuticals, and minor surgery (Fleming & Gutknecht, 2010). The medical schools in the United Kingdom do not offer courses in the clinical aspects of alternative medicine. However, it is integrated into the curriculum of several unconventional medical schools. Teaching is primarily theoretical, emphasizing communicating with alternative medicine practitioners (Tabish, 2008).

In 2010, in two separate monographs, the WHO provided the standards for training naturopaths (WHO, 2010a) and osteopaths (WHO, 2010b). In the United States and Canada, practitioners of naturopathic medicine take professional board exams as primary care general practice physicians. Currently, 15 states and two territories in the United States and several provinces in Canada, Australia, and New Zealand require licensure for naturopathic physicians (Fleming & Gutknecht 2010). Many osteopaths, dentists, nurses, and other HCPs also practice naturopathic medicine. They are employed in hospitals, clinics, community health centers, and private practices to provide individual and family health care.

The various naturopathic organizations have differing perspectives on the scope of practice, and different practitioners take different approaches to diagnosis and treatment. Naturopathic practitioners treat both short bouts of illness and chronic conditions, but their emphasis is on preventing diseases and educating patients. A conventional naturopath may prescribe medication to suppress symptoms and perform minor surgeries, but naturopaths emphasize the use of natural healing agents and collaborate with traditional medicine counterparts. On the other hand, traditional naturopaths do not use pharmaceutical agents but will search for alternative approaches to restore health that is not confined to curing illnesses. (WebMD, 2020).

The efficacy and safety of naturopathy are a matter of debate in the existing literature. Dunne and associates (2005) underscore the conundrum by stating that "documenting the safety and efficacy of naturopathic interventions presents significant challenges … naturopathic practice is distinguished by treatments individualized to a patient's physical condition and environmental circumstances, requiring combination therapies adjusted over time as guided by patient response." In response to this challenge, the NIH in 2002 funded more than 1200 researchers in a 2-year effort to develop the collaborative infrastructure required to examine the theory and practice of naturopathic medicine. The pace of development and overall research output from this effort is slow and inconsequential – RCTs are few. A leading naturopathic researcher, Britt Marie Hermes, in 2016, failed to confirm whether naturopathy is safe and effective.

In 2019, Myers and Vigar investigated the current state of evidence for using naturopathic medicine. The researchers identified 9859 studies for screening, but only 33 met the study inclusion criteria. The 33 studies reflect a range of mainly chronic clinical conditions and were conducted in the United States (11), Canada (4), Germany (6), India (7), Australia (3), United Kingdom (1), and Japan (1). The authors concluded that whole-system, multi-modality naturopathic medicine "effectively treats cardiovascular disease, musculoskeletal pain, type 2 diabetes, polycystic ovary syndrome, depression, anxiety, and a range of complex chronic conditions" (Myers & Vigar, 2019).

As the potential for harm does exist within the scope of practice of naturopathy, licensure in the United States requires that adverse medical events be reported to the federally mandated National Practitioner Databank. Over 10 years (1992–2002), 1805 licensees filed 173 complaints with the state licensing boards, and the board initiated 31 disciplinary actions. The punitive measures range from probation to fines or censure (Dunne et al., 2005). Some naturopathic treatments, such as homeopathy, Rolfing, and iridology, are widely considered quackery or pseudoscience. William Jarvis, inter-alia states, "non-scientific health care practitioners, including naturopaths, use unscientific methods and deception on a public who, lacking in-depth health care knowledge, must rely upon the assurance of providers. Quackery not only harms people, but it also undermines the ability to conduct scientific research, and should be opposed by scientists" (Jarvis, 1992). Furthermore, naturopathic practitioners are criticized for their "pervasive culture of patient blaming" where "when something doesn't work for the patient. The patient is not experiencing all of the positive effects and zero side effects that are promised with the therapy.

It's never because the therapy doesn't work; it's because the patient didn't do something right" (Andras, 2016).

Homeopathy Homeopathy is an alternative therapy that utilizes highly diluted preparations in tablet form to stimulate the body's natural healing process. A homeopath (Doctor of Homeopathy) will match the most appropriate medicine to patients based on their specific symptoms. It is a medical theory and clinical practice system that employs the smallest doses of a material that causes symptoms to trigger the body's self-healing response. Homeopathic practitioners hypothesized that one could select therapies by how closely symptoms produced by a remedy match the patient's disease signs. The phenomenon is called the "principle of similars." Because the ingredients of homeopathic remedies are in the minute, potentially non-existent material dosages, there is pessimism in the scientific world about its effectiveness (Tabish, 2008).

Many homeopaths assert that Hippocrates originated in about 400 BC by prescribing a small dose of mandrake root to treat mania itself; a more massive amount of mandrake root produced mania. Egyptian and Greek physicians use bloodletting as a first-line treatment for diseases (a migraine, fever, and hypertension) before all other therapies. In the absence of different remedies for hypertension, bloodletting could potentially have a salutary effect in temporarily reducing blood pressure by decreasing blood volume. Given that hypertension is very often asymptomatic and not diagnosed without modern methods, this effect was unintentional. At the time, physicians would open a vein with a lancet or sharpened piece of wood, and blood would flow out into a waiting receptacle. The practice continued in Europe until the end of the eighteenth century. The actual use of bloodletting was harmful to patients in the overwhelming majority of cases. New treatments and technologies edged out bloodletting by the late 1800s, and prominent physicians began to discredit the practice. Today, "phlebotomy" draws blood for laboratory analysis or blood transfusion or in sports for blood doping purposes. Therapeutic phlebotomy refers to withdrawing blood in specific cases like hemochromatosis, polycythemia vera, and porphyria cutanea tarda to reduce the number of red blood cells.

The roots of homeopathy are traced to a German physician Samuel Christian Hahnemann who lived from 1755 to 1843. Mainstream physicians during his era used bloodletting and purging and administered complex mixtures, such as Venice treacle, made from 64 substances, such as opium, myrrh, and viper's flesh, to treat diseases. Hahnemann rejected the practices extolled for centuries and advocated that the therapies are irrational and inadvisable. He proposed using single drugs at lower doses and promoting an immaterial, vitalistic theory of living organisms' function. He averred that diseases have spiritual, as well as physical, causes. Hahnemann came across a publication that claimed that the quinine-containing Peruvian bark (chinchona) cured malaria and coined the term homeopathy while translating a Scottish physician's medical treatise chemist William Cullen into German. Skeptical of Cullen's theory of using cinchonas to treat malaria and using himself as a subject, Hahnemann ingested a pellet of Peruvian bark. He began to feel feverish, shivering, joint pain, exhausted, desperately thirsty, and agitated – all of which he recognized as symptoms of malaria. From this experience, Hahnemann postulated that all effective drugs produce symptoms in healthy individuals similar to those they treat. This opinion is consistent with the "law of similars" proposed by ancient physicians. The pioneer of pharmacology, Paracelsus, declared in the sixteenth century that small doses of "what makes a man ill also cures him" (Hargrave, 2021).

Specialist pharmacies typically prepare homeopathic remedies using a careful dilution process and "succussion" (a specific form of vigorous shaking). Homeopaths further dilute "mother tincture" with lactose or alcohol, one part to 10 (written as "x" or one part to 100 (written as "c"). When vigorously shaken, these tinctures yield a one x or 1c dilution. Homeopath pharmacies can dilute these tinctures further 2x or 2c, 3x or 3c, and so forth. Any dilution is indicated for treatment, but the most commonly used is the 6x, 12x, 30x 6c, 12c, and 30c tinctures. Homeopaths believe the more diluted the substance, the more potent the healing powers. The homeopathic remedies prescribed are based on the patient's symptoms and for no more than 2 or 3 days. Some patients take only one or two doses of the remedies before they feel well; others may need more than one or two doses. If treatment fails, homeopaths believe the medications may be illegal.

The homeopathic practice is criticized as unethical. Scientists believe the mechanisms of action of homeopathic remedies are not only scientifically implausible, but the laws of physics preclude them. The mechanism of action of ultra-high dilutions in the human body is yet to be fully explained by scientists. However, laboratory experiments have repeatedly demonstrated that homeopathically prepared substances cause biological effects in animal models. The United States jurist Oliver Wendell Holmes Jr. (1841–1935) failed to reproduce the symptoms reported by Hahnemann following ingestion of cinchona Peruvian bark. Hahnemann's "law of similars" is still a postulate rather than an actual law of nature. Subsequent scientific work shows that Peruvian cinchona bark cures malaria because it contains quinine, which kills the Plasmodium falciparum parasite that causes sickness; its mechanism is unrelated to its symptoms cinchonism.

With the global popularity of homeopathy and market globalization, safety and the quality of care have become a significant concern because many of the raw materials and medicines in homeopathic products come from different countries. In 2009, in the Lombardy region of Italy, with 10 million people, about 20% of the population regularly uses homeopathic medicines. Still, almost 60% of them use them occasionally for their health and well-being more than 34% use homeopathic medicines for self-healing. The Regional Government of Lombardy collaborated with the WHO to develop a guideline that ensures that homeopathic products meet minimum global standards and high quality. The document produced by the WHO discussed the challenges for quality control of homeopathic medicines, quality control issues for homeopathic medication, and regulation regarding homeopathic medication. The document is ideal for promoting citizens' awareness about the safety and quality of homeopathic medicine (World Health Organization, 2009).

A 2012 National Health Interview Survey (NHIS) in the United States found that 5 million American adults and 1 million children used homeopathy in the previous year (Clarke et al., 2015). Although about 1.8% of children used homeopathy, only 0.2% of children went to a homeopathic practitioner. Most adults who used homeopathic products in the United States self-prescribe them for colds and musculoskeletal pain (NCCIH, 2018). In 2016, the U.S. Federal Trade Commission (FTC) announced it would hold over-the-counter homeopathic drugs to the same efficacy and safety standard as those for other similar products. And vendors must have reliable and valid scientific evidence that FTC requires for health-related claims, including claims on its use in treating specific conditions. In December 2017, the FDA proposed a new risk-based enforcement approach to homeopathic products that called for more scrutiny of products with the most significant risk for vulnerable populations, those intended for preventing or treating severe and life-threatening diseases and conditions, and those that are not taken by mouth or rubbed on the skin (NCCIH, 2018).

Back in time, the science of homeopathy was stoutly refuted based on the assessment that it lacks biological plausibility. The use of homeopathy is controversial because some of its key concepts are inconsistent with fundamental scientific concepts. It is difficult to explain in scientific terms how homeopathy products containing little or no active ingredient can have any meaningful physiological effect. Thus, the investigation of homeopathy products creates significant clinical challenges. Scientists cannot confirm what is listed on the label, nor have they developed objective measures that produce physiological effects in the human body for extremely dilute products (Kirby, 2002). Moreover, homeopathic treatments are individualized, and there is no uniform prescribing standard for homeopathic practitioners. There are hundreds of homeopathic remedies defined in various dilutions for thousands of symptoms.

A 2015 comprehensive assessment of homeopathy's efficacy and safety by the Australian National Health and Medical Research Council concluded that no reliable evidence that homeopathy is beneficial for any health condition (NCCIH, 2018). Certain homeopathic formulations called "nosodes" or "homeopathic immunizations" are promoted as substitutes for conventional immunizations. However, the CDC and NCCIH concluded no credible scientific evidence to support such claims.

Conventional HCPs and scientists have long considered homeopathy a sham, pseudoscience, and the mainstream medical community regard it as quackery (Tuomela, 1987; Smith, 2012; Baran et al., 2014; Ladyman, 2013; Ernst, 2002). Overall, the studies did not find the homeopathic remedies to be any more effective than a placebo – consistent with the lack of any biologically plausible pharmacological mechanism. Some clinical trials produced positive results, but recent systematic reviews suggest that the positive findings are chance, flawed research designs, and reporting bias.

A treatise published by the Americans for Homeopathy Choice in 2018 claimed: "thousands of studies and 200 years of clinical experience have shown that homeopathy is effective in treating a wide variety of conditions." They cited five studies that evaluated homeopathic medicines' effectiveness to bolster the view that homeopathy is effective. The first study cited is the *Journal of Rheumatology*, 2004; 43

(5):577–82. The double-blind three-month study compared patients with fibromyalgia treated with homeopathy with those treated with a placebo. Those treated with homeopathy showed significantly better outcomes than the placebo group. The improvements were also noticeable in other symptoms not related to the study. They attributed the latter finding to the belief that homeopathy treats the whole person, not just specific symptoms.

The second study cited by the Americans for Homeopathy Choice is also a randomized, double-blind, placebo-controlled trial that evaluated whether patients with severe sepsis in an intensive care unit who received homeopathic treatments would have a higher survival rate. The study was published in the *Journal of the Faculty of Homeopathy* 2005, 94(2): 75–80. The study findings revealed that long-term survival at 180 days was 76% for patients treated with homeopathy versus 50% for those treated with a placebo ($p < 0.05$).

The third study is a randomized, double-blind, placebo-controlled crossover study among children with attention deficit hyperactivity disorder treated with homeopathic treatment. The study was published in the *European Journal of Pediatrics*. 2005; 164 (12):758–67, and the findings revealed statistically significant differences in behavior and cognitive functions following homeopathy. The fourth study cited is a meta-analysis based on three RCTs published in the *Pediatric Infectious Disease Journal* 2003; 22 (3):229–34 that investigated the effectiveness of homeopathy in managing childhood diarrhea. The findings confirmed that individualized homeopathic treatment decreases the duration of acute childhood diarrhea. The fifth study cited by the Americans for Homeopathy Choice is an RCT published in *Cancer* 2001; 92 (3):684–90, which investigated the effectiveness of a homeopathic medication (Traumeel®) to treat chemotherapy-induced chemotherapy stomatitis in children undergoing stem cell transplantation. The researcher presented no objective finding, but they concluded that the homeopathic medicines "can significantly reduce the severity and duration of chemotherapy-induced stomatitis in children undergoing bone marrow transplantation."

In the United Kingdom, a 2010 House of Commons Science and Technology Committee report concluded that homeopathic products perform no better than placebos. The principles on which homeopathy is based are "scientifically implausible." The report also indicated that the "like cures like" focus is "theoretically weak" and that this is the "settled view of medical science." There's no evidence to support the homeopathic thesis that substances that cause specific symptoms can also help treat them. Nor is there any empirical evidence to support the idea that diluting and shaking substances in water can turn those substances into medicines. The tenets behind homeopathy philosophy are not accepted by mainstream medicine and are not consistent with long-accepted principles on how the physical world works. Conventional orthodox medicine and scientists consider homeopathy a sham, pseudoscience, and quackery (NHS, 2018a, b).

Homeopathic remedies are generally considered safe, and the risk of a severe adverse side effect is negligible. Although many homeopathic products are highly diluted, some products labeled as homeopathic contain essential active ingredients that can cause side effects or drug interactions with catastrophic health consequences. A 2012 systematic review by Kirby concluded that some homeopathic products contain heavy metals like mercury or iron that are not highly diluted and could cause serious adverse effects (Kirby, 2002). Some liquid homeopathic products contain alcohol at higher levels than conventional drugs. Although homeopathic practitioners expect some patients to experience "homeopathic aggravation" (a temporary worsening of existing symptoms after taking a homeopathic prescription), researchers have not found much evidence of this phenomenon in clinical studies. Moreover, research on homeopathic aggravations is limited.

In 2015, the FDA warned consumers not to use over-the-counter asthma products labeled as homeopathic because of no reliable study on its safety and effectiveness (FDA Center for Food Safety and Applied Nutrition (n.d.)). In 2017, the FDA alerted consumers that some homeopathic teething tablets had excessive amounts of the toxic substance belladonna. In 2019, FDA withdrew its compliance policy guide (CPG 400.400) on "Conditions Under Which Homeopathic Drugs May Be Marketed" because it is no longer consistent with the risk-based approach to regulatory and enforcement action. Revised draft guidance called "Drug Products Labeled as Homeopathic" was reissued by the FDA for public comment. Since FDA does not approve homeopathic drug products, it is reasonable to assume they have not met the standards for safety, effectiveness, and quality (NCCIH, 2018; United States Food and Drug Administration, 2020).

The NCCIH, in 2018, warned consumers not to use homeopathy to replace proven conventional care or postpone the visit to orthodox healthcare professionals. Mothers should not substitute homeopathic products for conventional immunizations and follow the recommended conventional immunization schedules for children and adults. Pregnant and nursing mothers or anyone should consult their healthcare providers before using a homeopathic product because they may pose a risk with untoward side effects or drug interactions (NCCIH, 2018).

About 25 homeopathic institutions exist in the United States, and most offer certification. No degree from any of the institutions provides a license to practice. However, some homeopaths are also mainstream conventional physicians. There are homeopaths licensed in virtually all health professions, including veterinarians. In many states, homeopathic practitioners must be licensed healthcare providers to practice homeopathy legally. The American Board of Homeotherapeutics recognizes MDs and D.O.s (Doctor of Osteopathic Medicine) specializing in homeopathy. Naturopaths study homeopathy as part of their medical training and are approved by the Homeopathic Academy of Naturopathic Physicians.

Aromatherapy For nearly 6000 years, the ancient Chinese, Egyptians, Indians, Greeks, and Romans utilized essential oils for therapeutic purposes. They used the essential oils in cosmetics, perfumes, and drugs for spiritual, therapeutic, hygienic, and ceremonial purposes.

Modern-day aromatherapy is traced back to 1928 when René-Maurice Gattefossé, a French chemist, discovered lavender oil's healing properties. He applied to a burn on his hand after an explosion in his laboratory. The bactericidal effect of essential oils promotes healing. He devoted his career to analyzing essential oils' chemical properties and systematically documented their usefulness in treating burns, skin infections, gangrene, and wounds in soldiers during World War I. By the 1950s massage therapists, nurses, physiotherapists, physicians/dentists, and beauticians began using aromatherapy.

In France, more than 1500 physicians trained to use essential oils as an alternative to antibiotics. Aromatherapy became popular in the United States in the 1980s when essential oils gained massage therapists' and alternative practitioners' attention. In 1990, Patricia Davis, who authored a book on aromatherapy, formed the National Association for Holistic Aromatherapy in Boulder, Colorado.

Aromatherapy is an alternative treatment that uses essential oils derived from volatile plant materials to alter a person's mind, mood, cognitive function, or health. The phrase "aroma" from Aromatherapy is Latin for "sweet odor" and Greek for "seasoning, any spice or sweet herb," in short, any fragrant substance with a distinctive, typically pleasant smell scent, fragrance, and perfume. However, the word "aroma" in aromatherapy is somewhat misleading because essential oils are not solely used as inhalants but can also be massaged into the skin or even taken orally (although this is less common). Essential oils are concentrated extracts made from the roots, leaves, or blossoms of plants. Each essential oil contains a mixture of active ingredients, and this mix determines the healing properties of the oil. The highly concentrated oils may be inhaled directly or indirectly or applied to the skin through massage, lotions, or bath salts.

Aromatherapy is applied through aerial diffusion as an environmental fragrance or aerial disinfection and by direct inhalation for treating respiratory disinfection, decongestion, expectoration, and psychological effects. Topical aromatherapy may occur through a massage, baths, compresses, therapeutic skin care, and oral ingestion. The latter is rare and usually takes place only under the supervision of a trained professional. Most topical and inhaled essential oils are safe to use and are sold over the counter or in stores, but they are often mislabeled. For this reason, the amount of essential oil contained in the bottle is unclear and may change in composition from dose to dose (if the oil is in capsules), and it is often doubtful whether it provides the remedy specified on the label. A qualified aromatherapist can determine which oils will be useful.

It is unwise to ingest essential oils because they are toxic and can be fatal when taken orally. Moreover, because they are highly volatile, essential oils should also not be applied near an open flame. Women in their first trimester of pregnancy and people with severe asthma or a history of allergies should avoid all essential oils.

Similarly, individuals with a history of seizures should avoid hyssop oil and avoid using essential oils near the eyes. Patients with high blood pressure should avoid stimulating essential oils, such as rosemary and spike lavender. Furthermore, patients with ovarian cancer receiving chemotherapy and estrogen-dependent breast should not use oils with estrogen-like compounds, such as fennel, aniseed, sage, and clary sage.

Aromatherapists emphasize that consumers should only use unadulterated essential oils, but the question of whether synthetic plant aromas can produce the desired therapeutic results is a hotly debated topic. Many aromatherapy practitioners recommend using authentic essential oils for topical use because synthetic products are more likely to have adverse reactions on the skin. However, the cost of essential oils is not cheap. Some rare agarwood oil teaspoons, some high-quality versions of commonly used essential oils, such as lavender, cost about $10–$20 per teaspoon. That seems pricey, and most patients in developing countries cannot afford it. That said, some aromatherapists insist that the price of essential oils is lower than the cost of many medication options (Jamrog, 2018).

Many aromatherapy proponents claim essential oils are safe when used as directed. Any essential oil safety depends on factors such as patient age, underlying health conditions, and medication and food supplement being used. It is crucial to consider the chemical composition and purity of the essential oil and the method of use, duration, and dosage. Pugle and Wilson (2019) provided safety guidelines for topical and oral use of different essential oils. The US FDA does not regulate essential oils used in aromatherapy. When oils are applied to the skin, they may elicit allergic reactions, skin irritation, and sun sensitivity (Bauer, 2020). Hence, further research is needed to determine how essential oils might affect children, pregnant, and breastfeeding women. Additionally, research is required to explore how essential oils might interact with prescribed medications and other treatments.

Regardless of the plant they are extracted from, aromatherapy oils must be administered carefully. When topically applied, contact with irritated or damaged skin must be avoided and particular attention paid to individuals with a history of contact with skin allergies. Consumers who are allergic to lavender and have skin irritability must avoid lavender aromatherapy (Koulivand et al., 2013). When the route of application is through the skin, the aromatherapist must dilute the essential oils at a concentration of 1.5%–3.0% in a carrier oil. If the contact also involves the face, the aromatherapist should increase the dilution to 0.2%–1.5% to prevent adverse reactions on the more sensitive skin.

Most importantly, consumers must avoid inhalation of large amounts of oils to prevent the triggering of seizures and bronchospastic episodes in predisposed individuals. Also, long exposures to oils should be avoided to avoid hypersensitivity (Antonelli & Donelli, 2020). Medical experts advise against the use of essential oil diffusers – a small household device that creates scented vapor – because diffusion in a public area can affect people differently (Johns Hopkins University, 2020).

Some oils promote physical healing, relieve swelling, or fight fungal infections. Some essential oils are used for therapeutic purposes because of their emotional value to enhance relaxation or enhance a room's pleasant smell and décor. For example, the essential oil derived from orange blossom contains ester, an active ingredient thought to induce a calming effect. The relaxing effect explains a bride's tradition in Western cultures carrying an orange blossom bouquet on the wedding day (Bauer, 2020). It is not entirely clear how aromatherapy and its products work. Bauer posits that it works by stimulating smell receptors in the nose, sending messages through the nervous system to the limbic system – the part of the brain that controls emotions.

Following an extensive review of the therapeutic on aromatherapy, Ali and associates concluded that it is a natural and non-invasive remedy that not only eradicates the disease symptoms but also rejuvenates the whole body by "regulating the physi-ological, spiritual and psychological upliftment for the new phase of life." It is rec-ommended to prevent and manage the acute and chronic phases of disease (Ali et al., 2015). Researchers at Johns Hopkins University found that certain essential oils can kill a type of Lyme bacteria better than antibiotics, but clinical trials in humans are mixed (Johns Hopkins University, 2020).

Aromatherapy enthusiasts claim essential oils, such as tea tree, have anti-microbial effects and effectively treat bacterial, fungal, or viral infections. However, there is still a lack of empirical evidence demonstrating their efficacy. Aromatherapy enthusiasts claimed their remedies have health benefits, including relief from anxi-ety and depression, nausea, insomnia, low appetite, dry mouth, and improved qual-ity of life, particularly for people with chronic health conditions, and enhanced sleep (Bauer, 2020; Johns Hopkins University, 2020).

An aromatherapy massage is quite popular in promoting relaxation and is one of the most commonly used CAMs in the United Kingdom. However, some detractors have cast doubts on the findings of available studies on which these recommenda-tions are based because the research designs are weak (Antonelli & Donelli, 2020). A few of the outcomes are summarized next.

A study of 8000 pregnant women in labor, provided with rose, lavender, and frankincense essential oils by qualified midwives, showed reduced anxiety and fear. Furthermore, women experienced less need for pain medications during delivery. In many women, peppermint essential oil relieves nausea and vomiting during labor (Simkin and Bolding, 2004).

Donelli and associates (2019) conducted a systematic review and meta-analysis of pooled data from six RCTs ($N = 448$) on the potential efficacy of lavender essen-tial oil massaged into the skin. The analysis produced a significant reduction of anxiety levels (Hedges' g = -0.66 [95% CI -0.97 to -0.35], $p < 0.0001$). The pri-mary limitation of this analysis was the low average quality of evidence from the included studies. Notably, confounding factors prevent quantifying the exact contri-bution to the observed anxiolytic effect of each treatment (body manipulation, lav-ender essential oil inhalation, and skin absorption, beneficial placebo effects like the rituality of the treatment). However, given that orally administered lavender essen-tial oil has a significant impact on anxiety levels and that, after the massage, its bioactive compounds (linalool and linalyl acetate) are detectable in the bloodstream (Jäger et al., 1992), it is reasonable to speculate that a useful anxiolytic and relaxing pharmacological role of this essential oil in aroma massage exists beyond the sole action of other treatment components (Donelli et al., 2019).

A systematic review and meta-analysis conducted by Yap and associates (2019) explored the anxiolytic effect of lavender essential oil taken as silexan® capsules compared to other comparators (i.e., placebo/paroxetine/lorazepam). They analyzed the data from five studies in which 524 subjects received silexan® 80 mg treatment, and 121 subjects received silexan® 160 mg. The findings indicated that silexan® 160 mg resulted in a higher decline in the Hamilton Anxiety Scale (HAMA) score than silexan® 80 mg, placebo, and paroxetine. The effect of silexan® 80 mg was the same as that of paroxetine. Overall, silexan® 160 mg was a more efficient treatment with a significant decline in anxiety score across other comparators. However, no improvements in anxiety scores were observed for the group that received lorazepam 0.5 mg compared to silexan® 160 mg, silexan® 80 mg, paroxetine 20 mg, and placebo.

Cheraghbeigi et al. (2019) and Bahrami et al. (2017) conducted a lavender essential oil aromatherapy massage clinical trial among elderly patients affected by cardiovascular diseases. The findings underscore the usefulness of lavender oil aromatherapy massage for anxiety, depression, mood status, and sleep quality. Another RCT by Lee (2005) also documented the beneficial effects of lavender aromatherapy hand massage on emotional and aggressive behavior in subjects with dementia. Her finding, along with evidence from the previously mentioned clinical trials, suggests an exciting role of aromatherapy hand massage in treating elderly patients with low quality of life (QOL) due to specific age-related diseases. A pilot study among 12 children with autism who received aromatherapy massage with lavender oil did not produce any significant change in their sleep pattern and quality (Williams, 2006). The minimal sample size in this study might have biased findings. Hence, further investigation is needed to demonstrate the real effect of the intervention in pediatric patients with neurodevelopmental disorders.

Other aromatherapy enthusiasts claim that essential oil with lavender oil can reduce pain for people with osteoarthritis of the knee, improve QOL for people with dementia, and reduce pain for people with kidney stones (Bauer, 2020). Overall, lavender essential oil massage is often recommended for symptomatic improvements of minor medical conditions characterized by chronic or sub-acute pain and low quality of life. A meta-analysis by Lakhan and associates (2016) found aromatherapy to be beneficial as an adjunct to conventional therapies in the management of musculoskeletal disorders. Another clinical trial involving 90 patients with knee osteoarthritis treated with lavender essential oil massage compared to another group massaged with a more inert substance like almond oil. The findings revealed the lavender essential oil aromatherapy massage is beneficial in reducing pain and improving functional status. Two clinical trials involving 32 patients with non-specific sub-acute cervical pain and 61 patients with lumbar pain received eight manual acupressure sessions with lavender oil. The results revealed significantly reduce pain and improve spine mobility (Koulivand et al., 2013).

Other pain-related conditions for which lavender oil aromatherapy massage appears to be significantly beneficial in managing the symptomatology are infantile colic (Çetinkaya & Başbakkal, 2012), dysmenorrheal (Bakhtshirin et al., 2015), and labor-induced pain (Ghiasi et al., 2019). Another study involving 118 elderly patients with chronic pain from non-malignant origin treated with lavender aromatherapy hand massage produced a significant decrease in pain intensity (Cino, 2014). Also, massage with lavender oil applied in tandem with routine treatment delivered symptomatic relief of pain among 70 patients with restless leg syndrome due to chronic kidney failure (Hashemi et al., 2015).

The evidence from an RCT conducted by Nasiri and associates underscores that lavender aromatherapy massage applied to treat knee osteoarthritis can significantly benefit compared to massage alone (Nasiri et al., 2016). The aromatherapist must consider the potential effect of lavender aromatherapy massage in managing pain concomitant with gynecological and pediatric conditions. Such intervention could decrease the use of common painkillers with minimal to no adverse events in these cohorts of patients. Along this line of reasoning, Antonelli and Donelli speculated that the analgesic effect of lavender oil application is due to its sedative compound, which has relaxing and anti-nociceptive properties following systemic absorption (Donelli et al., 2019; Koulivand et al., 2013).

In the hospice and palliative care setting, aromatherapy and its products are commonly used to treat various conditions – to enhance mood, relieve pain, and promote a sense of relaxation and calm. Under the name "aromatherapy," many lotions, candles, and beauty products are available in health spas and stores. Unfortunately, many contain synthetic fragrances that do not have the therapeutic substances found in essential oils. A recent systematic review by Armstrong and associates investigated the alleged role of aromatherapy massage in cancer palliative care. Their findings suggest that aromatherapy, reflexology, massage, and building a supportive relationship with the clinician who delivers such treatments can enhance patients' well-being and coping capacity dealing with the disease burden (Armstrong et al., 2019). Armstrong explained the findings by speculating that although the level of evidence for the efficacy of aromatherapy and massage in cancer palliative care may not be substantial, the intervention is safe and valuable in modulating patients' quality of life.

In a Cochrane systematic review published on the same topic, Fellowes and associates (2004) drew similar conclusions. They suggested that aromatherapy massage can exert some short-term benefits on the psychological well-being of patients living with cancer. Armstrong and associates (2019) investigated the effects of foot massage with lavender oil among 100 hospitalized patients (50% of whom receiving artificial ventilation) treated for severe conditions in an intensive care unit. The findings suggest that foot massage with lavender oil elicits several physiological responses (blood pressure, heart rate, respiratory rate, and wakefulness) in the short term, including decrease pain (Armstrong et al., 2019). Another study by Soden et al. (2004) treated 42 patients living with cancer in the hospice setting with a lavender oil aromatherapy massage. In the short term, the intervention improved the patients' sleep quality but did not produce long-term benefits.

Antonelli and Donelli (2020) proffered several reasons to explain these findings based on the weak research design surrounding the use of lavender oil aromatherapy massage compared to massage alone. The studies' threats to internal validity include the high level of heterogeneity and risk of bias within and across the studies reviewed and the less than optimum sample size in the clinical trials. Additionally, the lack of meaningful qualitative outcome measures and the potentially less pronounced sedative, analgesic, and relaxing action of lavender oil in such patients limits the study's external validity. The findings notwithstanding, the authors recommended that considering the nature of the intervention (easy to administer and generally safe) vis-à-vis the potential short-term benefits relating to the QOL of patients with incurable diseases, it is worthwhile to investigate the topic further to define the effect size better.

Evidence from clinical trials investigating lavender-based interventions (inhalation, oral administration, and aroma massage) for anxiety and relaxation indicated that the safety data are poorly presented or not reported in most studies. Based on available reports, lavender oil is considered safe, with only mild and reversible side effects. However, adverse side effects have been reported for oral consumption of encapsulated essential oil. An observational study describes three pre-pubertal male subjects (ages 7–10 years old) who developed gynecomastia after local applications of products containing both lavender and tea tree oils. The gynecomastia resolved after discontinuation of the intervention. Based on this finding, further studies are needed to understand better the modality's safety profile among different pediatric patients.

In 2019, the Michigan Health System provided a summary of nine studies on the efficacy of aromatherapy in palliative care. Three of the nine studies used different essential oils to treat anxiety and depression associated with cancer. The first clinical trial studied the effects of massage alone compared to massage with Roman chamomile essential oil among 103 patients living with cancer. Two weeks post-intervention, the group with massage with essential oil observed decreased anxiety and improved symptoms, but the group who only had massage did not experience the same benefit. Another study of 58 patients with various varieties of cancers completed six aromatherapy sessions. Post-treatment, the patients showed a decrease in anxiety and depression compared to baseline.

An RCT reported the effects of inhalation aromatherapy on anxiety during radiation therapy. The researchers randomly assigned 313 patients to lavender, bergamot, or cedarwood essential oils groups. There were no differences reported in depression or anxiety between the three groups. The fourth study provided essential oil through a diffuser overnight to newly diagnosed patients with acute myeloid leukemia undergoing intensive chemotherapy. The patients were offered the choice of lavender, peppermint, or chamomile. Three weeks later, the patients' sleep pattern and overall well-being improved, and the reduction was also observed in tiredness, drowsiness, appetite, depression, and anxiety.

Radioactive iodine used in oncology often damages patients' salivary glands. Thus, in this patient population, increased saliva production during treatment may decrease damage to salivary glands. To test this hypothesis, an RCT divided the study participants into two groups: one group of patients inhaled a mixture of lemon and ginger essential oils. The other group was provided a placebo. The group that inhaled the combination of lemon and ginger essential oils had increased saliva production compared with the placebo group that had no significant change. In one of the studies, the investigators provided women receiving chemotherapy for breast cancer with inhaled ginger essential oil. Post-treatment, the women experienced decreased acute nausea, but vomiting or chronic nausea remains the same.

The researchers provided children and adolescents at the time of stem cell infusion with inhaled bergamot essential oil. Post-intervention, the study participants reported an increase in anxiety level and nausea but no effect on pain. In a study of adult patients at the time of stem cell infusion, they were provided tasting or sniffing sliced oranges or inhaling an orange essential oil. The study revealed that tasting or sniffing sliced oranges was more effective at reducing nausea, retching, and coughing than inhaling an orange essential oil.

In another study, women undergoing breast biopsies were assigned randomly to receive lavender-sandalwood or orange-peppermint essential oil drops placed on a felt tab and attached to their hospital gown or no scent on the felt tab. The findings revealed that the women who received the lavender-sandalwood aromatherapy tab had less anxiety compared to women who received the orange-peppermint aromatherapy tab or no scent tab. The ninth study evaluated the effect of inhaled lavender essential oil, eucalyptus essential oil; on the pain experienced by patients with cancer having a central venous catheter- port. The patient group who inhaled lavender essential oil reported less pain (Michigan Health System, 2019). Although the findings reported above appear promising, they should be consumed with tepid skepticism because none of the nine studies have been published in a peer-reviewed scientific journal.

Currently, 35 aromatherapy training schools exist in the United States and six in Canada. The training is limited to certificate programs. There is presently no board certification or license for aromatherapists. State law does not regulate aromatherapy, and no licensure is required to practice. Practitioners often combine aromatherapy training with a license in other health disciplines such as massage therapy, nursing, acupuncture, or naturopathy. The two professional organizations with national educational standards for aromatherapists are the National Association for Holistic Aromatherapy (www.naha.org) and the Alliance of International Aromatherapists (www.alliance-aromatherapists.org). The schools that offer certificate programs approved by the National Association for Holistic Aromatherapy are available at https://naha.org/index.php/education/approved-schools/. The Canadian Federation of Aromatherapists (www.cfacanada.com) certifies aromatherapists in Canada. The International Federation of Aromatherapists website (www.ifaroma.org/) provides a list of international aromatherapy programs (Michigan Health System, 2019).

Spirituality Among all the CAM treatments, prayer is the most commonly used. Spirituality is the way we find meaning, hope, comfort, and inner peace in our life. Some people find spirituality through religion; others find it through music, art, connection with nature, or in one's values and principles. Nathan (2017) opined, any religion without spirituality is like tea without sugar, and there is no religion without spirituality. According to the New Testament, spirituality refers to the "life force" and man's religious experience, which comes from God and illuminates the committed child. Among Christians, spirituality is the direct relationship with God and is the expression of man's response and the interpretation of God's experience. Anyone can apply spirituality to any religious system and see it manifest in action.

Religion and spirituality are critical aspects of health and well-being. Some studies have demonstrated a connection between one's beliefs and sense of well-being and have proposed a body, mind, and spirit connection (Puchalski, 2001). Some medical experts postulated that positive thoughts, comfort, and strength gained from religion, meditation, or prayer could positively promote well-being and healing. Improving one's spiritual health may not cure an illness, but it may help one feel better, prevent some health problems, and help one cope better with illness, stress, or death (Familydoctor.org, 2017). Although prayer and other spiritual practices are used in different cultures worldwide as complementary therapy in health care, scientific investigation of these practices has only recently begun. It is currently unclear if spirituality intervention is beneficial, and the specific diseases that are amenable to them are unsettled. The recently published studies that evaluated the impact of spirituality intervention in particular disease conditions are presented below.

The impact of spirituality on health has been studied in three major areas: mortality, coping, and recovery (Puchalski, 2001). Several cross-sectional studies suggest that people who have regular spiritual practices tend to live longer (Strawbridge et al., 1997). Koenig and associates (1997) tracked the interleukin-6 (IL-6) levels of 1700 older adults who regularly attended church – IL-6 is a group of cytokines expressed by white blood cells (leukocytes), with high levels associated with an increased incidence of disease. Koenig and associates found a weak correlation between IL-6 and religious attendance that other covariates could not explain, such as depression and adverse life events. Older adults who attended church were half as likely to have elevated levels of IL-6. Their findings suggest that older adults who regularly attend religious services have healthier immune systems. Although the mechanism of the effect remains unknown, the authors speculated that "religious commitment may improve stress control by offering better coping mechanisms, richer social support, and the strength of personal values and worldview."

Several studies have documented that patient who are spiritually inclined tend to have a more positive outlook and a better quality of life. For example, Yates and associates (1981) found that patients with terminal cancer who found comfort from their religious and spiritual beliefs were more satisfied with their lives, were happier, and had less pain. Spirituality is a critical component of the "existential domain" reflected in quality-of-life scores – a meaningful personal existence, fulfillment of life goals, and a feeling that life to that point had been worthwhile. High scores on the existential domain are correlated with good QOL for patients with terminal chronic disease (Cohen et al., 1995). Blacks in the United States with chronic conditions generally acknowledge the relationship between spirituality and their overall health and sought mobile health monitoring and intervention opportunities (Thomas-Purcell et al., 2020). Based on these studies, Puchalski (2001) posited that patients who are spiritual might better utilize their beliefs in coping with illness, pain, and life stresses.

The relationship between spirituality and pain perception has been widely investigated. For example, Brady et al. (1999) found that spiritual well-being is correlated to enjoying life even with symptoms, including pain. McNeill and associates found that personal prayer was the most commonly used non-pharmacological strategy for pain modulation by patients on admission in the hospital setting – 76% of the study sample reported using prayer to cope, 66% use intravenous pain medication, 62% use pain injections, 33% use relaxation, 19% use touch, and 9% use massage (McNeill et al., 1998).

Many studies have also reported that spiritual beliefs can help patients cope with the disease and face death compos mentis. A study by Roberts and associates interviewed 108 women with gynecologic cancer and asked them, "what helped you cope with your diagnosis" 93% mentioned spiritual beliefs, and 75% stated that religion had an essential place in their lives, and 49% indicated that they had become more spiritual after their diagnosis (Roberts et al., 1997). Among the 90 patients who are HIV-positive, Kaldjian and associates found that those who are active spiritually had less fear of death and less guilt (Kaldjian et al., 1998).

A Gallup International Institute in New Jersey, United States, conducted a national survey asking people what concerns they would have if they were dying. The top two issues mentioned by the study respondents were finding companionship and spiritual comfort. Surprisingly, advance directives, economic/financial/social concerns were not on the top list. The most common spiritual reassurances mentioned were "beliefs that they would be in the loving presence of God or a higher power, that death was not the end but a passage and that they would live on through their children and descendants" (Nathan Cummings Foundation et al., 1997). Cook and Wimberly (1983) found that 80% of parents (N = 145) whose children had died of cancer received comfort from their religious beliefs 1 year later and had a better physiologic and emotional adjustment. Furthermore, 40% reported a strengthening of their religious commitment a year before their child's death.

Several observational studies found that spiritual commitment tends to enhance recovery from illness and surgery. For example, Harris and associates discovered that patients who had received a heart transplant and participated in religious activities complied better with follow-up treatment and had higher physical functioning 12 months post-surgery. They also had higher self-esteem, less anxiety, and fewer health worries. The authors posited that "people who don't worry as much tend to have better health outcomes…and spirituality enables people to worry less, to let go and live in the present moment" (Harris et al., 1995).

The power of positive thinking and hope is linked to spirituality. For example, a study published in the Journal of the American Medical Association revealed that 35% (range 16%–60%) of patients benefited from receiving a placebo treatment for different symptoms such as pain, cough, drug-induced mood change, headaches, seasickness, or the common cold (Beecher, 1955). It is now well known that the placebo effects have three primary components – patients' positive beliefs and expectations, healthcare professionals, positive beliefs and expectations, and a good relationship between the two parties (Benson, 1996).

Benson (1990) found that 10–20 min of transcendental meditation performed twice a day produced decreased metabolism, heart rate, respiratory rate, and slower brain waves. The meditation was beneficial in treating chronic pain, insomnia, anxiety, hostility, depression, premenstrual syndrome, and infertility. It was a useful complementary treatment for patients with cancer or HIV. He concluded: "To the extent that any disease is caused or made worse by stress, to that extent evoking the relaxation response is an effective therapy."

Several well-designed studies in the last two decades have explored the effectiveness of spirituality in different patient populations. For example, Moritz et al. (2006) investigated the efficacy of a home study-based spirituality program on mood disturbance in emotionally distressed patients. The researchers randomly assigned 165 patients with mood disturbance [score of >40 on the Profile of Mood States (POMS)] to three groups – a spirituality group (8-week audiotaped spirituality home-study program), a mindfulness meditation-based stress reduction group (8 weeks of attendance at facilitated classes), and a wait-list control group (no intervention for 12 weeks). Mood disturbance was measured with the POMS; QOL was measured with a short-form health survey with 36 questions (SF-36). The outcome measures – POMS and the SF-36 – were completed at baseline, 8 weeks, and 12 weeks. After the 8-week intervention, the mean POMS score improved by 45.7% (−43.1) for the spirituality group, 26.3% (−22.6) for the meditation group, and 11.3% (−10.3) for the control group (p < 0.001 for spirituality vs. control group; p < 0.05 for spirituality vs. meditation group. The improvement in the SF-36 score was 14.4 (48.6%) for the spirituality group, 7.1 (22.3%) for the meditation group, and 4.7 (16.1%) for the control group (p < 0.001). The post hoc test comparing the spirituality and control group is statistically significant (p = 0.029). At 12 weeks, the POMS and SF-36 scores were significantly different from baseline measures for the spirituality group.

An RCT by Wiriyasombat and associates (2011) investigated the efficacy of doctrine-based programs on spiritual well-being, coping, and sleep quality. A sample of 79 Thai Buddhist elders in southern Thailand was randomly allocated to three groups: Group one (n = 31) practiced Vipassana meditation, group two (n = 23) practiced chanting, and group three (n = 25) constitutes the control group. Aside from demographics, other outcome measures (Family Status and Religious Experiences, Thai Elderly Spiritual Well-being Scale, Thai Elderly Coping Scale, and Thai Elderly Sleep Quality Scale) were collected from each study participants at four-time frames – baseline, at one, two, and four months after the intervention program. The outcome measures of the elders in the control group did not change during the three time frames. The spiritual well-being of the elders who practiced meditation improved significantly during the four time frames. Those who practiced chanting also showed a significant improvement in spiritual well-being at 2 months and 4 months post-intervention. The three groups showed significant changes in coping during three of the five time frames. Both the meditation group and the chanting group showed better coping than the control group. Compared to the control group, both the meditation and chanting group's sleep quality improved 4 months after completing their invention. The findings suggest that HCPs can utilize Vipassana meditation and chanting to promote spiritual well-being, coping, and sleep quality of Thai elders.

McCauley and associates (2011) conducted another RCT in 2011 to determine whether a spiritually based intervention can improve perceived health status. The investigators assigned 100 adults with chronic illness into Spiritual or Educational standard cardiac risk reduction intervention groups. The two groups were shown a 28-min video and provided a workbook to complete over 4 weeks. The study participants were 90% Christian, 62% of women had an average of three chronic illnesses, and a mean age of 65.8 ± 9.6 years. At baseline and 6 weeks later, the study participants completed a questionnaire that assesses psychosocial and health outcome measures. At baseline, frequent daily spiritual experiences were associated with being African American ($p < 0.05$), with co-morbidities ($p < 0.01$), and increased pain ($p < 0.01$). Energy decreased significantly ($p < 0.05$) in the educational group and increased in the Spiritual group. However, the improvements observed in pain, mood, and health perceptions, illness intrusiveness, and self-efficacy were not statistically ($p > 0.05$) significant.

An RCT conducted by Olver and Dutney (2012) investigated whether researchers could measure the impact of intercessory prayer on the spiritual well-being and QOL of patients with cancer. At a cancer center in South Australia, the investigators recruited 999 patients and randomly assigned them into two groups. The experimental group had the Christian intercessory prayer added to the usual prayer lists that the control group had. The researchers administered the Functional Assessment of Chronic Illness Therapy-Spiritual Well-being questionnaire to measure spiritual well-being and QOL at two time frames – baseline and 6 months later. The experimental group showed significant improvement in the spiritual well-being ($p = 0.03$), emotional well-being ($p = 0.04$) and functional well-being ($p = 0.06$) as compared to the control group. Study participants randomly allocated to the experimental group showed small but significant improvements in spiritual well-being.

Another RCT by Amir and associates (2015) investigated the efficacy of a spiritual-based intervention on patients' spiritual well-being with leukemia. The researchers randomly allocated 64 adult patients with leukemia into experimental and control groups. The experimental group had a spiritual-based intervention that included supportive presence and support for religious rituals for 3 days. Both groups completed the Palutzian and Ellison Spiritual Well-being Questionnaire at baseline and following the intervention. The findings revealed a significant difference in the experimental group's spiritual well-being scores before and after the intervention ($p < 0.001$), but no difference was found in the control group. In addition, the experimental group's post-intervention mean spiritual well-being score was significantly higher ($p < 0.001$, $F = 63.303$) than the control group. Thus, the CAM intervention implemented in this study promoted the spiritual well-being of patients with leukemia. The finding suggests that clinicians should apply a holistic care approach that includes spirituality-based intervention in managing refractory diseases such as leukemia.

Ochoa et al. (2018) examined the plausible differences between Hispanic and non-Hispanic white cancer survivors on health, social support, spirituality, and the potential mediating roles of mental health and emotional distress on general health perceptions. This national cross-sectional study analyzed the data ($N = 7778$; 693 were Hispanic and 7085 were non-Hispanic whites) from the American Cancer Society's Study of Cancer Survivors-II and compared sociodemographic and medical characteristics between the two groups to identify significant covariates. Overall, the Hispanics had poorer health and more likely to have co-morbidities such as diabetes and depression than non-Hispanic whites. The findings revealed that spiritual belief was fully mediated through mental health. Still, emotional distress did not directly affect general health perceptions, nor did it mediate the effects of spiritual belief and social support on general health perceptions. Instead, there was a mediated effect of social support on general health perceptions.

Park and associates (2018) explored the relationships between the four core dimensions of R/S (beliefs, behaviors, identity, and coping) and three health behaviors (fruit/vegetable intake, physical activity, and maintenance of a healthy weight) among 172 women who survived breast cancer. Their findings revealed that both spiritual identity and religious coping were positively correlated to fruit and vegetable intake, while private prayer was only marginally positively correlated. Both service attendance and religious identity (marginally) were associated with less physical activity, while private prayer was positively correlated. Finally, the BMI was positively correlated with afterlife beliefs and private prayer.

A recent quasi-experimental (pre- and post-test with the control group) research design study by Darvishi et al. (2020) investigated the efficacy of spirituality intervention on spiritual well-being, self-esteem, and self-efficacy in patients on hemodialysis. Twenty-four convenience sample patients were allocated randomly into experimental and control groups. The experimental group had twelve 60-min sessions of spiritual therapy twice a week. Post-treatment, their spiritual health scores increased from 39.32 ± 3.38 to 43.40 ± 2.82, self-esteem increased from 42.65 ± 2.61 to 45.90 ± 3.88, and self-efficacy from 40.99 ± 2.19 to 44.65 ± 2.58. The experimental group changes were statistically significant compared with the control group ($p < 0.01$). The authors concluded that a holistic spiritual therapy implemented by an interdisciplinary team can be a beneficial intervention to improve patients' spiritual well-being, self-esteem, and self-efficacy on hemodialysis.

Another recent quasi-experimental study by Hajibabaei et al. (2020) evaluated existential-spiritual psychotherapy's efficacy with cognitive-behavioral therapy on women's QOL with chronic disease. A convenience sample of 43 women with multiple sclerosis was randomly assigned into three groups: a cognitive-behavioral intervention and an existential-spiritual intervention, and the control group. The dependent variables (QOL and meaning in life) were measured at pre-test, post-test, and 5-months follow-up time frames. The control group's findings revealed no difference in life scores, but the existential-spiritual intervention ($p = 0.027$) and cognitive-behavioral therapy groups improved significantly ($p = 0.039$). Both mental ($p = 0.014$) and physical functioning ($p = 0.013$) health dimensions of QOL increased dramatically in the two intervention groups. The women in the existential-spiritual intervention group showed a more significant change in some aspects of meaning in life (search for purpose) and QOL (role physical and role emotional, pain and energy) compared to women in the cognitive-behavioral intervention group. However, the cognitive-behavioral intervention group displayed better improvements on two subscales (physical function and health distress). Overall, the existential-spiritual intervention resulted in more positive gains in some aspects of meaning in life and quality of life.

Park and Lee (2020) recently tested the hypothesis as to whether religiousness/spirituality (R/S) may blunt the decline in symptoms and QOL in patients with congestive heart failure (CHF). The researchers tracked four mental and physical outcome measures (depressive symptoms, positive states of mind, mental health-related quality of life, and physical health-related quality of life) among 191 patients (122 males; mean age = 68.6 years) with CHF at baseline and 6 months later. After controlling for demographics and baseline health status, higher spiritual peace levels, and social support, each uniquely increased positive states of mind. However, only social support predicted improved physical health-related quality of life. In addition, neither spiritual peace nor social support predicted change in mental health-related quality of life, and only spiritual peace predicted reduced levels of depressive symptoms during the 6 months post-intervention. The authors concluded that their findings revealed that "R/S may play an important role distinct from social support in promoting well-being in people with CHF."

Kahrizeh and associates (2020) conducted a quasi-experimental (a pre-test-post-test design with a control group) study to evaluate the effectiveness of spiritual, religious interventions on anxiety, depression, and adjustment to parental divorce among female high school students. A convenience sample of 28 female high school students whose parents had divorced in Malayer, Iran, was randomly allocated into a spiritual-religious intervention group and a control group. The findings revealed that the spiritual-religious intervention implemented significantly improve anxiety ($F = 24.22$, $p < 0.05$), depression ($F = 4.50$, $p < 0.05$), and facilitate adjustment to parental divorce ($F = 6.75$, $p < 0.05$).

Several research studies have addressed whether patients want their HCPs to show concern about their spiritual beliefs. For example, a survey conducted in 1996 by the ICR Research Group in the United States found 65% of patients surveyed felt that it was appropriate for physicians to discuss their spiritual beliefs. Sadly, only 10% indicated their physician had previously had such a discussion with them (McNichol, 1996).

Another study at the University of Pennsylvania in the United States found that 66% of patients with pulmonary diseases agreed that a physician's conversation about their spiritual beliefs would strengthen their trust in their physician. For patients whose spirituality was important, 94% of them wanted their physicians to address their spiritual beliefs and be sensitive to their values system. And for patients whose spirituality was not important, 50% of them felt that their physicians should at least discuss their spiritual beliefs when diagnosed with a terminal illness (Ehman et al., 1999).

In 2001, Puchalski contended that understanding patients' spirituality is quite valuable to HCPs because it "may be dynamic in the patient's understanding of the disease. Religious convictions may affect healthcare decision-making. Spirituality may be a patient need and maybe necessary inpatient coping. A sense of the patient's spirituality is integral to whole-patient care."

Global Demand for the Use of CAM

The demand for CAM is increasing all over the world. About 50% of the general population in developed countries uses CAM. In the Western Pacific region, between 40% and 60% of the population uses CAM to treat various diseases (WHO, 2002a; WHO, 2002b). In Hong Kong, about 60% of the population consults with CAM practitioners. CAM is gaining widespread acceptance in Australia, France, and Canada with 46%, 49%, and 70% of the population, respectively, using CAM (WHO, 2002a; Amzat & Abdullahi, 2008). Almost 40% of the physicians in the United Kingdom make a CAM referral (WHO, 2002a). In Chile and Colombia, about 71% and 40% of their populations, respectively, have used CAM (Amzat & Abdullahi, 2008). Because of these developments, the WHO acknowledged traditional medicine's contributions to healthcare delivery in developing countries (WHO, 2000; 2001; 2002a). For example, traditional healers in developing countries provide disease prevention services, treat non-communicable diseases, and manage mental and gerontological health problems (WHO, 2001). There is also increasing evidence that traditional medicine is beneficial in managing chronic illnesses (Thorne et al., 2002). In addition, several medical schools in the United States now include CAM content in the curriculum (Wetzel et al., 1998). So, perhaps the essential questions are: What is responsible for the growing demands for CAM globally? And what is responsible for the sudden interest in evaluating the effectiveness of CAM?

Some factors are responsible for the upsurge in CAM use and the increased interest in assessing the efficacy of CAM globally. Research has shown that some CAM treatments, such as acupuncture and herbs, are beneficial in a broad spectrum of diseases, some of which may not be effectively managed using the conventional approach. The poor accessibility to allopathic medicines contributed to the widespread use of traditional medicine in developing countries, especially in low households. A WHO and Health Action International study in 36 low- and middle-income countries found that large sections of the population cannot afford their drugs (Cameron et al., 2008). For instance, in Africa, the ratio of traditional healers to the people is 1:500 compared to 1:40,000 physicians (Abdullahi, 2011). The majority of the physicians/dentists in Africa practice in urban centers. Consequently, for millions of rural dwellers, the native healers remain their only healthcare providers.

Frass et al., in 2012, conducted a systematic review of the acceptance of CAM among the general population and HCPs. They found that the prevalence rates of CAM use worldwide were between 5% and 74.8%. German-speaking countries use homeopathy and acupuncture more. The general population most commonly used chiropractic manipulation, homeopathy, herbal medicine, and massage. Gender, age, and education are viable predictors of CAM utilization; women, the middle-aged, and more education were associated with higher use. CAM utilization is common for back pain, severe headache or migraine, depression, insomnia, and stomach or intestinal illnesses. Medical students (18.2%), compared to nursing and pharmacy students (44.7%), were the most critical toward CAM utilization. Medical students also had the least consultation with a CAM practitioner (10%). This study demonstrated increased utilization of CAM between 1990 and 2006 in all the countries investigated. The researchers found geographical differences and differences between the general population and medical personnel (Frass et al., 2012).

James et al. (2018) conducted a systematic search of original articles that examined traditional medicine and CAM (TCAM) utilization in Sub-Saharan Africa between January 1, 2006 and February 28, 2017. The publications identified were diverse but generally of low quality. The review revealed a relatively high use of TCAM alone or conventional medicine in both the general population and for specific health conditions. Compared with non-TCAM users, TCAM users are more likely to be from low socioeconomic and educational status. At the same time, there were inconsistencies in age, sex, spatial location, and religious affiliation between the two groups. In addition, most TCAM users (55.8%–100%) fail to disclose the preparations they are using to their healthcare providers for fear of receiving improper care, a negative attitude, and a lack of inquiry about TCAM use from healthcare providers.

CAM Utilization in the United States

The demand for dietary supplements in the United States is rapidly growing annually. A landmark study in 1993 found that more than one-third of Americans had sought CAM therapies. In 1990, Americans made more visits to CAM providers than to primary care physicians. Consumers spent more than $13 billion out-of-pocket for CAM visits. Demand for CAM services continues to grow at an alarming rate. Another 2001 survey found that nearly 70% of Americans have used at least one CAM therapy in their lifetime, making it one of the fastest-growing sectors within American health care. Although the utilization of CAM services, such as acupuncture, chiropractic, and naturopathy, remained stable on a percentage basis from 1993 to 1998, the use of dietary supplements surged (Nahin & Straus, 2001). Vitamin and mineral supplement use has soared in the United States since the 1970s (Bender et al., 1992; Subar & Block, 1990). By 2002, the sales of dietary supplements increased to over $18.7 billion per year, with herbs/botanical supplements accounting for $4.3 billion in sales (NBJ's Annual, 2003).

In 2002, 36% of Americans in the past 12 months, 50% in a lifetime, reported using some form of alternative therapy, such as Yoga, meditation, herbal treatments, and the Atkins diet. Most Americans (54.9%) used CAM in conjunction with conventional medicine to treat and prevent musculoskeletal conditions and other ailments linked with chronic and recurring pain. Comparatively, women more than men are more likely to use CAM with the most substantial gender difference observed in mind-body therapies, including prayer for health reasons. When the prayer was considered an alternative treatment, the utilization data increased to 62.1%. Twenty-five percent of the study participants who use CAM do so because a medical professional recommended it. A 1998 telephone survey of 1209 British adults shows that around 20% of the sample used alternative therapies in the past year.

A 2012 National Health Interview Survey (Clarke et al., 2015) in the United States found the top ten commonly used CAM services to be natural products (17.7%), deep breathing (10.9%), Yoga, Tai Chi or Qi Gong (10.1%), chiropractic or osteopathic manipulation (8.4%), meditation (8%), massage (6.9%), special diets (3.0%), homeopathy (2.2%), progressive relaxation (2.1%), and guided imagery (1.7%). Natural products are sold as dietary supplements, and they include vitamins and minerals, and probiotics, herbs (also known as botanicals). They are readily available to consumers over the counter and widely marketed. The most commonly used natural product was fish oil.

The increased utilization of CAM in the United States is often attributed to dissatisfaction with conventional treatment's high cost and perceived impersonal and ineffective treatment offered by orthodox practitioners. Patients are empowered to decide the healthcare services compatible with their values and spiritual beliefs and the nature of their illness. There is also the strong appeal that CAM services are "natural," "non-artificial," "pure," and "non-synthetic." Presently, the number of stores that sell herbal supplements and "organic" food instead of "processed "foods has increased, particularly in major centers and cities nationally. In 2007, $34 billion was spent to seek "natural" means to good health.

In 1994, 60% of physicians in the United States recommended CAM to their patients. About 50% of the physicians who responded to the survey acknowledged that they used CAM themselves. More health insurance plans now cover acupuncture, chiropractic, and Ornish Heart Program (which has a basis in Yoga and nutrition). Presently, herbs and supplements are not regulated in the United States, and pharmacies are experiencing a tremendous surge in demand for these alternative remedies. Between 1991 and 1996, the market for over-the-counter natural medications (including herbs and supplements) doubled. Over 70% of health management organizations reported an increase in requests for CAM. About 56% of the survey respondents requested acupuncture treatment, 45% consulted chiropractors, 25% asked for massage therapists, 21% used acupressure and biofeedback, 8% used hypnotherapy, and 4% used reflexology (Landmark Healthcare, 1996).

CAM is still controversial in the United States – there are advocates and detractors or critics. The barriers to the use of integrative medicine are beginning to fall or, at least, are becoming less difficult to overcome. The assimilation of diverse cultures in the West brings once-distant healing practices to the forefront, and more Americans are turning to integrative medical care than ever before. Growing consumer demand for CAM services prompts the movement toward integrative medicine. Increasingly, well-designed research studies in alternative healing practices are evaluated for effectiveness and safety. Presently, alternative medicine is not included in the medical school curriculum, but complementary medicine services are available to some patients and hospitals. However, several medical schools now teach CAM content in their curriculum. In 1998, 64% of US medical schools offered at least one course in CAM.

Investigators should use the same scientific methods to assess CAM therapies' effectiveness and safety. When considering consulting a CAM practitioner, and during the first visit, the consumers should ask the following pertinent questions:

1. What adverse effects are to be expected?
2. What are the risks related to this therapy?
3. What benefits can be expected from this therapy?
4. Do the known benefits outweigh the risks?
5. Will therapy affect conventional treatment?

6. Is this therapy part of a clinical trial?
7. If so, who is the sponsor of the research?
8. Will your health insurance cover the therapy?
9. The education and credential of the CAM practitioner
10. Is the practitioner licensed? Check on the state licensing board, whether the practitioner is licensed, and the number of disciplinary actions reported (Michigan Health System, 2019).

Conclusion

It is essential to fully understand the effectiveness and safety of any CAM treatment before combining it with conventional medicine. CAM enthusiasts must do their homework by discussing all treatment options with their HCPs to rule out possible drug interactions. They must search for empirical evidence, not anecdotal, personal stories. If news or advertisement about a CAM treatment or product appears only in mass media but not in scientific journals, it is probably not safe to use. Most importantly, if a CAM treatment or product promises to cure too many diseases, the advertisement is likely fraudulent. The word "natural" is often used by CAM practitioners and in their advertisements to entice but does not indicate the treatment or product is effective or safe. For example, poisonous mushrooms are natural, but they are not safe. Many herbal remedies and dietary products act as drugs in the body, causing significant adverse effects. Be careful not to give a nutritional or herbal product to a child because they metabolize drugs and nutrients differently. Therefore, they need different doses than adults. Before using any CAM treatment or product, it is always prudent to ask questions about safety. A summary of the primary CAM professions and occupations is presented in Table 6.1 in the Appendix of this chapter.

Case Study
Select any complementary and alternative medicine modality of your choice and evaluate its safety using the following guidelines:

1. Has the research supporting the CAM treatment been published in peer-reviewed journals, and is there useful safety data to support the therapy?
2. What is the goal of the procedure?
3. Does the CAM treatment or product work in combination with or replace a standard treatment?
4. If this therapy is used instead of conventional medicine, will it delay standard procedure?
5. Could this delay in receiving standard treatment be harmful?
6. Will the CAM treatment or product affect the chances of receiving treatment later?
7. Is it possible to have an adverse reaction to the CAM treatment or product?
8. Are the ingredients listed for natural products and supplements accurate and free of any contamination?
9. Is the CAM practitioner licensed?

Appendix

Table 6.1 An overview of the primary complementary and alternative medical professions and occupations

Profession	Origin	Progenitor	Treatment philosophy	Treatment modalities	Precautions	Education/Licensure in the United States
Traditional Chinese Medicine (TCM)	China 200 BC	Chinese immigrant since mid-nineteenth century	Yin and Yang, principal meridian and five elements philosophy	Shiatsu massage, acupuncture, acupressure, moxibustion, cupping, and herbs	Herbal products poorly labeled. Contain Aristolochic acid. No herbs if pregnant or nursing	35 oriental programs. No licensure requirement
Massage Therapy – MT	Linked to TCM 4000 years	Swedish massage introduced to the United States (US) in the 1850s	Through its physiological effects by stimulating the release of endorphins, boost energy, generate electrical signals that stimulate circulation	Over 100 different types of massage, aromatherapy, craniosacral, lymphatic, myofascial, reflexology, Rolfing, shiatsu, sports, trigger point	Relatively safe treatment. Pain or soreness. Caution during pregnancy. Check blood sugar if diabetic	Certified MTs complete 500 hrs. Take national board exams, licensed or registered in 29 states
Acupuncture Therapy – LAc	Linked to TCM 200 BC	Popular after President Nixon visited China in 1972	Ying and Yang, principal meridian and five elements philosophy	Different approaches to the use of needle acupuncture. French energetic, Korean, Japanese, auricular, myofascial, electro-	Same as TCM. In addition, ensure only disposable needles are used; HIV	Duration of training varies widely. Most states require licensure

Chiropractic – DC (Doctor of Chiropractic)	China/Greece written in 2700 B.C. and 1500 B.C. Hippocrates; 460 to 357 B.C.	In 1895, Daniel David Palmer founded the Chiropractic profession in Davenport, Iowa	Metaphysical and ritualistic believes and practices. Vertebral subluxation leads to interference with an innate intelligence Detection and correction of vertebral subluxation via adjustment	Spinal manipulation + Exercise, massage, ice packs, moist heat, nutritional supplements, acupuncture, homeopathy, herbal remedies, and biofeedback	Minor aches, stiffness, tiredness, and severe adverse effects such as stroke (rare); 1 out of three million manipulations	Four years of education. Chiropractors are licensed in all 50 states; 17 chiropractic colleges
Ayurveda	It was developed in India more than 3000 years ago	Dhanvantari, the physician to the gods in Hindu mythology, is the progenitor	Ayurveda focuses equally on the body, mind, and spirit and strives to restore the individual's innate harmony using diet, exercise, meditation, herbs, massage, exposure to sunlight, and controlled breathing. Ayurveda follows a traditional diet and engages in regular detoxes believed to rid toxins' body and mind and ultimately prevent illnesses.	Traditional diet and regular detoxifications to get rid of body and mind toxins and ultimately prevent illnesses	Ayurvedic products are potentially toxic and many of the formulations contain lead, mercury, and arsenic	Ayurvedic medicine is not regulated in the United States – No state currently requires a license to practice

(continued)

Table 6.1 (continued)

Profession	Origin	Progenitor	Treatment philosophy	Treatment modalities	Precautions	Education/ Licensure in the United States
Osteopathy (Osteo D.) and Osteopathic Medicine (DO)	Dates back to nineteenth century. Hippocratic in the fourth century BC	Osteopathy philosophy was developed in 1874 by Andrew Taylor still, a Missouri physician and surgeon	Classical osteopaths – Strive to find the cause of disease by understanding the patient's body, mind, and spirit – Man is triune; "total" body adjustment structural. Osteopathic physicians indict strains and vertebra subluxation. Cranial osteopaths feels a rhythm at the lines between the skull bones and evaluates the quality of that rhythm, and applies subtle, indirect force to enhance its movement and pulsation	Osteopaths outside the United States – manipulation, nutrition, and lifestyle modifications Osteopathic medicine, DO, regular physician in the United States; prescribe medication and uses all technology used by MDs for diagnosis. DO may manipulate the spine and peripheral joints	With manipulation – Minor aches, stiffness, tiredness, and severe adverse effects such as stroke (rare); 1 out of three million manipulations	Four years of medical school education. DOs are licensed in all 50 states; In 1896, Vermont became the first state to license DOs 26 DO schools; 70,000 DOs in the U. S

Naturopathy – ND	Linked to Hippocrates the Greek physician who lived 2400 years ago	Benedict Lust, MD, from Germany, immigrated to the United States in 1896. In 1902, he established an Institute in New Jersey	Conventional NDs prescribe medication to suppress symptoms Traditional naturopaths sought natural approaches to restore health, not simply cure illness. They treat disease without pharmaceuticals or surgery but strives to find the cause of disease by understanding the patient's body, mind, and spirit – Man is triune: Three in one – Like Dr. still	Nutritional/dietary treatment – Detoxification, herbal/ homeopathic medicine, acupuncture, hydrotherapy, spirituality, lifestyle and psychological Counseling. Patients are partners in their health care, so lifestyle changes (sleeping, eating, and exercise habits) may be recommended	High doses of nutrients and herbs may cause toxicities and drug-herb interactions. Significant dietary changes can undermine good health (especially in the very young, the elderly, and those with certain medical conditions, such as diabetes)	By 1920 over 10,000 ND practitioners and 20 colleges established in the United States. Today, only five colleges in the United States; two colleges in Canada

(continued)

Table 6.1 (continued)

Profession	Origin	Progenitor	Treatment philosophy	Treatment modalities	Precautions	Education/ Licensure in the United States
Aromatherapy	Ancient Chinese, Indians, Egyptians, Greeks, romans used essential oils in cosmetics, perfumes, and drugs	In 1928, René-Maurice Gattefossé, a French chemist, discovered the healing properties of lavender oil when he applied it to treat a burn on his hand after an explosion in his lab. The bactericidal effect of the oil promotes the healing	The active ingredients in an essential oil determine its healing properties. Some oils promote physical healing – Relieve pain, swelling, bactericidal effect, relaxation/ calming effect. Stimulate positive emotions through the limbic system. Ideal in hospice and palliative care settings	*Aerial diffusion*: For environmental fragrance/ disinfection *Direct inhalation*: For respiratory disinfection, decongestion *Topical applications*: Massage, baths, or in the form of compresses, therapeutic skincare *Oral ingestion (rare)*: Use only under the supervision of a trained professional	Essential oils are highly volatile and flammable never use near an open flame. Avoid use near the eyes. Never ingest e. oils unless a trained AT advises. Oils sold in stores are often mislabeled. Some are toxic and could be fatal. Cancer patients receiving chemotherapy, Women in the first trimester, severe asthmatics, history of hypertension, seizures should avoid hyssop oil.	Training is at three levels supervised by the National Association for holistic aromatherapy: Level 1: 30 h Level 2: 200 h Level 3: Certification 35 training schools in the United States, 6 in Canada. No degree program, no licensure, and no board certification

Homeopathy					
Hippocrates, in about 400 BC, prescribed a small dose of mandrake root – Which in larger doses produced mania. In the sixteenth-century Paracelsus posited that small doses of "what makes a man ill also cures him."	In 1807, German physician, Samuel Hahnemann, gave homeopathy its name and expanded its principles in the late eighteenth century (1755–1843). In 1825, Hans Birch Gram established homeopathy in the United States and rapidly gained popularity	Substance which causes symptoms when taken in large doses can be used in small amounts to treat the same symptoms. Homeopaths espouse The "like cures like" and dilution and succussion principles-remedies are diluted and then "succussed," or shaken, in order to increase their potency. The repeated dilution and succussion is called potentization	Homeopathic remedies selected is based on the patient symptoms Health-food stores and some pharmacies sell homeopathic remedies for a variety of problems. Remedies are usually taken for no more than 2 or 3 days, though some people require only one or two doses before starting to feel better. If a remedy fails, it may be because it was the wrong substance for the set of symptoms.	Some homeopathic products contain heavy metals like mercury or iron that are not highly diluted and can cause serious adverse effects Some liquid homeopathic products contain alcohol at higher levels than conventional drugs. Homeopaths expect some patients to experience "homeopathic aggravation" – Temporary worsening of existing symptoms after taking a homeopathic remedy	Today, United States has 5 naturopathic schools and 16 homeopathy institutions. The majority of medical schools offer courses on homeopathy. Primary care physicians take introductory courses in homeopathy Homeopaths are not regarded as "doctors" without an MD degree

References

Abdullahi, A. A. (2011). Trends and challenges of traditional medicine in Africa. *African journal of traditional, complementary, and alternative medicines: AJTCAM*, 8(5 Suppl), 115–123. [online]. Available at: https://www.ncbi.nlm.nih.gov/pmc/articles/PMC3252714/. Accessed: 27 Nov 2020.

Ali, B., Ali Al-Wabel, N., Shams, S., Ahamad, A., Alam Khan, S., & Anwar, F. (2015). Essential oils used in aromatherapy: A systemic review. *Asian Pacific Journal of Tropical Biomedicine*, 5(8), 601–611. [online]. Available at: http://www.sciencedirect.com/science/article/pii/S2221169115001033. Accessed 10 Dec 2020.

Americans for Homeopathy Choice. (2018). *The evidence for homeopathy's safety and effectiveness*. [online]. Available at: https://homeopathychoice.org/wp-content/uploads/2018/09/Evidence-Supporting-Homeopathy-REVISED-FINAL.pdf. Accessed 30 Nov 2020.

Amir, M., Mahboube, G., Tahereh, M. G., Mahnaz, K., & Fariba, T. (2015). A study on the efficacy of spirituality-based intervention on spiritual well being of patients with leukemia: A randomized clinical trial. *Middle East Journal of Cancer, 6*, 97–105. [online]. Available at: https://www.semanticscholar.org/paper/A-Study-on-the-Efficacy-of-Spirituality-Based-on-of-Amir-Mahboube/45ed549c8679482702c76d1c8519db6cdd2899dd?sort=relevance. Accessed 10 Dec 2020.

Andras. (2016). Episode #050, feat. Britt Hermes. *The European skeptics podcast*. [online]. Available at: https://theesp.eu/podcast_archive/episode_050_britt_hermes.html. Accessed 29 Nov 2020.

Antonelli, M., & Donelli, D. (2020). Efficacy, safety and tolerability of Aroma massage with Lavender essential oil: An Overview. *International Journal of Therapeutic Massage Bodywork, 13*(1), 32–36. [online]. Available at: https://www.ncbi.nlm.nih.gov/pmc/articles/PMC7043716/. Accessed 10 Dec 2020.

Armstrong, M., Flemming, K., Kupeli, N., Stone, P., Wilkinson, S., & Candy, B. (2019). Aromatherapy, massage and reflexology: A systematic review and thematic synthesis of the perspectives from people with palliative care needs. *Palliative Medicine, 33*(7), 757–769. https://doi.org/10.1177/0269216319846440

Augustyn, A. (2021). Ayurveda medical system. *Encyclopaedia Britannica*. [online]. Available at: https://www.britannica.com/science/Ayurveda. Accessed 5 May 2021.

Bahrami, T., Rejeh, N., Heravi-Karimooi, M., Vaismoradi, M., Tadrisi, S. D., & Sieloff, C. (2017). Effect of aromatherapy massage on anxiety, depression, and physiologic parameters in older patients with the acute coronary syndrome: A randomized clinical trial. *International Journal of Nursing Practice, 23*(6), e12601. https://doi.org/10.1111/ijn.12601

Bakhtshirin, F., Abedi, S., YusefiZoj, P., & Razmjooee, D. (2015). The effect of aromatherapy massage with lavender oil on severity of primary dysmenorrhea in Arsanjan students. *Iran Journal Nursing Midwifery Research, 20*(1), 156–160. [online]. Available at: https://www.ncbi.nlm.nih.gov/pubmed/25709705. Accessed 10 Dec 2020.

Balkrishna, A. & Misra, L.N. (2017). Ayurvedic plants in brain disorders: the herbal hope. *Journal of Traditional Medicine & Clinical Naturopathy, 6*, 1–9. [online]. Available at: https://www.omicsonline.org/open-access/ayurvedic-plants-in-brain-disorders-the-herbal-hope.php?aid=89160. Accessed 29 Nov 2020.

Balogun, J. A. (1999). Acupuncture: A rebuttal. *Disability and Rehabilitation, 21*(3), 137–138. [online]. Available at:https://www.researchgate.net/publication/271077361_Balogun_JA_1999_Editorial_introduction_The_effects_of_acupuncture_electroneedling_and_transcutaneous_electrical_stimulation_therapies_on_peripheral_hemodynamic_functioning_Acupuncture_a_rebuttal_Disab

Balogun, J. A., Biasci, S., & Han, L. (1998). The effects of acupuncture, electroneedling and transcutaneous electrical stimulation therapies on peripheral haemodynamic functioning. *Disability and Rehabilitation, 20*, 41–48. [online]. Available at: https://www.researchgate.net/publication/13737763_The_effects_of_acupuncture_electroneedling_and_transcutaneous_electrical_stimulation_therapies_on_peripheral_haemodynamic_functioning

Baran, G. R., Kiana, M. F., & Samuel, S. P. (2014). Science, pseudoscience, and not science: How do they differ?. Chapter 2: Science, pseudoscience, and not science: How do they differ? *Healthcare and biomedical technology in the 21st century.* Springer, pp. 19–57. https://doi. org/10.1007/978-1-4614-8541-4_2. ISBN 978-1-4614-8540-7.

Bauer, B. A. (2020). *What are the benefits of aromatherapy?* [online]. Available at: https:// www.mayoclinic.org/healthy-lifestyle/consumer-health/expert-answers/aromatherapy/ faq-20058566. Accessed 10 Dec 2020.

Beecher, H. K. (1955). The powerful placebo. *Journal of American Medical Association, 159,* 1602–1606.

Bender, M. M., Levy, A. S., Schucker, R. E., & Yetley, E. A. (1992). Trends in prevalence and magnitude of vitamin and mineral supplement usage and correlation with health status. *Journal of American Dietetic Association, 92,* 1096–1101. [online]. Available at: https://pubmed.ncbi. nlm.nih.gov/1512368/. Accessed 16 Mar 2021.

Benson, H. (1990). *The relaxation response* (Reissue ed.). Avon.

Benson, H. (1996). *Timeless healing: The power and biology of belief.* Simon and Schuster.

Brady, M. J., Peterman, A. H., Fitchett, G., Mo, M., & Cella, D. (1999). A case for including spirituality in quality-of-life measurement in oncology. *Psycho-Oncology, 8,* 417–428.

Cameron, A., Ewen, M., Ross-Degnan, D., & Laing, R. (2008). Medicine prices, availability, and affordability in 36 developing and middle-income countries: A secondary analysis. *The Lancet.* 373(9659):240–249. [online]. Available at: https://pubmed.ncbi.nlm.nih.gov/19042012/. Accessed: 27 Nov 2020.

Carnes, D., Mars, T. S., Mullinger, B., Froud, R., & Underwood, M. (2010). Adverse events and manual therapy: A systematic review. *Manual Therapy, 15*(4), 355–363. https://doi. org/10.1016/j.math.2009.12.006

Çetinkaya, B., & Başbakkal, Z. (2012). The effectiveness of aromatherapy massage using lavender oil as a treatment for infantile colic. *International Journal Nursing Practice, 18*(2), 164–169. https://doi.org/10.1111/j.1440-172X.2012.02015.x

Cheraghbeigi, N., Modarresi, M., Rezaei, M., & Khatony, A. (2019). Comparing the effects of massage and aromatherapy massage with lavender oil on sleep quality of cardiac patients: A randomized controlled trial. *Complementary Therapy Clinical Practice, 35,* 253–258. https:// doi.org/10.1016/j.ctcp.2019.03.005

Cino, K. (2014). Aromatherapy hand massage for older adults with chronic pain living in long-term care. *Journal Holistic Nursing, 32*(4), 304–313. https://doi.org/10.1177/0898010114528378

Clarke, T. C., Black, L. I., Stussman, B. J., Barnes, P. M., & Nahin, R. L. (2015). *Trends in the use of complementary health approaches among adults: The United States, 2002–2012. National health statistics reports; no 79.* Hyattsville: National Center for Health Statistics. [online]. Available at: https://www.nccih.nih.gov/research/trends-in-the-use-of-complementary-health-in-the-united-states-20022012. Accessed 10 Dec 2020.

Cohen, S. R., Mount, B. M., Strobel, M. G., & Bui, F. (1995). The McGill quality of life questionnaire: A measure of quality of life appropriate for people with advanced disease. A preliminary study of validity and acceptability. *Palliative Medicine, 9,* 207–219.

Cook, J. A., & Wimberly, D. W. (1983). If I should die before I wake: Religious commitment and adjustment to death of a child. *Journal of the Scientific Study of Religion, 22,* 222–238.

Darvishi, A., Otaghi, M., & Mami, S. (2020). The effectiveness of spiritual therapy on spiritual well-being, self-esteem and self-efficacy in patients on hemodialysis. *Journal of Religion and Health, 59*(1), 277–288. https://doi.org/10.1007/s10943-018-00750-1

Davidson, K., & Tinsley, G. (2020). *What is the Ayurvedic detox, and does it work?* [online]. Available at: https://www.healthline.com/nutrition/ayurvedic-detox. Accessed 29 Nov 2020.

Degenhardt, B. F., Johnson, J. C., Brooks, W. J., & Norman, L. (2018). Characterizing adverse events reported immediately after osteopathic manipulative treatment. *Journal of the American Osteopathic Association, 118*(3), 141–149.

Devitt, M. (2018). *Research finds acupuncture effective for chronic pain.* [online]. Available at: https://www.aafp.org/news/health-of-the-public/20180521acupuncture.html. Accessed 10 Dec 2020.

Donelli, D., Antonelli, M., Bellinazzi, C., Gensini, G. F., & Firenzuoli, F. (2019). Effects of lavender on anxiety: A systematic review and meta-analysis. *Phytomedicine, 65.* https://doi.org/10.1016/j.phymed.2019.153099.153099

Dunne, N., Benda, W., Kim, L., Mittman, P., Barrett, R., Snider, P., & Pizzorno, J. (2005). Naturopathic medicine: What can patients expect? *Journal of Family Practice, 54*(12), 1067–1072. [online]. Available at: https://www.mdedge.com/familymedicine/article/61947/naturopathic-medicine-what-can-patients-expect. Accessed 29 Nov 2020.

Ehman, J. W., Ott, B. B., Short, T. H., Ciampa, R. C., & Hansen-Flaschen, J. (1999). Do patients want physicians to inquire about their spiritual or religious beliefs if they become gravely ill? *Archives of Internal Medicine, 159,* 1803–1806.

Elmer, G. W., Lafferty, W. E., Tyree, P. T., & Lind, B. K. (2007). Potential interactions between complementary/alternative products and conventional medicines in a Medicare population. *Annals of Pharmacotherapy, 41*(10), 1617–1624. [online]. Available at: https://www.medscape.com/viewarticle/564019. Accessed 27 Nov 2020.

Ernst, E. (2002). A systematic review of systematic reviews of homeopathy. *British Journal of Clinical Pharmacology, 54*(6), 577–582. https://doi.org/10.1046/j.1365-2125.2002.01699.x

Ernst, E. (2007). Adverse effects of spinal manipulation: a systematic review. *Journal of the Royal Society of Medicine, 100*(7), 330–338. [online]. Available at: https://www.ncbi.nlm.nih.gov/pmc/articles/PMC1905885/. Accessed 30 Nov 2020.

Fan, K. W. (2005). National Center for Complementary and Alternative Medicine Website. *Journal of Medical Library Association, 93*(3), 410–412. [online]. Available at: https://www.ncbi.nlm.nih.gov/pmc/articles/PMC3307506/. Accessed 10 Dec 2020.

FDA Center for Food Safety and Applied Nutrition. (n.d.). *Dietary supplements.* [online]. Available at: https://www.sciencedirect.com/topics/agricultural-and-biological-sciences/center-for-food-safety-and-applied-nutrition. Accessed 10 Dec 2020.

Fellowes, D., Barnes, K., & Wilkinson, S. (2004). Aromatherapy and massage for symptom relief in patients with cancer. *Cochrane Database Systematic Review, 3,* CD002287.

Fleming, S. A., & Gutknecht, N. C. (2010). Naturopathy and the primary care practice. *Primary Care: Clinics in Office Practice, 37*(1), 119–136. [online]. Available at: https://www.ncbi.nlm.nih.gov/pmc/articles/PMC2883816/citedby/. Accessed 29 Nov 2020.

Food and Drug Administration. (2008). *Use caution with Ayurvedic products.* [online]. Available at: https://www.fda.gov/consumers/consumer-updates/use-caution-ayurvedic-products. Accessed 29 Nov 2020.

Frass, M., Strassl, R. P., Friehs, H., Müllner, M., Kundi, M., & Kaye, A. D. (2012). Use and acceptance of complementary and alternative medicine among the general population and medical personnel: A systematic review. *Ochsner Journal, 12*(1), 45–56. [online] Available at: https://www.ncbi.nlm.nih.gov/pmc/articles/PMC3307506/. Accessed 10 Dec 2020.

Ghiasi, A., Bagheri, L., & Haseli, A. (2019). A systematic review on the anxiolytic effect of aromatherapy during the first stage of labor. *Journal of Caring Science, 8*(1), 51–60. https://doi.org/10.15171/jcs.2019.008

Goertz, C., & Coulter, I. (2019). *Efficacy of chiropractic care for back pain: A comparative effectiveness controlled trial evaluated the addition of chiropractic care to usual medical care for patients suffering from low back pain.* Remedy Health Media, LLC, pp. 64–65 [online]. Available at: https://www.practicalpainmanagement.com/treatments/manipulation/efficacy-chiropractic-care-back-pain-clinical-summary. Accessed 27 Nov 2020.

Goertz, C., et al. (2018, May 18). Effect of usual medical care plus chiropractic care vs usual medical care alone on pain and disability among US service members with low back pain. *Journal of the American Medical Association Network Open*; ePub.

Guha, A. & Cameron, M. E. (2016). *Is Ayurvedic medicine safe?* [online]. Available at: https://www.takingcharge.csh.umn.edu/explore-healing-practices/ayurvedic-medicine/-ayurvedic-medicine-safe-0. Accessed 29 Nov 2020.

Hajibabaei, M, Kajbaf, MB, Esmaeili, M, Harirchian, MH, Montazeri, A. (2020) Impact of an existential-spiritual intervention compared with a cognitive-behavioral therapy on quality of life and meaning in life among women with multiple sclerosis. Iranian Journal of Psychiatry;15(4):322-330. [online]. Available at: http://search.ebscohost.com/login.aspx?direct=true&AuthType=sso&db=ccm&AN=146015160&site=ehost-live. Accessed 10 Dec 2020.

Hargrave, J. G. (2021). Paracelsus. *Encyclopedia Britannica*. https://www.britannica.com/biography/Paracelsus

Harris, R. C., Dew, M. A., Lee, A., Amaya, M., Buches, L., Reetz, D., & Coleman, C. (1995). The role of religion in heart-transplant recipients' long-term health and well-being. *Journal of Religion and Health, 34*(1), 17–32.

Hashemi, S. H., Hajbagheri, A., & Aghajani, M. (2015). The effect of massage with lavender oil on restless leg syndrome in hemodialysis patients: A randomized controlled trial. *Nursing Midwifery Studies, 4*(4), e29617. https://doi.org/10.17795/nmsjournal29617

Heid, M. (2017). *Are chiropractors legitimate?* [online]. Available at: https://time.com/4282617/chiropractor-lower-back-pain/. Accessed 27 Nov 2020.

Hensel, K. L., Roane, B. M., Chaphekar, A. V., & Smith-Barbaro, P. (2016). PROMOTE study: Safety of osteopathic manipulative treatment during the third trimester by labor and delivery outcomes. *Journal of the American Osteopathic Association, 116*(11), 698–703. https://doi.org/10.7556/jaoa.2016.140

Hermes, M. (2016). *Is Naturopathic medicine safe and effective? Leading naturopathic researchers cannot even say.* [online]. Available at: https://www.science20.com/profile/britt_hermes. Accessed 29 Nov 2020.

Ingraham, P. (2020). *The chiropractic controversies: An introduction to chiropractic controversies like aggressive billing, treating kids, and neck manipulation risks.* PainScience.com. [online]. Available at: https://www.painscience.com/articles/does-chiropractic-work.php. Accessed 27 Nov 2020.

Jäger, W., Buchbauer, G., Jirovetz, L., & Fritzer, M. (1992). Percutaneous absorption of lavender oil from a massage oil. *Journal Society of Cosmetic Chemistry, 43*(1), 49–54.

James, P. B., Wardle, J., Steel, A., et al. (2018). Traditional, complementary and alternative medicine use in sub-Saharan Africa: A systematic review. *British Medical Journal Global Health, 3*, e000895. [online]. Available at: https://gh.bmj.com/content/3/5/e000895. Accessed 10 May 2021.

Jamrog, K. A.. (2018). The effectiveness of aromatherapy. *New Hampshire Magazine* [online]. Available at: https://www.nhmagazine.com/the-effectiveness-of-aromatherapy/. Accessed 10 Dec 2020.

Jarvis, W. T. (1992). Quackery: A national scandal. *Clinical Chemistry, 38*(8B Pt 2), 1574–1586. [online]. Available at: https://pubmed.ncbi.nlm.nih.gov/1643742/. Accessed 29 Nov 2020.

Johns Hopkins Medicine. (2020) *Acupuncture.* [online]. Available at: https://www.hopkinsmedicine.org/health/wellness-and-prevention/acupuncture. Accessed 10 Dec 2020.

Johns Hopkins University. (2021). *What is Ayurveda?* [online]. Available at: https://www.hopkinsmedicine.org/health/wellness-and-prevention/ayurveda#:~:text=Ayurveda%2C%20a%20natural%20system%20of,translates%20to%20knowledge%20of%20life. Accessed 5 May 2021.

Kahrizeh, M., Saberi, M., & Bashirgonbadi, S. (2020). Effect of spiritual-religious interventions on anxiety, depression, and adjustment to parental divorce in female high school students. *Health, Spirituality and Medical Ethics Journal, 7*(2), 2–8. https://doi.org/10.29252/jhsme.7.2.2

Kaldjian, L. C., Jekel, J. F., & Friedland, G. (1998). End-of-life decisions in HIV-positive patients: The role of spiritual beliefs. *AIDS, 12*, 103–107.

Kirby, B. J. (2002). Safety of homeopathic products. *Journal of Royal Society of Medicine, 95*(5), 221–222. [online]. Available at: https://www.ncbi.nlm.nih.gov/pmc/articles/PMC1279671/. Accessed 30 Nov 2020.

Koenig, H. G., Cohen, H. J., George, L. K., Hays, J. C., Larson, D. B., & Blazer, D. G. (1997). Attendance at religious services, interleukin-6, and other biological parameters of immune function in older adults. *International Journal of Psychiatry Medicine, 27*, 233–250.

Koithan, M. (2009). Introducing complementary and alternative therapies. *Journal of Nursing Practice, 5*(1), 18–20.

Kootenaycolumbiacollege. (2018). The *Chinese medicine meridian system*. [online]. Available at: https://kootenaycolumbiacollege.com/the-chinese-medicine-meridian-system/. Accessed 29 Nov 2020.

Koppelman, M. H. (2018). *Acupuncture: An overview of scientific evidence*. [online]. Available at: https://www.evidencebasedacupuncture.org/acupuncture-scientific-evidence/. Accessed 10 Dec 2020.

Koulivand, P. H., Ghadiri, M. K., & Gorji, A. (2013). Lavender and the nervous system. *Evidence Based Complementary Alternative Medicine*. https://doi.org/10.1155/2013/681304.681304

Ladyman, J. (2013). Chapter 3: Towards a demarcation of science from pseudoscience. In M. Pigliucci & M. Boudry (Eds.), *Philosophy of pseudoscience: Reconsidering the demarcation problem* (pp. 48–49). University of Chicago Press. ISBN 978-0-226-05196-3.

Lakhan, S. E., Sheafer, H., & Tepper, D. (2016). The effectiveness of aromatherapy in reducing pain: A systematic review and meta-analysis. *Pain Research Treatment, 8158693*.

Landmark Healthcare. (1996) [online]. Available at: https://www.dnb.com/business-directory/company-profiles.landmark_healthcare_services_inc.73f61c765d6254b624e620831a893906.html. Accessed: 27 Nov 2020.

Lee, S. Y. (2005). The effect of lavender aromatherapy on cognitive function, emotion, and aggressive behavior of elderly with dementia. *Journal Korean Academic Nursing, 35*(2), 303–312. https://doi.org/10.4040/jkan.2005.35.2.303

Lee, D. Y. W., Li, Q. Y., Liu, J., & Efferth, T. (2021). Traditional Chinese herbal medicine at the forefront battle against COVID-19: Clinical experience and scientific basis, *Phytomedicine, 80*. [online]. Available at: https://doi.org/10.1016/j.phymed.2020.153337. Accessed 29 Nov 2020.

Licciardone, J. C., & Aryal, S. (2013a). Prevention of progressive back-specific dysfunction during pregnancy: An assessment of osteopathic manual treatment based on Cochrane Back review group criteria. *Journal of the American Osteopathic Association, 113*(10), 728–736. https://doi.org/10.7556/jaoa.2013.043.

Licciardone, J. C., Minotti, D. E., Gatchel, R. J., Kearns, C. M., & Singh, K. P. (2013b). Osteopathic manual treatment and ultrasound therapy for chronic low back pain: A randomized controlled trial. *Annals Family Medicine, 11*(2), 122–129. https://doi.org/10.1370/afm.1468

Lucas, K. H. (2006). *The interaction of CAM and prescription heart medications*. [online]. Available at: https://www.uspharmacist.com/article/the-interaction-of-cam-and-prescription-heart-medications. Accessed 27 Nov 2020.

Mandal, A., & Cashin-Garbutt, A. (2019). *How effective is acupuncture?* [online]. Available at: https://www.news-medical.net/health/How-Effective-is-Acupuncture.aspx

McCauley, J., Haaz, S., Tarpley, M. J., Koenig, H. G., & Bartlett, S. J. (2011). A randomized controlled trial to assess effectiveness of a spiritually-based intervention to help chronically ill adults. *International Journal of Psychiatry in Medicine, 41*(1), 91–105. https://doi.org/10.2190/PM.41.1.h

McNeill, J. A., Sherwood, G. D., Starck, P. L., & Thompson, C. J. (1998). Assessing clinical outcomes: Patient satisfaction with pain management. *Journal of Pain Symptomatology Management, 16*, 29–40.

McNichol, T. (1996). The new faith in medicine. *USA Today Weekend*; 4–5 (survey conducted February 1996 by ICR Research Group).

Michigan Health System – UMHS. (2019) *Aromatherapy with essential oils (PDQ®): Integrative, alternative, and complementary therapies – Patient information*. [online]. Available at: https://www.uofmhealth.org/health-library/ncicdr0000458089

Moritz, S., Quan, H., Rickhi, B., et al. (2006). A home study-based spirituality education program decreases emotional distress and increases quality of life -- a randomized, controlled trial. *Alternative Therapies in Health and Medicine, 12*(6), 26–35. [online] Available at: https://pubmed.ncbi.nlm.nih.gov/17131979/

Myers, S. P., & Vigar, V. (2019). The state of the evidence for whole-system, multi-modality naturopathic medicine: A systematic scoping review. *Journal of Alternative Complementary Medicine, 25*(2), 141–168. [online]. Available at: https://www.ncbi.nlm.nih.gov/pmc/articles/PMC6389764/. Accessed 29 Nov 2020.

Nasiri, A., Mahmodi, M. A., & Nobakht, Z. (2016). Effect of aromatherapy massage with lavender essential oil on pain in patients with osteoarthritis of the knee: A randomized controlled clinical trial. *Complementary Therapy Clinical Practice, 25*, 75–80. https://doi.org/10.1016/j.ctcp.2016.08.002

Nathan, U. (2017). Religion verses spirituality. *The Nigerian Voice*. [online]. Available at: https://www.thenigerianvoice.com/news/256218/religion-verses-spirituality.html Accessed 18 Mar 2021.

Nathan Cummings Foundation, Fetzer Institute, George H. Gallup International Institute. (1997). *Spiritual beliefs and the dying process, a report on a national survey*. The George H Gallup International Institute.

National Cancer Institute. (2021). *Complementary and alternative medicine*. National Institutes of Health. [online]. Available at: https://www.cancer.gov/about-cancer/treatment/cam. Accessed 27 July 2021.

National Center for Complementary and Integrative Health- NCCIH. (2019). *Traditional Chinese medicine: What you need to know – What is the bottom line?* [online]. Available at: https://www.nccih.nih.gov/health/traditional-chinese-medicine-what-you-need-to-know. Accessed 27 Nov 2020.

National Center for Complementary and Integrative Health- NCCIH. (2020). Ayurvedic medicine: *In depth*. [online]. Available at: https://www.nccih.nih.gov/health/ayurvedic-medicine-in-depth. Accessed 29 Nov 2020.

NBJ's Annual Industry. (2003). Overview VIII. *Nutrition Business Journal, 8*, 1–9.

NCCIH. (2018). *Homeopathy*. [online]. Available at: https://www.nccih.nih.gov/health/homeopathy. Accessed 30 Nov 2020.

NHS. (2018a). *Homeopathy*. [online]. Available at: https://www.nhs.uk/conditions/homeopathy/. Accessed 30 Nov 2020.

NHS. (2018b). *Safety and regulation: Osteopathy*. [online]. Available at: https://www.nhs.uk/conditions/osteopathy/safety/. Accessed 30 Nov 2020.

Nielsen, S. M., Tarp, S., Christensen, R., Bliddal, H., Klokker, L., & Henriksen, M. (2017). The risk associated with spinal manipulation: An overview of reviews. *Systems Review, 6*(1), 64. https://doi.org/10.1186/s13643-017-0458-y

Noll, D. R., Degenhardt, B. F., & Johnson, J. C. (2016). Multicenter osteopathic pneumonia study in the elderly: Subgroup analysis on hospital length of stay, ventilator-dependent respiratory failure rate, and in-hospital mortality rate. *Journal of the American Osteopathic Association, 116*(9), 574–587.

Ochoa, C. Y., Haardörfer, R., Escoffery, C., Stein, K., & Alcaraz, K. I. (2018). Examining the role of social support and spirituality on the general health perceptions of Hispanic cancer survivors. *Psycho-Oncology, 27*(9), 2189–2197. https://doi.org/10.1002/pon.4795

Olver, I. N., & Dutney, A. (2012). A randomized, blinded study of the impact of intercessory prayer on spiritual well-being in patients with cancer. *Alternative Therapies in Health & Medicine, 18*(5), 18–27. [online]. Available at: https://pubmed.ncbi.nlm.nih.gov/22894887/

Osteopathic Medical Foundation. (n.d.) *Principles of osteopathy*. [online]. Available at: http://www.omfmichiana.org/principles-osteopathy. Accessed 16 Mar 2021.

Painter, F. M. (2020). *Stroke and chiropractic*. [online]. Available at: https://chiro.org/Stroke/. Accessed 30 Nov 2020.

Park, C. L., & Lee, S. Y. (2020). Unique effects of religiousness/spirituality and social support on mental and physical Well-being in people living with congestive heart failure. *Journal of Behavioral Medicine, 43*(4), 630–637. https://doi.org/10.1007/s10865-019-00101-9

Park, C. L., Waddington, E., & Abraham, R. (2018). Different dimensions of religiousness/spirituality are associated with health behaviors in breast cancer survivors. *Psycho-Oncology, 27*(10), 2466–2472. https://doi.org/10.1002/pon.4852

Puchalski, C. M. (2001). The role of spirituality in health care. *Proceedings of Baylor University Medical Center, 14*(4), 352–357. https://doi.org/10.1080/08998280.2001.11927788

Pugle, M., & Wilson, D. R. (2019). Are essential oils safe? 13 things to know before use. *Healthline.* [online]. Available at: https://www.healthline.com/health/are-essential-oils-safe#topical-use. Accessed 10 Dec 2020.

Roberts, J. A., Brown, D., Elkins, T., & Larson, D. B. (1997). Factors influencing views of patients with gynecologic cancer about end-of-life decisions. *American Journal of Obstetrics and Gynecology, 176*(1), 166–172.

Sarker, M. R. (2014). Therapeutic efficacy and safety of traditional Ayurvedic medicines: Demands for extensive research and publication. *Journal of Homeopathic Ayurvedic Medicine, 3*, e113. https://doi.org/10.4172/2167-1206.1000e113. [online]. Available at: https://www.omicsonline. org/open-access/therapeutic-efficacy-and-safety-of-traditional-ayurvedic-medicines-demands-for-extensive-research-and-publications-2167-1206.1000e113.php?aid=27099#:~:text=Tradit ionally%2C%20Ayurvedic%20medicines%20are%20very,their%20therapeutic%20effectiveness%20and%20safety. Accessed 29 Nov 2020.

Schroeder, S., Burnis, J., Denton, A., Krasnow, A., Raghu, T. S., & Mathis, K. (2017). Effectiveness of acupuncture therapy on stress in a large urban college population. *Journal of Acupuncture and Meridian Studies, 10*(3), 165–170. [online]. Available at: https://www.sciencedirect.com/ science/article/pii/S2005290116301224. Accessed 10 Dec 2020.

Seffinger, M. A. (2018). The safety of osteopathic manipulative treatment. *The Journal of the American Osteopathic Association, 118*, 137–138. https://doi.org/10.7556/jaoa.2018.031

Simkin, P., & Bolding, A. (2004). Update on nonpharmacologic approaches to relieve labor pain and prevent suffering. *Journal of Midwifery and Women's Health, 49*(6) [online]. Available at: https://www.medscape.com/viewarticle/494120_11. Accessed 10 Dec 2020.

Sinay, D. (2019) Electroacupuncture. *Healthline.* [online]. Available at: https://www.healthline. com/health/electroacupuncture. Accessed 11 Apr 2020.

Smith, K. (2012). Homeopathy is unscientific and unethical. *Bioethics, 26*(9), 508–512. https://doi. org/10.1111/j.1467-8519.2011.01956.x

Soden, K., Vincent, K., Craske, S., Lucas, C., & Ashley, S. (2004). A randomized controlled trial of aromatherapy massage in a hospice setting. *Palliative Medicine, 18*(2), 87–92. https://doi. org/10.1191/0269216304pm874oa

Strawbridge, W. J., Cohen, R. D., Shema, S. J., & Kaplan, G. A. (1997). Frequent attendance at religious services and mortality over 28 years. *American Journal of Public Health, 87*, 957–961.

Subar, A. F., & Block, G. (1990). Use of vitamin and mineral supplements: Demographics and amounts of nutrients consumed. The 1987 Health Interview Survey. *American Journal of Epidemiology, 132*, 1091–1101. [online]. Available at: https://pubmed.ncbi.nlm.nih. gov/2260541/. Accessed 16 Mar 2021.

Tabish, S. A. (2008). Complementary and alternative healthcare: Is it evidence-based? *International Journal Health Science (Qassim), 2*(1), V–IX. [online]. Available at: https://www.ncbi.nlm.nih. gov/pmc/articles/PMC3068720/. Accessed 10 Dec 2020.

Taylor, D. M., Walsham, N., Taylor, S. E., & Wong, L. (2006). Potential interactions between prescription drugs and complementary and alternative medicines among patients in the emergency department. *Pharmacotherapy, 26*, 634–640. [online]. Available at: https://www.medscape. com/viewarticle/542437. Accessed 27 Nov 2020.

The Osteopathic Cranial Academy. (2018). *History of osteopathy.* [online]. Available at: https:// cranialacademy.org/patients/history-of-osteopathy/. Accessed 16 Mar 2021.

Thomas-Purcell, K., Ibe, T. A., Purcell, D., Quinn, G., & Ownby, R. (2020). Exploring spirituality and technology receptivity among a sample of older Blacks to inform a tailored chronic disease self-management health intervention. *Patient Relative Outcome Measurement, 11*, 195–207.

[online]. Available at: https://www.ncbi.nlm.nih.gov/pmc/articles/PMC7553651/. Accessed 10 Dec 2020.

Thorne, S., Paterson, B., Russell, C., & Schultz, A. (2002). *Complementary/alternative medicine in chronic illness as informed self-care decision making.* Int J Nurs Stud;39(7):671–83. [online]. Available at: https://pubmed.ncbi.nlm.nih.gov/12231024/. Accessed: 27 Nov 2020.

Tuomela, R. (1987). Chapter 4: Science, protoscience, and pseudoscience. In J. C. Pitt & P. Marcello (Eds.), *Rational changes in science: Essays on scientific reasoning* (*Boston studies in the philosophy of science*) (Vol. 98, pp. 83–101). https://doi.org/10.1007/978-94-009-3779-6_4. Springer.

Turner, RC, Lucke-Wold, BP, Boo, S, Rosen, CL, Sedney, CL. (2018). The potential dangers of neck manipulation and risk for dissection and devastating stroke: An illustrative case and review of the literature. *Biomedical Research Review, 2*(1). https://doi.org/10.15761/BRR.1000110. [online]. Available at: https://www.ncbi.nlm.nih.gov/pmc/articles/PMC6016850/citedby/. Accessed 30 Nov 2020.

University of California, San Francisco. (2020). *Complementary and alternative medicine.* [online]. Available at: https://memory.ucsf.edu/treatments-stays/medications-dementia/complementary-alternative-medicine. Accessed 27 Nov 2020.

University of Minnesota. (2016). *Is TCM evidence-based and safe?* [online]. Available at: https://www.takingcharge.csh.umn.edu/tcm-evidence-based-and-safe. Accessed 29 Nov 2020.

US Food and Drug Administration. (2020). *What is homeopathy?* [online]. Available at: https://www.fda.gov/drugs/information-drug-class/homeopathic-products. Accessed 30 Nov 2020.

ValueMD. (2005). *List of countries where US-trained osteopaths are recognized.* [online]. Available at:https://www.valuemd.com/osteopathic-medicine/29288-list-countries-trained osteopaths-recognized.html. Accessed 26 Feb 2020.

Vick, D. A., McKay, C., & Zengerle, C. R. (1996). The safety of manipulative treatment: Review of the literature from 1925 to 1993. *Journal of the American Osteopathic Association, 96*(2), 113–115.

Vickers, A., & Zollman, C. (1999). The manipulative therapies: Osteopathy and chiropractic. *BMJ, 319*(7218), 1176–1179. https://doi.org/10.1136/bmj.319.7218.1176. [online]. Available at: https://www.ncbi.nlm.nih.gov/pmc/articles/PMC1116959/citedby/. Accessed 30 Nov 2020.

WebMD. (2020). *What is naturopathic medicine?* [online]. Available at: https://www.webmd.com/balance/guide/what-is-naturopathic-medicine#1. Accessed 29 Nov 2020.

Wetzel, M., Kaptchuk, T. J., Haramati, A., Eisenberg, D. M. (2003). Complementary and alternative medical therapies: Implications for medical education. *Annals of Internal Medicine*,138(3):191–6. [online]. Available at: https://www.researchgate.net/publication/10925936_Complementary_and_alternative_medical_therapies_Implications_for_medical_education. Accessed: 27 November 2020.

WHO (2000). *Traditional and modern medicine: Harmonizing the two approaches Western Pacific Region.* Geneva: World Health Organization.

WHO (2001). *Promoting the role of traditional medicine in health systems: A strategy for the African region Harare, WHO Regional Office for Africa, Harare, 2001* (document reference AFR/RC50/9).

WHO (2002a). *WHO Traditional medicine strategy 2002–2005.* Geneva: World Health Organization.

WHO (2002b). *Traditional Medicine-Growing needs and potential.* Geneva: World Health Organization.

WHO (2010a). *Benchmarks for training in traditional/complementary and alternative medicine: Benchmarks for training in naturopathy.* [online]. Available at: https://www.who.int/medicines/areas/traditional/BenchmarksforTraininginNaturopathy.pdf. Accessed 29 Nov 2020.

WHO (2010b). *Benchmarks for training in traditional/complementary and alternative medicine: Benchmarks for training in osteopathy.* [online]. Available at: https://www.who.int/medicines/areas/traditional/BenchmarksforTraininginOsteopathy.pdf. Accessed 30 Nov 2020.

Williams, T. I. (2006). Evaluating effects of aromatherapy massage on sleep in children with autism: A pilot study. *Evidence Based Complementary and Alternative Medicine, 3*(3), 373–377. https://doi.org/10.1093/ecam/nel017

Wiriyasombat, R., Pothiban, L., Panuthai, S., Sucamvang, K., & Saengthong, S. (2011). Effectiveness of Buddhist doctrine practice-based programs in enhancing spiritual well-being, coping and sleep quality of Thai elders. *Pacific Rim International Journal of Nursing Research, 15*(3), 203–218. [online]. Available at: http://search.ebscohost.com/login.aspx?direct=true&AuthType=sso&db=ccm&AN=104686039&site=ehost-live. Accessed 10 Dec 2020.

World Health Organization. (2009). *Safety issues in the preparation of homeopathic medicines.* [online]. Available at: https://www.who.int/medicines/areas/traditional/Homeopathy.pdf. Accessed 30 Nov 2020.

Yap, W. S., Dolzhenko, A. V., & Jalal, Z. (2019). Efficacy and safety of lavender essential oil (Silexan) capsules among patients suffering from anxiety disorders: A network meta-analysis. *Science Report, 9*, 18042. [online]. Available at: https://doi.org/10.1038/s41598-019-54529-9https://www.nature.com/articles/s41598-019-54529-9. Accessed 10 Dec 2020.

Yates, J. W., Chalmer, B. J., St James, P., Follansbee, M., & McKegney, F. P. (1981). Religion in patients with advanced cancer. *Medical Pediatric Oncology, 9*, 121–128.

Zhang, X. Y., Li, Y., Liu, D., Zhang, B., & Chen, D. (2019). The effectiveness of acupuncture therapy in patients with post-stroke depression: An updated meta-analysis of randomized controlled trials. *Medicine (Baltimore), 98*(22), e15894. [online]. Available at: https://www.ncbi.nlm.nih.gov/pmc/articles/PMC6708961/citedby/. Accessed 10 Dec 2020.

Chapter 7
Complementary and Alternative Medical Practice in Nigeria

Learning Objectives

After reading this chapter, the learner should be able to:

1. Trace the origin of the major disciplines associated with complementary and alternative medicine in Nigeria
2. Discuss the demand for utilization of complementary and alternative medical practices in Nigeria
3. Identify centers in Nigeria where complementary and alternative medical practitioners are available and institutions where they are trained

Introduction

Since the inception of the republic, Nigeria's federal government has shown some interest in integrating traditional medicine into the healthcare system. The first democratically elected government under President (Dr.) Nnamdi Azikiwe, in 1966, authorized the University of Ibadan to research the medicinal properties of local herbs, to standardize and regulate traditional medicine practice in the country. In 2000, a proposal was put forth by the federal government to establish the Traditional Medicine Council of Nigeria to facilitate the practice and development of traditional medicine and to oversee the training and regulation of traditional medicine to protect the population from deception, fraud, and incompetence. The federal government empowers the Medical and Dental Council of Nigeria (MDCN) to cooperate with state boards of traditional medicine by enforcing the Federal Traditional Medicine Board Act's policies and guidelines. Areas of collaboration include the establishment of model clinics, botanical gardens, herbal farms, and traditional medicine manufacturing units throughout the country (Ailemen, 2020). Additional proposed responsibility of the MDCN includes collaboration with agencies and parastatals within and outside Nigeria with the same objectives.

Many analysts believe the shortcomings of the Western-style health system in Nigeria led to the evolution of several complementary and alternative medical (CAM) disciplines (Oshikoya et al., 2008). However, the problems facing the Nigerian health system are myriad. They include the inadequate number of hospitals to provide quality health services, lack of authentic medication, long queues in the hospitals/clinics, limited surveillance/medical intelligence systems to effectively curtail epidemics, corruption, and inadequate funding (Ajao, 2017). The existing literature on the Nigerian health system contains limited information on the origin of CAM disciplines. Aside from traditional Chinese medicine (TCM) and homeopathy, the precise date of importation of the other CAM disciplines into the country is unknown. Although the organizations representing the CAM disciplines received tacit recognition by the federal government and the Medical and Dental Council of Nigeria (MDCN), the attention lacks legislative imprimatur. The MDCN presently regulates only chiropractic and osteopathy disciplines.

The CAM practitioners often adopt aggressive marketing strategies in print and electronic media to promote their products, which are also freely available on the open market. The advertisement and publicity notwithstanding, the CAM practitioners in Nigeria are not well known by the healthcare professionals (HCPs) and the public (Oshikoya et al., 2008). Currently, the scope of practice, training, utilization, and clinical expertise provided by these emerging occupations deserves a comprehensive review in this book. This chapter traces the origin of CAM practices within the Nigerian health system. It also describes the emerging developments within three complementary medical systems – acupuncture, chiropractic, and osteopathy – and seven alternative medical systems such as traditional Chinese medicine, Ayurveda, naturopathy, homeopathy, aromatherapy, spirituality, and African traditional medicine.

In this chapter, the term "complementary medicine" refers to medical practices used together with conventional (orthodox) western medicine – for example, the use of acupuncture to treat pain and the side effects associated with cancer treatment. The term "natural," "traditional," and "alternative" medicines are the healthcare practices outside of conventional medicine utilized by individual cultures throughout the world.

The Evolution of Complementary and Alternative Medical Systems in Nigeria

The various governments since independence have shown varying degrees of interest in integrating traditional medicine into the healthcare system. A watershed event occurred during Major General Obasanjo's military rule, in 1977, with the establishment of the Nigeria Institute of Medical Research and charged to conduct medical research of public health importance. Another significant landmark development occurred in 1997, when General Sani Abacha created the Nigeria Natural Medicine Development Agency (NNMDA) with the specific mission to develop and promote natural medicine, indigenous herbs, and non-medication healing systems. Additionally, the NNMDA was empowered to contribute to job creation, socioeconomic growth, and the promotion of traditional medicine practitioners (TMPs) in the country (NNMDA, 2020).

Another milestone development occurred in 2017, when President Muhammadu Buhari's administration created the Center for Research in Traditional Complementary and Alternative Medicine (CRTCAM). Subsequently, the Federal Ministry of Health (FMH) (FMH, 2007) charged CRTCAM with the dual mission to implement the World Health Organization's (WHO's) policy on integrating the TMPs into the health system and collaborating with the Nigerian Council of Physicians of Natural Medicine (NCPNM). The CRTCAM was housed administratively within the Nigeria Institute of Medical Research established in 1977 to conduct medical research of public health importance (CRTCAM, 2019).

The NCPNM, formed in 1993, was registered with the Corporate Affairs Commission (CAC) in 1997. Among the primary achievements of NCPNM is establishing the National College of Natural Medicine (NCNM) in Lagos in 2004 (Odunsi, 2013). The NCPNM has its Association of Physicians of Complementary and Alternative Medicine recognized by the FMH. It registered with CAC in July 2011 as an MDCN *continuing professional development* provider. In 2005, the MDCN recognized the NCPNM as the umbrella body representing alternative medicine practitioners in Nigeria. The NCPNM is an affiliated body of the Nigerian Association of Physicians of Traditional Medicine and the Nigerian Association of Physicians of Alternative Medicine (NCPNM, 2020).

The primary functions of the NCNM are to provide full and part-time courses in CAM as stipulated by the Medical Practitioners Act. It offers continuous professional development seminars, certificate, diploma, bachelors, masters, and doctoral degree programs in African traditional medicine, acupuncture, homeopathy, osteopathy, chiropractic, and naturopathy. Also, the NCNM evaluates foreign-trained CAM practitioners' credentials and promotes research and development in natural and traditional medicine. To date, it has produced over 100 graduates (NCPNM, 2020).

In 2009, the FMH took over NCNM and remained the Federal College of Complementary and Alternative Medicine (FEDCAM). The College was closed by the National Universities Commission (NUC), in 2010 due to non-adherence to regulations. The primary mission of FEDCAM is to offer certificate and diploma programs for TMPs and not to offer undergraduate or postgraduate degree programs (Vanguard, 2013; Punch 2020; Lawal, 2019). As of 2020, 32 practitioners of CAM – in homeopathy, naturopathy, osteopathy, acupuncture, and chiropractic – have been trained and registered and licensed by the MDCN. The FMH is reorganizing FEDCAM in collaboration with the University of Benin to establish a CAM Institute. The FMH also proposes setting up CAM clinics to make the services available to state ministries' health departments and the public (Punch 2020).

Besides the FEDCAM campuses in Lagos, Abuja and Sokoto, there are other CAM institutions in the country (Table 7.1).

Although the NCPNM recognizes the other institutions, the NUC and the Medical Rehabilitation Therapist (Registered) Board of Nigeria (MRTB) do not accredit the academic programs offered by the CAM institutions in the country. This situation is awkward because the FMH approves the acupuncture institutions to provide ordinary and higher national diplomas and certificate programs. But the existing institutions go beyond the authority granted them by the FMH and are offering PhD programs. The federal government statutorily recognizes only the NUC to accredit institutions offering undergraduate and postgraduate degree programs. This conflicting development is confusing to the public, students and stakeholders. President Buhari's administration must do something urgently to resolve the unwarranted rivalry and stalemate between the FMH and the NUC.

Table 7.1 Complementary and alternative medical institutions in Nigeria

Serial #	Name of institution	Name of proprietor/ provost	Ownership
1	Pan African Homeopathic Medical College, Oguta, Imo State	Dr. Nkem Okafor	Private
2	National College of Natural and Alternative Medicine, Lagos	Bishop (Dr.) M.A. Atilade	Private
3	Nigerian Institute of Homeopathy, Enugu	Prof. E. Ugo	Private
4	Lummar International College of Alternative Medicine, Enugu	Prof. Okoro Akpa	Private
5	Adewale Afonja College of Health Sciences and Complementary and Alternative Medicine, Buari, Kwara State	Dr. Adewale Afonja	Private
6	Modem College of Homeopathy and Alternative Medicine, Uyo, Akwa Ibom	Dr. Umoreh	Private
7	Lagos State College of Health Technology, Yaba, Lagos	Dr. K. Moyo	Public
8	Kwara State University, Malete, Kwara State	Dr. Sawya	Public
9	O/B Osteopathic Training Center/African College of Osteopathy and Chiropractic, Lagos	Dr. O. Obankole	Private
10	Cyrllic College of Holistic Health Sciences and Alternative Medicine	Dr. C. Omisande	Private
11	Bodunrin Oluwa Institute of Manual Manipulative Medicine	Dr. Bodunrin Oluwa	Private
12	Havillah Institute of Holistic Health Science, Delta	Dr. Joseph Akpile	Private
13	Integrative Holistic Medical Institute	Prof. Osmond Onyeka	Private
14	Green Center Academy of Natural Medicine, Lagos	Long Green Int. Ltd.	Private
15	Nigerian College of Natural Medicine, Lagos	Ministry of Science and Technology	Public
16	Royal College of Traditional Medicine, Shagamu	Dr. Sunday Oladenide	Private
17	African College of Traditional Medicine, Abeokuta	Dr. S.O. Soyoye	Private

Alternative medical training institutions exist in all of the six geopolitical zones of the country. Of the 17 institutions, three are public institutions, while the remaining 14 institutions are private (Table 7.1). The ordinary national diploma and certificate are the entry-level education in CAM. The ordinary diploma program lasts for 3 years (six semesters) and the certificate for 2 years (four semesters). The higher national diploma program, which includes a specialty option, lasts 2 years (four semesters). In the CAM educational programs, a semester consists of 15 contact weeks of classroom and clinical instruction, examinations, quizzes, and tests. The programs incorporate supervised clinical and community-based experiences, which last for 12 weeks in an academic year.

Utilization of Complementary and Alternative Medicine Treatments in Nigeria

Globally, the use of CAM is surging, but the utilization varies significantly from 7% in high-income countries to 80% in developing countries (Oshikoya et al., 2008). The WHO indicated that 80% of the emerging world's population relies on traditional medicine for their healthcare needs. At least 70% of the people in Germany and Canada have tried CAM at least once. In Ethiopia, 90% of the population use herbal remedies as their primary health care (Mahomoodally, 2013). For over a decade, several studies have investigated the utilization of CAM in Nigeria. As expected, the utilization varies widely among the different patient groups, as shown by the literature summarized below:

Herbal medicine, spiritual healing, aloe vera, medicinal tea, and nutritional supplements are mostly used CAM in Ni Awodele geria (Amira and Okubadejo 2007; Ogbera et al., 2010; Onyiapat, 2011; Oreagba, 2011; Okoronkwo et al., 2014; Li et al., 2020, Awodele et al. 2014). The CAM users reported benefits of pain and constipation relief, feeling of good health, reduced swelling, and wound healing (Ezeome and Anarado, 2007; Oke and Bandele, 2004). Nevertheless, some CAM users also experience mild to moderate adverse side effects (Oreagba et al., 2011; Okoronkwo et al., 2014; Busari and Mufutau, 2017; Aliyu et al., 2017; Oche et al., 2018). Many CAM users combine their remedies with Western medicine and are often reluctant to disclose them to their HCPs for fear of criticism or stigmatization. Coincidentally, many HCPs do not ask their patients if they are using CAM.

In 2007, Ezeome and Anarado investigated the prevalence, patterns, and factors influencing the use of CAM in Nigeria. They interviewed 160 (43% men and 57% women; ages 13–86 years) patients with breast, urogenital, and gastrointestinal cancer at the University of Nigeria Teaching Hospital (UNTH) Enugu between June 2003 and September 2005. Sixty-five percent of the patients have used CAM during their cancer illness, and 35% have not used any form of CAM, and more than 21% of users reported various side effects. The most commonly used CAMs were herbs (52%), faith/prayer healing (49%), aloe vera (23%), Forever Living Products®

(16%), medicinal tea (14%), and Blackstone® (13%). Of the patients who used CAM, over 23% were satisfied, but 68% were not. Most CAM users (67%) did not observe any benefit from the treatment, but 25% experienced some specific benefits. Eight-seven percent of the CAM users plan to use Western medicine instead of CAM, while 10% plan to combine both CAM and orthodox medicine. Most CAM users (80%) will not use it in the future or recommend it for cancer treatment. The majority of the study participants (56%) did not discuss their use of CAM with their physician because they did not ask (Ezeome and Anarado, 2007).

In another study published in 2007, Amira and Okubadejo studied the frequency and pattern of CAM utilization among 225 patients with essential hypertension at the Lagos University Teaching Hospital. The sample consisted of 90 (40%) men and 135 (60%) women with a mean age ± SD at 55.1 ± 12.4 years. Approximately 39% of the respondents used CAM, and herbal products were the most commonly used. Of those who used herbs, the most frequently used was garlic (69.3%), followed by native herbs (25%), ginger (23.9%), bitter leaf (*Vernonia amygdalina*) (9.1%), and aloe vera (4.5%); 2.5% of the respondents used spiritual therapy.

The following year, in 2008, Oshikoya et al. interviewed 318 parents of children with chronic health conditions who presented consecutively to the pediatric neurology, respiratory and hematology clinics at the Lagos State University Teaching Hospital (LASUTH), Ikeja. The majority (84%) of the patients were already using different CAMs, either alone or in combination with other CAMs. Approximately 31% of the patients (epilepsy – 38%, sickle cell anemia – 36%, and asthma – 25%) used CAMs; 16% discontinued their CAMs 6 months before the study. The most frequently used CAM were biological products (58%), followed by alternative medical systems (27%) and mind-body interventions (14%), and 7.1% of the patients reported adverse reactions. Seventy-six percent of the parents who used CAM for their children indicated family members, friends, and neighbors influenced them. Eighty-five (85%) parents were willing to discuss the use of CAM, but their physicians did not ask them (Oshikoya et al., 2008).

Algebra et al., in 2010, evaluated the frequency and pattern of CAM utilization among 263 patients with diabetes mellitus at the Lagos State University Teaching Hospital and the General Hospital Gbagada in Lagos State. The participants' age ranges from 28 to 80 years – the mean (SD) was 60 (10.7) years. The prevalence of CAM utilization was 46%, with the female to male ratio at 2:1. The CAM users were older than non-CAM users ($p = 0.006$). The primary CAM used were biological-based therapies that include bitter leaf (*Vernonia amygdalina*), aloe vera, garlic, ginger, and local herbs, and 94% of the study sample adhered to the prescribed medications.

In 2011, another cross-sectional study from UNTH investigated the use of CAM among urbanites from three local governments. The study participants (N = 732; 37.2% males and 62.8% females) ranged from 18 to 65 years. Approximately 85% of them have used CAM, while 15% have not previously used any CAM. Utilization ranges from one to 20 different types, but biological products were the most commonly used product, followed by prayer/faith healing. The major reasons for using

CAM are their "natural" state and health promotion and wellness benefits (Onyiapat et al., 2011)

Oreagba and associates in 2011 also investigated the general knowledge of the benefits and safety of herbal medicines utilization among Lagos urban dwellers ($N = 388$). The findings revealed that 12 herbs (crude or refined) were used alone or in combination with other herbal medicines. Approximately 67% of the sample used herbal medicines. Thirty-five percent of the respondents used "Agbo Jedi-Jedi" herbal preparation, followed by "agbo-iba" (28%) and Oroki herbal mixture® (9%). Seventy-eight percent of the respondents indicated family and friends had a marked influence on their herbal medicine use. About 50% of the sample considered herbal medicine safe, even though 21% experienced mild to moderate adverse effects.

The study by Tamuno in 2011 sets out to investigate the use of traditional medicines among patients (67% women and 33% men) with HIV infection receiving antiretroviral (ARV) drugs at the Aminu Kano Teaching Hospital. Of the 430 patients, 64% were married and 40% had at least two sexual partners. Approximately 28% used traditional medicine before the commencement of antiretroviral therapy (ART), but only 4% used ARV and traditional medicine concurrently. The widespread use of traditional medicine by patients living with HIV/AIDS should concern clinicians and policymakers.

Another study from UNTH in 2014 found that 85% of adults have used CAM products, and 79% found the treatment beneficial. Only 30% of the CAM users complained of adverse reactions, and 63% cannot identify the actual adverse effect experienced. The most commonly used CAM was biological remedies and spiritual therapy. The usual route of administration was oral, recitation, and reading. About 40% of adult CAM users combine it with orthodox medicine (Okoronkwo et al., 2014).

Busari and Mufutau, in 2017, investigated the prevalence, pattern, and tolerability of CAM among patients with sickle cell disease who received treatment at the Lagos University Teaching Hospital. The cross-sectional study consisted of 200 patients (56.5% males and 87; 43.5% were females), ranging in age from 1 to 10 years old; Mean (SD) = 18.8 ± 14.39 years. Approximately 89% of the study respondents used CAM; 63% used biological (herbal) remedies, followed by alternative medical systems (21%) and mind-body interventions (12%). Family members, friends, and neighbors recommended CAM to 85% of the study respondents. The products were well tolerated, as only 19% of the patients abandoned their CAM. There was no statistically significant difference ($p > 0.05$) in the proportion of CAM users and non-users (45.76% vs. 52.17%), between those who experienced two or more crises (51.41% vs. 34.78%), and those with stable hemoglobin concentration below and greater than 7 g/dL (15.81% vs. 8.69%). Surprisingly, the CAM non-users (91.30%) significantly spend more money monthly on prescription medicine (₦3000 or $15) than CAM users (4.51%) ($p < 0.001$).

In 2017, Aliyu and associates evaluated the prevalence of CAM use among 240 patients (mean age = 45 ± 13.7 years) with cancer at Usman Danfodiyo University Teaching Hospital (UDUTH) Sokoto. Approximately 66% of the sample used

CAM – prayer was the most common modality (30.8%), followed by herbal therapy (28.3%). The majority of CAM users (64.2%) did not derive any benefit from the treatment but rather reported adverse effects such as nausea and vomiting (52.5%) and diarrhea (44.2%). Most physicians (87.4%) were not aware of their CAM use because the physicians did not ask them. The male gender and absence of comorbidities were the significant predictors of the CAM used.

In 2018, Oche and associates investigated the use of traditional medicine (type not specified in the study) and determine the factors associated with its use among 271 patients living with HIV/AIDS on highly active ART at the UDUTH, Sokoto. Only 4.2% of the sample had used traditional medicine before, of whom 5% were women and 3% were men (p = 0.399). Only one of the respondents had side effects following traditional medicine utilization, and the most common reason for its use was too much weight loss (Oche et al., 2018).

Li and associates (2020) interviewed 748 adult women from Ibadan communities between 2013 and 2015. Their findings revealed the overall utilization of traditional medicine was 81.6%. Ibo and Hausa women were significantly less likely to use traditional medicine than the Yoruba women were. Furthermore, educated women were less likely than their non-educated peers to have used traditional medicine – the most prominent effect was among women with secondary education (Li et al., 2020).

Many of the CAM users in Nigeria use them purposely to treat or prevent diseases, improve their quality of life, and promote and maintain good health. Unfortunately, many HCPs in the country are not familiar with CAM practices and products, and often patients do not discuss utilization with their HCPs because they are not asked (Ezeome and Anarado, 2007; Oshikoya et al., 2008; Aliyu et al., 2017). The CAM systems currently practiced in Nigeria are discussed below.

Acupuncture

Several institutions in Nigeria offer ordinary and higher national diplomas, certificates, postgraduate diplomas, and PhD programs in acupuncture and other CAM disciplines. The institutions that provide the training in acupuncture and CAM disciplines are mostly in the major cities. Thirty-six of the acupuncturists in the country trained abroad; 18 practices in Lagos, six in Abuja, three in Oyo, two in Anambra state, two in Niger state, and the remaining five are in the other states (Vconnect, 2010a). Many of the acupuncturists also provide naturopathy, reflexology, and moxibustion treatments (Lagos Acupuncture Services, 2016). Besides the 36 acupuncturists who trained abroad, another 20–25 physiotherapists trained in the country as an acupuncturist. The Nigeria Society of Physiotherapy has a sub-specialty acupuncture therapy group (Fig. 7.1). Bayero University, Kano, presently offers a certificate course in basic dry needling techniques for physiotherapists but plan to extend admission to other HCPs (Sokunbi, 2020). A few other HCPs in Nigeria (physicians and nurses) received their acupuncture training abroad.

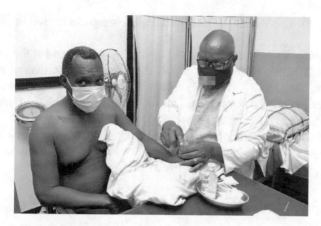

Fig. 7.1 A physiotherapist who trained in traditional Chinese medicine treats a patient with acupuncture needles (Photograph used with permission of Paschal Mogbo)

Chiropractic

At the inception of the MRTB in 1988, chiropractors trained abroad were registered along with the other medical rehabilitation professions like physiotherapy, occupational therapy, speech therapy, and clinical audiology. However, in 2000, the chiropractors left the MRTB and migrated to join the MDCN (Edet, 2013). Today, there are less than 20 chiropractors who trained abroad. It is estimated that about 1200 chiropractors are needed to serve Nigeria optimally. The majority of the chiropractors in Nigeria train at the government-approved alternative medical training institutions (NCNM/FEDCAM), but the MRTB does not register them. There is presently no government recognized chiropractic association in Nigeria (The Chiropractic Diplomatic Corps 2019; World Federation of Chiropractic, 2019).

In 2005, the WHO published the minimum requirements for chiropractic education program and the licensing guidelines to practice the profession (WHO, 2005). Internationally, chiropractic education is governed by the Council on Chiropractic Education International (CCEI) and is recognized by the WHO and the World Federation of Chiropractic as the accrediting agency for chiropractic schools worldwide. The current members are the Council on Chiropractic Education in Australia, the Canadian Federation of Chiropractic Regulatory and Educational Accrediting Boards, the Council on Chiropractic Education in the United States, and the European Council on Chiropractic Education (CCEI, 2018). The CCEI does not recognize the graduates of the NCNM/FEDCAM.

Osteopathy

As of 2005, the MDCN registers osteopathic physicians trained in the United States as medical practitioners (ValueMD, 2005). The MDCN now recognizes all the universities in the United States that offer the doctor of osteopathy (DO) degree

(MDCN, 2018). The MRTB registers traditional osteopaths trained in other parts of the world.

There are less than 50 osteopaths in Nigeria, mostly trained at the government-approved NCNM/FEDCAM institutions. As of 2018, the International Labor Organization, the global labor czar, recognized DO and MD who trained in the United States as licensed physicians. This recognition is probably an important factor in the decision of the Association of Medical Councils of Africa (AMCA) in approving the DO to practice in 15 African member countries. The decision does not affect the DO practicing in the country since Nigeria is not an AMCA member state. Lastly, alternative medical systems will be discussed next.

Traditional Chinese Medicine

The traditional Chinese medicine (TCM) debuted in Nigeria on June 6, 2018, when a team of experts from the Jiangxi University of Traditional Chinese Medicine conducted a workshop sponsored by the Chinese Government in Lagos. In his keynote address, the Consulate General of the People's Republic of China in Lagos, Deputy Consul General Duan Zhongqi, enumerated some of the advantages of TCM. They include the curative effect, safe medication, flexible mode of service, low cost, and the potential to treat malaria cheaply. Zhongqi confirmed the Chinese government's plans to establish a TCM hospital and university in Nigeria (Obinna 2018; Gbenga-Mustapha, 2018).

In developing countries, TCM is widely promoted and applied because of its affordability and availability. There are less than 100 Chinese herbal medicine practitioners in Nigeria (Chinese Medicine in Nigeria, n.d.; VConnect, 2018). But Chinese herbal products are widely sold and unregulated by the federal government (Nigeria Alternative Medicine, n.d.). This situation compromises the health and well-being of the Nigerian people. Some Chinese herbs contain harmful chemicals and should not be used unsupervised, especially during pregnancy and by nursing mothers.

Chinese herbal products sold over the counter are often poorly labeled, and essential information on their composition is usually not provided. Some products contain other drugs not included on their labels. For example, some Chinese herbal creams recommended for eczema contain steroid medications. Some Chinese herbal medicines include aristolochic acid, often implicated in kidney failure and even cancer. Callaway (2012) uncovers poisonous herb called *Ephedra* and the woody vine *Aristolochia which* contains aristolochic acid, which can cause kidney and liver damage and bladder cancer. He postulated that the medicinal use of the herb is responsible for the high rates of bladder cancer in Taiwan. Evidence-based research studies on TCM are needed to establish the mechanism of its action, effectiveness, cost, as well as possible hazards associated with its use and safety.

Ayurveda

Ayurveda products are available and widely promoted in Nigeria on several websites. Several centers and consulting health firms in the country provide coordinated overseas referral services for people and practitioners in need of Ayurveda treatment. Ayurveda practitioners are reachable online, and their products are sold unregulated. There is no known training institution and organization for Ayurveda in Nigeria. The few practitioners trained outside the country, and the occupation currently does not have a regulatory body.

Naturopathy

There are a few naturopathic centers in Nigeria, but the profession is not widely known. The Institute of Naturopathy Healthcare, located at 23 Isheri Rd., Ojodu-Berger, Lagos, offers a certificate course in natural medicine, a diploma in natural medicine, and an advanced diploma in naturopathy, quantum analyzer course, a certificate in meta-therapy, and a certificate in wave therapy. The Institute was established in 2000 by Dr. Macfonse Osmond (Naturopathy Healthcare, n.d.). Another Institute was established by Dr. Essien, managing director of Acupuncture Health Centre, located at 6 Debartho/18 Agoro Kessington Street, Amuwo Odofin, Lagos. He specializes in acupuncture, naturopathy, and reflexology. Another naturopathy practitioner is Dr. Olawale Qazeem, CEO of Olaking Naturopathic Clinic, located at 318 Sagamu Road, Aiyelala Bus Stop, Odogunyan, Ikorodu, Lagos. He uses various natural methods such as herbology, diet, and nutrition, acupressure. Dr. Emeka Mokeme, a naturopathic physician and the founder of Emmy Forever Healthcare and Research Centre, is located at 16 Ope Oluwa Street, Aduke House, Agege, Lagos. He specializes in natural medicine, health and wellness, and holistic nutrition.

Homeopathy

Although the homeopathy profession was introduced to Nigeria over six decades ago, it is relatively not well known compared to other occupations imported to the country at the same time. In 1961, the All-Nigeria Homeopathic Medical Organization was formed. The late Dr. I. Okogeri, the King of the Afikpo Kingdom, who trained as a physician in London, was the first to practice homeopathy in 1962. Other homeopathy practitioners in the country received their training in India and Germany through correspondence courses or self-taught.

In 1972, the Congress of Homoeopathic Medicine was formed in conjunction with the Nigerian College of Homeopathic Medicine, which has 30 practitioners on its register. The East Central State government recognized the Association, and both practitioners and laypersons admitted to practice homeopathy (Nwusulor, 2006). There are about 2000 lay practitioners and 167 homeopathic medicine practitioners in Nigeria (VConnect, 2010b). The Association has no journal of its own (WholeHealthNow, 2019).

The Nigerian Institute of Homoeopathy, a private school, was established in 1980 and currently has fellows, regular, associate, and student members. The Institute trains homeopathic physicians, homeopathic pharmacists, and homeopathic nurses. It also offers postgraduate diplomas, masters, and PhD programs in homeopathy (Nigerian Institute of Homoeopathy, 2012). The Institute has a special consultative recognition by the United Nations Department of Economic and Social Affairs (Nwusulor, 2006), but its professional programs are presently not recognized by the NUC. The MDCN is contemplating introducing homeopathy into the country's healthcare delivery system (WHO, 2018).

Aromatherapy

The origin of aromatherapy in the country is unknown. Many of the practicing aromatherapists also trained in other alternative healing systems, such as massage or chiropractic. Aromatherapy is relatively unknown by the public, and even by the HCPs in Nigeria.

Spirituality

Before colonization by the British, traditional worship of ancestral deities was the norm and spiritual practice in Nigeria. Every tribe had its unique way of life in terms of spirituality and acknowledgment of cultural identities. However, modern-day religious traditions have made traditional worship less relevant. Nigeria is a secular state equally divided between the mostly Muslim north and the predominantly Christian south. The country is a multi-religious society where both traditional and modern religions co-exist. Regular practitioners are believed to have spiritual healing powers (Ohaja et al., 2019). Ezekwesili-Ofili and Okaka (2019) provided the following examples of spiritual-based methods that are peculiar to Nigeria.

1. *Spiritual protection* is elicited by using talisman, charm, amulets, body marks, and a spiritual bath to drive away evil spirits.
2. *Sacrifices* of animals such as dogs and cats are slaughtered or buried alive at midnight to save the patient from dying.
3. *Spiritual cleansing* using animal blood or water/whisky/wine is poured from the patient's head to toe at specific times for several days.

4. *Appeasing gods* through sacrifice and/or libation practice when the patient's disease is perceived to be caused by a curse or violation of taboos. The religious leader or priest appeases the ancestors or spirits with specific items such as spotless animals (dove, cat, dog, goat, and fowl), local wine, cola nut, eggs, and white, red, or black clothing.

5. *Exorcism* is performed by a religious leader or a priest who can expel demons or evil spirits from the patient or the possessed places. The occasion is accompanied by dancing to the beating of drums, singing, and sometimes flogging or stroking the patient with animal tails and other objects to chase out the spirit. *Exorcism* is not limited to Africa but also in ancient Babylonian, Greek, and the Middle East.

6. *Libation* is the pouring of local wine on the ground or objects followed by chanting or reciting invocations and supplications.

A global survey conducted in 2015 by the PEW Research Group revealed that Nigeria is the second most religious country after Pakistan. The survey asked the participants the question, "how important is religion to you"? The participants' affirmative responses by country were Pakistan 98%, Nigeria 90%, Brazil 74%, Turkey 70%, United States 54%, Russia 18%, France 13%, Japan 10%, and China 2%. There is a mismatch between Nigeria's image as a highly religious country and the behavior of its citizens abroad. For example, a United Nations Office on Drugs and Crime survey ranked Nigeria the fourth most notable user of marijuana in the world (United Nations Office on Drugs and Crime, 2014). This global perception further damages the image of the country.

Besides perception, religion is a booming business in Nigeria. As baseball is America's pastime, so is religion Nigeria's hobby. Nigeria has the highest number of church buildings and the highest number of church denominations in the world (Ohuabunwa, 2018). Moreover, Nigeria takes pride in having the largest church auditorium in the world – The Dunamis' Glory Dome in Abuja is a 100,000-seater capacity edifice complex (PM News, 2018). The Pentecostal churches at which about 40 million Nigerians worship are among the most luxurious and thriving business empires (Ikenwa, 2019).

About a quarter of Nigerian Christians are Catholic, three quarters are Protestant, and a few other Christian denominations and Orthodox Christians. Protestants include the Church of Nigeria of the Anglican Communion, African Church, Assemblies of God Church, Nigerian Baptist Convention, The Synagogue, Church of All Nations, Redeemed Christian Church of God, Winners' Chapel, and the Christ Apostolic Church (the first *Aladura* Movement in Nigeria). Others are the Deeper Christian Life Ministry, Christ Embassy, Evangelical Church Winning All, Mountain of Fire and Miracles, Commonwealth of Zion Assembly (COZA), *Aladura* Church (indigenous Christian churches, especially prevalent among the Yorubas and Igbos), evangelical churches, and the Seventh-day Adventist. The Yoruba Christians are primarily Anglican. The Igbos are predominantly Catholic, while Edo's Assemblies of God, imported into the country by Augustus Ehurie Wogu and his associates at Old Umuahia.

The Nigerian Baptist Convention has about 3 million members and over 300,000 Early Pentecostal Apostolic Church parishes (Christ Apostolic Church, Apostolic Church, Celestial Church, Cherubim, Seraphim Church, etc.), and with 4.2 million adherents. Also, there are about 380,000 New Apostolic Church parishes with 6.5 million believers. The Roman Catholic Church Archdioceses are in Abuja, Onitsha, Benin City, Calabar, Ibadan, Lagos, and Owerri, with about 19 million members as of 2005. Roman Catholic Cardinal Francis Arinze is a Nigerian. The churches of Nigeria's Ecclesiastical provinces are in Lagos, Ibadan, Ondo, Bendel, Niger, Delta, Owerri, Abuja, Kaduna, and Jos, with about 17 million members (FamilySearch, 2020).

The notable churches in Nigeria, their founder, current pastor, year of establishment, and head office location are presented in Table 7.2.

Critics assert that mega-churches exploit Nigerians' faith in a country with the highest number of people living in extreme poverty (Facsar, 2018). In general, high-income countries tend to be less religious; an exception to that generalization is the United States. The pertinent question is, has religion helped the development of Nigeria?

In the 1980s, religious and spiritual health centers emerged as a significant CAM practice when the public hospitals began to lose their appeal due to their neglect by the government and the high cost associated with the Western-style healthcare system. Surprisingly, the utilization of religious and spiritual health centers cuts across socioeconomic strata. Those who patronize religious and spiritual health centers complement the services with other forms of orthodox health care. On the other hand, religious extremists rely entirely on this form of care for their health needs. Although religious and spiritual healers constitute a fraction of health providers, their influence is growing and attracting customers from all social strata.

After an extensive review of the spirituality literature, Asakitikpi (2019) inferred that "the general tendency of discussing traditional medicine as monolithic and unspecialized is grossly misleading and gives the erroneous impression that traditional medical practitioners are static in their knowledge and do not in any way improve upon the existing knowledge they received during their training." No empirically based study has been conducted to identify the health outcomes of the services provided by religious and spiritual practitioners in Nigeria.

Herbal Medicine

Herbal medicine is a form of alternative medical system that is indigenous to the African people. The practice of traditional medicine has been in existence before the arrival of allopathic medicine imported into Africa by the colonial masters. Today, herbal remedies are the dominant form of healthcare service in Nigeria, particularly in rural areas. Herbal medicines are very cheap compared to Western drugs, which are not affordable for most people. people. Sadly, the Nigerian government and the institutions of higher learning and research centers in the country have not effectively utilized these natural resources. Three universities in the country are offering or at advanced stages of developing programs in herbal medicine. In 2018,

Table 7.2 The list of the mega-churches in Nigeria

Serial #	Church name	Founder	Current general president/overseer	Year established	Headquarter
1	Redeemed Christian Church of God	Rev Josiah Akindayomi	Pastor Enoch Adeboye	1952	Lagos State
2	Living Faith Church Worldwide	David Oyedepo	David Oyedepo	1981	Ota, Ogun state
3	Christ Apostolic Church	Joseph Ayo Babalola	Pastor A.O. Akinosun	1918	Ibadan
4	Church of Nigeria	Henry Townsend	Nicholas Okoh	1842	Badagry
5	The African Church	Jacob Kehinde Coker	Emmanuel Josiah Udofia	1901	Lagos
6	Christ Embassy	Chris Oyakhilome	Chris Oyakhilome	1990	Lagos State
7	Deeper Christian Life Ministry	William Kumuyi	William F. Kumuyi	1982	Lagos State
8	Cherubim and Seraphim	Moses Orimolade Tunolase	Prophet Solomon Adegboyega Alao	1925	Lagos
9	Mountain of Fire and Miracles	Dr. Daniel Olukoya	Dr. Daniel Olukoya	1989	Yaba
10	The Apostolic Church Nigeria	Leader Joseph Shadare	Gabriel Olutola	1931	Lagos State
11	The Lord's Chosen	Lazarus Muoka	Lazarus Muoka	2002	Mushin
12	Roman Catholic Church	Portuguese traders	Ignatius Ayau Kaigama	Fifteenth century	Kaduna
13	The Synagogue	Late T. B. Joshua	Late T. B. Joshua	1987	Ikotun, Lagos
14	Church of the Lord	Josiah Ollunowo Ositelu	Adeleke Adejobi	1930	Ogere
15	Celestial Church of Christ (Aladura)	Samuel Biléhou Joseph Oshoffa	Rev. Arthur Nzekwu	1947	Cotonou
16	Methodist Church Nigeria	British missionaries	Prelate Samuel Chukwuemeka Kanu Uche, JP	1842	Marina/ Lagos State
17	Nigerian Baptist Convention	Southern Baptist Convention missionaries	Rev. Samson Olasupo Ayokunle	1850/1914	Ibadan
18	Salvation Ministries	Pastor David Ibiyeomie	David Ibiyeomie	1997	Port-Harcourt
19	Royal House of Grace International Church	Apostle Zilly Aggrey	King-David Zilly Aggrey	1992	Port-Harcourt

(continued)

Table 7.2 (continued)

Serial #	Church name	Founder	Current general president/overseer	Year established	Headquarter
20	ECWA/SIM Church[a]	Walter Gowan, Thomas Kent and Roland victor Bingham	Rev. Dr. Stephen Panya Baba	December 4, 1893	Jos

Source: Ikenwa, (2019)

[a]https://ecwanationwidegist.wordpress.com/2017/12/11/history-of-evangelical-church-winning-allecwa/#:~:text=It%20all%20started%20in%201893,by%20God%20for%20that%20purpose

the University of Medical Sciences, Ondo City, introduced a Bachelor's degree program in herbal medicine, while Samuel Adegboyega University, Ogwa, Edo State, planned to introduce a higher certificate program in herbal medicine. The University of Ibadan had already approved and commenced a Master and Ph.D. programs in African Traditional Medicine at its Institute of African studies. A course in herbal medicine is also offered through the Department of Pharmacy at the University of Ibadan (Nigerian Scholars, 2018).

At the outbreak of the coronavirus disease 2019 (COVID-19) pandemic in 2020, Madagascar's President touted the efficacy of an herbal drink made in his country to cure the coronavirus. The well-advertised cocktail was made from the *artemisia* plant – a local plant used in Africa as an antimalarial remedy. Despite having no scientific proof to substantiate the claim, many African countries from Tanzania to Liberia and Nigeria imported the brew.

On September 4, 2020, a Nigerian professor of biotechnology at the University of Jos, Innocent Ogbonna, claimed he had developed a more potent herbal cocktail with an artemisinin content of 4.8% compared to the 1.1% found in Madagascar's *artemisia annua* plant species. He also claimed that COVID-19 patients treated with his research team's herbal cocktail used as syrups and teas were able to recover. An infectious disease physician from the University of Jos, Dr. Nathan Shehu, cautioned that further testing is warranted before using the herbal remedy on a large scale to treat COVID-19 (Ettang, 2020).

For the herbal remedies from Nigeria to gain global recognition, double-blind, randomized controlled studies are needed to support their therapeutic effectiveness and safety claims. If they are found efficacious and safe, herbal cocktails from Nigeria will become a credible alternative to Western medicines. This topic is discussed in greater detail in Chapter 8 of this book.

Conclusion

This chapter chronicles the evolutionary development of the CAM disciplines in Nigeria. Although the federal government's interest in integrating traditional medicine into the healthcare system dates back to 1966, the pace of development has been slow due to poor execution and limited coordination between the FMH and the NUC. The Nigerian traditional medicine policy launched in 2007 expects both the traditional and allopathic medicine practitioners to practice in tandem to deliver high-quality health care. Traditional medicine enthusiasts anticipate an overall decrease in Western drug utilization, but this goal is yet to be realized.

Case Study: Clinical Observation and Interview Project

This case study will enable students to independently explore a CAM modality.

Select one of the following alternative therapies:

1. Therapeutic Touch
2. Herbal medicine and natural products – dietary supplements
3. Spirituality
4. Hypnotherapy
5. Yoga
6. Tai Chi and Qi gong
7. Meditation: Visualization, guided imagery, and progressive muscle relaxation
8. Mindfulness meditation or transcendental meditation
9. Music therapy
10. Pet therapy
11. Shamanic healing
12. Native American Medicine (http://wholehealthchicago.com/2009/05/07/native-american-medicine/)
13. Brazilian traditional medicine
14. Traditional herbal medicine in Bolivia, South America
15. Haitian traditional medicine
16. Korean traditional medicine
17. Mongolian traditional medicine
18. Tibetan traditional medicine
19. Unani traditional medicine
20. Siddha traditional medicine

Develop a questionnaire to obtain first-hand information about some of the facts gleaned from the literature review from an individual familiar with the CAM. The questionnaire must include knowledge of traditional medicine and ethnobotanical or ethnomedicinal plants.

A short paragraph describing the topic along with two (2) references is sufficient to obtain approval. Following approval by the instructor, the student will conduct an in-depth review of the literature on the topic and contact a facility or clinic that employs the CAM philosophy. It is the student's responsibility to set up the observation experience. During the visit, which must last a minimum of 2 h, the student will observe a practitioner's treatment session and conduct a brief interview with the practitioner and client. Present a detailed review of literature on the topic and also include their clinical observation visit experience. The four-page (essay) paper must address the following issues:

1. Treatment philosophy
2. History of the CAM
3. Mechanism of action/Effect of treatment
4. Treatment procedures
5. Disease conditions for which it is recommended (Indications)
6. Precautions
7. Education and certification of practitioners
8. Supporting research demonstrating or refuting clinical effectiveness
9. Clinical Observation Visit or Interview

References

Ailemen, A. (2020). FG approves bill for the establishment of council for traditional, alternative and complementary medicine practice in Nigeria. Business Day. [online]. Available at: https://businessday.ng/health/article/fg-approves-bill-for-establishment-of-council-for-traditional-alternative-and-complementary-medicine-practice-in-nigeria/ (Accessed: 10 December 2020).

Ajao, T.D. (2017) Nigeria's first University of Medical Sciences. *Vanguard*. November 26. [online]. Available at: https://www.vanguardngr.com/2017/11/nigerias-first-university-medical-sciences/. Accessed 26 Feb 2020.

Aliyu, U. M., Awosan, K. J., Oche, M. O., Jimoh, A. O., & Okuofo, E. C. (2017). Prevalence and correlates of complementary and alternative medicine use among cancer patients in Usman danfodiyo university teaching hospital, Sokoto, Nigeria. *Nigerian Journal Clinical Practice, 20*(12), 1576–1583. https://doi.org/10.4103/njcp.njcp_88_17. [online]. Available at: https://pubmed.ncbi.nlm.nih.gov/29378990/. Accessed 26 Nov 2020.

Amira, O. C., & Okubadejo, N. U. (2007). Frequency of complementary and alternative medicine utilization in hypertensive patients attending an urban tertiary care centre in Nigeria. *BMC Complement Altern Med, 7*, 30. [online]. Available at: https://doi.org/10.1186/1472-6882-7-30. Accessed 16 Dec 2020.

Asakitikpi, A. E. (2019). Healthcare coverage and affordability in Nigeria: An alternative model to equitable healthcare delivery. *IntechOpen*. https://doi.org/10.5772/intechopen.85978. [online]. Available at: https://www.intechopen.com/books/universal-health-coverage/healthcare-coverage-and-affordability-in-nigeria-an-alternative-model-to-equitable-healthcare-delive. Accessed 16 Dec 2020.

Awodele, O., Amagon, K. I., Wannang, N. N., & Aguiyi, J. C. (2014). Traditional medicine policy and regulation in Nigeria: An index of herbal medicine safety. *Current Drug Safety, 9*, 16–22. [online]. Available at: http://www.eurekaselect.com/118337/article. Accessed 26 Feb 2020.

Busari, A. A., & Mufutau, M. A. (2017). High prevalence of complementary and alternative medicine use among patients with sickle cell disease in a tertiary hospital in Lagos, South West, Nigeria. *BMC Complementary Alternative Medicine, 7*, 17(1), 299. [online]. Available at: https://pubmed.ncbi.nlm.nih.gov/28592256/. Accessed 26 Nov 2020.

Callaway, E. (2012). Screen uncovers hidden ingredients of Chinese medicine. *Nature*. [online]. Available at: https://www.nature.com/articles/nature.2012.10430#citeas. Accessed 12 June 2021.

Centre for Research in Traditional Complementary and Alternative Medicine – CRTCAM. (2019). [online]. Available at: https://nimr.gov.ng/centre-for-traditional-complementary-and-alternative-medicine/. Accessed 26 Feb 2020.

Chinese Medicine in Nigeria. (n.d.). [online]. Available at: https://www.businesslist.com.ng/category/chinese-medicine. Accessed 26 Feb 2020.

Councils on Chiropractic Education International – CCEI. (2018). [online]. Available at: https://www.cceintl.org/. Accessed 26 Feb 2020.

Edet, B. (2013). *Making a living curing backache.* [online]. Available at: https://www.dailytrust.com.ng/making-a-living-curing-backache.html. Accessed 26 Feb 2020.

Ettang, I. (2020). *Nigerian biotechnologist touts potent herbal COVID-19 treatment.* [online]. Available at: https://www.voanews.com/covid-19-pandemic/nigerian-biotechnologist-touts-potent-herbal-covid-19-treatment. Accessed 10 Dec 2020.

Ezekwesili-Ofili, J. O., & Okaka, A. N. C. (2019). Herbal medicine in African traditional medicine. *IntechOpen.* https://doi.org/10.5772/intechopen.80348. [online]. Available at: https://www.intechopen.com/books/herbal-medicine/herbal-medicines-in-african-traditional-medicine. Accessed 10 Dec 2020.

Ezeome, E. R., & Anarado, A. N. (2007). Use of complementary and alternative medicine by cancer patients at the University of Nigeria Teaching Hospital, Enugu, Nigeria. *BMC Complementary and Alternative Medicine, 7,* 28. [online]. Available at: https://www.ncbi.nlm.nih.gov/pubmed/17850665. Accessed 26 Feb 2020.

Facsar, F. (2018) Nigerian Pentecostal megachurches a booming business. *DW.Com.* [online]. Available at: https://www.dw.com/en/nigerian-pentecostal-megachurches-a-booming-business/a-45535263. Accessed 26 Feb 2020.

FamilySearch. (2020) *Nigeria church records.* [online]. Available at. https://www.familysearch.org/wiki/en/Nigeria_Church_Records. Accessed: 26 February 2020.

Federal Ministry of Health of Nigeria (2007). *Traditional medicine policy for Nigeria.* [online]. Available at: https://www.medianigeria.com/functions-of-federal-ministry-of-health-nigeria/http://www.eurekaselect.com/118337/articlehttps://www.ncbi.nlm.nih.gov/pmc/articles/PMC3252714/. Accessed 26 Feb 2020.

Gbenga-Mustapha, O. (2018). *Traditional Chinese medicine varsity coming.* [online]. Available at: https://thenationonlineng.net/traditional-chinese-medicine-varsity-coming/. Accessed 26 Feb 2020.

Ikenwa, C. (2019). *List of top 10 biggest churches in Nigeria today 2021.* [online]. Available at: https://nigerianinfopedia.com.ng/list-top-10-biggest-churches-in-nigeria-today/. Accessed: 26 Mar 2021.

Lagos Acupuncture Services. (2016). [online]. Available at: https://www.finelib.com/cities/lagos/health/alternative-medicine-practitioners/acupuncture. Accessed 26 Feb 2020.

Lawal, S. (2019). Nigeria: Govt takes steps to promote alternative medicine. *Vanguard* [online]. Available at: https://allafrica.com/stories/201912060178.html. Accessed 26 Nov 2020.

Li, S., Odedina, S., Agwai, I., Ojengbede, O., Huo, D., & Olopade, O. I. (2020). Traditional medicine usage among adult women in Ibadan, Nigeria: a cross-sectional study. *BMC Complementary Medicine Therapy, 20,* 93. [online]. Available at: https://www.ncbi.nlm.nih.gov/pmc/articles/PMC7083039/. Accessed 26 Nov 2020.

Mahomoodally, M. F. (2013). Traditional medicines in Africa: An appraisal of ten potent African medicinal plants, *Evidence-Based Complementary and Alternative Medicine*; ID 617459 [online]. Available at: https://doi.org/10.1155/2013/617459. Accessed 26 Nov 2020.

Medical and Dental Council of Nigeria –MDCN. (2018). [online]. Available at: http://www.mdcnigeria.org/RecognizedSch.htm. Accessed 26 Feb 2020.

Naturopathy Healthcare. (n.d.) *Institute of Naturopathy Healthcare.* [online]. Available at: http://www.naturopathyhealthcare.com/index.html. Accessed 26 Feb 2020.

Nigeria Alternative Medicine. (n.d.) [online]. Available at: https://www.finelib.com/health/alternative-medicine. Accessed 26 Feb 2020.

Nigeria Natural Medicine Development Agency – NNMDA. (2020). [online]. Available at: http://nnmda.gov.ng/. Accessed 26 Feb 2020.

Nigerian Council of Physicians of Natural Medicine – NCPNM. (2020). [online]. Available at: g http://www.ncpnmfct.com.ng/. Accessed 26 Nov 2020.

Nigerian Institute of Homoeopathy. (2012). [online]. Available at: https://www.digitaldreamstudios.net/nihedu/Membership.html. Accessed 26 Feb 2020.

Nigerian Scholars. (2018). *3 Nigerian universities to start offering degree programmes in herbal medicine.* [online]. Available at: https://nigerianscholars.com/school-news/universities-start-degree-herbal-medicine/. Accessed 26 Nov 2020.

Nwusulor, E. E. (2006). Homeopathy: The Nigerian experience. *Homeopathy, 95*(2), 105–107. [online]. Available at: https://www.sciencedirect.com/science/article/abs/pii/S1475491606000117?via%3Dihub. Accessed 6 Apr 2021.

Obinna, C. (2018, July 2). Traditional Chinese medicine debuts in Nigeria. *Vanguard Newspaper.* [online]. Available at: https://www.vanguardngr.com/2018/07/traditional-chinese-medicine-debuts-nigeria/. Accessed 26 Feb 2020.

Oche, M. O., Sadiq, U. A., Oladigbolu, R. A., & Chinna, K. (2018). Prevalence and factors associated with the use of traditional medicines among human immunodeficiency virus and acquired immunodeficiency syndrome patients in Sokoto, Nigeria. *Annals of African Medicine, 17*(3), 125–132. [online]. Available at: https://pubmed.ncbi.nlm.nih.gov/30185681/. Accessed 26 Nov 2020.

Odunsi, W. (2013). *MDCN shuts alleged fake College of Medicine in Lagos.* [online]. Available at: https://dailypost.ng/2013/08/10/mdcn-shuts-alleged-fake-college-of-medicine-in-lagos/. Accessed 26 Nov 2020.

Ogbera, A. O., Dada, O., Adeyeye, F., & Jewo, P. I. (2010). Complementary and alternative medicine use in diabetes mellitus. *West African Journal of Medicine, 29*(3), 158–162. [online]. Available at: https://doi.org/10.4314/wajm.v29i3.68213

Ohaja, M., Murphy-Lawless, J., & Dunlea, M. (2019). Religion and spirituality in pregnancy and birth: The views of birth practitioners in Southeast Nigeria. *Religions, 10*(2), 82. [online]. Available at: https://www.mdpi.com/2077-1444/10/2/82/htm. Accessed 26 Feb 2020.

Ohuabunwa, S. (2018). *Nigeria: High on religiosity, low on spirituality* [online]. Available at: https://www.vanguardngr.com/2018/11/nigeria-high-on-religiosity-low-on-spirituality/. Accessed 26 Feb 2020.

Oke, D. A., & Bandele, E. O. (2004). Misconceptions of hypertension. *Journal of the National Medical Association, 96*(9), 1221–1224.

Okoronkwo, I., Onyia-pat, J. L., Okpala, P., Agbo, M. A., & Ndu, A. (2014). Patterns of complementary and alternative medicine use, perceived benefits, and adverse effects among adult users in Enugu urban, southeast Nigeria. *Evidence Based Complement Alternative Medicine, 14*, 239372. [online]. Available at: https://www.hindawi.com/journals/ecam/2014/239372/. Accessed 26 Feb 2020.

Onyiapat, J. E., Okoronkwo, I. L., Ngozi, P., & Ogbonnaya, N. P. (2011). Complementary and alternative medicine use among adults in Enugu, Nigeria. *BMC Complementary Alternative Medicine, 11*, 19. [online]. Available at https://bmccomplementmedtherapies.biomedcentral.com/articles/10.1186/1472-6882-11-19. Accessed 26 Nov 2020.

Oreagba, I. A., Oshikoya, K., & Amachree, M. (2011). Herbal medicine use among urban residents in Lagos, Nigeria. *BMC Complementary Alternative Medicine, 11*, 117. [online]. Available at https://doi.org/10.1186/1472-6882-11-117. Accessed 26 Nov 2020.

Oshikoya, K. A., Senbanjo, I. O., Njokanma, O. F., & Soipe, A. (2008). Use of complementary and alternative medicines for children with chronic health conditions in Lagos, Nigeria. *BMC Complementary and Alternative Medicine, 8*, 66. [online]. Available at: https://link.springer.com/article/10.1186%2F1472-6882-8-66. Accessed 26 Feb 2020.

PM News. (2018). *Photos: World's largest church auditorium in Abuja.* [online]. Available at: https://www.pmnewsnigeria.com/2018/11/26/photos-worlds-largest-church-auditorium/. Accessed 26 Feb 2020.

Punch. (2020). *College inducts 37 complementary medicine practitioners.* [online]. Available at: https://healthwise.punchng.com/college-inducts-37-complementary-medicine-practitioners/. Accessed 26 Nov 2020.

Sokunbi, G. (2020). Personal communication. Professor, Department of Physiotherapy, Faculty of Allied Health Sciences, Bayero University, Kano.

Tamuno, I. (2011). Traditional medicine for HIV infected patients in antiretroviral therapy in a tertiary hospital in Kano, Northwest Nigeria. *Asian Pacific Journal of Tropical Medicine, 4*(2), 152–155. [online]. Available at: https://doi.org/10.1016/S1995-7645(11)60058-8. Accessed 26 Feb 2020.

The Chiropractic Diplomatic Corps. (2019). [online]. Available at: http://www.chiropracticdiplomatic.com/. Accessed 26 Feb 2020.

United Nations Office on Drugs and Crime. (2014). *World Drug Report* 2014. [online]. Available at: https://www.unodc.org/wdr2014/en/previous-reports.html. Accessed 26 Feb 2020.

ValueMD. (2005). *List of countries where US-trained osteopaths are recognized.* [online]. Available at: https://www.valuemd.com/osteopathic-medicine/29288-list-countries-trained-osteopaths-recognized.html. Accessed 26 Feb 2020.

Vanguard. (2013). *Fed college of alternative medicine not illegal – Provost.* [online]. Available at: https://www.vanguardngr.com/2013/08/fed-college-of-alternative-medicine-not-illegal-provost/. Accessed 26 Nov 2020.

Vconnect. (2010a). Best acupuncture professionals in Nigeria. [online]. Available at: https://www.eastacupunctureva.com/. Accessed 26 Feb 2020.

VConnect. (2010b). *Best homeopathic medicine professionals in Nigeria.* [online]. Available at: https://www.vconnect.com/nigeria/list-of-homeopathic-medicine_c288?page=1. Accessed 26 Feb 2020.

VConnect. (2018). *Quality Chinese herbal medicine professionals in Nigeria.* [online]. Available at: https://m.vconnect.com/nigeria/list-of-chinese-herbal-medicine-vendors search_p24142?page=1. Accessed 26 Feb 2020.

WHO. (2005). [online]. Available at: https://www.who.int/medicines/areas/traditional/Chiro-Guidelines.pdf. Accessed 26 Feb 2020.

WHO. (2018). *Essential medicines and health products information portal.* A World Health Organization Resource. [online]. Available at: http://apps.who.int/medicinedocs/en/d/Jh2943e/4.32.html#Jh2943e.4.32. Accessed 26 Feb 2020.

WholeHealthNow. (2019). *Homeopathy.* [online]. Available at: http://www.wholehealthnow.com/homeopathy_pro/nigeria.html. Accessed 26 Feb 2020.

World Federation of Chiropractic. (2019). [online]. Available at: https://www.wfc.org/website/. Accessed 26 Feb 2020.

Chapter 8
Emerging Developments in Traditional Medicine Practice in Nigeria

Learning Objectives

After reading this chapter, the learner should be able to:

1. Discuss the origin of African traditional medicine (ATM)
2. Describe the World Health Organization's roles, the Nigerian Traditional Medicine Practice Act 575, and the Nigerian Traditional Medicine Policy in promoting traditional medicine
3. Contrast the treatment philosophy of orthodox medicine and ATM
4. Articulate the current status of traditional medicine in Nigeria
5. Discern the different specialties in traditional medical practice in Nigeria
6. Explain the reasons for the growing use of herbal remedies
7. Enunciate the indications and treatment approach used by the practitioners of ATM
8. Discuss the contemporary practice and prospect of ATM in the healthcare system
9. Describe the roles of the Nigerian Institute for Pharmaceutical Research and Development in the production of pharmaceutical agents in Nigeria
10. Discuss the efficacy and safety of ATM

Introduction

The World Health Organization (WHO) defined traditional medicine as "the sum total of the knowledge, skills, and practices based on the theories, beliefs, and experiences indigenous to different cultures, whether explicable or not, used in the maintenance of health, as well as in the prevention, diagnosis, improvement or treatment of physical and mental illnesses" (WHO, 2000a). WHO defined a traditional healer as "a person who is recognized by the community where he or she lives as someone competent to provide health care by using the plant, animal and mineral substances and other methods based on social, cultural and religious practices" (WHO, 2000b). Before Europeans' arrival on the continent, Africans received their health care primarily from traditional medicine practitioners. Today, between 80% and 90% of Nigerians still receive healthcare from traditional medical practitioners (Offiong, 1999).

A survey study from Benin in 1988 found three traditional medicine sign-posts for every Western-style medical clinic. The popularity of traditional medicine, some experts opined, is due to acceptability, low cost, compatibility, safety, and suitability in treating chronic diseases (Okigbo & Mmeka, 2006). Other factors proposed include: (1) the anxiety about the adverse effects of chemical drugs, (2) improved access to health information, (3) the changing values and reduced tolerance of paternalism, and (4) increased cases of chronic diseases which many patients believe are not responsive to western medicine (WHO, 2002a; Thorne's et al., 2002). Besides the issue of accessibility, traditional medicine challenges how cultural heritages are preserved and respected. The utilization of traditional medicine is in line with the socio-cultural and environmental conditions of the people who use it (Owumi, 2002). For example, Igbo women from Ibibio indigenous healers in Akwa Ibom State use traditional medicine for: (1) diseases that had failed to respond to initial treatment, (2) health conditions stigmatized at communities of origin, and (3) health conditions thought to have resulted from supernatural causes (Izugbara et al., 2005).

In the developing world, including Nigeria, the practice of traditional medicine preceded technology-driven orthodox medical practice. While Western-style medical practice is hinged on the "germ theory," the traditional African medicine practitioners (TMPs) view the etiologies of illnesses from both natural and supernatural perspectives. The TMPs were stigmatized and marginalized by the Europeans, which denied the indigenous knowledge systems the chance to systematize and develop. In some cases, as in South Africa, TMPs were out rightly banned for believing that disease and illness are due to "witchcraft." In the Western-style medical paradigm, witchcraft is considered as "backward," "superstition," and "dark continent."

Traditional medicine is an alternative medical system that serves a unique role within the Nigerian healthcare system. Although the scientific literature has witnessed a surge in the number of publications on traditional remedies from Nigeria, there is limited information on the country's emerging developments and promising medicinal plants. This chapter chronicles the origin and evolutionary developments and challenges associated with traditional medicine in Nigeria. The chapter also examines the traditional medicine occupations, including their treatment philosophies and treatment approaches. Finally, the chapter analyses the emerging practice trends, future traditional medicine, including breakthroughs in pharmaceutical product development in Nigeria, efficacy, and traditional medicine safety.

Genesis of Traditional Medicine

The origin of traditional medicine is as old as the history of humanity. Through trial and error, African traditional religious scholars assert that Adam discovered the herbs in the Garden of Eden have medicinal value and power (Ekeopara & Ugoha, 2017). The tropical and subtropical climate in Africa makes the plants accumulate important secondary metabolites through evolutionary means of surviving in a hostile environment. The continent has a tremendous share of intense ultraviolet rays from the tropical sunlight and numerous pathogenic microbes, including several bacteria, fungi, and viruses. Several scientists have postulated that African plants accumulate chemo-preventive substances more than plants from the northern hemisphere. Interestingly, of all species of *Dorstenia* (Moraceae), only the *Dorstenia mannii* Hook.f – a perennial herb growing in the tropical rain forest of Central Africa – contained more biological activity than related species (Mahomoodally, 2013).

Africa is the cradle of humanity with a rich biological and cultural diversity but marked by regional differences in healing practices. Before Europeans' arrival on the continent, Africans in rural and urban communities received their health care primarily from traditional medicine practitioners called ethnomedicine or folk medicine practitioners, or natural healers. However, the traditional medicine remedies used varies within the 54 African countries. In Nigeria, the alternative medicine practitioners that predate the introduction of allopathic medicine include herbalists, native doctors, native healers, medicine men, and witch doctors. They are called *Babalawo's, Adahunse*, or *Onisegun* among the Yoruba-speaking people, *Abia ibok* among the Ibibio community, *Dibia* among the Igbo, *Boka* among the Hausa-speaking people, and *Sangoma* or *Nyanga* among South Africans (Cook & Sangomas, 2009).

The process of modernization in Nigeria, some scholars argued, is intrinsically linked to Europeans' influence, particularly in the areas of health care and education (Offiong, 1999). Between 1840 and 1860 marked a profound and rapid transformation with the discovery of *Quinine* to treat malaria in the world's most endemic region. The era marked the modern healthcare system, one of the many "legacies" of Western colonization in Nigeria.

African traditional medicine (ATM) is the oldest and arguably the most assorted of all therapeutic systems. Africa has over 216 million hectares of forest and up to 45,000 species, of which 5000 species are used for medicinal purposes. Today, the continent has one of the highest deforestation rates globally, with a loss of 1% per annum through deforestation. Africa has the highest endemism rate, with the Republic of Madagascar ranked number one, while the continent contributes nearly 25% of global trade in biodiversity. Despite the abundant biodiversity, Africa produces only a fraction of the international drugs sold for commercial purposes (Mahomoodally, 2013). Factually, Africa provides about 60,000 of the global higher plant species but sadly contributes less than 8% of the 1100 drugs placed on the market worldwide (Dzoyem et al., 2013).

Over the last three decades, high-income countries have seen a steady increase in the use of complementary and alternative medicine (CAM) including herbal remedies. In low-income countries, particularly in Africa, traditional medicine is the primary source of healthcare delivery in spite of Western civilization's influence and availability of modern technology and allopathic medicine. Over 80% of the population in Asia, Latin America, and Africa use traditional medicine in meeting their primary healthcare needs because it is an easily accessible and affordable source of health care (Gouws, 2018).

The evolution of traditional medicine in Nigeria led to various categories of healing methods. The traditional medical practitioners (TMPs) use natural herbs for healing bodily, spiritual, emotional, and psychological disorders. Both orthodox and traditional systems of health care now exist in the country, with the primary objective of maintaining good health by preventing, managing, and curing diseases. Although this chapter presents the traditional system, it should not be construed as an endorsement by the author. Instead, the author recommends the use of orthodox medicine when available. This position is based on the fact that many of the statements espoused by TMPs are conjectural and not supported by evidence-based research.

Today, between 80% and 90% of Nigerians receive their health care from TMPs. In many rural areas, the TMPs are the main or sole healthcare provider – they are culturally accepted, easily accessible, and affordable (Offlong, 1999; Okoronkwo et al., 2014). Orthodox Western health care in the country remains inaccessible due to the high cost and concentration of health facilities in urban centers. To address these issues, the federal government, in 2007, formulated a national policy governing the regulation and practice of traditional herbal medicine as part of a comprehensive healthcare system designed to ensure safety and effectiveness.

The World Health Organization's Role in Promoting Traditional Medicine

For over five decades, the World Health Organization (WHO) has advocated using traditional medicine and provided guidelines on deploying it within the primary healthcare system. Since early 1970, the WHO recognized the TMPs as the backbone of any primary healthcare system and recommended its integration into the conventional (orthodox) healthcare system. The WHO first espoused the importance of traditional medicine at the historic Almaty (formerly Alma-Ata) Congress held in Kazakhstan (formerly Kazakh Soviet Socialist Republic) on September 6–12, 1978. Subsequently, the WHO crafted a global declaration and framework for achieving the targeted goal of rendering excellent healthcare services for all by the year 2000.

In 1993, the WHO further validated the importance of traditional medicine and published several monographs on the quality, safety, and effectiveness of medicinal plants and herbal remedies. Notable among the many publications is the document titled: *"Promoting the Role of Traditional Medicine in Health Systems: A Strategy for the African Region,"* adopted in Ouagadougou, Burkina Faso, on August 31, 2000, by the WHO Regional Committee for Africa. The declaration on traditional medicine is recognized in the statement of the *"Decade of African Traditional*

Medicine" (2000–2010) that was adopted in Lusaka, Zambia, in July 2001, by the African heads of state.

The first WHO's Congress on traditional medicine held in Beijing, China, from November 7–9, 2008, provided the framework for integrating traditional medicine into national healthcare systems worldwide (Stafford, 2010). The Beijing Declaration identified six primary articles on the knowledge of traditional medicines, treatments, and practices and created an action plan by calling on each nation to formulate national policies, regulations, and standards on safety and effective use of traditional medicine. Each country should develop traditional medicine based on research and innovation consistent with the global plan of action adopted at the 61st World Health Assembly in 2008. Governments should partner with international organizations and other stakeholders in implementing the global strategy and plan of action and establish systems for the qualification, accreditation, or licensing of traditional medicine practitioners to enhance their knowledge and skills based on national requirements. The communication between orthodox healthcare workers and traditional medicine practitioners should be strengthened, and appropriate training programs established for healthcare workers/students, and scientists (WHO, 2008).

Twelve years after the first WHO's Congress, many of the 193 sovereign member states and governing bodies have adopted several traditional medicine resolutions. The United Kingdom, European Union, Australia, China, India, Japan, Malaysia, and Korca have integrated the WHO's national policies on traditional and herbal medicines into their healthcare system. The implementation is not the same in all the countries, but they all have a similar framework for ensuring the safe use of herbal medicines within their healthcare system. In these countries, herbal products are now readily available in departmental and drug stores. In Nigeria, the goal as stated in the national health policy is that herbal remedies will be available in the foremost hospitals alongside conventional drugs when the two traditional and Western medicine systems are fully integrated into the healthcare system (Awodele et al., 2014; Nwafor, 2017).

Over the past two decades, the WHO has partnered with several African countries to develop several safe and effective herbal medicines. The foremost global health organization has funded clinical trials in 14 African nations leading to marketing authorization for 89 traditional medicine products, which have met the international standard for registration, and 43 have been listed in the national essential medicine directory. These products are now used to treat malaria, opportunistic infections related to HIV, diabetes, sickle cell disease, and hypertension.

In Nigeria, many TMPs claim they have a cure for coronavirus disease but will not disclose the ingredients in their remedies (Fig. 8.1). The WHO at the fiftieth session of the Regional Committee for Africa meeting held on May 4, 2020, at Congo-Brazzaville, officially recognized the potential role of herbal plants such as *Artemisia annua* – also known as sweet wormwood, sweet annie, sweet sagewort, annual mugwort, or annual wormwood – as possible treatments for COVID-19 and calls for rigorous scientific investigation into its efficacy and side effects (WHO, 2020). The WHO is currently collaborating with several African research institutions to investigate Madagascar's herbal cocktails from the *artemisia* plant acclaimed

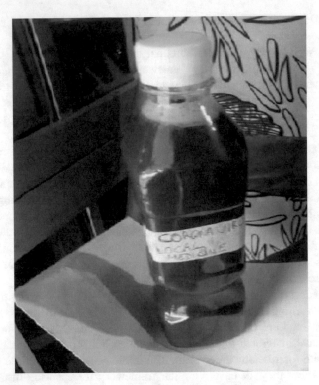

Fig. 8.1 A traditional medicine for COVID-19 bought at Ile-Ife market. (Photograph used with permission of Bamidele Solomon)

to be potent in treating COVID-19 (Ettang, 2020). In the interim, several intellectuals in Nigeria claimed they had developed herbal remedies and vaccines to prevent COVID-19 (Surperformance, 2020). Beyond the claims made in the lay media on the "miracle cure" of the herbal products, no randomized control experimental design study has been published in a peer-review journal that supports any of the claims. The confusion created in the lay press prompted the WHO to warn that many herbal remedies are touted on social media as efficacious in treating COVID-19 without rigorous research to ascertain their safety and efficacy. The use of such herbal remedies, the WHO cautioned, can put the public in danger by giving a false sense of security and distraction from the known effective public health strategies that can curtail the spread of the virus (WHO, 2020).

Common Medicinal Plants in Nigeria

Several studies from Nigeria have evaluated the effectiveness of medicinal plants in the management of various conditions that include treatment of opportunistic infections associated with HIV/AIDS and COVID-19 (Christian, 2009; Abdullahi, 2011;

Ettang, 2020; Adebowale, 2020; Surperformance, 2020; The Africa Report 2020). TMPs use medicinal plants as home remedies to treat various diseases, and at least 522 medicinal plant species have been identified (Weintritt, 2007; Falodun and Imieje, 2013; Iwu, 2014; Ozioma and Chinwe, 2019; Adodo and Iwu, 2020; Olawale, 2021).

Table 8.1 The popular Nigerian medicinal plants and their uses

Serial #	Medicinal plant	Local name	Properties	Indications[a]
1	Moringa plant (*Moringa Oleifera*)	Miracle tree	Rich in amino acids, minerals, and vitamins A, C, and E and has antioxidants' properties – fight free radicals and molecules that cause cell damage, inflammation, and oxidative stress, antibacterial and antimicrobial properties	Anemia, arthritis (rheumatism), asthma, cancer, constipation, diabetes, diarrhea, epilepsy, fluid retention, headache, heart problems, high blood pressure, intestinal spasms, kidney stones, stomach pain and ulcers, thyroid disorders, infections (bacterial, fungal, viral, and parasitic infections), and abscesses
2	Bitter leaf (*Vernonia Amygdalina*)	Ewuro (Yoruba), Onugbu (Igbo), Shiwaka (Hausa)	Detoxification and antipyretic properties	Stomach ache, malaria, typhoid fever, diarrhea, hypertension, diabetes, sexually transmitted infections, pneumonia, eczema, ringworm, prostate cancer, dysuria, insomnia, fertility
3	Aloe vera	Eti erin (Yoruba)	Anti-inflammatory properties – cosmetic and medicinal uses	Hair and scalp moisturization and treatment. Skin irritations and rashes, dermatitis, psoriasis, oral mucositis, mouth ulcers, canker sores, ulcer, dental plaque, burn injuries, constipation, diabetes
4	Basil (*Ocimum gratissimum*)	Scent leaf, Efirin (Yoruba), Daidoya (Hausa), Nchanwu (Igbo)	Laxative effect	Diarrhea, dysentery, stomach ache, vomiting, colon pains, earache, cold and catarrh, cough, fever, malaria, aiding digestion, relief bloating, ringworm, oral infections, and fungal infections

(continued)

Table 8.1 (continued)

Serial #	Medicinal plant	Local name	Properties	Indications[a]
5	Girdle pod (*Mitracarpus Scaber*)	Irawo Ile (Yoruba), Gudugal (Hausa) Obuobwa or Ogwungwo (Igbo)	Antibacterial and antimicrobial properties	Skin infections such as scabies, dermatoses, ringworm, body aches, headaches, toothaches, arthritic, pains, amenorrhea, hepatitis, and sexually transmitted infections
6	Ringworm bush or candle plant (*Senna Alata*)	Ogalu (Igbo), Asunrun Oyinbo (Yoruba)	Antibacterial, antifungal, anti-inflammatory, anti-tumor, analgesic, diuretics, and laxative properties	Fungal infections of the skin, ringworm, scabies, parasitic skin infections, filarial worms, eczema, constipation, diarrhea, intestinal parasites, uterus problems, biliousness, and hypertension
7	Wild lettuce	Efo Yarin (Yoruba)	Healing, relaxant, sedative, anti-oxidative, analgesic, euphoric, antitussive and diuretic properties	Arthritic pain, colic pain, joint pain, muscle pain, muscle spasms, relieve uterine cramps during menstruation, bronchitis, whooping cough, headaches, migraines, sexual disorders, nymphomania, premenstrual syndromes such as anxiety, uneasiness, and pain, skin itching, irritation, or minor skin infection, atherosclerosis, and urinary tract problems
8	Mint leaf	Ewe minti (Yoruba)	Analgesic, antipyretic properties	Aid digestion, stomach ache, abdominal cramps, fever, morning sickness, nausea, and vomiting, nausea. Also use in cosmetic products such as toothpaste, air freshener, shampoo, peppermint spray, or oil
9	Water leaf (*Talinum fruticosum*) – Philippine or Florida spinach	Gbure (Yoruba), Ebe-dondon (Edo)	Boosts the immune system, enhances brain activity, diuretics, high concentration of oxalic acid	Malaria, lethargy, diarrhea, hepatitis, and liver enlargement, gout, kidney disorders, and rheumatoid arthritis

Table 8.1 (continued)

Serial #	Medicinal plant	Local name	Properties	Indications[a]
10	Alligato pepper/ grain of paradise (*Aframomum melegueta.* K. Schum (Zingiberaceae)	Ataare (Yoruba), Amaka – Oseoji (Igbo) – chitta, gyan'dammar yaji (Hausa) Erhie (Urhobo)	Rich in high fiber and tannin and reduces inflammation, natural aphrodisiac, increases thermogenesis	Promote wound healing, burns, gastrointestinal disorders such as ulcers, diarrhea, stomach pains, intestinal worms, diabetes, strong erectile dysfunction (ensuring delayed discharge), weight loss, and improves women libido as the nerve endings are stimulated more
11	Zobo leaf Hibiscus Sabdariffa	Zoborodo (Hausa) Used to prepare the local drink known as Zobo	Contains polyphenol	Prevent skin and prostate cancer, and treat hyperlipidemia and hypertension

Sources: Weintritt, 2007; Falodun & Imieje, 2013; Olawale, 2021
[a] No published randomized controlled study to support these claims

The popular Nigerian medicinal plants and their uses are summarized in Table 8.1. TMPs prepare herbal products in powder form, which could be swallowed or taken with pap (cold or hot) or any drink or rubbed into cuts made on the body with a sharp knife. They are prepared by soaking in the water or local gin and decanted before drinking it. The concoction could also be boiled in water and allowed to cool before use. Herbal products are also produced in the form of: (1) native soap and used for bathing; such locally produced "medicated soaps" are commonly used to treat skin diseases; (2) pomades or ointments and pastes in a medium of palm oil or shea butter; or (3) pounded yam with soup which the patient consumes. Herbal preparations are also administered as an enema (Adesina, 2005).

Besides the medicinal plants mentioned in Table 8.1, Falodun and Imieje (2013) highlighted other plants grown in Nigeria that have demonstrable promising pharmacological results. They include: Boophone (*Boophone disticha*), Goat weed (*Ageratum conyzoides L Compositae*), Garlic (*Allium sativum*) L.Liliaceae, Echinacia (*Echinacea angustifolia, Echinacea pallida, Echinacea purpurea*), Feverfew (*Chrysanthemum parthenium*), Gawo (*Faidherbia albida*), German Chamomile (*Matricaria chamomilla*), Ginger (*Zingiber officinale*), Grapefruit (*Naringenin*), Green tea (*Camelia sinensis*), Morinda citrifolia (*Noni*), Black cumin (*Nigella sativa*), Pawpaw (*Carica papaya L Caricaceae*), Rauvolfia serpentina, Rose hips, Saw Palmetto, Shiitake mushrooms (*Lentinus edodes*), and St. John's wort.

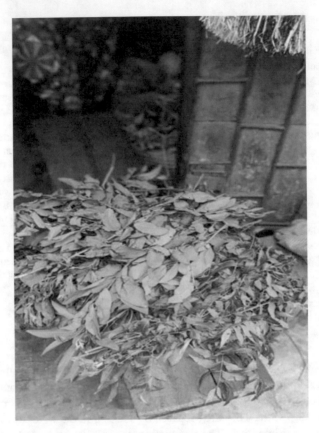

Fig. 8.2 Assorted leaves of medicinal plants (Cocoa, Mango, and *Dongoyaro*) on display for sale at Oyingbo market in Lagos. (Photograph used with permission of Paschal Mogbo)

In addition, the bark, leaves, and seeds of the Neem tree, also known as *Dongoyaro* in Nigeria (Fig. 8.2), contain chemicals that might help reduce blood sugar levels, prevent pregnancy, kill bacteria, prevent mouth plaque formation, and heal ulcers in the digestive tract (WebMD, 2021a). It is used to treat tooth plaque, gum disease (gingivitis), lice, and insect repellant, but there is limited empirically based evidence to support these uses.

Lemongrass (*Cymbopogon citratus*) (Fig. 8.3) is another common medicinal plant in Nigeria with antioxidant properties that can boost red blood cell levels and fight free radicals. It contains inflammation-fighting compounds such as chlorogenic acid, isoorientin, and swertiajaponin (Wilson & Nall, 2018). Lemongrass remedies are commonly taken orally as herbal tea, or the powder added to food or applied directly to the skin. TMPs claim it can relieve anxiety and pain, reduce swelling and fever, improve sugar levels, lower cholesterol, prevent infection, boost oral health, and stimulate the uterus and menstrual flow. As a cautionary note, there is limited empirical evidence in the literature to support this recommendation. In the industrial setting, lemongrass is used as a fragrance in deodorants, soaps, cosmetics, and in making vitamin A and natural citral (WebMD, 2021b).

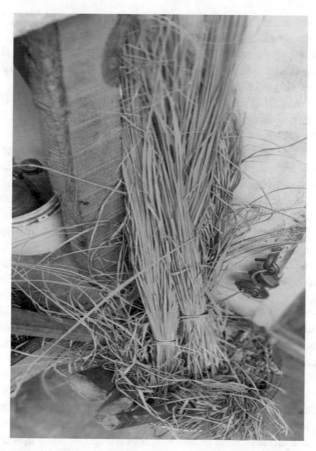

Fig. 8.3 Lemongrass (*Cymbopogon citratus*) on display for sale at Oyingbo market in Lagos. (Photograph used with permission of Paschal Mogbo)

In the last decade, over a dozen studies were identified in the literature that investigated the medicinal plants used by TMPs in the different parts of Nigeria. The pertinent findings from the studies are presented next. Idu and associates (2010) investigated the medicinal plants sold in Abeokuta. The study identified 60 medicinal plant species, and most of the herbal remedies were in dried form and sold alone or in combination with other plants. They are used to treat malaria, hypertension, typhoid, jaundice, hyperthermia, skin irritations, dysentery, anemia, gonorrhea, cough, measles, and fibroid. The researchers suggest the need to encourage domestication and cultivation of medicinal plants and implement conservation measures to ensure a sustainable source of medicinal plants.

Oreagba and associates (2011) assessed the use and knowledge of the benefits and safety of herbal medicines among urban dwellers in Lagos. The majority (66.8%) of the study participants (N = 388) used 12 herbal remedies (crude or refined) alone or with other herbal medicine to treat malaria (20.8%) and diabetes

(16.2%). The most frequently used herbal preparation is *agbo jedi-jedi* (35%), followed by *agbo-iba* (27.5%) and *Oroki* herbal mixture® (9%). Family and friends influenced 78.4% of the study participants who use herbal medicine. Herbal remedies were considered safe by 50% of the study participants, even though 20.8% experienced mild to moderate adverse effects.

Ajibesin et al. (2012) surveyed TMPs and community elders (N = 460) to determine the medicinal plants used in Rivers State. The study identified 188 medicinal plant species representing 169 genera and 82 families commonly used herbal remedies. The most popular genera were *Ipomoea* and *Citrus*, providing four species each. The most important species that showed the highest Fidelity level value were *Ageratum conyzoides* L. (Asteraceae) (100%) and *Tridax procumbens* L (Asteraceae) (100%). The researchers obtained the highest informant consensus factor value of 0.99 for the essential categories of dermal and digestive disorders, including fever and malaria. The leaves were the most used plant part (42%), while decoction was the primary method of drug preparation (36%).

Adachukwu and colleagues in 2014 investigated the medicinal plants used by TMPs in the Eastern region of Nigeria. The findings revealed that most of the plants identified were Angiosperms growing in the wild. Some of them were cultivated, and the others developed in the wild. The highest proportion of plant parts used to treat ailments were leaves and roots. All the plants identified contain phytochemical agents: alkaloids, tannins, flavonoids, saponnins, glycosides, phenolic compounds, and phytosterols.

Idu and colleagues in 2014 investigated the medicinal plants used by 50 TMPs from Idoma in Benue State. The findings pinpointed 63 plants belonging to 36 families and provided their botanical names, diseases treated, plant parts used, mode of administration, and their pharmaceutical forms. Among the plants identified were *Azadirachta indica*, *Telferia occidentalis*, and *Ocimum gratissimum*, which are used to treat common ailments such as malaria, anemia, and stomach upset.

A nationwide study by Chukwuma and associates (2015) interviewed members of the National Association of Nigerian Traditional Medicine Practitioners (NANTMP), Nigerian Traditional Medical Association, and the Nigerian Union of Medical Herbal Practitioners, to identify the medicinal plants used for cure and prevention of disease. The study identified 127 herbal plants used in the management of different ailments. The authors noted that medicinal plants play vital roles in the Nigerian healthcare sector, but TMPs are not fully recognized. And the federal government is yet to adequately contribute positively to the conservation and sustainable use of the flora species in the country.

An investigation of the medicinal plants used to treat rheumatism by Amahor people in Edo State was conducted by Erhenhi in 2016. The findings identified three plant species – *Dysphania ambrosioides* Taub, *Spondias mombin* L, and *Pterocarpus soyauxii Jacq* belonging to the family Amaranthaceae, Anacardiaceae, and Fabaceae – were used to treat rheumatism. When analyzed, the plants contained several phytochemicals such as alkaloid, saponin, flavonoid, phenol, tannin, terpenoid, steroid, and anthraquinone at moderate concentration. The herbal remedies were prepared with leaves, stem, bark, and root with other materials such as fresh palm fruits and native chalk.

In 2016, Monier and Abd El-Ghani investigated the medicinal plants used by TMPs in the different parts of Nigeria. The study identified 325 species and 95 families of medicinal plants used to treat various diseases. Fabaceae has the highest species (42), followed by Asteraceae (22), Euphorbiaceae (20), Acanthaceae (13), and Apocynaceae (12). The highest genera were Euphorbia (6 species), followed by Cola and Hibiscus with five species each, Albizia, Acacia, Combretum, and Ficus with four species each, Acalypha, Allium, Clerodendrum, and Cleome with three species each. The findings also revealed that traditional medicinal practices have wide acceptability, probably because Nigerians believe in their effectiveness. The therapeutic utilization varied widely; the plant parts used include leaves, roots, stem, bark, fruits only, or in combination with two or more in a species or with those of other species.

Following standard protocol, Gini and colleagues in 2016 collected herbal samples from urban and rural locations in eight states. They analyzed the sample for efavirenz, nevirapine, lopinavir, darunavir, ritonavir, atazanavir, tenofovir, FTC (Emtricitabine), and 3TC (Lamivudine). Out of 138 herbal samples, the analysis found the three (2%) samples from Jos and Ibadan contained antiretrovirals – tenofovir (0.2 ng/mg powder). FTC (0.0065 ng/mg powder) was detected in one sample from Jos. Two samples from Ibadan also contained FTC (0.123 and 0.00049 ng/mg powder) and tenofovir (0.2 and 1.6 ng/mg powder), one of these also contained 3TC (0.25 ng/mg powder). The study also interviewed 742 patients who are HIV-positive attending Rural Hospital, Idong, and three urban Antiretroviral Therapy (ART) facilities – Specialist Hospital Gombe, Faith Alive Foundation Clinic Jos, and Dalhatu Araf Specialist Hospital Lafia. Mothers were interviewed for information on pediatric patients. Of the 742 study participants (aged 2–91 years), the investigators found the prevalence of herbal medicine use was 41.8%. Of the patients who took herbal medicine, 54.9% did so before diagnosed as HIV positive; 54.1% did so to cure HIV; only 5.5% of the patients believed they are cured, and 46.1% reported herbal medicines were of no help. About half (54.1%) obtained their herbal preparation from TMPs and 35.1% from city drug vendors. Regardless of educational or employment status, there was wide use of herbal medicines across all ages and genders. In over half the patients using herbal products, the use preceded starting ART and continued during ART use. The overwhelming majority (82.2%) of the patients who used herbal medicines were also receiving ART. The investigators noted the lack of regulation and standardization of herbal remedies and argue strongly for a follow-up study to confirm their findings in other settings and understand if antiretroviral contamination negatively impacts ART programs through the generation of drug resistance.

A prospective cross-sectional study by Okoh and Enabulele (2017) investigated the prevalence of herbal medicine use and self-medication practices among patients at a tertiary dental healthcare center in Benin city. About 24.4% of the study participants (N = 119) had used an herbal product before the study. Plant roots and leaves soaked in alcohol were used by 17.1% of those who used herbal products. There was a statistically significant relationship between the level of education and herbal remedies utilization. Almost half of the participants had self-medicated before presentation at the dental clinic. The drugs used include analgesics and antibiotics. The most commonly reported painkillers were paracetamol and diclofenac, while the most commonly used antibiotic was ampiclox.

Abubakar and associates (2017) investigated the medicinal plants used to treat diabetes mellitus in Zaria. Twenty-two TMPs and herb vendors participated in the survey study. The researchers identified 26 species of plants belonging to 18 families. Herbal remedies were mainly prepared from freshly collected plants, while decoction was the primary method of preparation. Leaves and stem bark formed the significant parts of plants for herbal preparations. The most frequently mentioned families were Malvaceae, Amaryllidaceae, Fabaceae, Moraceae, Myrtaceae, Anarcadiaceae, Meliaceae, and Combretaceae, while leaves, stem bark, and roots were the most frequently used plant parts.

Mephors and associates (2017) determined the medicinal plants used for cancer treatment in two local government areas – Adamasingba (North-West) and Ogbomoso (South) – in Oyo State. TMP, herbalists, elders, and herb sellers (N = 31) were interviewed with semi-structured questionnaires. The study identified 87 plant species belonging to 57 families used as traditional remedies for treating five different types of cancers. Caesalpiniaceae was the most dominant family with seven species, followed by Meliaceae, Euphorbiaceae, Lamiaceae, Annonaceae, Mimosoideae, and Moraceae with four species each. The most frequently mentioned plants in the recipes proffered by respondents were *Aframmomum melegueta* and *Dysphania ambrosioides*. The study provides an inventory of Southwest Nigerian plants with anti-cancer potential that could be investigated as cancer chemotherapeutic agents.

Coolborn and Adegbemisipo (2018) investigated the herbal plant use by TMPs in Ekiti State to prevent and cure diabetes. Twenty-three plant samples were identified and they include: *Anacardium occidentale* (Cashew), *Anthocleist djalonesis* (Cabbage tree), *Bridelia ferruginea* (Ira), *Carica papaya* (Pawpaw), and *Vernomia amygdalina* (Bitter leaf). All 23 plants are readily available in the herbarium, but their uses and preparation are unknown to many people. In preparing the herbal products, the tree is mostly (43%) used, followed by shrubs (30%), and climber group of plants (13%) is least used. The 23 plants identified belong to 18 families, where Leguminosae contributes 12%, Anacardaceae, Apocynaceae, and Cucurbitaceae contribute 8% each, and other 14 families shared one species each. The flower and fruits of plants are primarily used for prevention, while other parts of the plants are for a cure. The TMPs package their remedies in concoction and decoction of plant part or combination of plant parts. For commercial purposes, the products are in smooth powder in well-packaged containers with instructions for use. Most of the plants identified are not used alone but in mixtures of one or two plant parts.

Ishiekwene et al. (2019) reviewed the literature on the consumption, nutritional values, micronutrient composition and medicinal use of selected leafy vegetables available in Nigeria. The study deduced that bitter leaf (*Vernonia amygdalina*), water leaf (*Talinum triangulare*), fluted pumpkin (*Telfairia occidentalis* Hook f.), *Moringa oleifera*, mint leaf, lemongrass, *Amaranthus hybridus* are cheap sources of macro and micronutrients, including fibers, minerals, and vitamins, yet, less than half of these indigenous vegetables are consumed. The vegetables examined all have natural medicinal properties.

Another survey study conducted in 2020 investigated the medicinal plants used to treat persons living with cancer in Sokoto (Malami et al., 2020). The investigators identified 67 species belonging to 31 families. *Acacia nilotica* was the most frequently cited specie (64%), followed by *Guiera senegalensis* (54%), *Erythrina sigmoidea* (34%), and *Combretum camporum* (30%). The barks (55.2%), roots (53.2%), and leaves (41.8%) are the most common parts of the plants used. The most frequently used modes of preparation are decoction (74.6%), powdered form (49.3%), and maceration (46.3%).

Therapeutic Values of Wild Animal Species

The primary ingredients and basis for traditional medicines are medicinal plants and wild animal species. The practice is widespread in Nigeria, where vendors and market stalls selling herbs, charms, and animal parts are common in rural and urban markets (Fig. 8.4). Many wild animal species and their products are used alone or with herbs. Animal parts are used to prepare the remedies to include bones, teeth, fat, glands, meat, hair, skin, tail, and fecal pellets. The medical disorders treated by animal remedies range widely from physical illnesses to mental and antenatal care.

In Nigeria, 23 wild animal species – 16 mammals, six reptiles, and a bird – are advertised and sold to cure and prevent diseases. Another 34 species are used for infertility treatments, and 33 species are used in potency and aphrodisiac medicines (Anonymous, n.d.). Whole animals or animal parts and fecal droppings of 26 species of wild animals are also used in traditional medicine preparations (Fig. 8.5).

The fat extracted from the Python is purported to have curative powers for several diseases. Also, the Manatee (family *Trichechidae,* genus *Trichechus*) are large, fully aquatic, primarily herbivorous marine mammals sometimes known as sea cows found in marshy coastal areas in Nigeria, and is used to treat rheumatism, boils, and backache. Similarly, oils from the Leatherback turtle are used to treat stroke, general body pains, skin diseases, and constipation. Elephant dung is also used to treat at least five various disorders. The giant snail, including the shell, the flesh, and body fluids, is used to treat hypertension, anemia, and convulsions in children (Anonymous, n.d.).

TMPs affirm the therapeutic value of insects. Among the Ijebu Remos in Southwest Nigeria, some insects, when combined with other ingredients, are used to prepare love medicine, spiritual protection, prevention and control of convulsion in children, and management of eye and ear problems. Additionally, arthropods are reportedly used to cure thunderbolt (*magnum*), child delivery (*igbebi*), bedwetting (*atole*), yellow fever (*iba Spanje*), and a host of many other ailments that TMPs declare cannot be treated with Western medicines and therapies (Lawal & Banjo, 2003, 2007). There is presently limited empirical research to support the safety and efficacy of these claims.

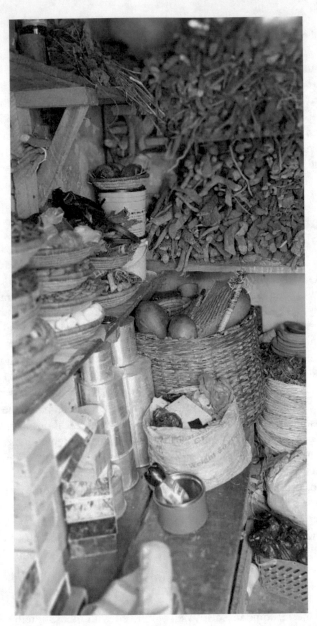

Fig. 8.4 A traditional medicine dealer store at Oyingbo market in Lagos. (Photograph used with permission of Paschal Mogbo)

Coincidentally, wild animal species are also used in biomedical research. Gorillas are taken to zoological gardens in developed countries and killed in some parts of Africa to obtain specimens for medical research. Furthermore, some wild animals are used in the production of modern drugs. For example, hemotoxin and

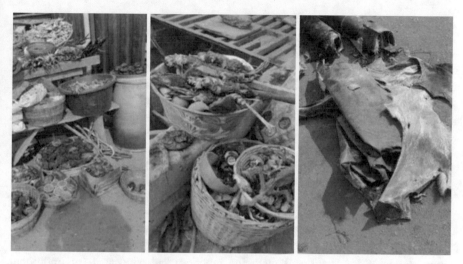

Fig. 8.5 Dry wild animal parts on display for sale at a market in Ibadan. (Photograph used with permission of Babatunde Adegoke)

neurotoxin venoms are used to treat hemophilia and as a sedative and pain killer, respectively (Anonymous, n.d.). Hemotoxin is produced by venomous animals such as pit vipers and vipers, while some living organisms produce neurotoxins for their protection from predators or for preying. Air pollution, pathogenic microorganisms, and some animals also make neurotoxin (Synapeducation, 2016).

In the 1900s, treatments for hemophilia include lime, bone marrow, inhaled oxygen, thyroid gland, hydrogen peroxide, and gelatin. By the 1930s, medical scientists discovered that diluting certain snake venoms caused blood to clot. The concept was used to manage patients with hemophilia (Henderson, 2017; Idaho Chapter of the National Hemophilia Foundation, 2021). Scientists at the University of Queensland in 2017 discovered that a small molecule in spider (tarantula) venom could significantly modulate pain when administered in combination with a low dose of opioid, making the dual treatment a promising new approach to pain management (The University of Queensland, 2017). In 2018, Mehra et al. presented a case report of snake venom use, by a 33-year-old man with a history of substance use for 15 years, as a replacement or additional agent to get high or as a substitute for opioids.

Major Milestones in the Development of Traditional Medicine in Nigeria

Nigerian Traditional Medicine Policy

Since the inception of the republic, Nigeria's federal government has shown genuine interest in integrating traditional medicine into the healthcare system. The first protest against traditional medicine's marginalization in Nigeria occurred when a group of native healers in 1922 insisted that their services be legally recognized. The government of President Nnamdi Azikiwe, in 1966, authorized the University of Ibadan to research the medicinal properties of local herbs to standardize and regulate traditional medicine practice in the country. Fourteen years later, in 1980, the Federal Ministry of Health (FMH) of President Shehu Shagari registered native healers and regulated their practice. The following year, in 1981, the National Council on Health approved the establishment of a National Traditional Healers Board made up of representatives of the federal and state governments. The Board is duplicated at the state levels.

Under the military government of General Muhammadu Buhari, a national traditional medicine development program was formed in 1997 at the behest of the National Technical Working Group on Traditional Medicine constituted by the FMH to develop a national policy on traditional medicine and the national code of ethics for the practice of traditional medicine. The federal government also established the Federal Traditional Medicine Board Decree, and promulgated the minimum standards for traditional medicine practice, and advocated for traditional medicine practice at all levels, including the National Council on Health (since 1997), Consultative Meetings of the Minister of Health and State Commissioners for Health and Local Government Chairmen (since 1999), and the Presidential Think Tank Forum (since 1999).

Three years later, the Traditional Medicine Council of Nigeria Act was proposed in 2000 by President Olusegun Obasanjo's administration to facilitate the practice and development of traditional medicine and establish guidelines for regulating the traditional medical practice and protecting the population from dishonesty, fraud, and incompetence. The FMH directed the Council to collaborate with the state boards of traditional medicine to ensure the guidelines and policies outlined in the Federal Traditional Medicine Board Act are followed. Additionally, the Council was empowered to collaborate with organizations within and outside Nigeria with similar objectives and establish model traditional medicine clinics, create botanical gardens, traditional medicine manufacturing units, and herbal farms in the country's six geopolitical zones. The government anticipated the efforts would create jobs in conservation, cultivation, and harvesting of medicinal plants and build up capacity in agroforestry, manufacturing, distribution, and marketing.

In 2004, President Olusegun Obasanjo's administration officially recognized traditional medicine as an essential component of the healthcare system, particularly at the primary care level (FMH, 2007, 2016). In 2007, Professor Eyitayo Lambo, as President Olusegun Obasanjo's Heath Minister, crafted a Nigerian traditional medicine policy per the WHO recommendation. The policy addressed legislation and regulation, strategy, system management, management information system, human resources development, technology, financing, conservation of the environment, biodiversity, knowledge, skills and culture; protection of intellectual property rights and indigenous knowledge, and how to foster partnerships between traditional and conventional medicine practitioners. The policy also mandates the curriculum of the TMPs to screen for disease and provide effective treatment within the healthcare system. The policy also requires the training programs for TMPs to be established at all national health system levels to ensure adequate human capacity in traditional medicine. The Nigerian traditional medicine policy also promotes traditional medicine stakeholders' interests, such as TMPs, researchers, regulatory agencies, policymakers, law enforcement agents, and business entrepreneurs (FMH, 2007). Professor Lambo also established the NANTMP in 2007. Over the years, the Association is bedeviled with leadership struggles and a lack of cooperation with the orthodox medical establishments.

African countries with national traditional medicine policies increased from 8 in 2000 to 39 a decade later in 2010. The number of African nations with strategic plans soared from 0 to 18 in 2010, and eight countries had training institutions for TMPs by 2010 (Asakitikpi, 2019). Despite the progress, the issue of sustainability is always a recurring theme in the African health systems. In Nigeria, healthcare sustainability is often influenced by a global capitalist perspective which encourages the government to boost the health budget to buy state-of-the-art equipment without a maintenance contract and purchase expensive allopathic medicines that an average Nigerian cannot afford. Many scholars have repeatedly emphasized the need for government to look inward and concentrate on producing and distributing traditional medication. The government should closely monitor the herbal remedies produced locally to ensure they meet global quality control standards. Such efforts will create jobs and foster knowledge in herbal science.

National Agency for Food and Drug Administration and Control

The Nigerian traditional medicine policy developed in 2007 empowered the National Agency for Food and Drug Administration and Control (NAFDAC) to regulate the production of vaccines and medicines and the herbal products used by the TMPs. Based on the guidelines formulated by the Traditional Medicine Practitioners Council, TMPs are empowered to control the appropriate Boards and Committees at the state and local government levels, respectively.

In 2014, the NAFDAC published the available ethnomedicinal supplements and extracts on the market but did not endorse them because of limited clinical trial data attesting to their effectiveness and safety. Cases of adverse reactions and herb-drug interactions following herbal medicine use are reported widely in Nigeria (Awodele et al., 2014). Presently, NAFDAC only publishes products tested for safety studies but has recently formed a Scientific/Expert Committee on verifying herbal medicine claims, particularly on safety, efficacy, and quality. The FMH encourages herbalists to register their herbal remedies with the NAFDAC. Unfortunately, as of 2014, NAFDAC recognized only about 20 of the many herbal remedies in circulation (Okoronkwo et al., 2014).

The 2018 Complementary and Alternative Medicine (Advertisement) Regulations oversee the advertisement of herbal products in the country. The Regulations also require all herbal remedies to be registered with NAFDAC before being imported, used, sold, manufactured, or advertised publicly. Advertisements must not state or imply in absolute terms that the herbal preparation is "safe" or has "guaranteed efficacy" or special status. It must not guarantee a cure or prevention of any disease and not claim or indicate a superlative function such as "most effective," "least toxic, "best tolerated," or another special status.

The label of herbal products is to specify the name and complete location address of the manufacturer and a detailed list of ingredients by their botanical or common names. The products must be handled and transported under conditions that prevent deterioration, contamination, spoilage, and breakage to ensure the product quality is maintained up to the time of delivery to the consumer. At the same time, the devices must conform to the standards of good manufacturing practice.

The Regulations also require that herbal product ads are accurate, complete, transparent, and promote credibility and trust of the general public and healthcare practitioners. All the statements or illustrations in labeling and ads must not mislead the public. Cautionary and disclaimer statements must be displayed on the package label and advertisement of herbal products (Ajayi, 2019).

Nigerian Herbal Pharmacopoeia

The first edition of the Nigerian herbal pharmacopeia was published in 2008 with the financial support of the WHO. The herbal pharmacopeia was developed by 16 experts who served on a special committee constituted by the FMH and chaired by Professor Iwu. The Committee's work received extensive publicity in the media and tremendous support within the FMH because there was a global appeal for herbal medicines. The herbal pharmacopeia listed 42 medicinal plants commonly used for therapeutic purposes in Nigeria. Twenty-two of the cultivated plants were indigenous plants, and 18 were imported into the country. The herbal pharmacopeia is the official documentation of medicinal plants and guides herbal production, quality control, and critical information on standardization, efficacy, and safety. Many medical experts averred, at the time, that Nigeria's herbal pharmacopeia would earn foreign exchange revenue by exporting herbaceous medicinal plants.

Regulation and Practice of Traditional Medicine in Nigeria

The Traditional Medicine Practice Act 575 was promulgated in 2000 by President Olusegun Obasanjo's administration to establish a Council to regulate the education and practice of traditional medicine and the sale of herbs and other products. The Council is expected to consult with the educational and research institutions and the Minister of Health on traditional medicine, and to collaborate with establishments involved in large-scale cultivation, preserve medicinal plants, and advise the Food and Drugs Board on the manufacturing, packaging, exportation, and importation of herbal medicine. The Traditional Medicine Practice Act 575 conforms with WHO's

Beijing Declaration that each nation has a national policy on CAM, including governmental regulation of the practice of traditional and herbal medicine. The legislation is also in tandem with WHO's recommendation about research on CAM and its application in primary health care (Stafford, 2010).

President Goodluck Ebele Jonathan's administration in 2013 established another new Committee to produce a curriculum for traditional medical practice education. Unfortunately, it took several years for the Committee to submit their report, which recommended integrating herbal medicine in the curriculum of all health disciplines offered in the Nigerian universities at different credentialing (diploma, degree, and MSc) levels. The FMH created a database and provided resources to license and track the TMPs in the country. The University of Ibadan currently offers Master's and PhD programs in African traditional medicine at its Institute of African Studies. It has also introduced herbal medicine into its medical school curriculum and plans to offer a professional certificate in herbal medicine (Nigerian Scholars, 2018). In 2018, a Department of Herbal Medicine was established at the University of Medical Sciences (UNIMED), Ondo City, to train the first set of professional herbal medicine practitioners in Nigeria (Fig. 8.6).

In 2017, President Muhammadu Buhari's administration introduced a bill to establish the Complementary and Alternative Medicine Commission and the Traditional Medicine Council of Nigeria. Both Bills passed the National House of Representatives on March 8, 2017. The consolidated Traditional, Complementary, and Alternative Medicine bill seek to encourage, promote, and regulate traditional medicine practice. The Traditional Medicine Council is charged with monitoring and creating acceptable standards in alternative and traditional medicine and eliminating quackery, which is pervasive among TMPs. The Council is governed by a Board of 12 members distributed as follows:

1. Five nominees by the NANTMP with at least one woman member.
2. Two nominees by the health minister, including the Director of the Traditional Medicine Services in the Health Ministry Division.

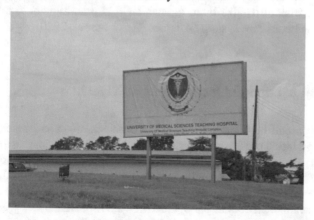

Fig. 8.6 The main entrance to the UNIMED Teaching Hospital, Ondo City. (Photograph used with permission from UNIMED PRO)

3. Two nominees from the research institutions and universities must be a pharmacist, and the other person is an expert in the preservation of biodiversity.
4. The Director of the Center for Scientific Research into Plant Medicine.
5. The Chief Executive of the Food and Drugs Board.
6. The Registrar who serves as the Secretary to the Council.

The President is mandated to appoint the members of the Board, and they can serve for two terms; maximum of 6 years (Awodele et al., 2014).

On April 4, 2018, the Traditional Medicine Division in the FMH was upgraded to a full-fledged Department of Traditional, Complementary, and Alternative Medicines by the Head of Service. The new Department was launched in July 2018 but received the formal approval at the 62nd regular meeting of the National Council on Health held at Asaba, Delta State from September 9–13, 2019. As defined in the 2014 National Health Act, the National Council on Health is the highest policymaking body on health matters in Nigeria. The membership comprises the Minister of Health, who is the Chairman of the Council, the Minister of State for Health, Commissioners for Health in the 36 States, and the Secretary of Health and Human Services Secretariat, at the federal capital territory.

In 2019, the Minister of Health in President Buhari's administration, Dr. Osagie Ehanire, delivered a keynote address titled *"Consolidating the Journey Towards Achieving Universal Health Coverage"* at the National Council on Health meeting. He provided updates on the 2014 National Health Act and developments on the 2016 National Health Policy, the Second National Strategic Health Development Plan (2018–2022), which drives the national health policy, and the Basic Healthcare Provision Fund. At the meeting, the National Council on Health approved creating a Department of Traditional, Complementary, and Alternative Medicines in each of the 36 states and the federal capital territory (FMH, National Council on Health Meeting Communique, 2019).

The Buhari's administration on October 21, 2020, introduced a bill to protect the intellectual property rights of CAM practitioners and take the occupations out of obscurity and institutionalize them to enable CAM practitioners to take an active role within the healthcare system (Ailemen, 2020; Igomu, 2020).

Traditional Medicine Occupations in Nigeria

The TMPs contend they can cure a host of diseases, such as cancer, psychiatric disorders, high blood pressure, cholera, venereal diseases, epilepsy, asthma, eczema, fever, anxiety, depression, benign prostatic hyperplasia, urinary tract infections, gout, even Ebola, as well as heal wounds and burns (Abdullahi, 2011; Adesina, 2005). There is limited evidence-based research to support the above claims. Like their orthodox medical counterparts, the TMPs also specialize and practice referral healthcare processes (Ekeopara & Ugoha, 2017). TMPs typically accept all non-complex cases and some complex cases after consultations. However, if there is no noticeable response to treatment after some trials, the practitioner will refer the patient to a specialist in that particular ailment. If the patient's family gives consent, the patient will consult with the specialist immediately. Also, where the medicinal plant for producing a specific remedy is not readily available, the TMP consults with a practitioner in a nearby community to get the plant or the preparation which another practitioner already makes. Evidence abounds that TMPs refer cases to conventional medical practitioners, especially when one exists nearby (Mafimisebi & Oguntade, 2010).

As a result of this development, some conventional medical practitioners now appreciate the knowledge and clinical skills of TMPs and occasionally discharge their patients, advising them to seek treatment from TMPs. They do this more often in mental health situations once convinced the case goes beyond the confines of western medicine. This development is a good omen to support the call for integrating the two medical systems. The primary specialization within the traditional medical practice in Nigeria is discussed next.

- *Herbalists:* In a typical traditional setting, the herbalists combine the orthodox physician's role with that of the pharmacist and the nurse. The herbalist is the general practitioner knowledgeable in the various aspects of healing and the functioning of the different organs of the body. He/she is expected to diagnose the patient's illness, treat, and predict the course of the treatment. The use of herbs for therapeutic purposes predates man and remains part of the cultural tradition in Nigeria. The herbalist cures diseases mainly by using fresh plants. When seasonal plants are to be used, the herbs are collected when available and are preserved by drying to eliminate moisture. Herbalists prepare an herbal concoction by grinding medicinal plants or parts of such plants (stem bark or root bark, whole root, stem, leaves, flowers, fruits, seeds), in conjunction with animal parts (small whole animal snails, snakes, chameleons, tortoises, lizards), inorganic residues (alum, camphor, salt) as well as insects, bees, and black ants.
- *Traditional Birth Attendants:* The WHO defines traditional birth attendants as health workers who assist pregnant mothers during childbirth and who acquired skills to deliver babies alone or collaborate with other birth attendants. In the Northern states, traditional birth attendants are primarily women, whereas, in the Southern states, both men and women are involved. Traditional birth attendants are usually old, and they see themselves as contributing their skills for the good of the community. Traditional birth attendants serve a prominent role in the healthcare system as they are responsible for 60–85% of births delivered in the country. They are trained to diagnose pregnancy and determine the position of the growing fetus. In rural areas, they provide pre- and post-natal care like midwives (Adesina, 2005).

Because of their experience, and their knowledge of childbirth, traditional birth attendants are trained to assist in orthodox medical practices. Highly experienced traditional birth attendants in some centers assist in obstetric and pediatric care to manage simple maternal and babyhood illnesses. With their extra hands, the orthodox medical practitioners can see more patients and provide broader coverage.

Thus, help to lower the high maternal and child mortality and morbidity rates in the rural areas (Adesina, 2005).

Childbirth by cesarean section is rare under the care of experienced traditional birth attendants. They routinely wash the womb or the vulva a few days before delivery, using some plant preparations now known to have muscle relaxant properties. To deliver a bridged baby, traditional birth attendants use incantations and encouraging words according to different religious and social or cultural beliefs of the patients. The incantations and encouraging words may include statements such as "we do not normally defecate through the head; we do not normally vomit through the anus. The route of delivery ordained by God should be followed" (Adesina, 1988). The traditional birth attendants will proceed to massage and press on the abdomen and work on the fetus. Traditional birth attendants use plant extracts and chemicals with muscle relaxant properties to assist in child deliveries.

- *Traditional Surgeon*: The traditional surgeons have no knowledge of anatomy, and they perform their skills without X-rays. While they are respected in rural areas, complicated surgery is better done in the hospital setting under septic conditions. Infection is a primary concern in all surgical procedures done by traditional surgeons. The techniques commonly undertaken by the traditional surgeon include:

  1. Cutting tribal marks into the cheeks and bellies, followed by rubbing charred herbal products into the bleeding marks to effect healing
  2. Male and female circumcision (clitoridectomy) with special knives and scissors. The bloodletting and wounds that result from these operations are usually treated with snail body fluid or pastes prepared from plants. These practices are, however, becoming extinct in the urban areas
  3. Whitlow of the toes or fingers are usually cut open and treated
  4. Piercing of ear lobes in children to allow the fixing of earrings
  5. Infected teeth are removed and treated with herbal medicines prepared in local gin
  6. Amputations are occasionally done with a very sharp knife after the patient is "anesthetized" to sleep with a potent narcotic concoction. The excision is achieved with the first stroke, and healing usually occurs within some 4 or 5 weeks after the stump is packed with suitable herbal preparation
  7. Cutting of the uvula (uvulectomy) to protect the patient from infections of the pharynx and the respiratory system. Traditional surgeons in the Northern states are versed in cutting off the epiglottis (upper end of the throat flap) to treat many illnesses (Adesina, 2005).

- *Bone Setters*: Bone setting (similar to orthopedic surgery) is the art of repairing fractures and treating other musculoskeletal injuries. Traditional bonesetters are trained in the art of aligning broken bones to ensure that they unite and heal properly (Adesina, 2005). Bone setters treat simple, compound, or complicated fractures resulting from motor accidents or falls from trees. Wounds associated with the fractures are usually cleaned and the bones aligned to prevent deformity. Bleeding is stopped by applying plant extracts, basil or cassava leaf extracts, or body fluid extracted from giant snails.

The use of banana leaves as lint is a common practice by bonesetters. Rigid splints made from bamboo are used to immobilize the fractures, while fresh or dry banana stem fibers (a fibrous plant) are used as a bandage. Various forms of tractions are applied in the management of the fractures of the lower limbs. Adjunct treatments include the use of radiant heat and the application of peppers to reduce inflammation and swelling. The occurrence of deformities is widespread.

An unusual ritual performed by bonesetters is selecting a chicken whose limb would be broken and re-set. The fracture of the chicken is treated in the same way as that of the patient. The chicken's response to treatment is used to indicate the patient's outcome and determine when to remove the wrapped rigid splints. At the same time, it is often asserted that bonesetters can arrest the deterioration of gangrenous limbs that may lead to amputation. Unfortunately, many patients are usually withdrawn from the hospital for treatment in the bone setter's clinics, with these unsubstantiated promises.

- *Rehabilitation:* Unlike the western healthcare system, the traditional health system has no organized skills development system for persons with disabilities to ensure they are gainfully employed. In the spirit of "being your brother's keeper rather than brother's killer," each family or community takes an active role in ensuring independence for their disabled persons. This communal social assistance called "Ubuntu philosophy" gives people living with disabilities a sense of belonging, creating a pleasing way of living through tradition, culture, norms, and taboos. People living with disabilities are accepted and recognized as part of the family or community and are supported to lead a functional and fulfilled life despite their apparent disability. With this kind of communal social support, every physically challenged person discovers ability in their disability. The accommodation provided by families and communities brings about mental, emotional, and psychological healing to the physically challenged person (Ekeopara & Ugoha, 2017).
- *Traditional Medicinal Ingredient Dealers*: These TMPs sell plants, animals, insects, and mineral oil used in making herbal preparations. Some TMPs indulge in preparing herbal concoctions or decoctions for the management or cure of febrile conditions or some other diseases common in women and children (Adesina, 2005).
- *Traditional Psychiatrists*: The traditional psychiatrist specializes in the treatment of persons with mental disorders/illness. Such persons are usually restrained from violent physical aggression by chaining them down to a rigid bar or clamping them down with wooden shackles. Those who are violent, considered to be demon-possessed, are usually caned or beaten into submission and then given herbal hypnotics or highly sedative herbal potions to calm them down. Such herbal preparations include extracts of the African *Hauwolfia*. Treatment and rehabilitation of people with mental disorders usually take a long duration.
- *Practitioners of Therapeutic Occultism*: These practitioners include diviners or fortune tellers, who may be seers, alfas, and priests. They use supernatural or mysterious forces, incantations, and prescribe rituals associated with the community's religious worship, and use all sorts of inexplicable agents to treat various diseases (Adesina, 2005). They are primarily consulted to diagnose diseases, pinpoint their causes, and possible treatment. Because of their reputed ability to

deal with unseen supernatural forces, therapeutic occultism practitioners are usually held in high esteem in the community. They are believed to have extrasensory perception and can see beyond humans. They receive telepathic messages and consult with oracles and spirit guides. Their activities include prayers, singing incantations, invocations, and the use of fetish materials to appease unknown gods. Diseases caused by supernatural forces are readily diagnosed and treated by these practitioners (Adesina, 2005; Ozioma & Chinwe, 2019). TMPs generally assert that their treatment outcomes are better than conventional medical care. Scientific investigation studies have not verified these claims.

Indications for Traditional Medicine

As reflected in Table 8.1, the TMPs in Nigeria often profess they have success treating a wide array of diseases that include cardiovascular disease, such as hypertension and stroke, with antihypertensive herbs, such as the *African Rauwolfia* and the *Negro coffee*. They also manage the nervous system's disorders, such as convulsions and insomnia with parrot's beak and the African Rauwolfia. They treat diseases of the digestive system, such as diarrhea and dysentery with the *Basil* plant. The TMPs also claim success in treating the endocrine system's conditions, such as diabetes, by using the leaves of the common *Periwinkle* or *Mormodica plants*. They manage the respiratory system's diseases, such as asthma and cough, with the *Lemongrass* plant and treat infections of the genitourinary system, such as gonorrhea and hematuria with the bush banana (*Marsdenia australis*).

The TMPs avouch they effectively treat wounds and dermatomycosis (*Craw-craw*) and illnesses associated with the ear, nose, and throat ache and sinusitis, with the *Resurrection* plant. They also maintain they manage diseases caused by microbes, viruses, insects, and infections and malaria with garlic, clove. The African *Mahogany* tree extracts are used to treat hernia, snake bite, arthritis, and gout by using the herbs alone or in admixture with animal parts and minerals.

Childhood leukemia and Hodgkin's disease are managed with *reserpine* extracted from the African or Indian *Rauwolfia*. Reserpine medicine is also used as a tranquilizer, and shea butter extracts as a nasal decongestant. Rheumatism is treated with plant extracts, such as *Vincristine* and *Vinblastine* isolated from the *Rose Periwinkle*, which is also used to treat childhood leukemia and Hodgkin's disease. Extract from the *Diosgenin* plant is also used to treat rheumatism and as an oral contraceptive (Adesina, 2005). Herbal remedies extracted from the *Rauvolfia vomitoria (Afzel), Vernonia amygdalina (Compositae), Ocimum gratissimum (Labiatae),* and *Allium sativum (Liliaceae)* plants are also used to treat malaria, diabetes, diarrhea, pyrexia, high blood pressure, gastrointestinal disorders, and as a general tonic (Amole, 2012).

Non-plant-based treatment used by TMPs includes bee venom for arthritis and the civet cat exudates for its anticonvulsant effects. The traditional birth attendants use plant extracts and chemicals to assist in child delivery because of their muscle relaxant properties (Ekeopara & Ugoha, 2017).

Traditional Medicine Treatment Philosophies

The philosophy of treatment by the TMPs differs substantially from that of the orthodox physician, which is based on the "germ theory." The TMPs believe that illness is due to spiritual or social imbalance, and they make a diagnosis through spiritual means. The treatment prescribed usually consisting of an herbal remedy that has healing abilities and symbolic or religious significance.

On the other hand, the orthodox medical practitioner treats the patient's disease using drugs or surgically removes the disease's cause. Instead, the traditional healers use a holistic approach by reconnecting the patient's "social and emotional equilibrium based on community rules and relationships. The traditional healers act as an intermediary between the visible and invisible worlds; between the living and the dead or ancestors, sometimes to determine which spirits are at work and how to bring the sick person back into harmony with the ancestors" (Abdullahi, 2011).

The herbal remedies produced by TMPs is usually the first line of treatment for 60% of Nigerian children with a high fever from malaria (WHO, 2002b). In many instances, patients use traditional and allopathic medicine simultaneously to alleviate suffering associated with disease and illness. Amira and Okubadejo (2007) reported that many patients with hypertensive receiving treatment at the tertiary health facility in Lagos also used traditional medicine.

Treatment Approach Utilized by Traditional Medical Practitioners in Nigeria

The treatment approach adopted by the TMPs is somewhat similar to that of the orthodox physician but without the use of sophisticated diagnostic equipment. The TMPs make a "diagnosis" by asking their clients to describe the symptoms and observe for "signs" of illness. The healer monitors clinical state changes, such as fever or abnormal rise in body temperature; jaundice manifested by the yellow eyes. Also, urine, palm, and fingers are suggestive of possible liver problems. Furthermore, the healer would probe their clients for any blood in the urine, coughing and vomiting blood, breathing difficulty, sneezing, swelling which may be minor and localized, general weakness of the body, and development of rashes and even pain? Experienced herbalists can readily differentiate constant or intermittent pains from sharp or dull ones and link them with specific diseases. The healer may ask for any history of seizures (often experienced in convulsions), diarrhea in poisoning cases, characterized by frequent stooling and vomiting and bleeding from the nose, mouth, gums, and teeth, from private parts, anus? (Adesina, 2005).

The common diseases or problems are diagnosed easily by TMPs based on the symptomatology of the condition. Following treatment, if the illness persisted, the client is referred to the practitioner of occultism (the diviner), who may consult various spirits, including his Oracle and prescribe appropriate rituals and make sacrifices to solicit the right answer. The occultists believe that diseases are caused by sorcery, ghosts, breach of taboo, spirit intrusion, and acts of God (Adesina, 2005). Western medical practitioners and scientists believe African traditional medicine defies scientific reasoning regarding objectivity, measurement, codification, and classification. Although there are indications that scientists can study the physical aspects of traditional medicine (i.e., the natural ingredients), the spiritual element is difficult to investigate (Oyelakin, 2009). The biggest challenge is how to accurately examine the religious aspect of traditional medicine, such as incantation; "Ọfọ."

Challenges in the Development of Traditional Medicine in Nigeria

Since independence, the various federal governments of Nigeria, including President Nnamdi Azikiwe, in 1966, have shown some interest in the development of traditional medicine with the primary purpose to integrate it into the healthcare system in line with the practice in China and India. Unfortunately, the lingering mutual distrust and animosity between the allopathic and the traditional medicine practitioners make this goal a pipe dream. Allopathic-trained physicians appear unwilling to cooperate with the traditional system of medical care in Africa.

Before traditional medicine is integrated into the healthcare system, their treatment modalities must overcome several obstacles. First, Phytomedicine must be widely taught in health professional programs to decrease the prejudice among practitioners who believe all traditional medicine to be ineffective. Equally, there is the need to change some traditional herbalists' belief that unprocessed natural herbs have an innate superiority and that their mystical aura will be destroyed by extraction and standardization (Raphael, 2011). Finally, another challenge that the FMH must overcome is to address the vast misinformation written to sell herbal products and the expression of personal opinions not substantiated by scientific evidence.

Critics assert that the TMPs lack the skills required to make the correct diagnosis of severe disorders and are often unwilling to accept the limitations of their knowledge and skills. And the products they prescribe lacks standard dosage and are not subjected to rigorous scientific investigation. Instead, their outcomes are based on anecdotal reports from the patients. As a result, critics contend that TMPs often inflate the "success" of their treatment procedures and products. The other criticisms include the traditional healers' assertion that they have divine and supernatural powers – a dubious belief system because scientists cannot verify through experimentation.

Another fundamental challenge in the development of traditional medicine is the widely reported cases of fake healers who take advantage of the public. Moreover, many charlatans practice in unsanitary conditions, and their herbal remedies are adulterated with dangerous metals. Sadly, the government has been incapable of controlling its dubious practices. In addition, the slow pace of development of traditional practice education at the university level is of concern. Except for the

University of Ibadan and the University of Medical Sciences at Ondo City with traditional medicine programs, the other 42 medical schools in the country have not included traditional medicine into their curriculum, as is the case in other parts of the world (Abdullahi, 2011).

To overcome the aforementioned challenges, the National Universities Commission and the FMH must be in constant dialogue to ensure the successful implementation of the national health policy's tenets. The FMH must ensure that herbalists conduct their work in a clean, hygienic environment and provide acceptable herbal manufacturing practices to prevent raw material and finished product contamination. The government must ensure the herbal products of the TMPs are stable and well-preserved, and properly labeled. Most importantly, the government must enforce uniform standards and monitor accurate dosing of herbal remedies. The herbalists must be required to correctly identify their medicinal plants and other ingredients used to prepare their products.

Emerging Training and Practice Trends and the Future of Traditional Medicine in Nigeria

The training and promotional aspects of traditional medicine help men inculcate good characters in the apprentices, making them responsible. The TMPs engage themselves in ministering healing to the sick and educating the apprentices. Apprenticeship is a system or practice of training the next generation of intending practitioners to acquire skills to help serve their communities (Ekeopara & Ugoha, 2017).

In the past, entry into traditional medicine practice was through a long apprenticeship period, through genealogy, or a call by a spirit. However, the training of TMPs is no longer exclusive to the family members, as institutes under the supervision and instructorship of literate healers are now emerging in different parts of the country. Also, the institutes encourage research into the medicinal properties of plants. A few successful TMPs in Nigeria receive their training from India, China, and other Asian countries where traditional medicine has gained international prominence (Adefolaju, 2011).

Some sociologists aver that TMPs have the knowledge and specialized skills to maintain their patients' health needs who believe that ailment does not come independently as something must be responsible for its occurrence. However, most modern traditional healers have deviated from this philosophical belief system because they now have advanced trado-medical skills and in-depth knowledge of herbs' pharmaceutical properties and the shared cultural perception of diseases in society (Owumi, 2002; Adefolaju, 2011).

Many TMPs in the country now use stethoscopes and other simple clinical instruments to ascertain "signs." Typical patients now commence treatment by obtaining a registration card, paying consultation fees, and having their blood pressures taken. Unlike in the past, a "feasting" ceremony is no longer required, but patients are now required to pay for their treatment at the time of discharge. In addition, the TMPs now use aggressive marketing strategies in print and electronic media, such as radio, television, and news magazines, to reach a wider audience and patronage. Also, they buy airtime to sponsor programs of greater public importance, like drama, football, and so forth, on radio and television. They also exhibit their products at various trade fairs organized to showcase new medical and technological developments.

Herbalists who usually rely on the collection of plants from the wild are now encouraged by the government to have their medicinal gardens and farms and grow some plants, especially those facing extinction from bush burning, drought, and urban development. Herbalists are also now encouraged by the federal government to undertake toxicity studies on their products in collaboration with scientists and recognized research institutions (FMH, 2007).

The "purist" TMPs believe that illnesses do not occur by chance, but some underlying forces are responsible for diseases. Most modern traditional healers have deviated from this belief system with the acquisition of herbs' pharmacological properties and the shared cultural views of diseases (Adefolaju, 2011). The modern literate TMPs have changed their herbal preparation by using sophisticated machines for transforming the plants and ingredients to soluble granules and tablets in clean and standard forms. The TMPs now package their products in capsules like conventional drugs and assign them suggestive names, such as Energy 2000®, Hero®, Vision 2010®, and Hyper 5000®. The products are also hygienically preserved in sachets labeled appropriately by specifying the manufacturer's names and address, preparation, and dosage, including the preservation methods and the diseases for which they are indicated (Adefolaju, 2011).

The assimilation of Christianity and urbanization has eroded the use of traditional medicine in the country. Furthermore, the increased contact of Nigerian youths with the global community through social media has made them abandoned the culture and jettisoned traditional medicine for allopathic medicine.

Indeed, modern-day technology and Western education have positively impacted the practice of traditional medicine in Nigeria. Surprisingly, the general public is now interested in comparing the effectiveness of TMPs with orthodox medical practitioners. Seizing on the public sentiment, the federal government should encourage TMPs to allow scientists to evaluate the efficacy and safety of their products – an area of collaboration that TMPs have over the years resisted for fear of losing their trade.

Breakthroughs in Pharmaceutical Products Development

Traditional herbal remedies are natural plant-derived products – such as phytomedicines, nutraceuticals, and cosmeceuticals – that are used to treat illness for centuries, but only recently did the WHO endorse them as CAM. The reason for the upsurge in the popularity of herbal remedies is multifaceted – the raw materials are available naturally in abundance, easily accessible, and affordable. However, the natural plant-derived products' therapeutic potential has been studied systematically within the last four decades.

The Nigerian Institute for Pharmaceutical Research and Development, established in 1987 as a parastatal by the Federal Government (order No. 33 Vol. 74) and Part B under the Science and Technology Act Cap 276, has developed herbal remedies to manage the sequelae associated with sickle cell anemia (NIPRISAN™) and a fixed-dose combination drug (NIPRIBOL) to treat Ebola virus disease. NIPRD reclaimed the NIPRISAN license, and the Attorney General of the Federation obtained trademark status and legal protection for its social and commercial production. NIPRD has also developed four remedies for treating malaria, fungal infection, diabetes, and immune-boosting. They are trademarked as NIPRIMAL, NIPRIMUNE, NIPRIFAN, and NIPRIDAB and patented with the Ministry of Commerce, Trade, and Investment. NIPRD is currently collaborating with the Institute of Human Virology at the University of Maryland to develop a phytomedicine to treat AIDS and enhance capacity-building in Nigeria (Muanya, 2018).

The International Centre for Ethnomedicine and Drug Development (InterCEDD), InterCEDD Health Products (IHP) makers, and their global partners have developed an herbal weight loss product made from local herbs, such as Moringa, Pigeon pea, and cocoa. The remedy is called "Flat Belly" and promises a flat belly within 3 months. No scientific research has validated this claim. The IHP has also developed another immune booster (Immunovit IHP), marketed as "a disease-fighting supplement and immunity" for a spectrum of ailments. They allege the immune booster combines the antioxidant properties of pomegranate fruits and the adaptogenic/immune-enhancing effects of Korean ginseng root extract and the health-restoring advantage of Ganoderma mushroom.

Similarly, IHP has also produced the *Vernonia Ocimum tea*, made from *Vernonia amaygdalina* (bitter leaf) and *Ocimum gratissimum* (scent leaf). InterCEDD Health Products created another product in partnership with the Neimeth Pharmaceuticals called "Physogen Plus," which contains bitter melon *(Momordica charantia)*, *Vernonia amaygdalina, Ocimum gratissimum*, and bitter kola *(Garcinia kola)*. InterCEDD is an affiliate of the Bioresources Development and Conservation Program, which is a non-governmental, non-profit organization (Muanya, 2018).

Established in 1953 due to the International Bank's recommendation for Reconstruction and Development (colloquially, the World Bank), the Federal Institute for Industrial Research has produced several nutraceuticals for decades, including an anti-sickling supplement made from a blend of two legumes and herbal onion spices. It has also provided ready-to-use therapeutic foods, such as low glycemic drinks, anti-lipidemic snacks, and Viola-Emilia Infusion tea. Furthermore, the Institute has developed herbal products from Neem, such as Neem soap, body lotion, toothpaste, oil, cream and mouthwash, herbal shampoo, and Shea butterfat. The Institute developed a refining process to remove the pale yellow from the crude Shea butterfat's dark color.

The Institute also developed a muscle relaxant, "Citrobalm," and an insect repellant from the refined product. The intermediate raw materials produce essential oil extraction (eucalyptus, lemon oil, and citronella) and protein sweeteners for the industrial sector. Paxherbals Laboratories and Research Center in Ewu, Edo State, produced "Pax Malatreat" to treat malaria. They also profess to have 34 herbal supplements already approved by the National Agency for Food Drug Administration and Control (NAFDAC). Paxherbals and Pax pharmaco-vigilance Centers in Lagos, Jos, and Owerri are the country's local herbal manufacturing firms. Their products are in fierce competition with competitors from Europe, China, India, and other Asian countries. In collaboration with the NNMDA and Irrua Specialist Teaching Hospital in Edo State, Paxherbals Laboratories and Research Center conducted a clinical trial to establish the efficacy of Pax Malatreat medication (Muanya, 2018).

The NMDA has produced mosquito repellant extracts from indigenous medicinal plants. Their future goal is to incorporate these extracts into the mosquito-treated nets presently made from pyrethroids, which are not very efficient in this clime. The NMDA mosquito repellant extract has a pleasant fragrance when rubbed on the skin. Adults, children, dogs, and other pets can use it to repel mosquitoes and flies (Muanya, 2018).

Efficacy of African Traditional Medicine

Many countries such as China, India and South Korea take much pride in their herbal remedies, a resource that TMP in Nigeria has been trying to explore for decades without undermining the power held by orthodox medical practitioners who largely hold the sway of the government. The TMPs have recently invested time and funds in producing home remedies that are acceptable to the poor than the elites, though government institutions are largely skeptical about the claims by herbal practitioners to have the cure for certain ailments such as HIV/AIDS and cancer (Musari, 2014). Studies on the efficacy, toxicity, interactions, and mechanisms of action of traditional African medicines are minimal (Gouws, 2018). Furthermore, there are presently no standardization and safety guidelines on the use of herbal medicine in Nigeria. The TMPs often assert that their products are very effective with no side effects compared to allopathic medicines, but credible double-blind controlled studies have not corroborated these assertions. Chinese traditional medicines have been extensively investigated for safety and therapeutic effects. This development is, in part, responsible for its popularity and the growing global market value. At present, China shares over $6 billion USD of the herbal products market globally, and Indian shares about $1 billion USD (Sarker, 2014). The appropriate question is why is it that Nigeria cannot harness its enormous and extensive herbal products to generate income like China and India? Insufficient scientific evidence on traditional medicine's therapeutic efficacy and safety may be one of the several reasons for this.

Despite the success of antibiotic discovery, infectious diseases are still the second leading cause of death globally. Unfortunately, resistance to antibiotics is among the significant public health challenges in the twenty-first century. Nigeria is blessed with a diverse collection of medicinal plants, and these plants are very rich in phytochemicals, which can be structurally optimized and processed into new drugs. Several herbal plants such as guava (*Psidium guajava*), ginger (*Zingiber officinale*), neem (*Azadirachta indica*), and moringa (*Moringa oleifera*) have been found to exhibit a broad range of antimicrobial activities, and they contain alkaloids, polyphenols, terpenes, and glycosides, with plausible therapeutic potentials.

The growing use of herbal remedies can be attributed partly to recent scientific evidence demonstrating their efficacy. For example, St. John's Worth is found to be useful for treating mild depression. Another reason for the growing popularity of herbal medicines is the general belief that they are more natural and safer than pharmaceutical products. Unfortunately, not all-natural products given by herbalists are safe. Some natural products that TMPs dispense are linked to serious illnesses ranging from allergy to liver or kidney malfunction to cancer and even death.

In evaluating the benefits of traditional medicine, scientists consider the cost-effectiveness and appropriate health outcome. In rural areas, TMPs readily provide access to health care, and the service they provide is cheap compared to western medicine. However, in severe and complex conditions, the care provided by TMPs is often ineffective and fraught with complications, which usually require more resource-intensive treatment by orthodox healthcare professionals. Indeed, allopathic medicine has its roots in herbal remedies, and many essential new drugs will likely be developed and commercialized in the future from the African biodiversity.

Fennell and associates about two decades ago uncovered that many African herbal plants have antibacterial, antifungal, anthelmintic, anti-amoebic, anti-schistosomal, antimalarial, anti-inflammatory, antioxidant, psychotropic and neuro-trophic properties. The active compounds isolated from the herbal remedies provided scientific validation for traditional medicine use (Fenneell et al., 2004). A decade later, Mahomoodally discovered the top ten promising African medicinal plants with short- and long-term potential to be developed as phytopharmaceuticals to treat and manage many infectious and chronic conditions. The ten plants are *Acacia Senegal*, *Aloe ferox*, *Artemisia herba-alba*, *Aspalathus linearis*, *Centella Asiatica*, *Catharanthus roseus*, *Cyclopia genistoides*, *Harpagophytum procumbens*, *Momordica charantia*, and *Pelargonium sidoides*. The medicinal plants are of particular interest because they form part of African herbal pharmacopeia with commercial importance from which modern phytopharmaceuticals have been derived (Mahomoodally, 2013).

In the same line of inquiry similar to Mahomoodally, Ugboko and associates recently identified the antimicrobial properties of some new compounds such as alloeudesmenol, hanocokinoside, orosunol, and 8-demethylorosunol, derived from herbal plants in Nigeria. They found them effective as an alternative therapy in combating multidrug-resistant pathogens' development and survival, coupled with curtailing some antibiotics' toxic effects (Ugboko et al., 2020).

In vitro and in vivo research and double-blind, randomized control studies in humans are desperately needed to establish the efficacy of the products used by the TMPs. Demonstration of their herbal formulations' effectiveness and safety will make the modalities acceptable to the international community's scientists and health professionals. In the case of adverse findings from the therapeutic efficacy and adverse-effects evaluation, the investigator should take appropriate steps to modify that specific preparation's formulation and doses until a positive outcome is achieved. When that occurs, scientists should disseminate their findings in reputable journals globally.

Scientific evaluation of the effectiveness and safety of spiritual-based methods is limited. The relevant spirituality studies are summarized in Chap. 6 of this book. Available data suggests intercessory prayers in the Christian tradition are generally safe, but efficacy and safety data are not available for Nigerian-based spiritual practices.

Safety of African Traditional Medicine

Because herbal remedies are not regulated, no warning information is provided to consumers that "too much of a good thing" could be dangerous (Gouws, 2018). Most herbal products are presently not tested for their safety and effectiveness. Some contain mercury, lead, arsenic and corticoids, poisonous organic substances in harmful amounts, and hepatic failure and death have been reported following herbal medicine's ingestion. Moreover, 25% of childhood blindness in Nigeria is associated with traditional eye medicines utilization (Raphael, 2011).

Although many of the herbal plants used by TMPs are widely assumed to be safe, sadly, some are potentially harmful. A few examples will be presented here. A publication in the *Journal of Ethnopharmacology* cited five studies that showed traditional medicine and many plants used as food to be potentially toxic, muta-genic, and carcinogenic in animals (Fenneell et al., 2004). In 2019, a case study reported the severe acute cholestatic hepatitis following intake of *Artemisia annua* tea by a patient as prophylaxis for malaria. On physical examination, the patient presented with jaundice, elevated transaminases, and indications of cholestasis (total bilirubin 186.6 µmol/L, conjugated bilirubin 168.5 µmol/L). Follow-up test with liver biopsy revealed portal hepatitis with lymphocytic infiltration of the bile ducts and diffuse intra-canalicular and intra-cytoplasmic bilirubinostasis, with no other identifiable etiologies of liver disease. Sequencing of genes encoding for hepatic transporters for bile acid homeostasis (BSEP, MDR3, and FIC1) found no genetic variants usually associated with hereditary cholestasis syndromes. The bilirubin levels normalized 3 months after the onset of the disease. Toxicology analysis of the *Artemisia annua* tea confirmed its ingredients *arteannuin b, deoxy-artemisin, campher*, and *scopoletin*. The authors conclude that "the use of artemisinin-derivatives for malaria prevention is ineffective and potentially harmful and should be discouraged" (Ruperti-Repilado et al., 2019). However, some scientists contend that herbal remedies poisoning usually occurs because it has been misidentified or incorrectly prepared and administered by inadequately trained personnel (Fenneell et al., 2004).

Kamsu-Foguem and Foguem (2014) investigated the safety of some popular medicinal plants used in African herbal remedies. They found that herbal remedies' adverse drug reactions are often due to a lack of understanding of their preparation and appropriate use. Some of the adverse effects they observed are associated with some herbal remedies from different parts of Africa including the following:

1. Gastrointestinal complaints (nausea, heartburn, diarrhea), skin rashes, and allergic (hypersensitivity) reactions.
2. Medullary aplasia, leucopenia, incoordination of movements, centrilobular hepatic, or hepatocellular necrosis.
3. Potentiation of diabetes mellitus (hyperglycemia), sometimes hypoglycemia, and confusions.
4. Chronic renal disease, acute kidney injury (acute tubular necrosis), hyperkalemia, a disturbed level of consciousness, convulsions, and liver failure, hepatic venous-occlusive disease, pulmonary injury, and thrombocytopenia.
5. Hepatotoxicity, cardiovascular diseases (hypertension, cerebrovascular ischemia, dilated cardiomyopathy, myocardial infarction, rhabdomyolysis, and thromboembolism), diabetes, amenorrhea, pseudoaldosteronism, duodenal ulcer, and hepatitis.

Mensah et al. (2019), after reviewing the literature on the toxicity of plants used in traditional medicine, inferred that some of the toxic plants are also used as poisons for hunting and as pesticides. For example, *Datura* is used as a tropane alkaloid, digitalis as cardiac glycosides, and *Pyrethrum* used as a pyrethrin insecticide. *Lantana Camara*, when used to treat malaria, is found in several animal species to be hepatotoxic. Similarly, *Momordica charantia*, an anti-diabetic and antimalarial plant used as an abortifacient in Ghana, can cause fatal hypoglycemia in children. Neurological disorders have been reported following a large intake of fresh *Bambusa vulgaris* leaves by horses. Mensah and associates infer that the toxicity of medicinal plants and even food is, for the most part, dependent on the amount or dose used. And an innocuous substance can be toxic at a high quantity, and patients can tolerate a very toxic substance at a high dose with untoward effects at a low dosage. Adverse reactions may arise from misidentification of the herbal plants and errors made by healthcare providers and patients. Prolonged use even at a tolerable dose may also be damaging to health.

Interactions between allopathic medicines and herbal remedies may increase or decrease either treatment's pharmacological or toxicological effects. Synergistic effects may also complicate some medications used for treating chronic diseases. An herbal remedy used to treat diabetes could cause hypoglycemia when taken in tandem with conventional anti-hyperglycemic drugs. Despite these concerning scenarios, many traditional medicine enthusiasts insist they are safe based on oral knowledge accumulated over several centuries (Fenneell et al., 2004; Gouws, 2018; Mensah et al., 2019). Given the seriousness of the side effects alleged by Kamsu-Foguem and Foguem (2014), it is irrational to describe the African herbal remedies to be safe.

Although there have been some breakthroughs in pharmaceutical product development in the country, there is a lack of clinical evidence showing that African herbal remedies are effective and safe for humans (Falodun & Imieje, 2013). In the absence of this information, African herbal plant users will remain skeptical about such remedies' value. This unfortunate situation denies Africans and the world the freedom to choose herbal plants that are potentially less costly and more accessible. More importantly, aside from efficacy, information about the safety of African herbal remedies is urgently required. The creation of a reporting system to facilitate the monitoring and evaluation of adverse drug events in Africa is warranted.

Conclusion

The number of publications on Nigerian traditional medicine has increased substantially in the last decade, but sadly, most of the publications are review articles and studies that lack scientific rigor. There is still a lack of a comprehensive compilation of promising medicinal plants. The number of double-blind controlled studies on therapeutic effectiveness and safety are few and far between. Such studies are needed for the global acceptability of traditional medicine practices in the country. The bioactive chemical composition of most herbal remedies has not been identified. This situation presents a public health challenge, and scientists should scale up research efforts in this area.

Case Study
Conduct a literature search on the efficacy and safety of traditional African medicine. Select five of the articles published, preferably in the last 3 years, and summarize the findings.

References

Abdullahi, A. A. (2011). Trends and challenges of traditional medicine in Africa. *African Journal of Traditional, Complementary, and Alternative Medicines, 8*(5 Suppl), 115–123. [online]. Available at: https://www.ncbi.nlm.nih.gov/pmc/articles/PMC3252714/. Accessed 10 Oct 2020.

Abubakar, U. S., Abdullahi, S., Ayuba, V., Shettima, K., Usman, S. H., & Ayuba, M. K. (2017). Medicinal plants used for the management of diabetes mellitus in Zaria, Kaduna state, Nigeria. *Journal of Pharmacy & Pharmacognosy Research, 5*(3), 156–164. [online]. Available at: https://jppres.com/jppres/pdf/vol5/jppres16.184_5.3.156.pdf. Accessed 10 May 2021.

Adebowale, N. (2020). *Coronavirus: Nigeria to receive Madagascar herbal medicine.* [online]. Available at: https://www.premiumtimesng.com/coronavirus/392324-coronavirus-nigeria-to-receive-madagascar-herbal-medicine.html. Accessed 10 May 2021.

Adefolaju, T. (2011). The dynamics and changing structure of traditional healing system in Nigeria. *International Journal of Health Research, 4*(2), 99–106. [online]. Available at: https://www.ajol.info/index.php/ijhr/article/view/73868. Accessed 10 October 2020.

Adesina, S. K. (2005). Traditional medical care in Nigeria. *OnlineNigeria.com* [online]. Available at: https://onlinenigeria.com/health/?blurb=574. Accessed 18 Mar 2021.

Adodo, A., & Iwu, M. M. (2020). *Healing plants of Nigeria: Ethnomedicine and therapeutic application.* [online]. Available at: https://www.routledge.com/Healing-Plants-of-Nigeria-Ethnomedicine-and-Therapeutic-Applications/Adodo-Iwu/p/book/9781138339828. Accessed 10 May 2021.

Ailemen, A. (2020). FG approves bill for the establishment of council for traditional, alternative and complementary medicine practice in Nigeria. *Business Day.* [online]. Available at: https://businessday.ng/health/article/fg-approves-bill-for-establishment-of-council-for-traditional-alternative-and-complementary-medicine-practice-in-nigeria/. Accessed 10 Dec 2020.

Ajayi, O. (2019). Traditional medicines and OTC products. *PharmaBoardroom.* [online]. Available at: https://pharmaboardroom.com/legal-articles/traditional-medicines-and-otc products-nigeria/. Accessed 10 May 2021.

Ajibesin, K. K., Bala, D. N., & Umoh, U. F. (2012). Ethnomedicinal survey of plants used by the indigenes of Rivers State of Nigeria. *Pharmaceutical Biology, 50*(9), 1123–1143. https://www.tandfonline.com/doi/full/10.3109/13880209.2012.661740. Accessed: 10 May 2021.

Amira, O. C., & Okubadejo, N. U. (2007). Frequency of complementary and alternative medicine utilization in hypertensive patients attending an urban tertiary care centre in Nigeria. *BMC Complementary and Alternative Medicine, 7*(30), 1–5.

Amole, O. (2012). The role of traditional medicine in primary health care. *Journal of Immunogenic Disorder, 1*, 2. [online]. Available at: https://www.scitechnol.com/role-of-traditional-medicine-in-primary-health-care-HBda.php?article_id=19. Accessed 10 Oct 2020.

Anonymous. (n.d.). *3.2.2 Physical and mental health.* [online]. Available at: http://www.fao.org/3/w7540e/w7540e0c.htm. Accessed 10 May 2021.

Asakitikpi, A. E. (2019). *Healthcare coverage and affordability in Nigeria: An alternative model to equitable healthcare delivery.* [online]. Available at: https://www.intechopen.com/books/universal-health-coverage/healthcare-coverage-and-affordability-in-nigeria-an-alternative-model-to-equitable-healthcare-delive. Accessed 10 Dec 2020.

Awodele, O., Amagon, K. I., Wannang, N. N., & Aguiyi, J. C. (2014). Traditional medicine policy and regulation in Nigeria: An index of herbal medicine safety. *Current Drug Safety, 9*, 16–22. [online]. Available at: http://www.eurekaselect.com/118337/article. Accessed 10 Oct 2020.

Christian, G. E. (2009). Digitization, intellectual property rights and access to traditional medicine knowledge in developing countries. The Nigerian experience. In *A research paper prepared for the International Development Research Centre (IDRC), Canada.* [online]. Available at: https://idl-bnc-idrc.dspacedirect.org/bitstream/handle/10625/41341/129184.pdf?sequence=1. Accessed 10 May 2021.

Chukwuma, E. C., Soladoye, M. O., & Feyisola, R. T. (2015). Traditional medicine and the future of medicinal plants in Nigeria. *Journal of Medicinal Plant Studies, 3*(4), 23–29. [online]. Available at: https://www.plantsjournal.com/archives/2015/vol3issue4/PartA/3-2-491.pdf. Accessed 10 May 2021.

Cook, C. T., & Sangomas, T. (2009). Problem or solution for South Africa's health care system. *Journal of the National Medical Association, 101*(3), 261–265.

Coolborn, A. F., & Adegbemisipo, A. A. (2018). *Medicinal vegetal use by traditional healers in Ekiti State of Nigeria for diabetes treatment.* [online]. Available at: http://www.ijccts.org/fulltext/17-1543510028.pdf. Accessed 10 May 2021.

Dzoyem, P., Tshikalange, E., & Kuete, V. (2013). 24 – Medicinal plants market and industry in Africa medicinal plant research in Africa. In *Medicinal plant research in Africa: Pharmacology and chemistry* (pp. 859–890). Elsevier Science & Technology Books.

Ekeopara, C. A., & Ugoha, A. M. (2017). The contributions of African traditional medicine to Nigeria's health care delivery system. *IOSR Journal of Humanities and Social Science, 22*(5), 32–43. [online]. Available at: www.iosrjournals.org. Accessed 10 Oct 2020.

Erhenhi, A. H. (2016). Medicinal plants used for the treatment of rheumatism by Amahor people of Edo State, Nigeria. *International Journal of Plant Research, 6*(1), 7–12. [online]. Available at: http://article.sapub.org/10.5923.j.plant.20160601.02.html. Accessed 10 May 2021.

Ettang, I. (2020). *Nigerian biotechnologist touts potent herbal COVID-19 treatment.* [online]. Available at: https://www.voanews.com/covid-19-pandemic/nigerian-biotechnologist-touts-potent-herbal-covid-19-treatment. Accessed 10 Dec 2020.

Falodun, A., & Imieje, V. (2013). Herbal medicine in Nigeria: Holistic overview. *Nigerian Journal of Science and Environment, 12*(1). [online]. Available at: http://universityjournals.org/journal/NJSE/article-full-text-pdf/f163b81. Accessed 10 May 2021.

Federal Ministry of Health. (2016). *National health policy 2016: Promoting the health of Nigerians to accelerate socio-economic development.* [online]. Available at: https://extranet.who.int/countryplanningcycles/sites/default/files/planning_cycle_repository/nigeria/draft_nigeria_national_health_policy_final_december_fmoh_edited.pdf. Accessed 10 Dec 2020.

Federal Ministry of Health National Council on Health Meeting. (2019). Communique issued at the end of the 62nd National Council on Health (NCH) meeting on September 9–13th at the Event Center, Asaba, Delta State. *Nursing World Nigeria.* [online]. Available at: https://www.nursingworldnigeria.com/2019/09/communique-issued-at-the-end-of-62nd-national-council-on-health-nch-meeting-federal-ministry-of-health#:~:text=The%20Council%20meeting%20which%20held,Maternal%20and%20Child%20Health%20in. Accessed 10 Oct 2020.

Federal Ministry of Health of Nigeria - FMH - (2007). *Traditional medicine policy for Nigeria.* [online]. Available at: https://www.medianigeria.com/functions-of-federal-ministry-of-health-nigeria/; http://www.eurekaselect.com/118337/article; https://www.ncbi.nlm.nih.gov/pmc/articles/PMC3252714/. Accessed 26 February 2020.

Fenneell, C. W., Lindsey, K. L., McGraw, L., & Staden, J. (2004). *Assessing African medicinal plants for efficacy and safety: Pharmacological screening and toxicology.* [online]. Available at: https://www.researchgate.net/publication/8385896_Assessing_African_medicinal_plants_for_efficacy_and_safety_Pharmacological_screening_and_toxicology. Accessed 10 Dec 2020.

Gini, J., Clayden, P., et al. (2016). *Nigerian herbal medicines widely used by HIV positive people can contain antiretrovirals.* [online]. Available at: https://i-base.info/htb/29847. Accessed 10 May 2021.

Gouws, C. (2018). Traditional African medicine and conventional drugs: Friends or enemies? *The Conversation.* [online]. Available at: https://theconversation.com/traditional-african-medicine-and-conventional-drugs-friends-or-enemies-92695. Accessed 10 Dec 2020.

Henderson, W. (2017). A brief history of hemophilia treatment. *BioNews Services.* [online]. Available at: https://hemophilianewstoday.com/2017/05/15/brief-history-hemophilia-treatment/. Accessed 11 May 2021.

Idaho Chapter of the National Hemophilia Foundation. (2021). *History of bleeding disorders.* [online]. Available at: https://idahoblood.org/bleeding-disorders/what-is-a-bleeding-disorder/history-of-bleeding-disorders.html. Accessed 11 May 2021.

Idu, M., Erhabor, J. O., & Efijuemue, H. M. (2010). Documentation on medicinal plants sold in markets in Abeokuta, Nigeria. *Tropical Journal of Pharmaceutical Research, 9*(2), 110–118. [online]. Available at: http://www.bioline.org.br/pdf?pr10013. Accessed 10 May 2021.

Igomu T. (2020) FEC approves establishment of alternative traditional medicines' council. [online]. Available at: https://healthwise.punchng.com/fec-approves-establishment-of-alternative-traditional-medicines-council/ Accessed: 18 March 2021.

Ishiekwene, I. C., Dada, T. E., Odoko, J., & Nwose, E. U. (2019). Promoting African indigenous vegetables and its medical nutrition properties: A mini-narrative review based on Ukwani communities of Delta State, Nigeria. *Integrative Food, Nutrition and Metabolism, 6*, 1–6. [online]. Available at: https://www.oatext.com/pdf/IFNM-6-256.pdf. Accessed 10 May 2021.

Iwu, M. M. (2014). Pharmacognostical profile of selected medicinal plants. In *Handbook of African Medicinal Plants*. CRC Press. [online]. Available at: https://www.routledgehandbooks.com/doi/10.1201/b16292-4. Accessed 10 May 2021.

Izugbara, C. O., Etukudoh, I. W., & Brown, A. S. (2005). Transethnic itineraries for ethnomedical therapies in Nigeria: Igbo women seeking Ibibio cures. *Health and Place, 11*, 1–14; *Journal of Nursing Practice, 5*(1), 18–20. [online]. Available at: https://www.ncbi.nlm.nih.gov/pmc/articles/PMC2754854/. Accessed 10 Oct 2020.

Kamsu-Foguem, B., & Foguem, C. (2014). Adverse drug reactions in some African herbal medicine: Literature review and stakeholders' interview. *Integrative Medicine Research, 3*(3), 126–132.

Lawal, O. A., & Banjo, A. D. (2007). Survey for the usage of arthropods in traditional medicine in Southwest Nigeria. *Journal of Entomology, 4*(2), 104–112. [online]. Available at: https://scialert.net/abstract/?doi=je.2007.104.1120. Accessed 10 Oct 2020.

Lawal, O. A., Banjo, A. D., & Junaid, S. O. (2003). A survey of ethnozoological knowledge of honeybees (Apis Mellifera) in Ijebu division of Southwest Nigeria. *Indilinga Africa Journal of Indigenous Knowledge System, 2*, 75–87. [online]. Available at: https://www.researchgate.net/publication/272331250_A_survey_of_the_ethnozoological_knowledge_of_honey_bees_Apis_mellifera_in_Ijebu_division_of_south_western_Nigeria. Accessed 10 Oct 2020.

Mafimisebi, T. E., & Oguntade, A. E. (2010). Preparation and use of plant medicines for farmers' health in Southwest Nigeria: Socio-cultural, magico-religious and economic aspects. *Journal of Ethnobiology and Ethnomedicine, 6*, 1. [online]. Available at: https://link.springer.com/article/10.1186/1746-4269-6-1#citeas. Accessed 10 May 2021.

Mahomoodally, M. F. (2013). Traditional medicines in Africa: An appraisal of ten potent African medicinal plant. *Evidence-Based Complementary and Alternative Medicine*. [online]. Available at: https://www.hindawi.com/journals/ecam/2013/617459/. Accessed 10 Dec 2020.

Malami, I., Jagaba, N. M., Abubakar, B. I., Muhammad, A., Alhassan, A. A., Waziri, P. M., Yahaya, I. Z. Y., Mshelia, H. E., & Mathias, S. N. (2020). Integration of medicinal plants into the traditional system of medicine for the treatment of cancer in Sokoto State, Nigeria. *Heliyon, 6*(9). [online]. Available at: https://www.sciencedirect.com/science/article/pii/S240584402031673X. Accessed 10 May 2021.

Mehra, A., Basu, D., & Grover, S. (2018). Snake venom use as a substitute for opioids: A case report and review of literature. *Indian Journal of Psychological Medicine, 40*(3), 269–271. [online]. Available at: https://www.ncbi.nlm.nih.gov/pmc/articles/PMC5968650/. Accessed 11 May 2021.

Mensah, M. L. K, Komlaga, G., Forkuo, A. D., Firempong, C., Anning, A. K., & Dickson, R. A. (2019). *Toxicity and safety implications of herbal medicines used in Africa*. [online]. Available at: https://www.intechopen.com/books/herbal-medicine/toxicity-and-safety-implications-of-herbal-medicines-used-in-africa. Accessed 15 Dec 2020.

Mephors, V. C., Ogbole, O. O., & Ajaiyeoba, E. O. (2017). Plants used in treatment of five cancers in two Local Government Areas in southwest Nigerian ethnomedicine. *Nigerian Journal of Natural Products and Medicine, 21*. [online]. Available at: https://www.ajol.info/index.php/njnpm/article/view/178092. Accessed 10 May 2021.

Monier, M., & Abd El-Ghani, M. (2016). Traditional medicinal plants of Nigeria: An overview. *Agriculture and Biology Journal of North America*. [online]. Available at: https://scihub.org/media/abjna/pdf/2016/09/ABJNA-7-5-220-247.pdf. Accessed 10 May 2021.

Muanya, C. (2018). *Nigeria advances in natural medicine*. [online]. Available at: https://allafrica.com/stories/201708310466.html. Accessed 10 Oct 2020.

Musari B. (2014) Nigeria: In search of legal backing for u.S.$120 billion herbal medicine sector. Guardian Newspaper. https://allafrica.com/stories/201411250581.html.

Nigerian Scholars. (2018) 3 Nigerian universities to start offering degree programmes in herbal medicine. [online]. Available at: https://nigerianscholars.com/school-news/universities-start-degree-herbal-medicine/. Accessed: 26 November 2020.

Nwafor, N. (2017, March 8). Bill to regulate, promote traditional medicine in Nigeria passes 2nd reading. *Vanguard*. [online]. Available at: https://www.vanguardngr.com/2017/03/bill-regulate-promote-traditional-medicine-nigeria-passes-2nd-reading/. Accessed 10 Oct 2020.

Offlong, D. A. (1999). Traditional healers in the Nigerian healthcare delivery system and the debate over integrating traditional and scientific medicine. *Anthropological Quarterly, 72*(3). [online]. Available at: https://www.questia.com/read/1P3-46950113/traditional-healers-in-the-nigerian-health-care-delivery. Accessed 10 Oct 2020.

Okigbo, R. N., & Mmeka, E. C. (2006). An appraisal of phytomedicine in Africa. *KMITL Science and Technology Journal, 6*(2), 83–94. [online]. Available at: http://citeseerx.ist.psu.edu/viewdoc/download?doi=10.1.1.533.5239&rep=rep1&type=pdf. Accessed 10 Oct 2020.

Okoh, M., & Enabulele, J. E. (2017). Herbal/traditional medicine use and self-medication among patients prior to seeking oral health care in a tertiary health facility in Nigeria. *Journal of Medical Research, 3*(3), 127–131. [online]. Available at: http://www.medicinearticle.com/JMR_20173_08.pdf. Accessed 10 May 2021.

Okoronkwo, I., Onyia-pat, J. L., Okpala, P., Agbo, M. A., & Ndu, A. (2014). Patterns of complementary and alternative medicine use, perceived benefits, and adverse effects among adult users in Enugu urban, Southeast Nigeria. *Evidence-based Complementary and Alternative Medicine, 14*, 239372. [online]. Available at: https://www.researchgate.net/publication/326519223_Unmasking_the_Practices_of_Nurses_and_Intercultural_Health_in_Sub-Saharan_Africa_A_Useful_Way_to_Improve_Health_Care. Accessed 10 Oct 2020.

Olawale, J. (2021). *List and uses of medicinal plants in Nigeria*. [online]. Available at: https://www.legit.ng/1163088-list-uses-medicinal-plants-nigeria.html;   https://www.legit.ng/1147611-yoruba-herbs-uses.html. Accessed 8 May 2021.

Oreagba, I. A., Oshikoya, K. A., & Amachree, M. (2011). Herbal medicine use among urban residents in Lagos, Nigeria. *BMC Complementary and Alternative Medicine, 11*, 117. [online]. Available at: https://www.ncbi.nlm.nih.gov/pmc/articles/PMC3252251/. Accessed 8 May 2021.

Owumi, B. E. (2002). The political economy of maternal and child health in Africa. In U. C. Isiugho-Abanihe, A. N. Isamah, & J. O. Adesina (Eds.), *Currents and perspectives in sociology*. Malthouse Press.

Oyelakin, R. T. (2009). Yoruba traditional medicine and the challenge of integration. *The Journal of Pan African Studies, 3*(3). [online]. Available at: https://www.questia.com/library/journal/1P3-1888144371/yoruba-traditional-medicine-and-the-challenge-of-integration.   Accessed   10 Oct 2020.

Ozioma, E. J., & Chinwe, O. A. N. (2019). Herbal medicine in African traditional medicine. *IntechOpen*. [online]. Available at: https://www.intechopen.com/books/herbal-medicine/herbal-medicines-in-african-traditional-medicine. Accessed 10 Dec 2020.

Raphael, E. C. (2011). Traditional medicine in Nigeria: Status and the future. *Research Journal of Pharmacology, 5*(6), 90–94. [online]. Available at: http://docsdrive.com/pdfs/medwelljournals/rjpharm/2011/90-94.pdf. Accessed 10 Oct 2020.

Ruperti-Repilado, F. J., Haefliger, S., Rehm, S., Zweier, M., Rentsch, K. M., Blum, J., Jetter, A., Heim, M., Leuppi-Taegtmeyer, A., Terracciano, L., & Bernsmeier, C. (2019). Danger of herbal tea: A case of acute cholestatic hepatitis due to *Artemisia annua Tea*. *Frontiers in Medicine, 6*, 221. https://doi.org/10.3389/fmed.2019.00221. [online]. Available at: https://www.frontiersin.org/article/10.3389/fmed.2019.00221. Accessed 09 Dec 2020.

Sarker, M. R. (2014). Therapeutic efficacy and safety of traditional Ayurvedic medicines: Demands for extensive research and publication. *Journal of Homeopathic Ayurvedic Medicine, 3*, e113. [online]. Available at: https://www.omicsonline.org/open-access/therapeutic-efficacy-and-safety-of-traditional-ayurvedic-medicines-demands-for-extensive-research-and-publications-2167-1206.1000e113.php?aid=27099#:~:text=Traditionally%2C%20

Ayurvedic%20medicines%20are%20very,their%20therapeutic%20effectiveness%20and%20 safety. Accessed 29 Nov 2020.

Stafford, L. (2010). *WHO congress passes Beijing declaration on traditional medicine.* [online]. Available at: http://scielo.sld.cu/scielo.php?script=sci_arttext&pid=S1028-47962010000100008. Accessed 10 Oct 2020.

Surperformance. (2020). *Coronavirus: Herbal cure found in Nigeria?* [online]. Available at: https://www.marketscreener.com/quote/stock/TOYOTA-MOTOR-CORPORATION-6492484/news/Coronavirus-Herbal-cure-found-in-Nigeria-30468415/. Accessed 10 May 2021.

Synapeducation. (2016). *What is the difference between neurotoxin and hemotoxin?* [online]. Available at: https://synapeducation.wordpress.com/2016/12/09/what-is-difference-between-neurotoxin-and-hemotoxin/. Accessed 10 May 2021.

The Africa Report. (2020). *Coronavirus: Madagascar's 'Covid-organics' born from local tradition.* [online]. Available at: https://www.theafricareport.com/27203/coronavirus-madagascars-covid-organics-born-from-local-tradition/. Accessed 10 May 2021.

The University of Queensland. (2017). *Taking the bite out of chronic pain with a new spider venom treatment.* [online]. Available at: https://imb.uq.edu.au/article/2017/07/taking-bite-out-chronic-pain-new-spider-venom-treatment. Accessed 11 May 2021.

Thorne, S., Paterson, B., Russell, C., & Schultz, A. (2002). Complementary/alternative medicine in chronic illness as informed self-care decision making. *International Journal of Nursing Studies, 39,* 671–683.

Ugboko, H. U., Nwiny, O. C., Oranus, S. U., Fatoki, T. H., & Omonhinmi, C. A.. (2020). Antimicrobial importance of medicinal plants in Nigeria. *The Scientific World Journal.* Article ID 705932. [online]. Available at: https://doi.org/10.1155/2020/7059323. Accessed 10 Dec 2020.

WebMD. (2021a). *Neem.* [online]. Available at: https://www.webmd.com/vitamins/ai/ingredient-mono-577/neem. Accessed 23 Apr 2021.

WebMD. (2021b). *Lemongrass.* [online]. Available at: https://www.webmd.com/vitamins/ai/ingredientmono-719/lemongrass. Accessed 23 Apr 2021.

Weintritt, J. (2007). The use of plants in traditional medicine in Nigeria. *Africana Bulletin. Warszawa, 60,* 119–131.

WHO. (2000a). *General guidelines for methodologies on research and evaluation of traditional medicine.* World Health Organization.

WHO. (2000b). *Traditional and modern medicine: Harmonising the two approaches.* Western Pacific, Region Geneva.

WHO. (2002a). *Traditional medicine strategy 2002–2005.* World Health Organization.

WHO. (2002b). *Traditional medicine – Growing needs and potential.* World Health Organization.

WHO. (2008). *Beijing declaration.* [online]. Available at: https://www.who.int/medicines/areas/traditional/congress/beijing_declaration/en/. Accessed 18 Mar 2021.

WHO. (2020). *WHO supports scientifically-proven traditional medicine.* [online]. Available at: https://www.afro.who.int/news/who-supports-scientifically-proven-traditional-medicine. Accessed 10 Dec 2020.

Wilson, D. R., & Nall, R. (2018). What are the health benefits of lemongrass tea? *Medical News Today.* [online]. Available at: https://www.medicalnewstoday.com/articles/321969. Accessed 23 Apr 2021.

Chapter 9
The Plight of Persons Living with Disabilities: The Visible Invisibles in Nigeria

Learning Objectives

After reading this chapter, the learner should be able to:

1. Explain the different types and the causes of disability
2. Describe the classifications and consequences of the disease
3. Discuss the International Classification of Impairments, Disabilities, and Handicaps and analyze the practical applications of the framework
4. Analyze the burden of disability in Nigeria
5. Articulate the challenges associated with disability
6. Defend the laws promulgated to protect the rights of people living with disabilities in Nigeria
7. Deconstruct the global dimensions and scope of disability
8. Discuss the actions that can be taken by the government to improve the quality of life of people living with disabilities in Nigeria

Introduction

Disability is an all-encompassing term for impairments, activity limitations, and participation restrictions. A disability is any condition of the body or mind (impairment) that makes it more difficult for the person to do certain activities (activity limitation) and interact with the world around them. An impairment is a clinical problem with body functioning or structure. An activity limitation is a difficulty experienced in executing a task or action, while a participation restriction is an issue experienced by an individual in involvement in life situations. Disability is not just a health problem, but it is also a challenging problem that reflects the features of a person's body and the society in which he or she lives. Disability is a component of the human condition with many disabilities not visible, and two people with the same disability cope differently.

Overcoming the challenges faced by people living with disabilities (PLWDs) requires interventions to remove environmental and social barriers (WHO, 2017). Yet only 26–55% of people who are disabled in developing countries receive the medical rehabilitation services that they need, and only 17–37% have the assistive devices (wheelchairs, prostheses, and hearing aids) that they need for mobility (Reproductive Epidemiology, n.d.). Treatment of the impairments associated with physical disabilities is one of the core functions of the medical rehabilitation team, including physicians, physiotherapists, occupational therapists, speech therapists, clinical psychologists, and social workers.

In Nigeria, it is common to find people with mental illness and those with physical disabilities roam the streets in the major urban centers begging for alms or hoarding goods. At dawn, they nomadically find shelter under the bridge or in uncompleted private and public buildings. This situation is unconscionable and a blemish on the image of the country. After all, the Nigerian culture prides itself as "our brothers' keeper."

PLWDs have needs similar to non-disabled people. They need life essentials, such as housing, employment, and access to affordable health care. Unfortunately, PLWDs have a narrow margin of health due to poverty and social annihilation. PLWDs may also be vulnerable to conditions such as urinary tract infections and pressure sores. They experience barriers in accessing the health and rehabilitation services they badly need. They are often socioeconomically disadvantaged with no access to educational resources and health care. In Nigeria, PLWDs are often stigmatized and excluded from the larger society's social, economic, and political affairs. The healthcare system has no social program designed to improve the quality of life of PLWDs and no designated department within the Federal Ministry of Health (FMH) to address their medical rehabilitation needs. In describing the debacle, one analyst called individuals with disabilities "visible but invisible people." Grass-root education of policymakers and the public are needed to bring about the much-needed change on the issues impacting PLWDs.

This chapter discusses the types and causes of disabilities, including the dimensions, scope, and burden of disability in Nigeria. It also analyzes the challenges of living with disabilities and relevant protection laws, recommendations for improving the quality of life, including learning accommodation for students with disabilities.

Types of Disabilities

Many different disabilities are subsumable into four broad categories: intellectual, physical, sensory, and mental illness.

Fig. 9.1 An ultrasound evaluation at UNIMED Teaching Hospital, Ondo City. (Photograph used with permission from UNIMED PRO)

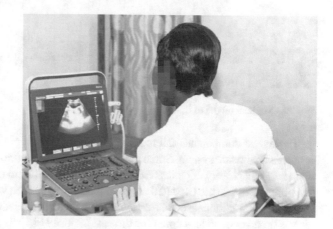

1. Intellectual disabilities include difficulty communicating, learning, and retaining information. They have Down syndrome, Fragile X syndrome, Prader-Willi syndrome, and developmental delays. A blood test and ultrasound scan (Fig. 9.1) performed at 12–13 weeks of pregnancy can predict the likelihood of Down syndrome (Pregnancy, Birth and Baby, n.d.).
2. Physical disability may affect temporarily or permanently a person's physical capacity and mobility. They include MS, cerebral palsy, spina bifida, brain or spinal cord injury, epilepsy, and muscular dystrophy. Ultrasound can diagnose congenital disabilities at 19–20 weeks of pregnancy, such as spina bifida, severe cardiac malformation, kidney problems, absence of part of a limb, and in some cases, cleft palate (Women's and Children's Health Network, 2018).
3. Sensory disabilities impact one or more senses: sight, hearing, touch, smell, taste, or spatial awareness. They include autism, blindness, and hearing loss.
4. Mental illness affects a person's thinking, emotional state, and behaviors. They include bipolar, depression, schizophrenia, and eating disorders.

The five primary disabilities in Nigeria are visual impairment, hearing impairment, physical impairment, intellectual impairment, and communication impairment (Umeh & Adeola, 2016).

Classification and Consequences of Disease

The difficulties in the classification of disease arise because of the inherent limitations in the medical model of illness (Fig. 9.2).

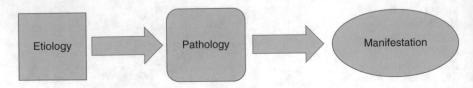

Fig. 9.2   Medical model of illness

The series' components fail to reflect the full range of problems that lead people to contact a healthcare system. Some consideration of the nature of the reasons for contact is therefore necessary. Sickness interferes with the ability to discharge those functions and obligations that are expected of us. In other words, when we are sick, we are unable to sustain the traditional social role and maintain cordial relationships with others. This view is broad enough to account for the vast majority of visits that are likely to be made in a healthcare system. It embraces life-threatening disease on the one hand and includes fewer medical experiences such as anxiety or the wish for advice and counseling. The only class of contact not incorporated in this approach is connections made in the absence of illness, such as attendances for prophylactic vaccination.

In 1980, the International Classification of Impairments, Disabilities, and Handicaps (ICIDH) was published by the World Health Organization (WHO) as a tool for classifying the consequences of disease and injuries and other disorders and their implications for individuals' lives. While ICIDH provides the underlying rationale for managing chronic conditions, critics expressed concern that it is limited in defining the impacts of the social and physical environment in the coping process. ICIDH has elicited philosophical debates, and its applications have included the design of population surveys at local, national, and international levels. It also includes other areas, such as assessing working capacities, demography, community needs assessment, town planning, and architecture.

ICIDH is used as a conceptual framework to explain the long-term consequences of diseases, injuries, or disorders and its use in personal health care, including early identification and prevention and mitigating environmental and societal barriers. ICIDH is also relevant to the study of healthcare systems in terms of evaluation and policy formulation. In several countries, the ICIDH framework has been used successfully by demographers, epidemiologists, health planners, policymakers, and statisticians in disability surveys at national, regional, and local levels.

A primary application of the ICIDH describes the circumstances of individuals with disabilities across a wide range of settings. It is applied often in the diagnosis, treatment, evaluation of treatment outcomes, and assessment of work abilities. The application of ICIDH in personal health care has come from nurses, occupational therapists, physicians/dentists, physiotherapists, and others working with a broad range of people, including older people, children and adolescents, and psychiatric patients. The ICIDH is also used to assess treatment outcomes in rehabilitation to facilitate communication between various health professionals and coordination of different types of care, type of staff required. It is used to identify the healthcare utilization patterns at the institutional level, the needs of PLWDs at the community level, place constraining situations in the social and physical environment, and formulate the policy decisions necessary for improvements in everyday life, including modifications of the material and social environment. In occupational health and employment, the ICIDH is used to make decisions on allowances, the orientation of individuals, and the terminology of handicaps for assessing working capacity.

Causes of Disabilities

Developments in medicine and technology in the nineteenth and twentieth centuries enhanced the understanding of disability. The medical model considers disability a biological dysfunction that creates impairments in body function and structure associated with different health conditions. Quite often, treatment is focused on a cure by professionals. In the 1970s, the medical model of disability was challenged and replaced by the social model of disability, which shifted attention from the medical aspects of disability and focused on the discrimination and social barriers faced by PLWDs.

Later, experts redefined disability as a societal problem rather than an individual problem, and solutions concentrated on removing obstacles and social change, not just a medical cure. The movement advocating for PLWDs, which began in the late 1960s in North America and Europe, was central to the change in understanding disability. The campaign has since garnered influence and is widespread throughout the world. Organizations for disabled people worldwide are focused on achieving full participation and providing equal opportunities for PLWDs by initiating the Convention on the Rights of Persons with Disabilities, which subsequently enhanced a shift toward a human rights model of disability (Gribble & Haffey, 2008).

Globally, low back pain (LBP) is the most common cause of functional disability and absence from work (Lidgren, 2003). LBP imposes a colossal socioeconomic impact on people, families, industry, and governments (Volinn, 1997), and a primary cause of morbidity worldwide (Hoy et al., 2012), including Nigeria with a prevalence rate ranging from 32.5% to 73.53% in the occupational setting (Bello & Bello, 2017). Treatment of LBP includes chiropractic, surgery, and physiotherapy (Fig. 9.3).

Many factors are responsible for disability, including malnutrition and disease, congenital malformation, environmental hazards, traffic, industrial accidents, civil conflict, and war. There is limited empirical data on the disability problem and the link between poverty and disability and malnutrition on health and intellectual development to design effective intervention programs. Medical rehabilitation has a critical role in fostering the independence of PLWDs and reducing human disability levels, but access to rehabilitation services for PLWDs is inadequate in Nigeria (Amusat, 2009).

Dimensions and Scope of Disability

Globally, about one in ten, or 650 million people, have a disability that substantially affects their daily lives. About 400 million people, 80% of the PLWDs in the world, live in developing countries. The population of PLWDs is growing because of their

Fig. 9.3 A physiotherapist treats a patient with chronic back pain with shortwave diathermy at a private practice clinic. (Photograph used with permission of Paschal Mogbo)

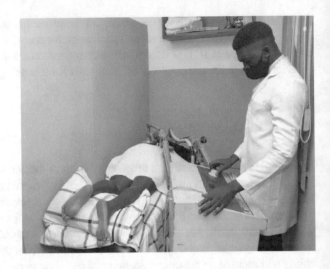

increased lifespan, and as people age, they are more likely to develop disabilities. In the United States, PLWDs are the largest minority group as their representation slowly surged from 11.9% in 2010 to 12.8% in 2016. Their distribution varies by state, employment, poverty, earnings, and health behaviors (Cornell University, 2019).

PLWDs are often socioeconomically disadvantaged with no access to educational resources and health care. COVID-19 has further increased the inequalities in health worldwide. The United States and the European Union chose first to prioritize vaccination for the elderly, healthcare workers, and people with severe co-morbidities (Okeenea, 2021). In Nigeria, PLWDs are often stigmatized and excluded from the larger society's social, economic, and political affairs. In describing the unsatisfactory situation, one analyst called individuals with disabilities in Nigeria "visible but invisible people" (Sango, 2013). Generally, PLWDs are perceived in Nigeria as possessed by devils or spirits and as punishment for past wrongdoing. Regrettably, these views are also embraced in many developing countries and traditional societies.

There are no reliable statistics on disability in Nigeria, therefore, a significant knowledge gap needs to be bridged (Amusat, 2009). A world report indicated that 25 million Nigerians have a disability, with 3.5 million having a significant social and physical functioning impairment (Sango, 2013; Eleweke et al., 2016). According to the United Nations, in 2004, the estimate of disability prevalence (%) in Nigeria is 0.5, and the years of health loss due to disability (YLDs per 100 persons) stand at 1312 (WHO, 2011; United Nations, 2017). In Africa, Ghana and Nigeria have two

Table 9.1 Global disability statistics

Serial #	Country	Raw number of people with disabilities (million)	As a % of population
Africa			
1	Nigeria	25	14.8
2	Ghana	5	18.2
3	Sierra Leone	0.5	7.8
		Asia	
4	Japan	5.8	4.8
5	China	83	6.4
6	India	70	5.6
		Europe	
7	Ukraine	2.7	6.0
		North America and South America	
8	Canada	3.8	13.7
9	Costa Rica	0. 5	10.5
10	United States	63.8	20.0
11	Brazil	16	8.0
		Oceania	
12	Australia	4.3	18.5

Source: WHO, 2011

of the highest rates of disability when PLWDs are expressed as a percentage of the population. In North America, the United States and Canada have the highest rates (Table 9.1).

The two major causes of physical disabilities are musculoskeletal in origin, including loss or deformity of limbs, osteogenesis imperfecta, muscular dystrophy, and neuromuscular due to cerebral palsy, spina bifida, poliomyelitis, stroke, head injury, and spinal cord injury (GPII DeveloperSpace, n.d.). In addition to complications from neonatal disorders, malaria, diarrheal, and lower respiratory infections (Statistica, 2021), road traffic accidents are among the primary causes of disability and death in Nigeria (Balogun & Abereoje, 1992). The primary causes of road traffic accidents are excessive speeding, dangerous overtaking and the impromptu pedestrian crossing on the highway, non-use of car seat belts, and disregard for highway codes.

The high burden of physical disability can be lowered considerably by preventing and treating the underlying causes with appropriate and timely medical care. The lack of state-of-the-art healthcare facilities has immensely contributed to the spread of infectious diseases which otherwise can be controlled or eradicated, as is the case in developed countries (Abang, 1988). The inadequate immunization coverage and poor maternal and neonatal care substantially contribute to the burden of disabilities in the country. Delayed and poor management of trauma at the health facilities and inadequate access to medical services are compounding factors as well (Fig. 9.4).

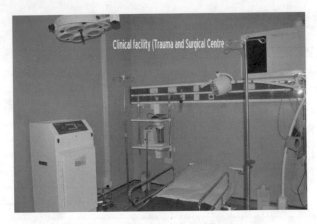

Fig. 9.4 The trauma and surgical unit at UNIMED, Ondo City. (Photograph used with permission from UNIMED PRO

The Burden of Disability in Nigeria

Globally, non-communicable diseases and injuries are increasing, while communicable, maternal, neonatal, and nutritional causes of disability-adjusted life years (DALYs) are declining. DALYs represent premature mortality (YLLs) and years of living with disability (YLDs) within a population. The YLDs are calculated by weighting the prevalence of different conditions based on severity. In Nigeria, malaria, HIV/AIDS, and lower respiratory infections had the highest ranking YLLs due to premature death in 2010. Out of the 25 leading causes of disease burden, as measured by DALYs, diarrheal showed the most substantial decrease, declining by 52% from 1990 to 2010 (Institute for Health Metrics and Evaluation, n.d.).

Overall, the three leading risk factors for the most disease burden are childhood underweight, household air pollution from solid fuels, and alcohol use. In 2010, the top risk factors for children under five and adults ages 15–49 years were childhood underweight and alcohol use, respectively. And in Nigeria, the five leading causes of YLDs are low back pain, iron deficiency anemia, major depressive disorder, malaria, and schistosomiasis. The three top causes of DALYs in 2010 were malaria, HIV/AIDS, and lower respiratory infections.

HIV/AIDS and road injury are the two conditions in the top ten causes of DALYs in 2010 and not 1990 (Institute for Health Metrics and Evaluation, n.d.).

Challenges of Living with Disabilities in Nigeria

Three-quarters of PLWDs in low- and middle-income countries are women (Nagarajan, 2016; Lime, 2018). African women and girls with disabilities experience various forms of abuse and physical violence that are often unreported.

Gender-based violence is more pernicious among women and girls with disabilities. They are less likely to seek help because they are usually not believed, and services are not accessible.

Developmental and physical disabilities are common (8.4%) in young women. Reproductive health issues such as puberty, sexuality, and menstruation are more complicated for teenagers with disabilities and their families due to concerns about menstrual hygiene, abuse risk, vulnerability, seizure pattern changes, and altered mood. Teenagers with disabilities have gynecologic healthcare needs similar to their peers without limitation, but they have unique needs related to their physical and cognitive challenges (Quint, 2014).

Because of their gender and disability, Nigeria women and girls find it more difficult to form relationships and get married. Society perceives them as unable to fulfill the traditional family roles of having sex, bearing children, cooking food, and caring for families. Although both women and men with disabilities face oppression, pervasive stereotypes, and misconceptions that worsen their lives, women have very different experiences. The unfortunate stereotypical words used in Africa to describe women with disabilities are asexual, hyper-sexual, and unattractive. Other demeaning terms used to describe African women with disability include infertile, useless, unemployable, stupid, abnormal, defective, not good wife material, suffering innocent, a burden to carry, and the will of God (Balogun, 2019; Nagarajan, 2016).

Given their social and economic vulnerability, women who are disabled are often sexually abused, sometimes resulting in pregnancies (WHO, n.d.; United Nations Population Fund n.d.). Hence, the right of PLWDs needs to be protected. The Republic of Malawi, a landlocked country located in Southeast Africa, took the lead in Africa to pass legislation in 2012 to protect the rights of persons with disabilities in response to the increasing cases of exploitation, violence, and abuse against women with disabilities (Disability Rights Funds, n.d.). Nigeria needs to enact a similar law.

The socioeconomically disadvantaged Nigerians have less access to education and health care, and they are more likely to become disabled by disease, illness, and injury. Similarly, because they do not have formal training, PLWDs are often unemployed, leading to abject poverty. PLWDs everywhere in the world want the same chance to participate fully and contribute to their communities. Unfortunately, they often lack the education needed for gainful employment and career mobility.

The stigma around mental health, learning difficulties, and depression are pervasive, and these issues are often not discussed. These concerning topics need to be addressed in Nigeria to achieve Article 16 of the United Nations Convention on the Rights of Persons with Disabilities, consistent with the Sustainable Development Goal 16 on peace and justice (DIWA, 2017). Compared to adults, children with disabilities are four times more likely to experience violence, and girls are more at risk than boys (Arroyo & Thampoe, 2018). For instance, people with albinism in Nigeria face discrimination, but they are tortured and murdered more horrifically. The 2012 National Policy on Albinism is intended to improve the status of persons with albinism by guaranteeing their equal access to education, health, social, political, and economic opportunities.

Due to poverty, 90% of children with disabilities do not attend school in Africa (Nagarajan, 2016). The problem is even direr as less than 5% of adults with disabilities have the requisite skill for reading or writing (Lime, 2018). Unfortunately, poverty is not going away anytime soon, and it is now occurring in unusual places. Extreme poverty is on the increase and gaining ground in nations previously taught to be making progress in eradicating the problem. Recently, Nigeria, one of the two wealthiest countries in Africa, has overtaken India as the world's largest concentration of extreme poverty. Today, over 87 million Nigerians live in extreme poverty, compared to 73 million Indians. In the next 12 years, Africans would make up nine out of every ten poor people in the world (Africa Educational Trust, n.d.).

A qualitative study by Eleweke and associates in 2016 revealed that PLWDs in Nigeria experience many challenges accessing essential services. The barriers to accessing critical services deprive PLWDs of the opportunity to enhance their potential for productive and contributing lives. Not much has been done over the years by the government to improve living standards for PLWDs. The biggest challenge facing the disabled is the superstitious belief system and the associated social stigma. Many Nigerians believe that a person's disability is due to a curse or reward for generational sins. Such views have made PLWDs to be treated with contempt and seen as inferior in society. There is a general perception that every disabled person is a beggar soliciting for alms. Consequently, they are not availed equal opportunities to demonstrate their potentials in nation-building.

A significant hurdle to the success of PLWDs in the country is the lack of vocational training facilities and programs, such as career guidance, professional training, and careful work placements designed to secure and retain employment. There is no concerted effort to provide vocational rehabilitation to ensure that disabled persons attain their full physical, social, mental, vocational, and economic capacity. Another challenge confronting PLWDs is employment discrimination. Employers often see them as less productive and prone to accidents. Without employment to earn a meaningful living, the future of the disabled remains uncertain. As a result of Western influences, the culture is shifting from communal and caring living to an individualistic lifestyle.

Global Effort to Enhance the Quality of Life of People Living with Disabilities

Following the 1978 Declaration of Alma-Ata, the WHO initiated community-based rehabilitation to foster the quality of life of PLWDs and families. While community-based rehabilitation was initially an approach designed to increase access to rehabilitation services in rural communities, it is now considered a multi-sectoral strategy to promote the social inclusion of PLWDs while combating the perpetual cycle of poverty. Implementation of community-based rehabilitation is through the combined efforts of individuals with disabilities, families, communities, relevant government and non-government health, education, vocational, social, and other services. The principal objectives of community-based rehabilitation are to:

1. Train family and community members on disability
2. Provide educational assistance and facilitate inclusive education through capacity-building with teaching staff and students and improving physical access
3. Refer PLWDs for specialized services that include surgery, physiotherapy, speech therapy, and occupational therapy
4. Provide assistive devices, such as walking sticks, crutches, wheelchairs, hearing aids, and glasses
5. Create employment opportunities by providing access to training, job coaching, and financial support for income-generation activities
6. Provide support for social events, including sports and recreation
7. Provide financial assistance for home modifications and education

In the physiotherapy literature, *community physiotherapy* or *community-based physiotherapy* is commonly used instead of community-based rehabilitation. Several outcome studies found community-based rehabilitation to be highly effective in enhancing the quality of life, providing access to care and promoting the rights and opportunities of PLWDs (Igwesi-Chidobe, 2012; Ibama et al., 2015; Mauro et al., 2014; Bongo et al., 2018; Rajan, 2017). The different components of community-based rehabilitation are presented in Fig. 9.5.

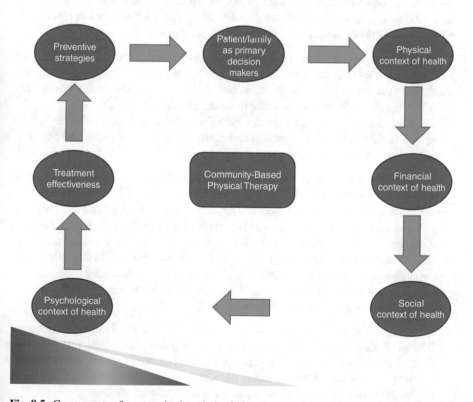

Fig. 9.5 Components of community-based physiotherapy

The Rights of People Living with Disabilities and Relevant Protection Laws

In 1993, General Sani Abacha's military government promulgated the Nigerian with Disability Decree, but characteristically, General Abdulsalami Abubakar's (1998–1999) government did not implement the decree. The Nigerian Senate in March 2009, under the civilian administration of Chief Olusegun Obasanjo, passed another Disability Bill, which prohibits discrimination and demands equal opportunities in all aspects of life for persons with disabilities. The Bill required all public buildings to be accessible for PLWDs and stipulated punitive actions for individuals and corporate organizations found to discriminate against PLWDs.

On September 24, 2010, President Goodluck Jonathan's administration ratified the United Nations Convention on the Rights of PLWDs and hosted the Africa Regional Community-Based Rehabilitation conference on October 7, 2010. These two seminal events placed disability on the national agenda, particularly among policymakers and civil societies, but the government did nothing in implementing any meaningful program for PLWDs. In 2015, another Disability Bill passed both chambers of the national assembly, but Jonathan failed to sign Bill. In the third attempt, the Discrimination Against PLWDs (Prohibition) Act was passed in 2017 and was signed to become law on January 23, 2019, by President Mohammadu Buhari. The legislation includes the following provisions:

1. Prohibition of discrimination based on disability and imposition of sanctions, including fines and sentences on individuals or organizations who fail to comply.
2. A five-year transitional period for public and private establishments to modify buildings and automobiles to make them accessible for PLWDs.
3. Establish a national commission for PLWDs to promote access to housing, education, and health care and receive complaints of rights violations and help victims seek legal redress, among other functions.

The Discrimination Against PLWDs (Prohibition) law is the first step in meeting Nigeria's obligations under the Convention on the Rights of PLWDs. The federal government would need to put adequate measures in place for its full implementation to ensure equal treatment and active participation of PLWDs across Nigeria. Despite the positive development, PLWDs continue to experience discrimination, are still excluded from the larger society, and encounter barriers in accessing various services. Also, other policy challenges remain. At the National level, several policies aligned to the Convention on the Rights of PLWDs have passed, but they are not yet fully implemented and include the following:

1. In 2016, the Federal Ministry of Education finalized the National Policy on Inclusive Education policy developed in collaboration with the National Education Research and Development Council, National Commission for Mass Literacy, Universal Basic Education Commission, and Disabled People's Organization after consultations at the state and national levels.

2. The 2014 National Health Act and the 2016 National Health Policy were established to provide the framework for developing, regulating, and managing national health systems and set standards for delivering services.
3. Establish National Commission for PLWDs to promote access to housing, education, and health care and receive complaints of rights violations and help victims seek legal redress, amongst other functions. The Commission is empowered to review rights violations and support victims to seek legal redress, among other duties. The new law and Commission is a welcome development since it took 9 years of relentless advocacy by disability rights groups and activists (Ewang, 2019).

Recommendations to Improve the Quality of Life of People Living with Disabilities

National Disability Strategy and Action Plan

Since the inception of the republic, the habilitation of PLWDs has not received the keen attention it deserves. Governments must develop a national disability strategy and action plan, establish clear lines of responsibility and mechanisms for coordination, monitoring, and reporting at all government levels, and regulate service provision by introducing service standards and monitoring and enforcing compliance with established standards. Additionally, the federal government must adopt national accessibility standards and ensure compliance in new buildings, transport, and information and communication standards and introduce measures to ensure that PLWDs are protected from poverty and benefit adequately from mainstream poverty alleviation programs. The federal government must include disability in national data collection systems, and wherever possible, provide disability-disaggregated data and implement communication campaigns to increase public knowledge and understanding of disability. The FMH must establish channels for people with disabilities and third parties to lodge complaints on human rights issues and laws that are not implemented or enforced (WHO (2011).

Address Stigma Against PLWDs

Stigma consists of three related problems – i*gnorance, prejudice, and discrimination* (Thornicroft et al., 2008). Therefore, specific anti-stigma action plans are needed to bring about positive change in society. Given the spectrum of the stigma associated with disability in Nigeria, the FMH must implement a multifaceted campaign to raise awareness about the problem. The strategy should include marketing and mass media campaigns on national television, print, radio, outdoor and online advertisement on social media. Furthermore, the government should initiate a grant program to fund grassroots intervention projects and local community events that will improve the quality of life of PLWDs. Civil society organizations, health professional students, teachers in training, and young people should challenge discrimination. The anti-stigma educational interventions should present factual information to correct misinformation or contradict negative attitudes and beliefs about disability. The campaigns should counter inaccurate stereotypes or myths about disability by replacing them with accurate information. The educational drives must be at local, state, and national levels (National Academy of Sciences, 2016).

Address the Barriers in Buildings

The government must make the owners of new multi-story buildings incorporate universal design systems (elevator, fire alarm, and sprinkler system) into their plans. It adds only around 1% to the total construction cost (WHO, 2011). This approach is cheaper than refitting such structures to an existing building, because of technical constraints making older buildings accessible requires flexibility, historic preservation issues, and variability in the owners' resources. Legal laws in the United States (Americans with Disabilities Act of 1990) and the Disability Discrimination Act of 1995 in the United Kingdom introduced terms such as "reasonable accommodations," "without undue hardship," and "technically infeasible." These terms provide acceptable ways to accommodate the constraints in existing building structures. The concept of "undue hardship," for example, allows flexibility for small businesses than for large corporations to make renovations that are costly because of the nature of existing building structures. Expanding the scope of buildings covered by-laws and standards after introducing the first stage of accessibility may be a better approach than making everything fully accessible at once.

In Nigeria, a strategic plan with priorities and a series of increasing goals can make the most of limited resources. First, policy and standards might treat construction in the rural areas differently from the urban centers and other types of buildings – focusing, perhaps, on access to the ground floor and then concrete on access to public toilets. After experimenting for a limited period with different approaches, more extensive standards might be introduced based on knowledge of what works based on the "progressive realization" strategy.

Address the Barriers of Roads

Given the unplanned nature of the roads in most cities and rural areas, transportation is an arduous task for PLWDs in Nigeria. The federal government must introduce accessible transportation as part of the comprehensive legislation on disability rights. The local government authorities must be made to identify strategies to improve the accessibility of public transport by applying universal design principles in the design and operation of public transport by removing physical barriers when renovating roads, bus stops, and stations.

The local governments must provide separate lanes and paths for PLWDs using tricycles, wheelchairs, bicycles and establish continuity of accessibility throughout the travel chain by improving pavements and roads and pedestrian access, installing ramps. The government can subsidize transport fares for the poor and PLWDs who may not afford them. Through public awareness campaigns using print, electronic and social media, the front-line staff and operators of public and private transport systems can teach passengers about priority seating for PLWDs.

National Policy on Educating Children with Disability

The federal government must develop a clear national policy to provide children with disabilities educational support guided by the necessary legal framework and adequate resources. After surveying the stakeholders to identify the level and nature of need, the educational institutions must provide proper support and accommodations. Some students may require only modifications to the physical environment to gain access, while others need more intensive instructional help. Educate teachers during training and through in-service workshops on their responsibilities toward children with special needs and build and improve their teaching of children with disabilities. Particular emphasis should be placed on teachers in rural areas, with fewer services for children with disabilities. Additional support services will be needed for some children with disabilities. Such support will require the expertise of special education teachers, counselors, and medical rehabilitation services. Teachers and schools should move away from a one-size-fits-all model toward flexible approaches that promote individualized education plans to ensure the students' individual needs are met.

Independent Living, Healthcare Access, and Vocational Training

On moral grounds, the governments must assist PLWDs in attaining full independence and providing them with employment to enable them to be productive members of society. The goal is to provide meaningful and happy life experiences that offer a sense of purpose and accomplishment. The level of impairment of the individual will determine the success of achieving these lofty objectives. Some PLWDs may not be able to live independently because of the severity of their disability.

Over 60 million Nigerians have mental disorders, and 80% of the cases are undiagnosed. The mental illness ranges from mood swings to extreme mental disorder cases – 20% of Nigerians have a severe mental disorder (Ugwuanyi, 2016). Without further delay, the government at federal, state, and local government levels must take responsibility for the care and well-being of PLWDs. Nigerians with mental disabilities must be institutionalized in a setting to receive psychiatric and counseling treatments. The plan must include vocational training to ensure PLWDs work and live independently in their communities (WHO, 2011; Joseph Rehabilitation Center, 2020).

Health System Reforms

The FMH must reform the health system to enable PLWDs to access center-based rehabilitation health care. The services include physiotherapy, occupational therapy, speech-language therapy, audiology, wheelchairs, prosthetics, and orthotics. Those with visual impairment must have access to computer-assisted aids to facilitate communication and learning. The government must establish vocational centers around the country where PLWDs can receive on-the-job training in the workplace. Furthermore, the government must provide service grants to private and non-governmental organizations to offer community living residential programs for adults with physical, developmental, and vision disabilities.

Training of Healthcare Professionals

Given the magnitude and scope of the people with mental illness in the country, it is imperative to expand the infrastructures needed to train professionals in the medical rehabilitation disciplines, including psychiatrists and clinical psychologists. The field of clinical psychology is still in its infancy in Nigeria and needs strengthening. The universities offering these programs must take the leadership role in making this happen. Prosthetists, orthotists (health providers trained in the fabrication of artificial limbs for people with lower and upper limb amputation), and biomedical engineers/technologists are in short supply. Their services can dramatically improve the quality of life of PLWDs.

The medical rehabilitation discipline's ongoing challenges are multifaceted, ranging from lack of physical and human resources to limited funding needed to offer world-class educational programs. The quality of education at the university level impacts the services provided for PLWDs. The federal government must adequately fund the various medical rehabilitation programs to attain global accreditation standards. For example, the quest for excellence in physiotherapy education was shaped several years ago by the worldwide standard that elevated the entry-level education from a baccalaureate to a clinical doctor of physiotherapy (DPT). The global paradigm shift led the Nigeria Society of Physiotherapy (NSP) and the Medical Rehabilitation Therapists (Registration) Board of Nigeria (MRTB) to submit a proposal to the National Universities Commission to transition to the DPT degree program. The proposal was approved in 2015, but as of December 2020, only one of the 13 universities in the country (Kaduna State University) offering physiotherapy program has initiated the DPT degree curriculum (Balogun, 2020).

Overcoming Barriers and Provision of Accommodation for Adult Students with Learning Disabilities

In Nigeria, the number of students with disabilities is unknown. For students with disabilities, finding a suitable institution can be challenging as no effort is made by the university authorities to provide accessibility and learning accommodation services. Some universities are making an effort toward offering accommodation to students with disabilities, particularly at the University of Jos, with the most significant number of blind students (Abang, 1988). However, addressing this issue is still not a priority in most higher institutions of learning.

The government must broaden the existing law for PLWDs to the education sector by mandating elementary and secondary schools and higher learning institutions to provide the necessary learning accommodation to be successful and become valuable members of society. The law must protect the students from overcoming barriers that limit daily living activities, walking, seeing, hearing, speaking, working, and performing manual tasks (United States Department of Justice and Civil Rights, 2019). The universal design principles must guide the policies of access to education. Many physical barriers are relatively straightforward to overcome by providing a ramp and changing the physical layout of classrooms.

All higher education institutions must have a Disability Unit within the Office of Student Services to coordinate and provide the appropriate services. The student must be made responsible for obtaining the required learning accommodation by providing necessary medical documentation of disability, including medical evidence of impairment of life activities, including learning to the Disability Unit. The educational counselor will review the validity of the documentation submitted and approve it if it has merit. Subsequently, the student seeking learning accommodation must meet with the teacher/instructor to provide the Disability Unit's approval letter that specifies the learning accommodation needed. If an instructor is hesitant to provide learning accommodation, the student must immediately contact the Disability Unit. The School Principal or Dean of Students will meet with the teacher/instructor to explain why the learning accommodation is necessary. The student must alert the teacher/instructor and the Disability Unit of any unanticipated learning problems as soon as they occur. Delayed action by the student will not provide the instructor with the adequate time needed for appropriate remediation efforts to occur.

Conclusion

The Nigerian government must address the recommendations discussed in this chapter to improve the quality of life of PLWDs and, ultimately, the healthcare system's quality of care. The procurement of state-of-the-art surgical and rehabilitative instruments and maintenance of a clean hospital environment will significantly reduce the number of physical disabilities and fatalities. Additionally, the Federal Road Safety Commission's medical patrol unit must be reformed to minimize physical disabilities arising from road traffic accidents. The federal government would need to fast-track the full implementation of the discrimination against persons with disabilities (prohibition) law to ensure their active integration into the larger society. All levels of government should take responsibility for the care and well-being of disabled persons by providing accommodation and accessible healthcare services. Furthermore, the government should fund private organizations to offer community living residential programs for adults with disabilities.

There is no one-size-fits-all solution to providing access and learning accommodation to students with disabilities. At a minimum, the buildings on campus must be outfitted for select accessibility and adaptive technology. Provision of learning accommodation is not about lowering academic standards or substantially changing the required course or graduation requirements. Examples of learning accommodation needed at tertiary institutions include priority registration, reduced course loads, substituting one system for another, providing note-takers or audio or video recordings of classes, providing auxiliary aids and services, personal attention, assistance with learning strategy, and study skill and extra testing time or offering an alternate testing location.

Interdisciplinary Team Clinical Case Study
The primary objective of this case study is to document the evaluation and management of a 30-year-old female patient with L4/5 spinal lesion resulting in paraplegia. The students from each of the professional disciplines in your College/Faculty must collaborate on this project to follow up with the patient for at least four visits to report treatment outcomes. This assignment must address the following issues:

1. *Social and Medical History* – Ask about the cause of the diagnosis, hospital admissions, major past illnesses, previous and current treatments
2. *Patient Evaluation* – Use the SOAP – Subjective, Objective, Assessment, Plan – format. Describe the various tests performed, including home and community need assessment to improve the patient's quality of life
3. *Interdisciplinary Team Treatment Plan* – Present short- and long-term treatment goals with objective and measurable criteria. Plan must include home and community modifications needed
4. *Interdisciplinary Team Treatment* – Observe the patient's response to treatment during the initial assessment and subsequent follow-up visit to the clinic. Describe patient response to treatment by appointment date. Record subjective and objective data (e.g., BP, HR, vital capacity, ROM, muscle power, pain rating, lab results, etc.) monitored during the visits.
5. *Treatment Outcome* – Present how the patient has responded to treatment. A graphical representation of any data collected will enhance the clarity of the presentation
6. *Conclusions* – Summarize how this clinical experience enhanced your knowledge about the other healthcare professions in the team

References

Abang, T. B. (1988). Disablement, disability and the Nigerian society. *Disability, Handicap & Society, 1*, 71–77. [online]. Available at: https://www.tandfonline.com/doi/citedby/10.108 0/02674648866780061?scroll=top&needAccess=true. Accessed 29 Mar 2021.

Africa Educational Trust. (n.d.). *Our work with people living with disabilities.* [online]. Available at: https://africaeducationaltrust.org/disability. Accessed 10 Oct 2020.

Amusat, N. (2009). Disability care in Nigeria: The need for professional advocacy. *AJPAR, 1*(1), 30–36.

Arroyo, C., & Thampoe, E. (2018). *Africa: Children and women with disabilities, more likely to face discrimination.* [online]. Available at: https://allafrica.com/stories/201808160405.html. Accessed 10 Oct 2020.

Balogun, J. A. (2019). Communicating research outcomes sensitively through consistent use of people-first language. *African Journal of Reproductive Health, 23*(2), 9. https://www. researchgate.net/publication/336498033_Communicating_Research_Outcomes_Sensitively_ Through_Consistent_Use_of_People-First_Language. Accessed 18 Mar 2021.

Balogun, J. A. (2020). Chapter 7: Emerging paradigms in healthcare education in Nigeria. In *Healthcare education in Nigeria: Evolutions and emerging paradigms.* Routledge Publication. [online]. Available at: https://www.routledge.com/9780367482091. Accessed 23 Dec 2020.

Balogun, J. A., & Abereoje, O. K. A. (1992). Pattern of road traffic accident cases in a Nigerian university teaching hospital between 1987 and 1990. *Journal of Tropical Medicine and Hygiene, 95*(1), 23–9. [online]. Available at: https://www.researchgate.net/publication/21414605_ Pattern_of_road_traffic_accident_cases_in_a_Nigerian_University_teaching_hospital_ between_1987_and_1990. Accessed 29 Mar 2021.

Bello, B., & Bello, A. H. (2017). A systematic review on the prevalence of low back pain in Nigeria. *Middle East Journal of Rehabilitation Health Studies, 4*(2), e45262. [online]. Available at: https://sites.kowsarpub.com/mejrh/articles/13146.html. Accessed 12 Apr 2021.

Bongo, P. P., Dzirun, G., & Muzenda-Mudavanhu, C. (2018). The effectiveness of community-based rehabilitation as a strategy for improving quality of life and disaster resilience for children with disability in rural Zimbabwe. *Jamba, 10*(1), 442. [online]. Available at: https://pubmed.ncbi.nlm.nih.gov/29955257/. Accessed 10 Oct 2020.

Cornell University. (2019). *2017 Disability status report.* [online]. Available at: https://www. disabilitystatistics.org/StatusReports/2017-PDF/2017-StatusReport_US.pdf. Accessed 10 Oct 2020.

Disability Rights Funds. (n.d.). *Disabled women in Africa.* [online]. Available at: http://disability-rightsfund.org/grantees/disabled-women-in-africa/. Accessed 10 Oct 2020.

DIWA. (2017). *Disabled women in Africa curbs violence against women and girls with disabilities.* [online]. Available at: http://www.diwa.ws/?p=101. Accessed 10 Oct 2020.

Eleweke, C., Jonah, E., & Ebenso, J. (2016). Barriers to accessing services by people with disabilities in Nigeria: Insights from a qualitative study. *Journal of Educational and Social Research, 6*(2), 113–124. [online]. Available at: http://pdxscholar.library.pdx.edu/cgi/viewcontent. cgi?article=1057&context=wll_fac. Accessed 10 Oct 2020.

Ewang, (2019) *Nigeria passes disability rights law: Offers hope of inclusion, improved access.* [online]. Available at: Human Rights Watch. https://www.hrw.org/news/2019/01/25/nigeria-passes-disability-rights-law. Accessed: 12 April, 2021.

GPII DeveloperSpace. (n.d.). *What is physical disability?* [online]. Available at: https://ds.gpii. net/content/what-physical-disability#:~:text=The%20two%20major%20categories%20 of,injury%20and%20spinal%20cord%20injury. Accessed 29 Mar 2021.

Gribble, J., & Haffey, J. (2008). *PRB – Reproductive health in sub-Saharan Africa.* [online]. Available at: https://www.prb.org/reproductivehealthafrica/. Accessed 10 Oct 2020.

Hoy, D., Bain, C., Williams, G., March, L., Brooks, P., Blyth, F., et al. (2012). A systematic review of the global prevalence of low back pain. *Arthritis and Rheumatism, 64*(6), 208–237. [online]. Available at: https://pubmed.ncbi.nlm.nih.gov/22231424/. Accessed 12 Apr 2021.

Ibama, A. S., Atibinye, D., & Obele, R. (2015). Community health practice in Nigeria – Prospects and challenges. *International Journal of Current Research, 01*(7), 11989–11992.

Igwesi-Chidobe, C. (2012). Obstacles to obtaining optimal physiotherapy services in a rural community in Southeastern Nigeria. *Rehabilitation Research and Practice*, Article ID 909675, 8. [online]. Available at: https://www.hindawi.com/journals/rerp/2012/909675/. Accessed 10 Oct 2020.

Institute for Health Metrics and Evaluation. (n.d.). *GBD profile: Nigeria. 2301 Fifth Ave., Suite 600 Seattle, WA 98121 USA*. [online]. Available at: http://www.healthdata.org/sites/default/files/files/country_profiles/GBD/ihme_gbd_country_report_nigeria.pdf. Accessed 10 Oct 2020.

Joseph Rehabilitation Center. (2020). *Community housing services for persons with disabilities*. [online]. Available at: http://www.josephrehabilitationcenter.com/. Accessed 10 Oct 2020.

Lidgren, L. (2003). The bone and joint decade 2000–2010. *Bulletin of the World Health Organization, 81*(9), 629. [online]. Available at: https://pubmed.ncbi.nlm.nih.gov/14710501/. Accessed 12 Apr 2021.

Lime, A. (2018). *Disability in Africa: I'm no longer ashamed of my disabled daughter*. [online]. Available at: https://www.bbc.co.uk/news/amp/world-africa-45220690. Accessed 10 Oct 2020.

Mauro, V., Biggeri, M., Deepak, S., & Trani, J. F. (2014). The effectiveness of community-based rehabilitation programmes: An impact evaluation of a quasi-randomized trial. *Journal of Epidemiology and Community Health, 68*(11), 1102–1108.

Nagarajan, C. (2016). *The abilities of women with disabilities*. [online]. Available at: https://thisisafrica.me/abilities-women-disabilities/. Accessed 10 Oct 2020.

National Academy of Sciences. (2016). *Ending discrimination against people with mental and substance use disorders: The evidence for stigma change*. [online]. Available at: https://www.ncbi.nlm.nih.gov/books/NBK384914/. Accessed 31 May 2021.

Okeenea. (2021). *Disabled people in the world in 2021: Facts and figures*. [online]. Available at: https://www.inclusivecitymaker.com/disabled-people-in-the-world-in-2021-facts-and-figures/. Accessed 31 May 2021.

Pregnancy, Birth and Baby, (n.d.). *Screening for down syndrome*. [online]. Available at: https://www.pregnancybirthbaby.org.au/screening-for-down-syndrome. Accessed 29 Mar 20201.

Quint, E. H. (2014). Menstrual and reproductive issues in adolescents with physical and developmental disabilities. *Obstetrics and Gynecology, 124*(2), 367–375.

Rajan, P. (2017). Community physiotherapy or community-based physiotherapy. *Health Promotion Perspective, 7*(2), 50–51. [online]. Available at: https://www.ncbi.nlm.nih.gov/pmc/articles/PMC5350549/. Accessed 10 Oct 2020.

Reproductive Epidemiology. (n.d.). [onlinc]. Available at: https://www.omicsonline.org/scholarly/reproductive-epidemiology-journals-articles-ppts-list.php; https://www.cdc.gov/reproductive-health/global/rhepi.htm. Accessed 10 Oct 2020.

Sango, P. (2013). *Visible but invisible: People living with disability in Nigeria*. [online]. Available at: https://books2africa.org/visible-but-invisible-people-living-with-disability-in-nigeria/. Accessed 10 Oct 2020.

Statistica. (2021). *Main causes of death in Nigeria 2019*. [online]. Available at: https://www.statista.com/statistics/1122916/main-causes-of-death-and-disability-in-nigeria/. Accessed 29 Mar 2021.

Thornicroft, G., Brohan, E., Kassam, A., et al. (2008). Reducing stigma and discrimination: Candidate interventions. *International Journal of Mental Health Systems, 2*, 3. [online]. Available at: https://doi.org/10.1186/1752-4458-2-3. Accessed: 31 May 2021.

Ugwuanyi, S. (2016, September 14). Over 60m Nigerians have mental disorder. *Daily Post*. [online]. Available at: https://dailypost.ng/2016/09/14/60m-nigerians-mental-disorder-health-commissioner/. Accessed 10 Oct 2020.

Umeh, N. C., & Adeola, R. (2016). African disability rights yearbook. *African Human Rights Law Journal*. ISSN: 2413–7138.

United Nations. (2017). Human functioning and disability. *United Nations Statistics Division – Demographic and Social Statistics*. [online]. Available at: https://unstats.un.org/unsd/demographic/sconcerns/disability/disform.asp?studyid=172. Accessed 31 May 2021.

United Nations Population Fund. (n.d.). *Sexual and reproductive health*. [online]. Available at: https://www.unfpa.org/sexual-reproductive-health. Accessed 10 Oct 2020.

US Department of Justice and Civil Rights. (2019). *Americans with disabilities act*. [online]. Available at: https://www.ada.gov/. Accessed 10 Oct 2020.

Volinn, E. (1997). The epidemiology of low back pain in the rest of the world. A review of surveys in low- and middle-income countries. *Spine, 22*(15), 1747–1754. [online]. Available at: https://pubmed.ncbi.nlm.nih.gov/9259786/. Accessed 12 Apr 2021.

WHO. (2011). *World report on disability 2011*. [online]. Available at: https://www.who.int/teams/noncommunicable-diseases/sensory-functions-disability-and-rehabilitation/world-report-on-disability; https://www.who.int/countries/nga/. Accessed 31 May 2021.

WHO. (2017). *World Bank and WHO: Half the world lacks access to essential health services, 100 million still pushed into extreme poverty because of health expenses*. [online]. Available at: https://www.who.int/news-room/detail/13-12-2017-world-bank-and-who-half-the-world-lacks-access-to-essential-health-services-100-million-still-pushed-into-extreme-poverty-because-of-health-expenses. Accessed 10 Oct 2020.

WHO. (n.d.). *Chapter six: Sexual violence*. [online]. Available at: https://www.who.int/violence_injury_prevention/violence/global_campaign/en/chap6.pdf. Accessed 10 Oct 2020.

Women's and Children's Health Network. (2018). *Ultrasound scan during pregnancy*. [online]. Available at: https://www.cyh.com/HealthTopics/HealthTopicDetails.aspx?p=438&np=459&id=2761#:~:text=Ultrasound%20can%20detect%20some%20types,some%20cases%20of%20cleft%20palate. Accessed 29 Mar 2021.

Chapter 10
A Comparative Analysis of the Health System of Nigeria and Six Selected Nations Around the World

Learning Objectives

After reading this chapter, the learner should be able to:

1. Enunciate the criteria and frameworks for measuring the performance of health systems.
2. Analyze the global ranking of the performance of health systems.
3. Discuss the global physician supply.
4. Contrast the significant strengths and challenges within the health systems of the United States, United Kingdom, Singapore, South Korea, Cuba, and Nigeria.
5. Compare the primary health outcome statistics for Nigeria with the United States, United Kingdom, Singapore, South Korea, and Cuba.

Introduction

Nigeria's health system is among the most inefficient in the world. In a 2000 World Health Organization's (WHO) study, Nigeria's overall health system performance ranked 187 out of 191 member states. The worst countries were the Democratic Republic of the Congo, Central African Republic, Myanmar, and Sierra Leone. The WHO's report described Nigeria's health system as "dysfunctional, ineffective, under-capitalized, costly, and inaccessible" (WHO, 2000). In another more recent study published in the *Lancet*, Nigeria ranked 140 of the 195 countries surveyed on healthcare access and quality index based on the number of deaths from 32 common preventable diseases, timeliness, and adequate health care (Fullman et al., 2018). Similarly, Nigeria has one of the worst infant and maternal mortality rates, the world's third-lowest life expectancy rate of 55 years, and the second-largest number of children with delayed growth (Onyeji, 2020; WHO, 2006, 2015, 2016).

One in every ten medications sold in Africa is adulterated. The problem is particularly rife in Nigeria, where primary hospitals and pharmacy outlets purchase their medicines at unsafe open-air drug markets (AXA.com, 2019). Because of the widespread dissatisfaction with private insurance plans and the healthcare system, 71% of Nigerians consequently embrace self-treatment options before consulting a physician. When they seek treatment, many deplete their savings and depend on money sent by family members in the diaspora or borrow money from a local merchant to pay for the services (AXA.com, 2019).

Over many years, Nigeria's health system has deteriorated further due to corruption, underfunding, waste, insufficient healthcare workers (HCWs), and ineffective leadership—factors described in more detail in Chapter 5 of this publication. The pertinent question is what lessons can Nigeria learn from other countries with high-performing health systems? This chapter sets out to identify the stellar health systems around the world that Nigeria can emulate to revitalize and invigorate its semi-comatose health system.

Operational Definitions

To fully understand the issues discussed in this chapter, it is appropriate to define the following basic terms:

1. A *system* is an arrangement of the different parts of an institution or organization and their interconnections that come together for a purpose.
2. *Health system* (also called the healthcare system) is a complex network of organizations or institutions delivering health services to citizens at the national levels. It is an organized structure within which workers, institutions, and organizations collaborate to garner and allocate resources to prevent and treat injuries and diseases. The different parts of a health system include the patients, families, communities, federal ministry of health (FMH), health professionals, and financing bodies (GAVI CSO Project, 2013). For any health structure to work effectively, certain fundamental conditions ranging from a well-managed civil service to an extensive communications system must be available.
3. *Health outcomes* are important events that occur as a result of an intervention. They can be measured clinically using physical examination measures, laboratory tests, imaging, and epidemiological indicators such as the number of hospitalizations prevented, the number of years people stay alive, and quality of life. They can also be measured from patients' self-report following an intervention (satisfaction, a decrease of pain or symptoms) or observed by the clinicians (such as gait or movement fluctuations). The purpose of measuring and comparing health outcomes is to achieve the following four goals: increase the consumers' experience of care provided, improve the health of population, decrease the

per capita cost of health care, and prevent clinician and staff burnout (ScienceDirect, 2020). Motivated by the stated four goals, organizations measure health outcomes to identify areas in which interventions could improve health care. Also, organizations monitor health outcomes to help reveal variations of health care, to provide evidence about interventions that work best for specific patients under certain circumstances, and to compare the effectiveness of various treatment procedures (Tinker, 2018).

Health Systems Performance Indicators

With burgeoning and aging populations, spiraling costs, and the recognition by most countries that constant vigilance and periodic healthcare reforms are necessary, interest in measuring the global performance of the health system is increasing. There are several criteria and frameworks for measuring the overall performance of health systems. They include mortality rate, the safety of care, patient experience, hospitalization readmissions, the effectiveness of care, timeliness of care, health status, responsiveness, efficient use of medical imaging, financial contribution, quality, efficiency, access, equity, patients satisfaction, quality of life, happiness index and healthy lives, governance and leadership, service delivery, adequate workforce, systems financing, access to essential medicines and vaccines, and information system among other measures. Chapter 2 of this book discusses these indicators of health system performance in greater detail.

Life expectancy is another critical criterion often used to measure the performance of a health system. As of 2019, Hong Kong (85.29), Japan (85.03), and Macao (84.68) are the top three countries with the highest life expectancy. They are followed by Switzerland (84.25), Singapore (84.07), Italy (84.01), Spain (83.99), and Australia (83.94). In all countries, females lived longer than men (Worldometer, n.d.).

In 2000, the WHO, for the first time, evaluated the performance of the health systems of its 191 member states using five indicators to track the overall level and equality of health and the responsiveness and financing of healthcare services. The three performance indicators monitored in the study were health status, responsiveness, and financial contribution. Health was operationally defined as the disability-adjusted life expectancy and was weighted 50% of the overall performance score. Responsiveness was defined as the speed of service, protection of privacy, and quality of amenities and weighted 25%, and financial contribution was weighted 25% (WHO, 2000). The overall health system performance analysis showed France, Italy, and San Marino on top, followed by Andorra, Malta, Singapore, Spain, Omar, and United Kingdom. However, the methodology used in the evaluation has been widely criticized that the WHO declined to repeat the study.

Aside from the WHO's 2000 study, other investigations on many countries' health systems have also emerged. In 2010, another study conducted by the Commonwealth Fund evaluated the health systems of seven high-income countries—Canada, the United Kingdom, Australia, Germany, the Netherlands, New Zealand, and the United States. Overall, the study ranked the United States the lowest on quality, efficiency, access, equity, and healthy lives. The most responsive healthcare system in ranking order is the United States, Switzerland, Luxembourg, Denmark, Germany, Japan, Canada, Norway, the Netherlands, and Sweden (Magarya, 2017).

Another health systems performance study undertaken by the WHO in 2017 assessed the overall quality of life in 80 different countries worldwide. The top five countries in the survey were Switzerland, Canada, United Kingdom, Germany, and Japan, and the five lowest-ranked nations were Lebanon (#76), Nigeria (#77), Algeria, Iran, and Serbia (#80). South Africa and Ghana ranked 38 and 68, respectively (WHO, 2017).

The first world happiness landmark study was published in 2012 by the United Nations Sustainable Development Solutions Network and ranked 156 countries by how happy their citizens perceived themselves (Helliwell et al., 2019). The survey measured happiness by posing the question: "Taken all together, how would you say things are these days; would you say that you are very happy, pretty happy, or not too happy?" The response to the question was coded on a Likert scale of 1, 2, or 3. The study is replicated annually, but besides happiness, it also focused on other themes. The 2012 report inferred that the quality of people's lives could be coherently, reliably, and validly assessed by various subjective well-being measures, collectively referred to then in follow-up reports as "happiness."

The 2016–2018 happiness data ranked Australia, United Kingdom, and the United States 11th, 15th, and 19th, respectively. Nigeria was rated 85th, and at the bottom were Afghanistan (154th), Central African Republic (155th), and South Sudan (156th). Togo was the biggest gainer in happiness level, moving up 17 places in the overall rankings from 2008 to 2015. The biggest loser was Venezuela, with a decrease in the happiness level by 2.2 points. Both domestic and foreign migrants' findings were generally positive. The rating of immigrant happiness is almost the same as the nonimmigrant population in the countries surveyed. The ten happiest nations in the overall rankings also constitute ten of the top eleven spots in immigrant happiness. Among American adolescents, happiness and life satisfaction increased between 1991 and 2011, suddenly declined after the first 2012 study. By 2016–2017, both adults and adolescents reported substantially less happiness than they had in 2012. Besides, low psychological well-being, including depression, suicide ideation, and self-harm, increased sharply among adolescents since 2010, particularly among girls and young women. Depression and self-harm also increased over this period among children and adolescents in the United Kingdom. Thus, at the same age, those born after 1995 (iGen) had markedly lower psychological well-being than those born in 1980–1994 (Millennials). The decline in happiness and mental health is paradoxical because violent crime and unemployment rates are low, and the income per capita has steadily grown over the last few decades. Several explanations have been offered to explain the decline in happiness, including decreases in social capital and social support, increases in obesity and substance abuse, and fundamental shifts in how children and adolescents spend their leisure time (Helliwell et al., 2019).

The 2019 world happiness report contained, in addition to its usual global ranking of the levels and changes in happiness in 156 countries, ranked 117 countries based on the happiness of the immigrants within and between countries. The survey focused on happiness and community: how satisfaction has evolved over the past decade and how information technology, governance, and social norms influence communities, conflicts, and government policies that have driven those changes. As of March 2019, Finland was ranked twice in a row, the happiest nation with the happiest immigrants and the happiest population overall. The next top-ranked countries are Denmark, Norway, Iceland, and the Netherlands. All the top countries rated tend to score high in income, healthy life expectancy, social support, freedom, trust, and generosity; the six critical variables are found to support well-being.

Workforce Supply

An adequate supply of HCWs is essential for any health system to provide comprehensive and quality care that will promote health, prevent and treat disease, reduce unnecessary disability and premature death, and achieve health equity for all citizens. In 2006, the WHO estimated a shortage of 4.3 million physicians/dentists, nurses, and other professionals worldwide. The deficit is more acute in developing countries due to the limited enrollment capacity of educational institutions. Because of international migration, physicians/dentists earn much more money and enjoy better working conditions in high-income countries. Paradoxically, many developed nations also report physician shortages, particularly in rural and other underserved areas. Needs exist and are growing in the United States, Canada, United Kingdom, Australia, New Zealand, and Germany (WHO, 2006).

Physician supply is the number of active physicians in the labor market in a healthcare system—it is determined by the number of students who graduated from medical schools and continue to practice in their country of origin. The number of physicians needed in a country depends on several different factors, such as the demographics, the number of other complimentary HCWs, the epidemiology of the local population, and the healthcare system's policies and goals. Suppose more physicians are trained more than needed when supply exceeds demand or too few physicians are produced and not retained. In that case, the poor and economically disadvantaged within the population may have difficulty accessing services.

Cuba tops the list of physician density in different countries worldwide with 591 physicians for every 100,000 people compared to Burkina Fossa with only five physicians to 100,000 people. Other top countries are Saint Lucia (517), Belarus (455), Belgium (449), Estonia (448), and Greece (438). At the bottom of the list are Tanzania, Malawi, and Niger, with only two physicians per 100,000 people, followed by Burundi, Ethiopia, Sierra Leone, and Mozambique, with three physicians per 100,000 people (Infoplease, 2007). Other highly ranked countries on the physician supply list include successor nations to the communist bloc, which generally had a sound (and cheap) health system, and the developed (capitalist) nations in Europe. Surprisingly, the United States, United Kingdom, the Netherlands, and Australia are not among the countries with the highest number of physicians per 100,000 globally. Switzerland is quite far down and behind other European countries such as Spain, Belgium, France, and Germany (Infoplease, 2007).

After a careful analysis of the literature mentioned earlier, 15 "shining" health systems were identified for further evaluation—United States, United Kingdom, Switzerland, Canada, Germany, Australia, South Korea, Cuba, the Netherlands, New Zealand, France, Japan, Finland, Singapore Taiwan (Fig. 10.1). In total, 6 of the 15 "shining" health systems (United States, United Kingdom, Singapore, South Korea, Taiwan, and Cuba) were selected for in-depth comparative analysis on several health outcome indicators.

United States

The United States, with 50 states and one district (Washington, DC), is the third-largest nation in the world based on population (330,954,637), land area (3,531,837 sq. miles), and the world's largest economy (Fig. 10.2). The GDP as a percentage of the world GDP in 2018 was 23.91%, compared to 24.07% in 2017 (Briney, 2019). The GDP for both years is lower than the long-term average of 29.09% (YCharts, n.d.). The United States is the most technologically advanced economy globally, primarily consisting of the industrial and service sectors. The government is a representative democracy with two legislative bodies—the Senate has 100 seats and the House of Representatives has 435 seats. The Executive branch consists of the President, the head of government, the judicial branch made up of the Supreme Court, court of appeals, district courts, and state and county courts.

The United States is one of the most advanced in medical technology, research, and healthcare facilities. It has pioneered several groundbreaking medical treatments and a global leader in health care innovation and health technology development, with market size of roughly $120 billion. The top nations poised to grow their health technology development sector are the United Kingdom, Canada, China, Germany, and India (Herper, 2011). While the United States continues to lead in biotechnology, other competing countries adopt new policies to expand their health care technology reach.

The healthcare system in the United States is a multi-payer system with three types of medical plans: Medicare, Medicaid, and private insurance. Medicare plan is for adults over 65 years, and specific categories of disabled persons and Medicaid is for low-income individuals and families. Private insurance is acquired from employers or self-purchased from open market chains. Medicaid and Medicare are government-funded programs, but they do not cover everyone. As of 2018, 27.9 million (8.5% of the population) adult Americans were uninsured, and 45% of these uninsured persons cite high medical insurance costs as the reason (Tolbert et al.,

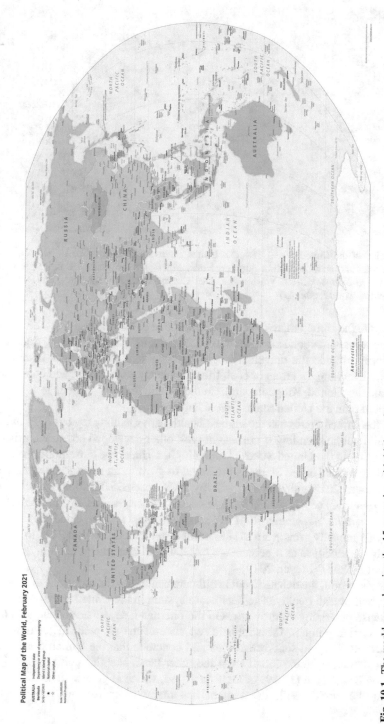

Political Map of the World, February 2021

Fig. 10.1 The world map showing the 15 countries with high-performing health systems. (Source: Political Map of the World, February 2021. *The World Factbook 2021*. Washington, DC: Central Intelligence Agency, 2021. https://www.cia.gov/the-world-factbook/)

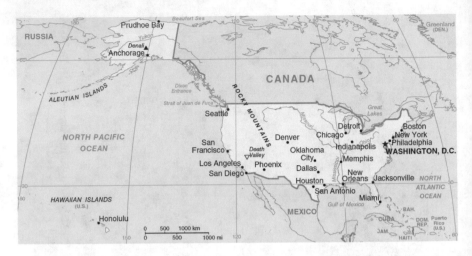

Fig. 10.2 Map of the United States. (Source: United States map showing the United States—including Alaska and Hawaii—within northern North America. Most major US cities are indicated. *The World Factbook 2021*. Washington, DC: Central Intelligence Agency, 2021 https://www.cia.gov/the-world-factbook/)

2020). Despite the United States' wealth, it is still one of the few high-income countries that do not guarantee medical care to all its citizens. The United Kingdom and Canada—both provide the universal single-payer system that provides insurance coverage for everyone. In terms of cost, life expectancy, complexity, and consumer satisfaction, the United Kingdom and Canada's single-payer system is a better health system than the United States (See Chapter 14).

Today, the United States has the highest health care spending (% of GDP) in the world. While public spending is consistent with other developed countries, private health spending in the United States is much higher. Under the current law, healthcare spending in the United States is projected to grow at an average rate of 5.5% per year between 2018 and 2027 and will, by 2027, reach $6.0 trillion. *Health care spending grew by 4.6% in 2018, reaching $3.6 trillion. As a share of the GDP, healthcare spending accounted for 17.7% in 2018. And it* is expected that health spending will annually grow from a 0.8% point faster than GDP from 2018 to 2027. Thus, health expenditure as a percentage of GDP will rise from 17.8% in 2019 to 19.4 percent by 2027 (Meyer, 2019).

Around the world, the debate about healthcare centers on the questions of access, efficiency, and overall quality. The healthcare system in the United States is a subject of intense polarizing controversy. On the one hand, supporters of the existing American system point to the sophisticated state-of-the-art medical technology, well-trained HCWs, and superb facilities and conclude that the United States has the best healthcare system globally. On the other hand, skeptics point to the high spending on health care (*17.8% of GDP in 2019*), which is greater than any other country in the world. Still, the system has many uninsured, uneven quality, administrative waste, and low overall healthcare quality. Critics also rebuke the United States' healthcare system as fragmented and inefficient.

In 2017, 7.9% (25.6 million) of Americans did not have health insurance. The number of insured surged to 8.5% (27.5 million) in 2018. The United States is among the few industrialized nations that do not guarantee access to health care for its population. However, the United States' healthcare system ranked number one in cost, sophistication, responsiveness, and innovation. The US health care's overall quality is rated 37th among the WHO's 191 member nations (WHO, 2000). The annual healthcare cost hit $3.6 trillion in 2018. Hospital costs alone (32.4%) were $387.3 billion, representing a 63% increase since 1997 (inflation-adjusted). About 26.4% was allocated for professional services (physicians, dentists, and other professions); 13.2% for retail, medical products (prescription drugs and all additional medical products); 7.0% for private health insurance administration; 5.2% for residential and personal care; and 4.8% for nursing care facilities and continuing care retirement communities (CMS.gov, 2019; HCT Advisor, 2018).

In the last four decades, health care per capita in the United States has increased 30-fold, from $355 in 1970 to $10,739 in 2017. In 2017 constant dollar amount, the increase was from $1797 in 1970 to $10,739 in 2017, about a sixfold increase. The amount surged to $11,172 per person in 2018 and is the most expensive compared to all other countries—the uninsured pay out of pocket for health care except during medical emergencies when care is provided without question. No one can be denied treatment regardless of the ability to pay.

The costs of treating the uninsured are passed on to the insured via cost-shifting, charity care, higher health insurance premiums, or taxpayers' pay through higher taxes. The federal government reimburses hospitals and other providers for providing uncompensated care and pays them through a matching fund process that empowers each state to enact legislation governing providers' reimbursement. Most of the uninsured are low-income families and often face substantial financial risks, including bankruptcy. They use the emergency room as the primary healthcare source because they have no other place to go. Unfortunately, hospital stays are the most expensive kind of healthcare service, accounting for 33% of all healthcare costs.

On the other hand, preventive care lowers healthcare costs by deterring diseases before requiring emergency room care. The four leading causes of death are preventable chronic diseases—heart disease (caused by poor nutrition and obesity), lung cancer, chronic obstructive pulmonary disease (both caused by smoking), and stroke. Sadly, the number of emergency room visits between 2005 and 2011 increased from 115 to 136 million because about 20% of adults use the emergency room each year (National Academy of Sciences, 2003).

The United States has 1.1 million physicians: 2.6 physicians per 1000 people ratios in 2017. Approximately 160,000 of the physicians are inactive, and 55,000 are unclassified. There are 200,000 dentists, 306,000 pharmacists, 2.86 million registered nurses, and over 5 million allied health professionals from 80 different disciplines. The dominant allied health professions are physical-and-occupational therapy, speech-language pathology, audiology, physician assistant, radiography, rehabilitation counseling, respiratory therapy, athletic training, medical sonography, and dietetics. The other occupations are cardiovascular perfusion technology, cytotechnology, dental hygiene, emergency medical technology, health administration, health information management, medical technology, nuclear medicine technology, optician, and radiation therapy technology. Allied health professionals account for 60% of all HCWs in the United States healthcare system. Their numbers substantially increased as healthcare jobs grew in 2010 from 15.6 to 19.8 million in 2020. Increasingly, many of the allied health disciplines now require bachelor's and graduate degrees to practice. Nurses are the most common occupation in the hospital setting, accounting for about 28% of hospital workers, and 21% of hospital jobs are nonclinical occupations such as office and administrative support workers. The hospital also employs physicians and dentists.

The health care industry in the United States has over 15 million establishments that vary in size, staffing patterns, and organizational structures. Hospitals constitute only 1% of the 15 million healthcare establishments, and about 75% of the establishments are offices of physicians, dentists, and other health practitioners. Hospitals are the largest single employer of HCWs, employing 39% of all health providers. There are different avenues for healthcare delivery—hospitals (general and specialty) and non-hospital-based facilities (nursing homes and community-based facilities, outpatient and other health facilities, government health departments, and the pharmaceutical industry). The nursing and residential care facilities employ about 20% of HCWs.

The general and teaching hospitals, which provide care for patients with various medical conditions requiring diagnosis and surgical/medical treatment, represent 87% of all hospitals. Only 13% of hospitals are specialist hospitals that provide care for patients with specific illnesses or conditions such as psychiatric illness, chronic disease, and rehabilitation. The nursing care facilities provide inpatient nursing, rehabilitation, and personal care to patients who need continuous care in activities of daily living (ADL) skills but do not require hospital services. About half of the nursing care establishment is for individuals with mental and developmental retardation and mental illness. Community-based residential care facilities provide 24/7 social and personal attention to children, the elderly, persons with disabilities, alcohol, drug rehabilitation centers, group homes, and halfway houses. The services provided at both facilities vary from skilled bedside nursing to ADL (bathing, dressing, providing meals, etc.) care.

Outpatient and health facilities employing HCWs include ambulance services, blood banks, clinical (medical), dental laboratories, family planning, home health services, opticians' establishments, poison control centers, and migrant health programs. Other facilities include community mental health and centers for individuals with particular problems (rehabilitation of the blind, deaf, physical disability, mental health problems) and specialized centers that provide inpatient/outpatient care, daycare, and 24-hour emergency, consultation, and educational services. Neighborhood health centers provide primary health care for people living in a particular geographic area within a city. Health Maintenance Organizations (HMOs) provide comprehensive services, including hospitalization, office visits, preventive checkups, and immunizations. Individuals and their employers using HMOs instead of the pay-as-you-go system pay a fixed monthly fee for all services, no matter how often they receive services. Health Practitioners' Offices employ HCWs of various kinds (physicians, dentists, therapist offices, and practices), depending on the clinical practice's size and patients served.

The health departments of the state and local governments control the spread of infectious disease, promote health education and immunizations, and safeguard the purity of food and water supplies. At the federal level, the Public Health Service of the Department of Health and Human Services oversees all citizens' health through the activities of the Centers for Disease Control and Prevention (CDC). The Occupational Safety and Health Administration of the Department of Labor enforces standards related to job health and safety. The Department of Agriculture's state-sponsored programs ensures that meat, poultry, and eggs are disease-free meet sanitary conditions. The Food and Drug Administration (FDA) monitors food safety, prescription drugs, and medical devices, and the army, navy, and air force and the Veterans Administration offer employment opportunities in every health occupation. The pharmaceutical industries manufacture prescription and over-the-counter medications and produce standard household health supplies and supplies used by hospitals and other health facilities. The primary care healthcare physicians (family practice and physicians in pediatric practice or internal medicine practice) focus on disease prevention to reduce health costs. It is generally less expensive to prevent problems or treat them in their earliest stages.

In some parts of the country, new health profession graduates are finding it difficult to find jobs. Similarly, low-income and overpopulated inner-city areas and under-populated rural areas cannot find enough HCWs to fill existing healthcare jobs. It is anticipated that hospitals will experience the slowest job growth within the healthcare industry because of government efforts to control hospital costs and increase the utilization of outpatient clinics and other alternative-care sites. It is also projected that the new technologies will create new job opportunities and training opportunities, and home care services will increasingly become essential.

Health care occupations create more jobs than any other sector of the economy. Health care employment will grow by 18% between 2016 and 2026—much faster than the average for all occupations, adding about 2.3 million new jobs. The projected growth, which is due to an aging population, will lead to a higher demand for healthcare services. The median annual wage for health care professionals and careers (such as physicians and surgeons, dental hygienists, and registered nurses) was $66,440 in May 2018, which was higher than the median annual wage ($38,640) in the economy. Vocational careers such as occupational therapy assistants, medical transcriptionists, and home health aides, in May 2018, have a median annual salary of $29,740, which is lower than the median yearly wage for all occupations in the economy.

Overall, health care in the United States is expensive, in part because of administrative costs which account for 8% of total national health expenditures, compared to only 1–3% in other countries. Healthcare providers in the United States have a higher "administrative burden" of time spent on insurance claims and clinical documentation (Sanger-Katz, 2019). However, they earn substantially more compared to their counterparts in other countries. For example, in 2018, United States' general physicians made an average of $218,173, which is significantly higher than the average pay for the generalists in many countries—the salary is $86,607 in Sweden and $154,126 in Germany (Papanicolas et al., 2018). The high wages in the United States are due to the longer duration spent during training and the higher education cost.

In the United States, complementary and alternative medicine (CAM) practitioners such as acupuncturists, chiropractors, homeopaths, hypnotherapists, and naturopaths are increasingly providing service. The increasing demand for CAM services is related to the general cynicism about conventional (orthodox) medical care and the noninvasive nature of the treatment.

United Kingdom

The United Kingdom has a total land area of 93,410 sq. miles and a population of 67,875,356 as of June 20, 2020, which is equivalent to 0.87% of the total world population (Fig. 10.3). About 83.2% of the population is urban (56,495,180 people in 2020). The population's median age is 40.5 years, and the average life expectancy in 2017 was 81.2 years, 78.5 years in the United States, and 82.5 years in Australia (Worldometer, 2020). Since 1922, the United Kingdom of Great Britain and Northern Ireland (United Kingdom) comprises four countries: England, Scotland, and Wales (which collectively make up Great Britain) and Northern Ireland (which is often described as a country, province, or region). Although the United Kingdom is a unitary sovereign nation, Northern Ireland, Scotland, and Wales have gained autonomy through devolution (NHS Workforce Statistics, 2020).

Health care in the United Kingdom is provided by the National Health Service (NHS), funded through general taxation, and managed by the Department of Health. Each country—England, Northern Ireland, Scotland, and Wales—operates its health system with different policies and priorities. The responsibility for purchasing healthcare services rests at the constituent country level: Primary Care Trusts in England, Health Boards in Scotland, local health groups in Wales, and Primary Care Partnerships in Northern Ireland. There is increasing private care and coverage use, with 12% of the population using additional private health insurance.

Public hospitals and private non-profit hospitals coexist with private for-profit hospitals. The hospitals are mainly publicly owned and independently operated and organized as hospital trusts with three hierarchical levels—community hospitals, district hospitals, regional or inter-regional hospitals, and several specialized hospitals offering advanced treatment. Primary care services are provided primarily by general practitioners who act as gatekeepers by providing access to secondary care services. About 3.1 million health care and social assistance employees make up 11% of national employment—1.4 million employed in the hospital sector, with 67% of all physicians working in hospitals.

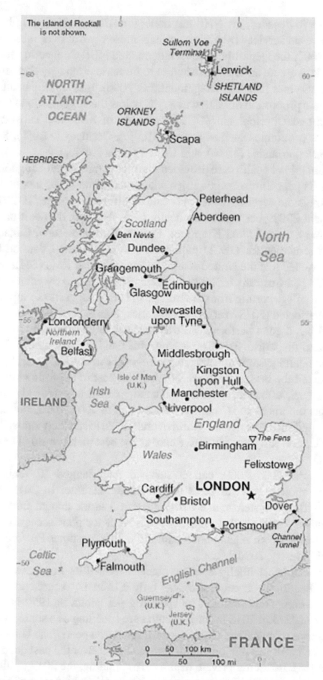

Fig. 10.3 Map of the United Kingdom. (Source: United Kingdom map showing the British Isles (including Northern Ireland) situated in the North Sea. *The World Factbook 2021*. Washington, DC: Central Intelligence Agency, 2021. https://www.cia.gov/the-world-factbook/)

In the last two decades, the NHS has undergone drastic changes in how it operates to improve its services by giving patients more control over their health care. On April 1, 2005, the Department of Health created NHS Connecting for Health—and charged it to create an IT infrastructure to increase efficiency and effectiveness in healthcare services (Healthmanagement.org, 2006). In 2013, the healthcare total expenditure as a proportion of GDP was 8.5%, below the Organisation for Economic Co-operation and Development (OECD) average of 8.9% and substantially less than their peer economies such as France (10.9%), Germany (11.0%), Switzerland (11.1%), the Netherlands (11.1%), and United States (16.4%).

The amount (%) of health care provided directly in the United Kingdom is higher than most of its peer European countries where insurance-based health care is provided with the state serving those who cannot afford insurance. In 2017, United Kingdom spent £2989 per person on health care, the second-lowest among seven cartels (United States, United Kingdom, France, Germany, Italy, Canada, Japan), but around the median for OECD members. The 2018 OECD data on health and social care revealed that the United Kingdom spent less per head (£3121) compared to France (£3471), Australia (£3892), Germany (£4057), and Sweden (£4877). The United Kingdom's departure from the European Union suggests the supply of medicines will be affected (NHS Workforce Statistics, 2020).

The NHS has a good performance track record when compared to other health systems around the world. The Commonwealth Fund in 2017 assessed the performance of the health system in selected high-income countries. Overall, the United Kingdom ranked the best globally and ranked the best in the following categories: care process (i.e., effective, safe, coordinated, patient-oriented) and equity. The three previous reports by the Commonwealth Fund in 2007, 2010, and 2014 ranked the United Kingdom the best in the world overall. In 2015, the Economist Intelligence Unit ranked United Kingdom palliative care as the best in the world (The Economist Group, 2021).

Conversely, in 2005–2009, cancer survival rates lagged 10 years behind in Europe, even though survival rates continued to increase. In 2015, the United Kingdom healthcare system ranked 14th out of 35 in the annual European health consumer index. Some analysts criticized the NHS for poor accessibility with an autocratic and top-down management style (Health Consumer Powerhouse, 2015; UK Medical Industry, 2020).

The NHS had substantially evolved since it treated its first patient on July 5, 1948, when healthcare expenditure was only £14bn but soared to £144.3bn in 2016–2017 at comparable rates. The spending per capita in 1950 is about £260, which grew to £2273 in 2018 money. Health care spending as a share of GDP in the United Kingdom is lower than many Western European peers. The United Kingdom spent just over 7% of its GDP on health care each year over the past decade (Duncan and Jowit, 2018). Including private health care spending, the 2017 total health care investment in the United Kingdom was 9.63% of GDP, higher than South Korea, Singapore, and Nigeria.

In the United Kingdom, access to health care is extensive compared to anywhere else in the world. Unlike the United States and, indeed, most countries, the NHS is a large and well-integrated health system, which tracks patients with their single

NHS number. However, the NHS contrasts with the United States, where the treatment provided depends on the physicians at a particular hospital and health insurance type. Scandinavian countries have similar health systems to the NHS but have a smaller population, far less diverse than the United Kingdom. The United Kingdom has the third-highest number of clinical trials worldwide after the United States and Germany (Boseley, 2018).

The United Kingdom and Canadian health systems are often criticized for the long waiting period needed to see a consultant and undergo any significant operation due to the system's micromanagement designed to control cost. In the last decade, thousands of United Kingdom-qualified physicians moved to the United States, Australia, New Zealand, and Canada, thus creating a physician workforce shortage which forced the government to have a liberal immigration policy to recruit foreign-trained HCWs. The NHS recruits globally to meet their personnel needs.

South Korea

South Korea is in the southern half of the Korean Peninsula in East Asia. It is mainly surrounded by water with a coastline along three seas—to the south is the East China Sea, to the east is the Sea of Japan, and to the west is the Yellow Sea (West Sea). It has a land border with North Korea, lying to the north with 238 kilometers (148 miles) of the border running along the Korean demilitarized zone. South Korea's landmass is approximately 38,623 square miles (Fig. 10.4). South Korea's republic is a presidential representative democracy with the president as the head of

Fig. 10.4 Map of South Korea. (Source: South Korea map showing major cities as well as parts of surrounding countries and water bodies. *The World Factbook 2021.* Washington, DC: Central Intelligence Agency, 2021. https://www.cia.gov/the-world-factbook/)

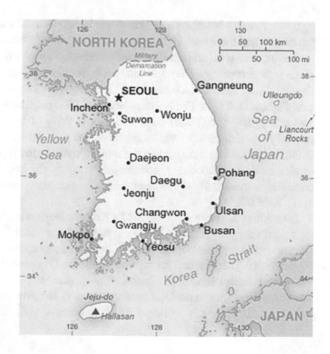

state of a multi-party system. The president exercises executive power, and the legislative role is vested in both the national assembly and the government. The judiciary is entirely independent of the legislature and executive arms of government and consists of the Supreme Court, constitutional court, and appellate courts. The constitution has undergone five major revisions since 1948, and the current sixth republic began in 1987 with the last major constitutional review. South Korea scored eight out of 10, making it the 23rd most democratic country in 2019 (KBS World Radio, 2018).

South Korea achieved universal health coverage for its citizens in 1989, just 12 years after introducing social health insurance. In early 2000, South Korea introduced two significant health care reforms: the merger of insurance societies into a single insurer system and the separation of drug prescription and dispensing (Kwon et al., 2015). The South Korean healthcare system is funded through the national health insurance scheme managed by the Ministry of Health and Welfare. Health care in South Korea is provided at no cost to all citizens. The private sector funds a significant portion of the health care, and South Korea ranked first among the OECD countries for access to health care (OECD, 2015).

In 2015, the South Korean health system was better than that of many other Asian countries and ranked among the world's best in quality (Kwon et al., 2015). Patient satisfaction with the healthcare system consistently has been among the highest globally and was rated, in 2015, the fourth most efficient healthcare system by Bloomberg. The South Korean national health insurance scheme covers 97% of the population, and foreign nationals enjoy the same access to their universal health care as the natives. The high insurance coverage, many scholars argue, is responsible for the impressive satisfaction with the health system (Numbeo, 2020; Du & Lu, 2016).

South Korea's healthcare system offers Western medicine and traditional oriental treatments and has excellent success in treating skin diseases. The hospitals are very well equipped, with an excellent (low) physician-to-patient ratio. The top four hospitals in the country—Seoul National University Hospital, the Samsung Medical Center, Asian Medical Centre, and Yonsei Severance Hospital—rank among the world's best facilities. The hospital beds per 1000 population in South Korea are 10, well above five for OECD countries. About 94% of hospitals (88% of beds) are privately owned, and private universities manage 30 of the 43 tertiary hospitals. Publicly owned universities run ten more. Payment for health care is on a fee-for-service basis and no direct government subsidy for hospitals. This arrangement encourages hospitals to expand and discourages community services (Chun et al., 2009).

Like many western nations, South Korea's healthcare system focuses more on treatment than prevention. Also, the system is famous for the one-stop medical tourism service that starts online at www.visitkorea.or.kr long before the patient leaves their country. The Council for Korean Medicine Overseas Promotion boasts over 30 top-quality health facilities. Simultaneously, there is plenty of government support and investment for the medical tourism sector (LaingBuisson International Limited, 2020). In 2013, nearly 400,000 medical tourists visited South Korea and were expected to rise to one million by 2020. Compared to the United States, major surgical procedures in South Korea are 30–84% cheaper (Health-Tourism.com, 2008). Some hospitals charge patients from abroad more than natives because they receive customized services such as airport pickup and translation costs.

South Korea's rapid growth and commercialization create environmental pollution in the larger cities, with a high incidence of chronic diseases. Despite universal coverage of the population, the high out-of-pocket (OOP) expenses have remained a key access issue. Koreans pay out-of-pocket for up to 20% of the cost for insured services in inpatient care, and differential cost-sharing is applied to outpatient care, depending on the health provider's level. The national health insurance provides some protection mechanisms, such as exemption from co-payments for the poor. There are also reduced co-payments for catastrophic illnesses like cancer. A ceiling on cumulative OOP payments depending on income and high OOP payments has remained a key access issue.

In South Korea, there is an adversarial relationship between private providers and the government (and the national health insurance system). Providers have been a stumbling block to meaningful health care reforms involving the prospective payment system. There has been a gradual rise in inequity in the country since the 1990s, and the surging aging population has had a substantial impact on the health-care system and health outcomes. The challenges facing the government include strengthening primary health care, reducing inequality in health coverage outcomes, and improving coordination between the long-term care facilities and hospitals to meet the needs of the growing aged population (Kwon et al., 2015).

Singapore

Singapore is a city and sovereign island nation located off the southern tip of Peninsular Malaysia in Southeast Asia. It is 279 square miles in dimension, with about six million people without rural or remote areas (Fig. 10.5). Singapore was, until 1959, a British colony when it offered free medical care through a system modeled on the United Kingdom's National Health Service. In 1959, the island became self-governing. Its political regime can be repressive. However, trust in the government is very high, and the government wields that power aggressively. In 2017, the Human Rights Watch stated that people who are critical of the government or the judiciary or speak critically about religion and issues of race frequently face criminal investigations or civil suits, often with crippling damages claims. Singapore is a "melting pot" as the world's most religiously diverse nation (Pew Research Center, 2014). Buddhism is the dominant religion (33.2%), followed by none (18.5%), Christianity (18.2%), Islam (14.0%), Taoism and folk religion (10.0%), and Hinduism (5.0%), and 0.6% of the population are Sikhism or other faith (Pew Research Center, 2014).

The Singaporean government has created and maintained a high-quality health-care system at a lower cost than any other high-income country in the world

Fig. 10.5 Map of Singapore. (Source: Singapore map showing major districts of this city-state surrounded by Malaysia and the Singapore Strait. *The World Factbook 2021*. Washington, DC: Central Intelligence Agency, 2021. https://www.cia.gov/the-world-factbook/)

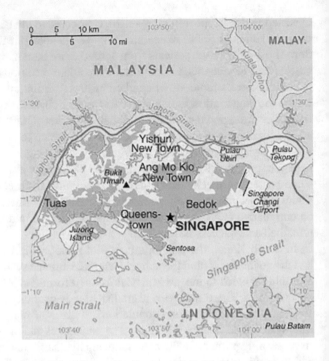

(Brookings.edu, 2016). However, an analyst skeptically opined that the Singaporean health system is among the best globally with a big caveat (Carroll, 2019). The 2014 United Nations' performance assessment ranked Singapore's health system number one out of 188 nations, and the United States trails behind at 24th. One healthcare technocrat affirmed that because of "bad politics" and unwillingness to compromise, the Democrats and Republicans in the United States spent the last decade arguing about providing insurance coverage to less than 10% of the uninsured population (Carroll, 2019). At the same time, Singapore was perfecting how to deliver care at a low cost and focusing on quality and efficiency (Advisory Board, 2019).

Health care in Singapore is a government-run universal health system with a robust private sector involvement. Financing healthcare costs is through a mixture of direct government subsidies, national health care insurance, compulsory savings, and cost-sharing. After independence, the country's new ruler introduced private insurance and healthcare providers. Singapore's employees pay around 37% of their salaries in mandated savings accounts spent on health care, housing, education, and insurance, with some contributed to employers (Skrybus, 2020). The country's progressive tax system has less poverty than other developed countries. The lower-income 20% of Singaporeans pay less than 10% of all taxes and receive more than 25% of all benefits. The wealthiest 20% spend more than half of all taxes and receive only 12% of the services.

The Ministry of Health manages the health system and ensures that everyone has access to different services quickly, cost-effectively, and seamlessly. All health facilities such as hospitals, medical centers, community health centers, nursing homes, clinics (including dental clinics), and clinical laboratories (including x-ray laboratories) are licensed under the Private Hospitals and Medical Clinics Act/ Regulations. As a result, Singaporeans have easy access to healthcare providers and hospitals (Ministry of Health, 2019).

Singapore's health outcomes are excellent because the system is well-designed and managed efficiently. The country has only been governing itself since about 1960, and power has been held by one party, partly because it has proven to be the most successful group of technocrats in human history. Singapore has evolved from a developing country in the 1950s to the third-highest per capita income today. Despite the country's wealth, only 15% of the citizens own cars because it is very costly. There are virtually no illegal drugs or gun crimes in the county because drug dealers are executed, and guns are outlawed. Cigarette and alcohol taxes are prohibitive by American standards (Klein, 2017). The school system throughout the country is comparable, and the government heavily subsidizes housing. Singapore is a health-conscious society, as smoking rates, alcoholism, drug abuse, and obesity are relatively low.

Singapore ranked sixth in the WHO's world's health systems performance evaluation in 2000. In 2014, Bloomberg ranked Singapore's healthcare system as the most efficient in the world. The Bloomberg Global Health Index of 163 countries ranked Singapore the fourth healthiest country globally and in Asia. In addition, Singapore ranked first on the Global Food Security Index. The Economist Intelligence Unit placed Singapore second out of 166 countries for health care outcomes. Many technocrats described Singapore as one of the most successful healthcare systems globally regarding both efficiency in financing and the results achieved in community health outcomes (Advisory Board, 2019; Brown, 2003; Carroll and Frakt, 2017; Lee, 2020). Their success is attributed to a combination of a firm reliance on medical savings accounts, cost-sharing, and government regulation (Tikkanen et al., 2020).

Singapore officially has a guest worker program for over 1.4 million foreigners, mainly in low-skilled, low-paying jobs. The jobs come with benefits and protections that are better than the workers' home countries. However, the guest workers are not qualified for the same services (such as access to the public health system) that citizens or permanent residents are entitled to. The guest workers' data are excluded intentionally from the national health metrics. The system is widely criticized for limited reliable health outcome data (Klein, 2017; Carroll, 2019).

Singapore is widely recognized for how it pays for its healthcare system but less noticed for its delivery system. The Singapore government controls and pays for much of the medical system itself. The hospitals are overwhelmingly public, and a large portion of physicians work directly for the state. Patients can only use their Medisave accounts to purchase preapproved medications that the government now subsidizes (Klein, 2017). Primary health care is provided mainly by the private sector at a low cost by over 1700 general practitioners. About 80% of the citizens use the service of general practitioners, and the rest use a system of 18 polyclinics managed by the government.

As health care services become more complicated and more expensive, more people migrate to the more efficient polyclinics and process as many patients as possible. The citizens are encouraged to use an online app to schedule appointments and pay for the service provided. About 45% of Singaporeans with chronic conditions utilize polyclinics. A major complaint is the wait time and lack of continuity. Physicians carry a heavy workload of about 60 patients a day and do not choose their physicians. The cost of care is relatively cheap—a visit costs 8 Singapore dollars (less than $6 US). A private physician charges three times the fee from a polyclinic, which is still more affordable than US hospitals. In 2014, Singapore spent $4047 per person on health care, which is slightly less than 5% of its GDP, while the United States spent $9403, representing 17% of the GDP (Healthline Media, 2015). Klein (2017) observed that Singapore spent $2752 per person on health care based on World Bank data in 2014. Health care spending per capita in Singapore, in 2015, declined to the United States $2000 level, which beats neighbors like South Korea, China, Malaysia, and Thailand but still lags behind Switzerland and United States, which allocated over US$8000 per capita spending (Singapore Business Review, 2020).

Only about 20% of Singaporeans select a private hospital for care, and 80% use the public hospitals that are heavily subsidized. Nearly half of the care provided in private hospitals is for noncitizens. Citizens, who select private hospitals, as care gets more expensive, often transfer to the public system. There is a more granular control of the healthcare delivery system. For example, in 1997, there were about 60,000 ambulance calls, but nearly half were for non-emergency services. This pattern of use led the government to institute a $185 fee for non-emergency services. The use of electronic health records is all connected, and data are shared between systems. For all its successes, Singapore's health system has its challenges. The population is aging rapidly, and the spending on health care, which is currently within the global average of 10%, is probably going to decline.

Policymakers in the country are worried about the rise of diabetes, unsustainable fee-for-service payments, and hospitals learning to game the system to make more money. They recognize that resources are lean, and not every medicine or device can be funded through the public health system. The government sets the prices, determines what subsidies are available, and strictly regulates the technology, drugs, and devices available and covered in public facilities. The government scrutinizes the latest and most remarkable technologies with a healthy skepticism of manufacturer claims. Also, government control applies to public health initiatives to ensure school lunches and meals served during government events are a healthy diet. Government campaign efforts encourage drinking water, and food choice labels are mandated. With control over its food importation, the government even got beverage manufacturers to reduce sugar content in drinks to a maximum of 12% by 2020 (Caroll, 2015).

Taiwan

Taiwan, also known as the Republic of China, is a small country with a population of 23,818,146 million in the eastern part of Asia that shares borders with the People's Republic of China to the northwest, Japan northeast, and the Philippines to the south

Fig. 10.6 Map of Taiwan.
(Source: Taiwan map
showing major cities of
this island in the Western
Pacific Ocean. *The World
Factbook 2021*.
Washington, DC: Central
Intelligence Agency, 2021
https://www.cia.gov/
the-world-factbook/)

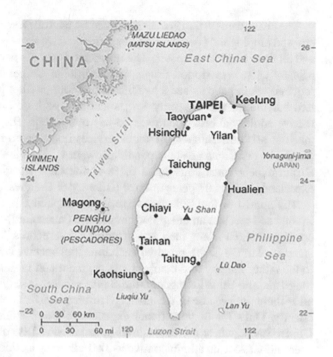

(Fig. 10.6). The Portuguese in 1544 named the island "Ilha Formosa" (Beautiful Island). Taiwan's main island has an area of 13,826 square miles, and Taipei is the capital and largest metropolitan area. The dominant religion is Buddhist (35.3%), Taoist (33.2%), and Christian (3.9%). Taiwan is among the most densely populated nations and is the most populous with the most robust economy, not a UN member. It is a representative democratic republic, where the head of state is the President and the Premier (President of the Executive Yuan) of a multi-party system. The legislative power is vested primarily by the parliament, and the government exercises executive control. The judiciary is independent of the legislature and the executive. The political system is dominated by the Kuomintang (KMT, "Chinese Nationalist Party"), which favors closer ties with mainland China, while the Democratic Progressive Party supports Taiwanese independence (Library of Congress, 2005; Mao Tse-tung, 1947).

In the last 60 years, Taiwan's economy has developed rapidly from an agricultural-based to an industrial-based economy. Taiwan is considered a developed country, ranking 15th in GDP per capita and ranked highly on political and civil liberties, health care, education, and human development (Library of Congress, 2005). In the 1980s, Taiwan was not yet a democracy, and about 40% of the citizens have no health insurance—many people were bankrupt when they have medical crisis. The ruling government at the time convened a high-profile committee to reform the healthcare system. In March 1995, they took a fractured and inequitable healthcare system and transformed it into a universal, affordable single-payer system. The one national health insurance plan, run by the government, covers every Taiwanese. The government modeled the system after Canada and the United Kingdom system (Scott, 2020).

The healthcare system is mainly funded by payroll-based deductions, with workers' and employers' contributions supplemented by some progressive income taxes and tobacco and lottery levies. The insurance coverage benefits cover hospital and primary care, prescription drugs, and traditional Chinese medicine. Co-pays are required when patients see a healthcare provider or fill a prescription or go to the ER, but the cost is generally low, about $12 or less. Lower-income Taiwanese receive additional breaks on their co-pay obligations. Higher-income citizens can take out private insurance for some services not covered by the single-payer program. The per capita health expenditures were US$752 in 2000 and $3047 in 2017. Health expenditures constituted 6.1% of the GDP in 2017, and the overall life expectancy was 84.07 years in 2020 ((Library of Congress, 2005).

The appeal of the Taiwan system is its simplicity. Every Taiwanese citizen is insured and receives an integrated circuit card (smart card)—NHI IC card—proof of coverage, which stores their health information/records. The patient provides the smart card to the health provider each time they receive health services. Compared to the rather lengthy and cumbersome payment and billing methods in the United States and the United Kingdom, the claims process is very rapid. The system operates efficiently because of the advanced information technology infrastructure in the country. Only 1% of operational expenditure is on administrative costs than the United States, where private insurers spend around 12% of overhead and hospitals spend about 25% on administrative work. Following a critical comparative analysis, Scott (2020) asserted that Taiwan's health care system is better under a single-payer than the American system.

Taiwanese have a high level of health-seeking behavior to take medicines or seek medical help frequently, even for minor ailments. The average outpatient department visit is 14 times per year per person. Because of the low co-pay and Taiwanese culture, the average number of physician visits per year in Taiwan is nearly twice that of other developed economies. Consequently, hospitals get crowded in Taiwan. The high cost-sharing in the United States makes patients skip necessary care of severe conditions. In 2002, Taiwan had 1.6 physicians and 5.9 hospital beds per 1000 population, with 36 hospitals and 2601 clinics. There is generally no waiting list, and patients can typically see any specialist of their choice during the usual working hours. The only exception is that a famous physician may have a waiting list for the appointment. The waiting list for elective surgical procedures is usually short as well. There is also a panel review system of medical records to keep healthcare costs down while maintaining healthcare quality. Payment for treatment procedures considered inappropriate by this specialist panel is denied.

Because of the easy accessibility to specialists, family physicians' gatekeeper role is relatively weak in Taiwan, where physicians believe they see too many patients every day. To ensure their incomes are maintained, it is common for physicians to consult with 50 patients in the morning, with each patient receiving no more than 5 minutes' duration. Such short contact time may result in poor patient-physician rapport and the inability to deal with complex cases in one visit.

Consequently, patients often attend for a second or third opinion, thus contributing to even higher patient volume and higher medical costs. Notwithstanding, 25 years after it was established, over 80% of Taiwanese are satisfied with their health system (Wu et al., 2010).

Cuba

Cuba is an island nation with a total land area of 41,097 sq. miles, located in the Caribbean Sea, where the Gulf of Mexico and the Atlantic Ocean meet. The population of Cuba is 11,326,783, which is equivalent to 0.15% of the world population. About 78% of the population is urban (Fig. 10.7). The median age is 42.2 years, and life expectancy is 79.1 years compared to 79.3 years in the United States. Since 1959, Cuba's political system is a Marxist–Leninist socialist ideology of the "one-state–one party" principle. The government created a national health system that provides free health for all its citizens. The government runs the health system—there are no private hospitals or clinics.

The Cuban healthcare system is often cited as one of Fidel Castro's legacy achievements. The system focuses heavily on a preventative medicine approach and offers the most straightforward annual physical to the most complex surgery, free of charge. In addition, dental care, medications, and even home visits from physicians are covered by their health system (Farouq, 2019). Given its impressive health outcome statistics, the United Nations Secretary-General Ban Ki-moon hailed the health system as "a model for many countries" (Warner, 2016).

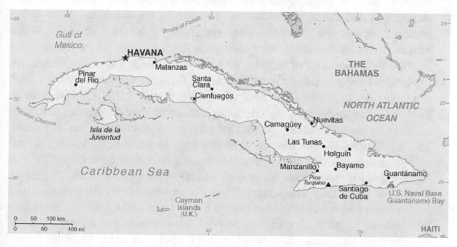

Fig. 10.7 Map of Cuba. (Source: Cuba map showing the island country in the Caribbean Sea. *The World Factbook 2021*. Washington, DC: Central Intelligence Agency, 2021 https://www.cia.gov/the-world-factbook/)

Cuban health system is highly structured, prevention-oriented, information-rich, innovative, and efficient (Gómez-Dantés, 2018). Cuba spends about 9403 dollars on health care, while it costs about 813 dollars per person in Cuba. The Cuban model is possible to replicate, but the United States is one of the few developed countries that still have not invested in a universal healthcare system (Farouq, 2019). As a result, the high health care cost in the United States does not yield corresponding high health outcomes. On the other hand, with less than a tenth of the United States' expenditures, Cuba has attained comparable results on many indicators, particularly life expectancy and infant mortality. Although Cuban HCWs have less access to technology and supplies, coverage is universal, and the system is mainly government-run, except for the black market and medical tourism.

Conversely, health care in the United States is not universal and consists of a disjointed patchwork, yet a well-resourced mixture of public and private providers and payers. The universal coverage in Cuba accounts for why it can do more with less (O'Hanlon and Harvey, 2017). The Cuba national health system consists of multiple levels:

1. The community-level consists of individuals and families.
2. The family physician-and-nurse team consists of physician and nurse teams that serve patients, families, and communities. They live above government-built family medicine offices, living directly in the communities they serve and providing care 24 hours a day. They biannually perform a neighborhood health assessment where community risk factors are identified and focus on improving the community's health. The team subsequently works to address any public health concerns and provide medical care. Clinically, family physician-and-nurse teams follow the continuous assessment and risk evaluation method, which monitors patients and their family health by evaluating medical history, current health, community, and home environments. The family physician-and-nurse teams make at least one yearly home visits to each family to assess their health. Those with chronic illnesses are seen at least every three months. These teams' roles combine the importance of focusing on both public health and clinical medicine.
3. Physicians refer patients to local polyclinics for more complex services, each serving a single geographic area of approximately 25,000–35,000 people. Polyclinics are community-based clinics that accommodate primary care specialists who are well-acquainted with the people and the communities they serve. The polyclinic staff provides services that include pediatrics, dental, ophthalmology, and behavioral health care. To ensure appropriate follow-up, they also communicate directly with the patient's family physician. Specialists support physicians when they are needed. They observe the social determinants and environment that affect the community's health and use the information to help their patients better. Each specialist supports 20–40 physicians-and-nurse teams.
4. The primary work team within the polyclinics supervises and assesses the family medicine offices' neighborhood and clinical health work.
5. Hospitals: Preventive medical care, diagnostic tests, and medication for hospitalized patients are free, but the patient pays for some health services. The items

paid for by patients who can afford it are outpatient drugs, hearing aid, dental and orthopedic appliances, crutches, and wheelchairs. These items are available at state stores at a low cost that is highly subsidized. For patients on low-income, these items are provided free of charge.

6. Medical Institute: Economic constraints and restrictions on medicines forced the Cuban health system to develop alternative medicine that is affordable and accessible to the population. The Cuban Ministry of Public Health in the 1990s recognized alternative medicine and integrated it with the Western medicine model.

At the dawn of the nineteenth century, modern western medicine has been in Cuba, and the first surgical clinic was established in 1823. Medical graduates in Cuba can address health issues and know when to refer to a higher level within the healthcare pyramid. They are committed to quality and equity within health care for their communities. The largest medical university in the world (Latin American School of Medicine) is in Cuba. As far back as the 1950s, the number of physicians in Cuba (per thousand of the population) ranked higher than Britain, France, and the Netherlands. In Latin America, Cuba ranked third after Uruguay and Argentina. However, there remained marked inequalities as most physicians worked in the cities and regional towns, and the rural areas, notably Oriente, were substantially worse.

The physician density in Cuba increased substantially from 9.2 physicians per 10,000 people in 1958 to 58.2 per 10,000 in 1999. In 2005, Cuba had 627 physicians and 94 dentists for every 100,000 people, and the United States had 225 physicians and 54 dentists for every 100,000 people. With 627 physicians and 94 dentists for every 100,000 people, Cuba surpassed the Central American isthmus with 123 physicians and 30 dentists for every 100,000 people. As of 2005, Cuba became the global leader in the ratio of physicians to the population with 67 physicians per 10,000 people compared with 43 for the Russian Federation and 24 for the United States (The World Bank, n.d.).

Besides having the highest physician to population ratio, Cuba also had the lowest infant mortality rate in Latin America. The mortality rate was the third-lowest in the world. In the 1960s, the government implemented a universal vaccination program that eradicated many contagious diseases, including polio, tetanus, diphtheria, and rubella. However, some diseases such as tuberculosis, hepatitis, and chickenpox increased during the economic hardship of the 1990s. By 2003, Cuba had the lowest HIV prevalence in the Americas and one of the world's lowest. By 2005, Cuba's epidemic was the smallest in the Caribbean.

Only a few countries around the world can surpass Cuba's 98% record of full immunization of children by the age of two, vaccinating them against 13 illnesses and providing antenatal care for 95% of pregnant women by the end of their first trimester with rates of infant mortality less than 5 per 1000 births. By the mid-1980s, Cuba had implemented universal access to primary care. The WHO recommended achieving the "Health for All" goal set at the 1978 international conference on primary care in Alma Ata. In 2012, Cuba ranked near the top of the countries on track to meet the MDGs focusing on the social determinants of health. The "Save the

Children" organization mentioned Cuba as the best among the Tier 2 less-developed countries on motherhood (Keck & Reed, 2012). In 2015, Cuba was the first country in the world to eliminate mother-to-child transmission of HIV and syphilis, a significant public health accomplishment (PAHO, 2015).

Abortion rates increased dramatically during the 1980s but were reduced by 50% by 1999. The rate declined to near the 1970s levels of 32.0 per 1000 pregnancies, which is still among the highest in Latin America. In the 1970s, the government implemented maternal and prenatal care programs to reduce the infant mortality rate. Between 2005 and 2010, Cuba had six deaths under age 5 per 1000 live births compared to eight in the United States. In 2013, infant mortality in Cuba was five deaths per 1000 live births compared with 5.9 in the United States and 4.8 for Canada (Jacobson, 2014; WHO, 2015, 2016) (Table 10.1).

In 2016, Cuba's infant mortality rate declined to 4.1 per 1000 live births, lower than the average for high-income countries (5.0 per 1000 live births). However, some critics noted that these statistics reflect the heavy-handed treatment of pregnant women and the possibility that the government may have falsified the outcome data. They also speculated that pregnant women with fetal abnormalities might have been forced to undergo abortions or forcibly placed under monitoring. And physicians have incentives to distort statistics, as a surge in infant mortality will cost them their jobs (Gómez-Dantés, 2018; Jacobson, 2014). In addition, several critical health outcome data for the Cuba health system, such as health expenditure per capita, happiness index, and the average response time for emergency calls, are not readily available in the open-access literature. Moreover, the country does not allow independent verification of its health outcome data (Gómez-Dantés, 2018; Jacobson, 2014).

In 2012, Cuba developed a new family medicine curriculum that expects the family physicians and nurses to be responsible for their patients' overall health, not just the treatment of disease and injury. The new medical curriculum increased contents in epidemiological and public health sciences (including social communication), emphasized service learning in the community, and introduced problem-based active learning methods. In addition, the faculty introduced clinical rotation early in tandem with the basic medical sciences (Keck and Reed, 2012).

Table 10.1 Critical healthcare indicators in Cuba compared with the United States

Health indicators	Cuba	United States
Infant mortality rate in 2013 (probability in dying by age 1 per 1000 live births)	5	5.9
Maternal mortality rate in 2015 (per 100,000 live births)	39	14
Mortality due to cancer, cardiovascular disease, diabetes, or chronic respiratory diseases (percent of population ages 30–70) in 2012	16.5%	14.3%
Total spending on health as percent of GDP in 2012	8.6%	17%
Per capita total expenditure on health at average exchange rate (US dollars) in 2012	$558	$8845

Source: NationMaster, 2021

The challenges within Cuba's health system include low pay for physicians, antiquated facilities in shoddy states needing repairs, inadequate equipment, the frequent absence of essential drugs, and concern regarding freedom of choice for both patients and physicians. Thus, while Cuba's healthcare outcomes resemble high-income countries, the hospital facilities indicate those in third-world countries. This health paradox one critic advocates could be diminished by modernizing the Cuban medical immigration laws that allow the physician to travel to developed countries to engage in technological exchange opportunities and contribute to the Cuban hospital's development (Lopez, 2019).

In 2002, the physician's average monthly salary was 261 pesos, 1.5 times the national mean. A physician's salary in the late 1990s was about US$15–20 per month in purchasing power and £52 a month in 2016 (Warner, 2016). Some HCWs prefer to work in the lucrative tourist industry where earnings can be much higher. Some Cuban physicians defect to other countries while sent on international missions. In the early 1990s, the loss of subsidies from the Soviets brought food shortages to Cuba. The regime refused to accept food donations, medicines, and money from the United States until 1993. Like the rest of the Cuban economy, the healthcare system has long suffered from severe material shortages caused by the US embargo.

Comparative Analyses

The subsequent section of this Chapter will address the question, what makes a sound health system? It will also compare and contrast the six countries' health outcome and performance ranking relative to one another and juxtapose it with Nigeria's ranking.

Health Outcome Indices

The purpose of this exploration is to compare health outcome indicators and service delivery costs in the six identified high-performing nations to gain insight into what Nigeria can learn from these countries. Of the six model health systems, Taiwan and South Korea's healthcare system topped the *global health care index* list published in 2020 by Numbeo. In the report, *health care* index estimates were defined as the status of systems health care professionals, equipment, staff, doctors, and cost. Surprisingly, the United Kingdom and United States healthcare systems ranked low at 13 and 30, respectively. South Africa's health system ranked 48 and Nigeria ranked number 86, while Venezuela ranked last at 93.

Table 10.2 summarizes the critical social-demographic and health outcome and performance data for Nigeria and the six shining model countries for comparative purposes. Singapore, representing only 0.08% of the world population, is the least populated and smallest landmass of the six countries. The overwhelming majority

Table 10.2 Health system outcomes in Nigeria and selected nations with high-performing health systems

Serial [a]	Social-demographic/health outcome/performance	Nigeria	United States	United Kingdom	S. Korea	Singapore	Taiwan	Cuba
1	Population (millions) as of 6/22, 2020	205,962,220	330,954,637	67,877,301	51,268,205	5,849,157	23,818,146	11,326,764
2	Percentage of the total world population (%) as of 6/22, 2020	2.64	4.25	0.87	0.66	0.08	0.31	0.15
3	Total land area (sq. miles)	351,650	3,531,837	93,410	37,541	270	13,672	41,097
4	Percentage of the population that is urban (%) as of 6/22, 2020	52.0	82.8	83.2	81.8	100	78.9	78.3
5	Percentage of people with health insurance coverage, 2018	1.1–3.1[a]	91.5	100	100	100	100	100
6	Life expectancy (years) in 2020	55.75[b]	79.11	81.77	83.50	84.07	80.6	79.18
7	Median age (years) in 2020	18.1	38.3	40.5	43.7	42.2	42.5	42.2
8	Physicians per 1000 people (2016–2018)[b]	0.4 (2018)	2.6 (2017)	2.8 (2018)	2.4 (2017)	2.3 (2016)	1.33 (2000)	8.4 (2018)
9	Health expenditure (% GDP)[c] in (2017)	3.76	17.06	9.63	7.60	4.44	6.1	11.71
10	Health expenditure per capital ($)[d] in (2017)	215	9536	4356	2556	3681	3047	N/A
11	WHO's 2000 ranking of overall health system performance	187	37	18	58	6	N/A	39
12	Happiness index[e] in 2020	4.724	6.940	7.165	5.872	6.377	6.455	N/A
13	Infant mortality rate (per 1000 live births) in 2017[f]	76	6	4	3	2	4	4
14	Maternal mortality ratio (per 100,000 live births) in 2017[g]	917	19	7	11	8	12	36

[a] https://www.ncbi.nlm.nih.gov/pmc/articles/PMC6326643/ and https://journals.plos.org/plosone/article?id=10.1371/journal.pone.0201833
https://www.census.gov/library/publications/2019/demo/p60-267.html#:~:text=The%20percentage%20of%20people%20with,in%20,201
[b] https://data.worldbank.org/indicator/SH.MED.PHYS.ZS
[c] https://data.worldbank.org/indicator/SH.XPD.CHEX.GD.ZS
[d] https://en.wikipedia.org/wiki/List_of_countries_by_total_health_expenditure_per_capita
[e] https://happiness-report.s3.amazonaws.com/2020/WHR20.pdf
[f] https://data.worldbank.org/indicator/SH.STA.MMRT
[g] https://data.worldbank.org/indicator/SH.STA.MMRT

(ranging from 78.3% in Cuba to 100% in Singapore) of the population of the six countries are urban dwellers. Only 52% of Nigerians live in the metropolitan area (Worldometer, 2020).

Of the six model countries, in 2020, Singapore had the highest life expectancy of 84.07 years, while it is only 55.75 years in Nigeria. The six model countries have an older population with a median age ranging from 38.3 years in the United States to 43.7 years in South Korea. The median age in Nigeria is only 18.1 years. In 2020, life expectancy in Cuba (79.18 years) was at parity with the United States (79.11 years), but Cuba had a lower infant mortality rate (4.0 deaths per 1000 live births) than the United States (6.0 deaths per 1000 live births) (Table 10.2). In 2013, Cuba had a lower infant mortality rate (4.76 deaths per 1000 live births) than the United States (5.90 deaths per 1000 live births). Between 2005 and 2010, Cuba had six deaths under age 5 per 1000 live births, compared to eight fatalities for the United States (Jacobson, 2014).

In 2017, Singapore, with meager investment in the health sector (only 4.40% share of the GDP), still had the lowest mortality rate (2 per 1000 live birth), and the United Kingdom had the lowest maternal mortality rate (7 per 100,000 live births) among the six model countries. Conversely, Nigeria, with a higher (6.10% share of the GDP) investment in health than Singapore, had one of the highest (poor) infants (76 per 1000 live births) and maternal (917 per 100,000 live births) mortality rates in the world. Critics bemoaned that the US life expectancy and high infant and maternal mortality rates did not justify the increased healthcare expenditure (Jacobson, 2014). In addition, O'Hanlon and Harvey (2017) noted that the United States spending on health does not provide "a bang for the buck" than Cuba's significant health indices.

The United States health system is transparent and patient-centered. Patients are empowered to ask questions, seek second opinions, and file complaints to recognized boards for arbitration. Countries with nationalized health systems adopt a more paternalistic approach to care with no providers and hospitals' choice. The US health system provides prompt consult with specialists and cutting-edge technology treatment supplied without unnecessary delay. Moreover, the United States leads the world in use of advanced equipment per capita—in MRI units per million population (25.9) and CT scanners per million (34.3).

The United States has some of the best outcomes globally for surviving a heart attack, stroke, and cancer. American women have a 63% likelihood of surviving at least 5 years after a cancer diagnosis than 56% for European women. The chance of survival is 66% for American men and 47% for European men. The United States offers better treatment of chronic disease than most countries in the world. In 2002, a German study found that US hospitals administered more state-of-the-art medicine than Europeans. For example, in 2002, 56% of Americans with high cholesterol took statins, but only 17–36% of Europeans took them. While 60% of the antipsychotic medication prescribed in the United States were of the newest brands, only 10% in Germany were new (Dhand, 2014; Lubin, 2010). The treatment of psychological disease is more prevalent in the United States than in most countries worldwide—American children are more likely to use psychotropic medication, and women commonly are on antidepressants.

In the WHO's 2000 global assessment of the performance of health systems, Singapore ranked the highest (#6), followed by the United States at 37th, Cuba at 39th, and Nigeria ranked 187 (worst) out of the 191 countries surveyed. In another health systems evaluation conducted in 2014, the United States ranked 50th out of 55 countries on life expectancy and healthcare spending. Only Jordan, Colombia, Azerbaijan, Brazil, and Russia ranked lower (Du & Lu, 2016). Furthermore, the 2020 world happiness data among the six model countries revealed that the British perceived themselves to be happier (7.165) than the Americans (6.940), Singaporeans (6.377), South Korean (5.872), and Nigerians (4.724) (Table 10.2).

The response time to an emergency call is one of the health outcome indicators used to judge health systems' performance. The responsiveness varies widely based on social and environmental factors. Social factors include the demand for transport, the request, traffic congestion, hospital location, population, etc. Ecological factors include road conditions, topography, and weather condition. The availability of essential life support infrastructures in risk situations involving humans and goods is the primary goal of emergency medical services (EMS). The EMS provides acute pre-hospital care for patients with illnesses and injuries. It has a crucial role in determining the quality of services offered to patients, minimizing the degree of lesions and the number of fatalities. The response time, which is the time between notification of an occurrence and the ambulance arrival at the scene, is the leading EMS service indicator. The ideal response time to emergencies recommended by WHO is less than 8 minutes, but only a few countries, such as South Korea, meet this benchmark. The average response time to emergency calls is 4.2 minutes in Seoul, South Korea, 5.2 minutes in five urban areas, and 7.6 minutes in the regions. Moreover, the average dispatch distance for emergency vehicles is 2.3 km in Seoul, 4.1 km in five metropolitan centers, and 7.1 km in the provinces. The dispatching distances and response times of cities are usually shorter than those of provinces.

The EMS law in the United States stipulates that 95% of emergency calls should be responded to within 10 minutes in urban centers and 30 minutes in rural areas. Similar standards exist in other parts of the world. For example, in London and Montreal, the criteria state that 95% of emergency calls be met within 14–10 minutes, 50 and 70% of emergency calls responded to within 8–7 minutes, respectively (Cabral et al., 2018). The average response time for emergency calls in the United States is 10 minutes, depending on the city and the type of emergency (Fritz, 2020). It is 12.5 minutes in the United Kingdom (BBC News, 2019) and 19.5 minutes in Africa (Cabral et al., 218). In Singapore, the average response time is 11.40 ± 4.88 minutes for an ambulance crew to reach a patient and 30.50 ± 10.62 minutes for the patient to get to the hospital after a call (Seow & Lim, 1993). In urban centers with more than one million inhabitants, the average response time in 2010 for Belo Horizonte in Brazil was about 21 minutes. In the town of São Paulo, in 2007, the response time was 27 minutes. In Vienna, Austria, the average response time in 2015 was 15 minutes; consider 10% dispersion of this value due to vehicles' heavy traffic and climatic conditions (Cabral et al., 2018). Long wait times for treatment are not an issue in the United States than in countries with a universal healthcare system (Blumberg, 2018).

Health Insurance Coverage

As the largest economy in the world since 1871, the United States exemplifies these four principles. The economy's size was $20.58 trillion in 2018 (nominal terms) and reached $22.32 trillion in 2020 (Silver, 2020). Despite the tremendous wealth, the United States does not guarantee accessible health care for its citizens. In 2018, 91.5% of Americans had health insurance coverage, lower than the 92.1% rate in 2017 (Berchick et al., 2019). United States health expenditure as a share of the GDP is expected to rise from 17.8% in 2015 to 19.9% by 2025. Spending on prescription drugs is projected to grow an average of 6.3% annually over the same time. The average American in 2018 spends nearly $4000 toward health care annually, and the number is expected to soar to more than $5000 by 2023 (Franck, 2018).

Between 2010 and 2012, about 79 million Americans, more than one in four—either lacked health insurance or were underinsured (Chokshi, 2014). To address these challenges, the 111th Congress in the United States enacted a good law called the Affordable Care Act (ACA), or colloquially known as Obamacare, to provide health insurance coverage for all Americans and protect consumers' preexisting medical conditions from being denied insurance. It was signed into law by President Barack Obama on March 23, 2010. From the start, because of bad politics, the ACA was highly controversial and passed through Congress without a single Republican vote, despite its economic and health outcomes merits. Republicans opposed the ACA proposals because they argued that it would bankrupt the nation, adversely impact the quality of care, increase tax and higher insurance premiums, and impose additional workload on HCWs and increase costs (Healthline, 2020). To advance their argument, at least on 70 different occasions, Republicans attempted but failed to repeal, modify, or curb the ACA (Riotta, 2017).

Several of the Republican skepticisms about the ACA were later found to be baseless. Within 5 years of the ACA's implementation, more than 16 million Americans, particularly young adults, the poor, people with disabilities, the unemployed, and individuals with low-paying jobs, obtained health insurance coverage. A decade after the ACA was initiated, objective evidence revealed that the landmark health legislation helped reduce the rate of growth of healthcare spending, which currently consumes nearly one-fifth of the United States' GDP. The most considerable savings were from the value-based payment programs, which created incentives for HCWs and hospitals to deliver high-quality care at a lowered cost (Buntin & Graves, 2020; Department of Health Policy (2020). Despite the savings outcome evidence, on June 26, 2020, President Trump's administration appealed to the Supreme Court to overturn the ACA (Stolberg, 2020).

On June 17, 2021, the United States Supreme Court, in a seven to two decision, turned down the latest effort by the Trump administration and the urging of 18 Republican state attorneys general to strike down the ACA as unconstitutional (Liptak, 2021). Before the Supreme Court's decision, the Biden administration reversed the Trump administration's Justice Department position. For now, the ACA remains the law of the land, and many legal scholars across the political spectrum view the argument against it as extremely weak (Center on Budget and Policy

Priorities, 2021). As a result of the decision by the United States Supreme Court, some 23 million Americans would now retain their insurance benefit.

In the last decade, many countries around the world had made great strides toward achieving universal health care. Unfortunately, over 95% of the population is uninsured in Nigeria, even though the country has a good healthcare law enacted on October 31, 2014, by former President Goodluck Jonathan (National Health Act, 2014). Ten years in the making, the law provided a legal framework for the regulation, development, and management of the health system, including access to primary care for vulnerable populations, such as persons with disabilities, women, children, and the elderly (National Health Insurance Scheme, 2020). The legislation made mandatory the provision of emergency health services by healthcare providers and health establishments. Failure to do so is a crime. Another notable provision of the law is the minister of health's authority to establish a framework for identifying individuals eligible for free health services (Goitom, 2014). Fifteen years after the enactment of good health law, sadly, because of a lack of political will and ineffective leadership at the national level, less than 5% of the population has health insurance coverage (Awosusi et al., 2015; Ifijeh, 2015; NOIPolls, 2017; Amu et al., 2018; Aregbeshola & Khan, 2018). Given that the United States spends about twice as much money on health care per capita as the average OECD country, 8.5% of the population is uninsured. Many Americans go bankrupt over medical bills; therefore, the US health system is not a "shining city on the hill" that Nigeria can emulate in health financing.

Achieving expanded health care and good health outcomes require efficient management of available resources by reducing duplication and waste. Shrank et al. (2019) estimated the cost of waste in the US healthcare system ranged from $760 to $935 billion, accounting for about 25% of the total healthcare spending. The waste is due to administrative costs that include time and resources devoted to billing, reporting to insurers, public programs, overtreatment, excess utilization of high-tech instrumentation, and overpayment totaling $266 billion a year (Frakt, 2019; Shrank et al., 2019). Other reasons for the health system's inefficiencies include failure to coordinate care, failures in processes that execute maintenance, administrative complexity, pricing failures (such as wide variations in charges for procedures and lack of transparency), fraud, and abuse (Martinez et al., 2016). Additionally, government regulations introduced inefficiencies serendipitously meant to reduce the number of patients a physician can consult due to increased time spent on documentation and public health issues. These initiatives have curtailed physicians/dentists' time available for direct patient care.

Health Expenditure

Aka (2020) argued that the four hallmarks of a sound health system are fair laws, adequate funding, acceptance of the principle that health care is a human right issue rather than a privilege, and good politics. These principles will be used as the guiding framework for the argument advanced within this comparative analysis.

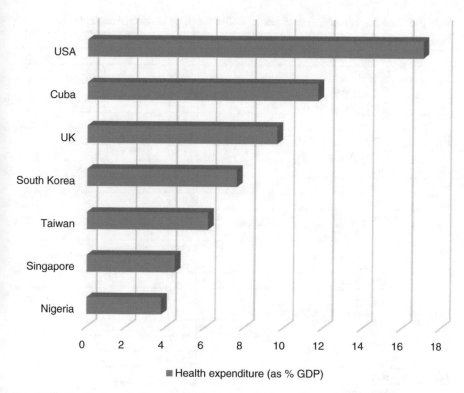

Fig. 10.8 Healthcare spending (as % of GDP) in Nigeria and the six model health systems. (Source: CIA, 2017)

Adequate funding is the "mother's milk" of any healthcare system and the key to healthcare access and good outcomes. Unfortunately, in some countries, high healthcare expenditure does not produce corresponding health outcomes. Again, the US health system exemplifies this paradox. The healthcare expenditure in the United States is the highest in the world. In 2017, healthcare expenditure (as % of GPD) in the United States was 17.06%, but only 11.71% in Cuba and 6.1% in Taiwan (Fig. 10.8). Yet, the two less advanced countries had better health outcome indicators than the United States.

Table 10.3 presents the global ranking of health spending as a proportion of the GDP in selected UN member countries worldwide. The health expenditure in Nigeria as a share of its GDP is relatively low compared to other countries globally. According to the Central Intelligence Agency (CIA) World Fact Book, Nigeria ranks 109th out of 191 countries on the GDP spent on health (CIA, 2017). Repeatedly, Nigeria falls short of its 2001 Abuja commitment to spend at least 15% of its budget on health while two African countries (Liberia and Sierra Leone) met this benchmark (NOIPolls, 2017). In 2019, the expenditure on health care in Nigeria declined further; only 3.9% was allocated to the health sector (Adegoke, 2019).

Table 10.3 Ranking of health expenditure (as a % of the GDP) in selected countries

Rank	Country	Expenditure as a % of the GDP
1	United States	17.90
3	Liberia	15.50
5	Sierra Leone	15.10
7	The Netherlands	12.40
	Cuba	11.70
10	Lesotho	11.60
13	Germany	11.30
26	Spain	9.60
30	United Kingdom	9.40
35	Malawi	9.20
37	Australia	9.10
42	South Africa	8.80
45	Togo	8.60
58	Uganda	8.00
	South Korea	7.60
109	Nigeria	6.10
123	Democratic Republic of the Congo	5.60
126	China	5.40
139	Cameroon	5.10
142	Egypt	5.00
148	Kenya	4.70
	Singapore	4.40
169	Bangladesh	3.60

Source: Central Intelligence Agency, 2017. *The World Factbook*: https://www.cia.gov/library/publications/the-world-factbook/

Philanthropy

Of the six model countries, Cuba ranks number one in providing humanitarian assistance to the global community. Cuba's healthcare system is globally reputed for giving medical aid in multiple countries and worthy of close study, particularly in developing countries. It has the highest supply of physicians in the world at 8.4 per 1000 people. On the other extreme, Nigeria only has 0.4 physicians per 1000 people. Education and health care are the two jewels in the Cuban crown because they offer more physicians to the developing world than the G8 countries combined (Lopez, 2019). Besides, they routinely provide free medical aid and services to the international community (especially third-world countries) following natural disasters.

Cuba currently exports essential health services and personnel: Over 25,000 Cuban physicians are in 68 countries worldwide. They typically served in crises such as the South Asian tsunami and the 2005 Kashmir earthquake. More than 20,000 children from Russia, Ukraine, and Belarus have traveled to Cuba to receive treatment for radiation sickness and psychologically based problems associated with the radiation disaster since the Chernobyl nuclear plant exploded in 1986. Following the 2005 Hurricane Katrina disaster, Castro offered to send 1500 physicians to provide humanitarian aid, but the US government rejected the offer. In 2020, over 2000 Cuban physicians served in South Africa, assisting with managing the coronavirus disease 2019 (COVID-19) pandemic. Cuban physicians also provide medical assistance in the Gambia, Guinea Mali, and Bissau.

Additionally, Cuba also exports personnel and medical products such as vaccines to Venezuela in exchange for subsidized oil. For more than two decades, Cuba has annually hosted about 20,000 medical tourists generating over $40 million for the economy. The health system operates specialized hospitals for patients and diplomats from Latin America, Europe, and Canada.

Although the United States healthcare system has poor health outcomes and struggles with inequity and access issues, there are several areas that the system is the envy of the world. An example is the humanitarianism towards the vulnerable population. United States hospitals are undoubtedly some of the most advanced, comfortable, and accommodating in the world. While in some countries, there are over a dozen patients in a single large room with difficulty separating men and women into different places—a fundamental compromise of human dignity. Despite the challenges associated with access to care, in emergencies, no American is denied treatment. A homeless patient admitted to the hospital with an acute health problem—such as a stroke, sepsis, or myocardial infarction—will receive better care than the elite in most countries worldwide. The university-affiliated hospitals in the United States lead the world in research and development. The achievements range the gamut from life-saving newest medications to high-tech invasive surgical procedures such as heart stents. American hospitals conduct the most clinical trials globally, leading to immediate access to advanced therapeutics (Dhand, 2014; Lubin, 2010).

Cost of Health Service Delivery

The cost of service and medication provided in the six countries assessed is the ultimate test of an affordable health system. The United States is well known for overspending on health care. The annual per capita spending was $9403 in 2019. It nearly doubled what other high-income countries spent (Blumberg, 2018). What sets the United States apart from other nations is the inflated prices for most services.

To allow for objective comparison of health service delivery cost globally, the WHO in 2010 published the average unit cost values for primary and secondary health care services for its 191 member states based on specific assumptions regarding the organization's health services and operational capacity (WHO, 2010). Singapore (1054/63), Switzerland (847/55), United States (834/53), and the Netherlands (732/48) had the highest cost for inpatient and outpatient health service deliveries among the 15 model countries. The most expensive inpatient and outpatient health service deliveries among the WHO member states are in Monaco (2724/128),

Luxembourg (1644/90), and Qatar (1447/80)—both inpatient and outpatient costs were reported in international dollars (purchasing power parities, PPP). As expected, the inpatient and outpatient health service deliveries for African nations are substantially cheaper than in high-income countries. It was 120/5 in South Africa, 24/4 in Nigeria, and only 5/1 in Niger. The hospitals in many African countries are overcrowded and environmentally unsanitary and reflect the nominal cost.

Aside from the inpatient and outpatient health service deliveries, the cost of hospital services and diagnostic tests in the United States is higher than in similarly situated high-income countries worldwide. In 2013, the average price for a coronary artery bypass graft surgery in the United States was $75,345, $15,742 in the Netherlands, and $36,509 in Switzerland. The average price for a computed tomography scan was $896 compared to $97 in Canada, $279 in the Netherlands, $432 in Switzerland, and $500 in Australia. An MRI costs $1145 in the United States, $350 in Australia, and $461 in the Netherlands (Blumberg, 2018). In 2017, an angioplasty procedure in the United States cost $32,200, $16,500 in New Zealand, $14,700 in Australia, $11,900 in UAE, but only $7400 in Switzerland, 9000 in South Africa, and $6400 in Holland (Hargraves and Bloschichak, 2019). An MRI scan in the United States costs $1420, but only $450 in the United Kingdom (Sanger-Katz, 2019).

The per capita expenditure on prescription drugs in the United States is $1011 a year. Sweden spends $351, while other nations such as France, the United Kingdom, and Australia pay about half the amount in the United States (Fig. 10.9). Despite the high cost of prescription medications, empirical evidence revealed that Americans are less reliant and use fewer prescription drugs and are more likely to use cheaper generic versions than their European counterparts (Haeder, 2019).

Prescription drugs in the United States cost an average of 56% more than in other high-income countries. For example, France's medication cost is only one-third of the United States' price and under two-thirds of Japan's. The prices for cardiovascular,

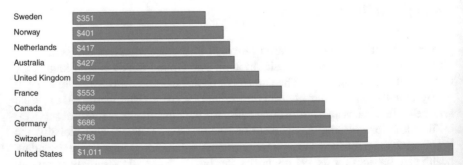

Fig. 10.9 The per capita expenses on prescription drugs in selected countries. (Reproduced from Haeder, S. F. (2019 Feb 7). Why the US has higher drug prices than other countries. *The Conversation.* https://theconversation.com/why-the-us-has-higher-drug-prices-than-other-countries-111256, licensed under the terms of the Creative Commons Attribution License (https://creativecommons.org/licenses/by-nd/4.0/). Source: The Commonwealth Fund Get the data

musculoskeletal, and nervous system drugs were among the cheapest in other high-income countries, averaging 80% less expensive than in the United States (Miller, 2020). For example, Herceptin injection, a critical breast cancer treatment, costs $211 in the United States but only $44 in South Africa (Papanicolas et al., 2018; Sanger-Katz, 2019). A 10 mL bottle of insulin in the United States costs $450, and a comparable bottle costs only $21 at the US-Canadian border. Given the price disparity, over 19 million Americans (8% of the population) annually import medication from Canada or other countries.

There are no government-controlled checks on prices in the United States, and the consumers bore the full brunt of the expensive cost for the development and production of new drugs. The costs are increased further by marketing expenses and profit accrued by all the pharmaceutical industry supply chain sectors. The lack of transparency within the industry creates conditions favorable to limited market competition and price maximization. The pharmaceutical supply chain is exceptionally skilled at finding regulatory loopholes that allow them to maximize profits by creatively expanding the duration of patents or having them reclassified as "orphan drugs" for rare diseases to preserve monopolies (Haeder, 2019).

In the United States, entrepreneurship among HCWs occasionally leads to abuse. Still, innovation and the use of cutting-edge technologies for evaluation and treatment are the bedrock of the private sector. The United States' health care is nonpareil because Americans embrace the idea that you get what you pay for. Upper-middle-class Americans can afford to pay for comprehensive health insurance to access the most extensive network of hospitals, specialists, and technology (Dhand, 2014; Lubin, 2010).

Manpower Shortage

More than one-quarter of all physicians (247,000) practicing in the United States trained abroad. The demand is expected to outpace supply, leading to a projected shortfall of between 46,100 and 90,400 physicians by 2025. These shortages are compounded by the fact that many physicians will be retiring in the next few years (American Immigration Council, 2018). Furthermore, more than 12% of the health care workforce in the United Kingdom is foreign nationals. The largest group of foreign physicians is from the European Union—56 physicians out of every 1000. Outside the European Union, there were 12,610 Indian and 4659 Pakistan physicians, followed by 2014 Egyptian and 1903 Nigerian physicians (Reality Check, 2019).

The largest number of nurses in the United Kingdom is from the Philippines (10,719) and India (6656), with smaller numbers from European Union countries such as Ireland (4608), Spain (3370), Portugal (3190), and Zimbabwe (2450)

(Reality Check, 2019). In 2018, the number of nurses from outside Europe soared from 2724 to 6157—a 126% increase. The primary attractive destinations for job opportunities by Nigerian healthcare professionals are the United Kingdom and the United States (NOIPolls, 2017).

Health Worker Remuneration

The world is increasingly becoming a global village with many highly skilled HCWs crossing national boundaries searching for better opportunities in other parts of the world. For healthcare professionals planning to relocate to another country for better career opportunities, it is crucial to be familiar with the remuneration. As shown in Fig. 10.10, the United States offers the highest pay for physicians and attracts the best HCWs globally (Rampell, 2009). Chapter 13 compares the salary for the major healthcare professions in Nigeria, the United Kingdom, and the United States.

Physicians in the United States and Europe are paid better than their counterparts in Africa. An outpatient and emergency physician in Ghana earn an annual gross salary of GH¢40,000, equivalent to ₦2, 863,163. The amount in naira is approximately ₦240 000 ($600) monthly salary (PayScale 2020). Similarly, Sierra Leone's physicians earn up to $2000 per month, translating to roughly ₦700 000. In contrast, physicians employed by the federal government receive a monthly salary of ₦195,000–₦220,000. Their peers in state government hospitals earn between ₦150,000 and ₦240,000. However, physicians employed by private hospitals are paid as low as ₦80,000 (GH¢1118) monthly (NOIPolls, 2017).

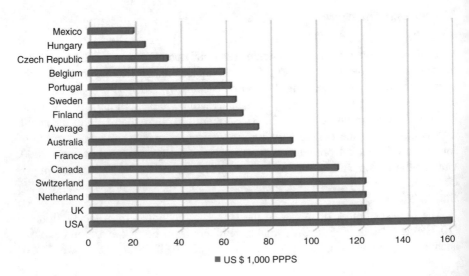

Fig. 10.10 Physician's salary in selected countries around the world (in US $1000 purchasing power parity scale). (Source: Kane et al., 2019)

Conclusion

After an exhaustive review of the literature, 15 stellar health systems worldwide were identified—United States, United Kingdom, Switzerland, Canada, Germany, Australia, South Korea, Cuba, the Netherlands, New Zealand, France, Japan, Finland, Singapore, and Taiwan. Subsequently, six countries (United States, United Kingdom, Singapore, South Korea, Taiwan, and Cuba) were selected for in-depth comparative analysis on several health indices. Of the six high-performing systems, Singapore had the highest life expectancy (84.07 years), while Cuba had the largest physician workforce (8.4 per 1000 people). The United States is the leader in innovation, health system responsiveness, and biotechnology development, with a market size of roughly $120 billion. Healthcare spending in the United States is the highest globally (17.9% of GDP), but 8.5% of Americans are uninsured. The system is among the poorest on several health indicators, such as life expectancy and infant/maternal mortality rates. Singapore had the lowest mortality rate (2 per 1000 live births), while the United Kingdom had the lowest maternal mortality rate (7 per 100,000 live births). Hospital services and diagnostic tests cost more in the United States than in other countries around the world.

The common elements among the six model health systems include a charismatic leader who can marshal a stable political system that will support and institutionalize universal health care, a functional national health insurance scheme backed by robust government funding. Other elements are a state-of-the-art nationalized health information system, a health service delivery that focuses on disease prevention rather than curative care, and an efficient administrative monitoring system to detect waste and corruption. Cuban health care, based on the *socialized medicine* payer system with primary care as its cornerstone, is the best adaptable and suitable for Nigeria.

Like Cuba, primary care is the cornerstone of the Nigerian health system. The government currently provides partially free health care in many states, and the government is the primary employer of HCWs in the country. The Cuban health care education's unique features can be integrated into the curricula and adapted to fit the Nigerian sociocultural milieu. After all, Singapore blended the best socialist and capitalist ideologies to create a growing and thriving health system. Indeed, Nigeria can do the same.

Case Study

Identify on the world map (see Fig. 10.11) the following 15 countries with stellar healthcare systems: United States, United Kingdom, Switzerland, Canada, Germany, Australia, South Korea, Cuba, the Netherlands, New Zealand, France, Japan, Finland, Singapore, and Taiwan.

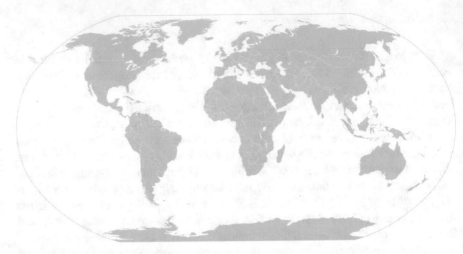

Fig. 10.11 World Map. (Source: Canuckguy (2021). Blank World Map. Adapted from File: "Political World" CIA World Factbook map 2005.svg, released under the terms of CC0)

References

Adegoke, Y. (2019, April 25). Does Nigeria have too many doctors to worry about a 'brain drain'? *BBC* Africa, Lagos. [online]. Available at: https://www.bbc.com/news/world-africa-45473036. Accessed 10 Oct 2020.

Advisory Board. (2019, May 17). Some call Singapore the best health system in the world. So how does it really work? *Advisory Board*. [online]. Available at: https://www.advisory.com/daily-briefing/2019/05/17/singapore. Accessed 10 Oct 2020.

Aka, C. (2020). Genetic counseling and preventive medicine in Bosnia and Herzegovina. *California Western International Law Journal, 50*(2), Article 2. [Online]. Available at: https://scholarly-commons.law.cwsl.edu/cwilj/vol50/iss2/2. Accessed 10 Oct 2020.

American Immigration Council. (2018, January). Foreign-trained doctors are critical to serving many U.S. communities. *Special report*. [online]. Available at: https://www.americanimmigrationcouncil.org/sites/default/files/research/foreign-trained_doctors_are_critical_to_serving_many_us_communities.pdf. Accessed 10 Oct 2020.

Amu, H., Dickson, K. S., Kumi-Kyereme, A., & Darteh, E. K. M. (2018). Understanding variations in health insurance coverage in Ghana, Kenya, Nigeria, and Tanzania: Evidence from demographic and health surveys. *PLoS ONE, 13*(8), e0201833. [online]. Available at: https://journals.plos.org/plosone/article?id=10.1371/journal.pone.0201833. Accessed 10 Oct 2020.

Aregbeshola, B. S., & Khan S. M. (2018). Predictors of enrolment in the national health insurance scheme among women of reproductive age in Nigeria. *International Journal of Health Policy Management, 7*(11), 1015–1023. [online]. Available at: https://www.ncbi.nlm.nih.gov/pmc/articles/PMC6326643/. Accessed 10 Oct 2020.

Awosusi, A, Folaranmi, T, & Yates, R. (2015). *Nigeria's new government and public financing for universal health coverage*. [online]. Available at: https://www.thelancet.com/journals/langlo/article/PIIS2214-109X(15)00088-1/fulltext. Accessed 16 Oct 2020.

AXA.com. (2019, May 24). Nigeria: Laying the groundwork for safe, quality healthcare. *AXA Magazine*. [online]. Available at: https://www.axa.com/en/magazine/nigeria-laying-the-groundwork-for-safe-quality-healthcare. Accessed 16 Oct 2020.

BBC News. (2019, March 15). *Police 999 response times almost double in seven years.* [online]. Available at: https://www.bbc.com/news/uk-england-manchester-47582743#:~:text=The%20 average%20response%20time%20for,2011%2C%20new%20data%20has%20revealed. Accessed 10 Oct 2020.

Berchick, E. R., Barnett, J. C., & Upton, R. D. (2019). Health insurance coverage in the United States: 2018. *US Census Bureau. Report Number P60-267 (RV).* [online]. Available at: https:// www.census.gov/library/publications/2019/demo/p60-267.html#:~:text=The%20percent-age%20of%20people%20with,in%20201. Accessed 10 Oct 2020.

Blumberg, Y. (2018). Here's the real reason health care costs so much more in the US. Sep 3. *CNBC LLC.* [online]. Available at: https://www.cnbc.com/2018/03/22/the-real-reason-medical-care-costs-so-much-more-in-the-us.html. Accessed 10 Oct 2020.

Boseley S. (2018) Getting results: *why NHS clinical trials are the envy of the world.* [online]. Available at: https://www.theguardian.com/society/2018/jul/05/nhs-clinicaltrials-other-countries-envious-getting-results. Accessed: 10 October 2020.

Briney, A. (2019). Geography of the United States of America. *ThoughtCo.* [online]. Available at: https://www.thoughtco.com/geography-the-united-states-of-america-1435745. Accessed 10 Oct 2020.

Brookings.edu. (2016). *Chapter 1: The Singapore healthcare system: An overview.* [online]. Available at: https://www.brookings.edu/wp-content/uploads/2016/07/affordableexcellence_chapter.pdf. Accessed 10 Oct 2020.

Brown, L. D. (2003). Comparing health systems in four countries: Lessons for the United States. *American Journal of Public Health, 93*(1), 52–56. https://doi.org/10.2105/ajph.93.1.52. [online]. Available at: https://www.ncbi.nlm.nih.gov/pmc/articles/PMC1447691/. Accessed 27 July 2021.

Buntin, M. B., & Graves, J. A. (2020). How the ACA dented the cost curve. *Health Affairs, 39*(3). [online]. Available at: https://www.healthaffairs.org/doi/abs/10.1377/hlthaff.2019.01478. Accessed 10 Oct 2020.

Cabral, E., Castro, W., Florentino, D., Viana, D., Junior, J., Souza, R., Rêgo III, A., Araújo-Filho, I., & Medeiros, A. (2018). Response time in the emergency services: Systematic review. *Acta Cirúrgica Brasileira, 33*(12). [online]. Available at: https://www.scielo.br/scielo. php?script=sci_arttext&pid=S0102-86502018001201110. Accessed 10 Oct 2020.

Canuckguy. (2021). *Blank world map.* [Image]. Retrieved from Wikimedia Commons: https:// commons.wikimedia.org/wiki/File:BlankMap-World.svg. Accessed 13 July 2021.

Carroll, A. E. (2019). *What can the US health system learn from Singapore?* [online]. Available at: https://www.nytimes.com/2019/04/22/upshot/singapore-health-system-lessons.html. Accessed 10 Oct 2020.

Carroll, A. E., & Frakt, A. (2017). The best health care system in the World: Which one would you pick? *New York Times.* [online]. Available at: https://www.nytimes.com/interactive/2017/09/18/ upshot/best-health-care-system-country-bracket.html. Accessed 27 July 2021.

Center on Budget and Policy Priorities. (2021). *Suit challenging ACA legally suspect but threatens loss of coverage for tens of millions.* [online]. Available at: https://www.cbpp.org/sites/default/ files/atoms/files/11-4-19health2.pdf. Accessed 19 Mar 2021.

Central Intelligence Agency (CIA). (2017). *The world factbook.* [online]. Available at: https:// www.cia.gov/library/publications/the-world-factbook/geos/tw.html. Accessed 10 Oct 2020.

Chokshi (2014) *Historians take note: What America looked like before Obamacare.* [online]. Available at: https://www.washingtonpost.com/blogs/govbeat/wp/2014/03/26/historians-take-note-what-america-looked-like-before-obamacare/. Accessed: 10 October 2020.

Chun, C. B., Kim, S. Y., Lee, J. Y., & Lee, S. Y. (2009). Republic of Korea: Health system review. *Health Systems in Transition, 11*(7), 1–184. [online]. Available at: https://www.euro.who.int/__ data/assets/pdf_file/0019/101476/E93762.pdf. Accessed 19 Mar 2021.

CMS.gov. (2019) National Health Expenditure Projections 2018–2027: *Forecast Summary 2018-2027 FINAL.pdf.* [online]. Available at: file:///C:/Users/Admin/AppData/Local/

Microsoft/Windows/INetCache/IE/AI96FJRO/Forecast%20Summary%202018-2027%20 FINAL.pdf. Accessed: 10 October 2020.

Department of Health Policy. (2020, March 2). *How the ACA dented the health care cost curve*. [online]. Available at: https://www.vumc.org/health-policy/affordable-care-act-effect-on-health-care-costs. Accessed 10 Oct 2020.

Dhand, S. (2014, August 5). 5 things that make US health care great. *KevinMD.com*. [online]. Available at: https://www.kevinmd.com/blog/2014/08/5-things-make-u-s-health-care-great. html. Accessed 10 Oct 2020.

Du, L., & Lu, W. (2016). *U.S. healthcare system ranks as one of the least-efficient: America is number 50 out of 55 countries that were assessed*. [online]. Available at: https://www.bloomberg. com/news/articles/2016-09-29/u-s-health-care-system-ranks-as-one-of-the-least-efficient. Accessed 10 Oct 2020.

Duncan, P., & Jowit, J. (2018). Is the NHS the world's best healthcare system? *Guardian News & Media Limited*. [online]. Available at: https://www.theguardian.com/society/2018/jul/02/is-the-nhs-the-worlds-best-healthcare-system. Accessed 19 Mar 2021.

Farouq, S. (2019). Cuba's healthcare system: A political, social, and economic revolution. *Berkeley Political Review*. [online]. Available at: https://bpr.berkeley.edu/2019/02/09/cubas-healthcare-system-a-political-social-and-economic-revolution/. Accessed 10 Oct 2020.

Frakt, A. (2019). The huge waste in the US health system – *The New York Times*. [online]. Available at: https://www.nytimes.com/2019/10/07/upshot/health-care-waste-study.html. Accessed 10 Oct 2020.

Franck, T. (2018, January 30). This chart of surging US health-care costs explains why these titans of business are getting involved. *CNBC Markets*. [online]. Available at: https://www.cnbc. com/2018/01/30/chart-of-surging-us-health-care-costs-explains-why-buffett-getting-involved. html. Accessed 10 Oct 2020.

Fritz, J. (2020, June 3). *What is the average police response time in the US?* [online]. Available at: https://www.safesmartliving.com/home-security/average-police-response-time/#:~:text=The%20average%20response%20time%20for,on%20the%20type%20of%20 emergency. Accessed 10 Oct 2020.

Fullman, N., et al., (2018). Measuring performance on the healthcare access and quality index for 195 countries and territories and selected subnational locations: A systematic analysis from the global burden of disease study 2016. *Lancet, 391*, 2236–2271. [online]. Available at: https:// www.thelancet.com/journals/lancet/article/PIIS0140-6736(18)30994-2/fulltext. Accessed 10 Oct 2020.

GAVI CSO Project. (2013). What are the health system building blocks? *Fact Sheet No. 5*. [online]. Available at: https://mail.google.com/mail/u/2/#inbox/KtbxLwgtBNMVMlDjFgwmTqZWWz FSGKqcDB?projector=1&messagePartId=0.1. Accessed 10 Oct 2020.

Goitom, H. (2014). *Nigeria: National health bill enacted*. [online]. Available at: https://www.loc. gov/law/foreign-news/article/nigeria-national-health-bill-enacted/. Accessed 10 Oct 2020.

Gómez-Dantés, O. (2018). Cuba's health system: Hardly an example to follow. *Health Policy and Planning, 33*(6), 760–761. [online]. Available at: https://academic.oup.com/heapol/article/33/6/760/5035053. Accessed 10 Oct 2020.

Haeder, S. F. (2019, February 7). Why the US has higher drug prices than other countries. *The Conversation US, Inc.* [online]. Available at: https://theconversation.com/why-the-us-has-higher-drug-prices-than-other-countries-111256. Accessed 10 Oct 2020.

Hargraves, J., & Bloschichak, A. (2019). International comparisons of health care prices from the 2017 iFHP survey. *Health Care Cost Institute Inc.* [online]. Available at: https://healthcostinstitute.org/in-the-news/international-comparisons-of-health-care-prices-2017-ifhp-survey. Accessed 10 Oct 2020.

HCT Advisor. (2018). *$3.67 Trillion: 2018 US healthcare spending by category*. [online]. Available at: https://hctadvisor.com/2018/01/3-67-trillion-2018-us-healthcare-spending-category/. Accessed 10 Oct 2020.

Health Consumer Powerhouse. (2015). *Outcomes in EHCI*. [online]. Available at: https://web.archive.org/web/20170606082345/http://www.healthpowerhouse.com/files/EHCI_2015/EHCI_2015_report.pdf. Accessed 19 Mar 2021.

Healthmanagement.org. (2006) *Health Departments*. [online]. Available at: https://web.archive.org/web/20061106183151/. http://www.ndad.nationalarchives.gov.uk/AH/21/detail.html Accessed: 10 October 2020.

Healthline. (2020). *The pros and cons of Obamacare*. [online]. Available at: https://www.healthline.com/health/consumer-healthcare-guide/pros-and-cons-obamacare. Accessed 10 Oct 2020.

Healthline Media. (2015). *Lessons the US can learn from Singapore's health system*. [online]. Available at: https://www.healthline.com/health-news/us-can-learn-from-singapore-health-system#1. Accessed 10 Oct 2020.

Health-Tourism.com. (2008). *Medical tourism to South Korea*. [online]. Available at: https://www.health-tourism.com/medical-tourism-south-korea/. Accessed 19 Mar 2021.

Helliwell, J. F., Sachs, J. D., & Leyva, G. (2019). *Happiness and community: An overview*. [online]. Available at: https://worldhappiness.report/. Accessed 10 Oct 2020.

Herper, M. (2011). *The most innovative countries in biology and medicine*. [online]. Available at: https://www.forbes.com/sites/matthewherper/2011/03/23/the-most-innovative-countries-in-biology-and-medicine/#16becbae1a71 and https://healthinformatics.uic.edu/blog/the-4-top-countries-for-health-tech-development/. Accessed 24 Oct 2020.

Human Rights Watch. (2017). *Singapore: Laws chill free speech, assembly*. [online]. Available at: https://www.hrw.org/news/2017/12/13/singapore-laws-chill-free-speech-assembly. Accessed 19 Mar 2021.

Ifijeh, M. (2015, November 12). Only five percent of Nigerians are covered by health insurance. *This Day Newspaper*. [online]. Available at: http://allafrica.com/stories/201511121412.html. Accessed 16 Oct 2020.

Infoplease. (2007). *Physicians per 100,000 people, by country*. [online]. Available at: https://www.infoplease.com/world/health-and-social-statistics/physicians-100000-people-country. Accessed 24 Oct 2020.

Jacobson, L. (2014). *Tom Harkin says Cuba has lower child mortality, longer life expectancy than US*. [online]. Available at: https://www.politifact.com/factchecks/2014/jan/31/tom-harkin/sen-tom-harkin-says-cuba-has-lower-child-mortality/. Accessed 10 Oct 2020.

Kane, L., Schubsky, B., Locke, T., Kouimtz, M., Duqueroy, V., Gottschling, C., Lopez, M., & Leoleli Schwartz, L. (2019). International physician compensation report 2019: Do US physicians have it best? *Medscape*. [online]. Available at: https://www.medscape.com/slideshow/2019-international-compensation-report-6011814. Accessed 10 Oct 2020.

KBS World Radio. (2018). *S. Korea ranks 23rd in annual democracy survey, N. Korea remains last*. [online]. Available at: https://world.kbs.co.kr/service/news_view.htm?lang=e&Seq_Code=150841. Accessed 19 Mar 2021.

Keck, C. W., & Reed, G. A. (2012). The curious case of Cuba. *American Journal of Public Health, 102*(8), e13–e22. https://doi.org/10.2105/AJPH.2012.300822. https://www.ncbi.nlm.nih.gov/pmc/articles/PMC3464859/.

Klein, E. (2017, April 25). Is Singapore's "miracle" healthcare system the answer for America? *Vox*. [online]. Available at: https://www.vox.com/policy-and-politics/2017/4/25/15356118/singapore-health-care-system-explained. Accessed 10 Oct 2020.

Kwon, S., Lee, T. J., & Kim, C. Y. (2015). *Republic of Korea health system review*. 5(4). Manila: World Health Organization, Regional Office for the Western Pacific. [online]. Available at: http://www.searo.who.int/entity/asia_pacific_observatory/publications/hits/hit_korea/en/. Accessed 10 Oct 2020.

LaingBuisson International Limited. (2020). *Healthcare in South Korea*. [online]. Available at: https://www.treatmentabroad.com/destinations/south-korea/healthcare-system-south-korea. Accessed 10 Oct 2020.

Lee, C. E. (2020). International health care system profiles: Singapore. *The Commonwealth Fund*. [online]. Available at: https://www.commonwealthfund.org/international-health-policy-center/countries/singapore. Accessed 27 July 2021.

Library of Congress. (2005). *Country profile: Taiwan*. [online]. Available at: https://web.archive.org/web/20150329124349/http://lcweb2.loc.gov/frd/cs/profiles/Taiwan.pdf.   Accessed   19 Mar 2021.

Liptak, A. (2021, June 17). Affordable care act survives latest supreme court challenge. *The New York Times*. [online]. Available at: https://www.nytimes.com/2021/06/17/us/obamacare-supreme-court.html. Accessed 17 June 2021.

Lopez, D. (2019). Modernizing the Cuban healthcare system by updating medical immigration rules. *Harvard Public Health Review, 22*. [online]. Available at: http://harvardpublichealthreview.org/cubanhealthcare/. Accessed 10 Oct 2020.

Lubin, G. (2010, March 10). 10 reasons why the US healthcare system is the envy of the world. *Business Insider*. [online]. Available at: https://www.businessinsider.com/10-reasons-why-the-us-health-care-system-is-the-envy-of-the-world-2010-3. Accessed 10 Oct 2020.

Magarya. (2017). *WHO ranks Nigeria 187 out of 190 in world health systems?* [online]. Available at: https://magarya.wordpress.com/2017/02/19/who-ranks-nigeria-ranks-187-out-of-190-in-world-health-systems/. Accessed 10 Oct 2020.

Mao Tse-tung. (1947). *Greet the new high tide of the Chinese revolution*. [online]. Available at: https://www.marxists.org/reference/archive/mao/selected-works/volume-4/mswv4_17.htm#bm7. Accessed 19 Mar 2021.

Martinez, J. C., King, M. P., & Cauchi, R. (2016). Improving the healthcare system: Seven state strategies. *National Conference of State Legislatures*. [online]. Available at: https://www.ncsl.org/Portals/1/Documents/Health/ImprovingHealthSystemsBrief16.pdf. Accessed 10 Oct 2020.

Meyer, H. (2019, February 20). Healthcare spending will hit 19.4% of GDP in the next decade, CMS projects. *Crain, Modern Healthcare*. [online]. Available at: https://www.modernhealthcare.com/article/20190220/NEWS/190229989/healthcare-spending-will-hit-19-4-of-gdp-in-the-next-decade-cms-projects; https://www.cms.gov/Research-Statistics-Data-and-Systems/Statistics-Trends-and-Reports/NationalHealthExpendData/Downloads/ForecastSummary.pdf. Accessed 10 Oct 2020.

Miller, E. (2020). U.S. drug price vs the world. *Drugwatch*. [online]. Available at: https://www.drugwatch.com/featured/us-drug-prices-higher-vs-world/. Accessed 10 Oct 2020.

Ministry of Health. (2019). *Singapore's healthcare system*. [online]. Available at: https://www.moh.gov.sg/home/our-healthcare-system. Accessed 10 Oct 2020.

National Academy of Sciences. (2003). *Uninsurance in America: Spending on health care for uninsured Americans: How much, and who pays?* [online]. Available at: https://www.ncbi.nlm.nih.gov/books/NBK221653/. Accessed 10 Oct 2020.

National Health Insurance Scheme. (2020). [online]. Available at: https://www.nhis.gov.ng/about-us/#. Accessed 10 Oct 2020.

National-Health-Act. (2014). *Federal Republic of Nigeria: Official Gazette; # 145 Vol 101. Oct 27*. [online]. Available at: https://nigeriahealthwatch.com/wp-content/uploads/bsk-pdf-manager/2018/07/01_-Official-Gazette-of-the-National-Health-Act-FGN.pdf.   Accessed   17 Dec 2020.

NationMaster. (2021). *Health Stats: Compare key data on Cuba & United States*. Available at: https://www.nationmaster.com/country-info/compare/Cuba/United-States/Health#2013. Accessed 26 July 2021.

NHS Workforce Statistics. (2020). [online]. Available at: https://digital.nhs.uk/data-and-information/publications/statistical/nhs-workforce-statistics/july-2020. Accessed 19 Mar 2021.

NOIPolls. (2017). *Emigration of Nigerian medical doctors: Survey report*. [online]. Available at: https://noi-polls.com/2018/wp-content/uploads/2019/06/Emigration-of-Doctors-Press-Release-July-2018-Survey-Report.pdf. Accessed 10 Oct 2020.

Numbeo. (2020). *Healthcare index by country 2020*. [online]. Available at: https://www.numbeo.com/health-care/rankings_by_country.jsp. Accessed 10 Oct 2020.

O'Hanlon, C. E., & Harvey, M. (2017). Doing more with less: Lessons from Cuba's healthcare system. *Rand Corporation Blog.* [online]. Available at: https://www.rand.org/blog/2017/10/doing-more-with-less-lessons-from-cubas-health-care.html. Accessed 10 Oct 2020.

OECD. (2002). *Nigeria.* [online]. Available at: https://www.oecd.org/countries/nigeria/1826208.pdf. Accessed 16 Oct 2020.

OECD. (2015). *Health at a glance 2015: OECD indicators.* [online]. Available at: https://read.oecd-ilibrary.org/social-issues-migration-health/health-at-a-glance-2015_health_glance-2015-en#page26; https://read.oecd-ilibrary.org/social-issues-migration-health/health-at-a-glance-2015-en#page4. Accessed 10 Oct 2020.

Onyeji, E. (2020, January 19). Analysis: Why Nigeria's vision 20:2020 was bound to fail. *Premium Times.* [online]. Available at: https://www.premiumtimesng.com/news/top-news/373321-analysis-why-nigerias-vision-202020-was-bound-to-fail.html. Accessed 16 Oct 2020.

Pan American Health Organization – PAHO. (2015). *WHO validates Cuba's elimination of mother-to-child transmission of HIV and syphilis.* [online]. Available at: https://www.paho.org/en/news/30-6-2015-who-validates-cubas-elimination-mother-child-transmission-hiv-and-syphilis. Accessed 10 Dec 2020.

Papanicolas, I., Woskie, L. R., & Jha, A. K. (2018). Health care spending in the United States and other high-income countries. *JAMA, 319*(10), 1024–1039. [online]. Available at: https://jama-network.com/journals/jama/article-abstract/2674671. Accessed 10 Oct 2020.

PayScale. (2020). *Average medical laboratory scientist salary in Nigeria: ₦732,503.* [online]. Available at: https://www.payscale.com/research/NG/Job=Medical_Laboratory_Scientist/Salary. Accessed 10 Oct 2020.

Pew Research Center. (2014). *Global religious diversity.* [online]. Available at: https://www.pewforum.org/2014/04/04/global-religious-diversity/. Accessed 19 Mar 2021.

Rampell, C. (2009, July 15). How much do doctors in other countries make? *Economix.* [online]. Available at: https://economix.blogs.nytimes.com/2009/07/15/how-much-do-doctors-in-other-countries-make/. Accessed 10 Oct 2020.

Reality Check. (2019, May 13). NHS staff shortage: How many doctors and nurses come from abroad? *BBC News.* [online]. Available at: https://www.bbc.com/news/world-48205445. Accessed 10 Oct 2020.

Riotta, C. (2017, July 29). GOP aims to kill Obamacare yet again after failing 70 times. *Newsweek.* [online]. Available at: https://www.newsweek.com/gop-health-care-bill-repeal-and-replace-70-failed-attempts-643832. Accessed 10 Oct 2020.

Sanger-Katz, M. (2019). *In the US, an angioplasty costs $32,000. Elsewhere? Maybe $6,400.* [online]. Available at: https://www.nytimes.com/2019/12/27/upshot/expensive-health-care-world-comparison.html. Accessed 10 Oct 2020.

ScienceDirect. (2020). *Health outcomes.* [online]. Available at: https://www.sciencedirect.com/topics/medicine-and-dentistry/health-outcomes. Accessed 10 Oct 2020.

Scott, D. (2020, Jan 13). Taiwan's single-payer success story – and its lessons for America. *Vox.* [online]. Available at: https://www.vox.com/health-care/2020/1/13/21028702/medicare-for-all-taiwan-health-insurance. Accessed 10 Oct 2020.

Seow, E., & Lim, E. (1993). Ambulance response time to emergency departments. *Singapore Medical Journal, 34*(6), 530–532. [online]. Available at: https://pubmed.ncbi.nlm.nih.gov/8153717/#:~:text=The%20information%20was%20obtained%20from,department%20after%20a%20995%20call. Accessed 10 Oct 2020.

Shrank, W. H., Rogstad, T. L., & Parekh, N. (2019). Waste in the US health care system estimated costs and potential for savings. *JAMA, 322*(15), 1501–1509. [online]. Available at: https://jamanetwork.com/journals/jama/article-abstract/2752664. Accessed 10 Oct 2020.

Silver, C. (2020). The top 20 economies in the world. *Investopedia.* [online]. Available at: https://www.investopedia.com/insights/worlds-top-economies/#:~:text=The%20U.S.%20has%20retained%20its,reach%20%2422.32%20trillion%20in%202020. Accessed 10 Oct 2020.

Singapore Business Review. (2020). *Singapore's healthcare expenditure to hit US$24.6b by 2020.* [online]. Available at: https://sbr.com.sg/healthcare/news/singapores-healthcare-expenditure-hit-us246b-2020. Accessed 10 Oct 2020.

Skrybus, E. (2020, June 11). How does Singapore's healthcare system work? Pacific Prime Singapore. *Health.* [online]. Available at: https://www.pacificprime.sg/blog/singapores-healthcare-system/. Accessed 10 Oct 2020.

Stolberg, S. G. (2020, June 26). Trump administration asks Supreme Court to strike down affordable care act. *New York Times.* [online]. Available at: https://www.nytimes.com/2020/06/26/us/politics/obamacare-trump-administration-supreme-court.html. Accessed 10 Oct 2020.

The Economist Group. (2021). *White paper – Quality of death index 2015.* [online]. Available at: https://www.eiu.com/industry/article/1413563125/white-paper-quality-of-death-index-2015/2015-10-07. Accessed 19 Mar 2021.

The World Bank. (n.d.). *Physicians (per 1,000 people) – Cuba.* [online]. Available at: https://data.worldbank.org/indicator/SH.MED.PHYS.ZS?locations=CU. Accessed 19 Mar 2021.

Tikkanen, R., Osborn, R., Mossialos, E., Djordjevic, A., Lee, G. A., & Earn, C. (2020). *International health care system profiles: Singapore.* [online]. Available at: https://www.commonwealthfund.org/international-health-policy-center/countries/singapore. Accessed 19 Mar 2021.

Tinker, A. (2018). *The top seven healthcare outcome measures and three measurement essentials.* [online]. Available at: https://www.healthcatalyst.com/insights/top-7-healthcare-outcome-measures. Accessed 10 Oct 2020.

Tolbert, J., Orgera, K., & Damico, A. (2020). Key facts about the uninsured population. *The Henry J. Kaiser Family Foundation.* [online]. Available at: www.kff.org/uninsured/issue-brief/key-facts-about-the-uninsured-population/. Accessed 10 Oct 2020.

UK Medical Industry. (2020). [online]. Available at: https://qabany.com/thai-restaurant-jgofdb/562g1y.php?3d782b=uk-medical-industry. Accessed 19 Mar 2021.

Warner, R. (2016). Is the Cuban healthcare system really as great as people claim? *The Conversation.* [online]. Available at: https://theconversation.com/is-the-cuban-healthcare-system-really-as-great-as-people-claim-69526. Accessed 10 Oct 2020.

WHO. (2000). *The world health organization's ranking of the world's health systems, by rank.* [online]. Available at: https://photius.com/rankings/world_health_systems.html. Accessed 10 Oct 2020.

WHO. (2006). The world health report. In *Working together for health* (pp. 1–15). World Health Organization.

WHO. (2010). *Economic analysis and evaluation team. Department of Health Systems Governance and Financing.* [online]. Available at: https://www.who.int/choice/cost-effectiveness/inputs/country_inpatient_outpatient_2010.pdf?ua=1. Accessed 10 Oct 2020.

WHO. (2015). *World health statistics. Part I: Global health indicators.* [online]. Available at: https://www.who.int/gho/publications/world_health_statistics/EN_WHS2015_Part2.pdf. Accessed 10 Oct 2020.

WHO. (2016). *Global health observatory (GHO) data: World health statistics 2016: Monitoring health for the SDGs.* [online]. Available at: https://www.who.int/gho/publications/world_health_statistics/2016/en/. Accessed 10 Oct 2020.

WHO. (2017). *World Bank and WHO: Half the world lacks access to essential health services, 100 million still pushed into extreme poverty because of health expenses.* [online]. Available at: https://www.who.int/news-room/detail/13-12-2017-world-bank-and-who-half-the-world-lacks-access-to-essential-health-services-100-million-still-pushed-into-extreme-poverty-because-of-health-expenses. Accessed 10 Oct 2020.

Worldometer. (2020). *Countries in the world by population.* [online]. Available at: https://www.worldometers.info/world-population/population-by-country/. Accessed 10 Oct 2020.

Worldometer. (n.d.). *Life expectancy of the world population.* [online]. Available at: https://www.worldometers.info/demographics/life-expectancy/. Accessed 10 Oct 2020.

Wu, T. Y., Majeed, A., & Kuo, K. N. (2010). An overview of the healthcare system in Taiwan. *London Journal of Primary Care (Abingdon), 3*(2), 115–119. [online]. Available at: https://www.ncbi.nlm.nih.gov/pmc/articles/PMC3960712/. Accessed 10 Oct 2020.

YCharts, (n.d.). *US GDP as % of world GDP: 23.91% for 2018.* [online]. Available at: https://ycharts.com/indicators/us_gdp_as_a_percentage_of_world_gdp. Accessed 10 Oct 2020.

Chapter 11
A Qualitative Investigation of the Barriers to the Delivery of High-Quality Healthcare Services in Nigeria

Learning Objectives

After reading this chapter, the learner should be able to:

1. Describe the scope and dimension of corruption in the Nigerian health system.
2. Discuss the impact of good leadership in managing the health system.
3. Analyze the seven significant themes identified as barriers to delivering affordable and high-quality healthcare services in Nigeria.

Introduction

A plethora of reviews and critique articles on the Nigerian health system have been published (Fajola et al., 2007; Tam, 2015; Ogbebo, 2015; Orekunrin, 2015; Okpani & Abimbola, 2015; Federal Ministry of Health – FMH, 2016; Julius, 2017; Ajao, 2017; Lopez, 2019; Asakitikpi, 2019; Scott-Emuakpor, 2010; Welcome, 2011). However, there is presently limited systematic research on the challenges associated with the delivery of high-quality care. Although the author identified 69 studies in the literature that investigated the challenges associated with managing specific diseases (HIV/AIDS, prenatal and maternal care, malaria treatment, etc.), only five studies examined the barriers to primary health care, technology utilization, and patient referral system.

Using a semi-structured interview, Ogaji (2016) explored patients' expectations using primary healthcare centers to promote quality assessment and care improvement. The qualitative study revealed 44 coded themes organized around five thematic areas cutting across the triad of structure, process, and outcome dimensions. The study provided insights into patients' beliefs and expectations from primary

© The Author(s), under exclusive license to Springer Nature Switzerland AG 2021   345
J. A. Balogun, *The Nigerian Healthcare System*,
https://doi.org/10.1007/978-3-030-88863-3_11

healthcare centers. It is recommended that patients' views be considered when selecting items to measure primary healthcare outcomes and performance.

Another qualitative study by Koce and associates (2019) explored patients' perceptions and experiences on the factors influencing their decision to self-refer to Nigeria's secondary healthcare facilities. The study identified several reasons why patients bypass the primary healthcare facilities in favor of the secondary care level. The primary reasons included patients' understanding of the health system, perceptions about the health providers, equipment/facilities, advice from relatives and friends, patients' expectations, access to health facilities, regulations/policies, medical symptoms, and perceptions of the severity of symptoms. They recommended evaluating the healthcare referral system and developing a contextual model applicable to individual settings based on their findings.

The same team of investigators (Koce et al., 2020) in another study explored the healthcare professionals' (HCPs) opinions on the factors that influence patient self-referral decisions and their suggestions on how primary health centers can retain patients. The respondents believed that healthcare providers' shortage was the primary reason patients self-refer to secondary and tertiary care centers. Other influencing factors for bypassing the primary health centers include lack of essential equipment, inequitable distributions of workforce and resources, and irregular opening hours. They recommended that physicians be made available within the health centers and collaboration between the different levels of care to prevent service delivery fragmentation.

Another qualitative study by Uzochukwu et al. (2020) assessed the capacity needs, policy areas of demand, and primary stakeholders' views on evidence-informed decision-making in Nigeria. The study respondents considered health technology assessment an essential and valuable tool in designing health benefits packages, developing clinical guidelines, and improving service. The three main areas that would immensely benefit from the application of health technology assessment were public health programs, medicines, and vaccines. The respondents perceived the availability and accessibility of health technology assessments as inadequate and limited. They expressed the need for evidence on health system financing, health service provision, disease burden, training support in research methodology, and data management.

A systematic study by Ephraim-Emmanuel and associates in 2018 investigated the quality of healthcare delivery in Nigeria. They analyzed 85 relevant articles that assessed treatment effectiveness, acceptability, efficiency, appropriateness, and equity. The study's findings revealed a myriad of factors for the low quality of health care, including declining government expenditure on health despite increasing healthcare needs and non-availability, non-functional, or insufficient essential medical equipment. Additional factors uncovered were inadequate health facilities, lack of necessary drugs, unavailability of prescribed medications, and long waiting times at the health facilities. Other factors include unfriendly, rude, and poor attitudes of HCPs toward patients, cost of healthcare services coupled with a high margin of out-of-pocket payment for health services over health insurance, the high price of full implementation of a hospital information system, inadequate power supply, and fragile infrastructures, corruption at all levels of governance. Also, unavailability or outright absenteeism and ongoing strike action by HCPs and non-compliance with required existing standards were responsible for the country's low healthcare quality.

Overall, there are limited systematic research studies on the challenges within the Nigerian health system. This chapter's primary objective is to uncover the barriers to delivering affordable and high-quality healthcare services in Nigeria.

Methodology

The author searched the literature using the PubMed database with the keywords: Nigeria, healthcare system, challenges/barriers, and qualitative studies. The search produced 73 "hits," but only four of the investigations (Ogaji, 2016; Koce et al., 2019; Uzochukwu et al., 2020) are relevant to the study's objectives. The author's experience as the pioneer physiotherapist at Mubi General Hospital in the defunct Gongola State (1977–1978) and physiotherapist at General Hospital, Ilorin, Kwara State (1978–1980); senior lecturer and vice-dean of the College of Health Sciences at Obafemi Awolowo University (OAU), Ile-Ifc, (1986–1991); and half a dozen visits to several Nigerian universities and hospitals between 2015 and 2019 provided the clinical and academic experiences needed to conduct this research. The trips to Nigeria included presenting two keynote speeches and three workshops to a diverse audience of professionals from different fields (Balogun, 2020).

The evaluation conducted by the author consists of unstructured interviews with 15 (ten men and five women) HCPs – four physicians, three physiotherapists, two radiographers, two nurses, two pharmacists, and two medical laboratory scientists (Fig. 11.1). The participants' average age was 40 years, and they had work

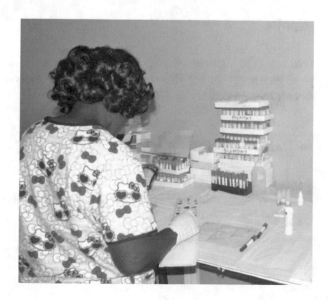

Fig. 11.1 A medical laboratory scientist at UNIMED Teaching hospital at work. (Photograph used with permission from UNIMED PRO)

experience ranging from four to 30 years. Before the interview, the study participants were reassured that their names and identities would not be divulged in any
publications that may emerge from the discussion. The unstructured interviews
were conducted in a natural conversation style and lasted between 20 and 25 minutes. The following seven primary questions were used as a guide to conduct the
interview, but the questions were modified to suit each participant's initial response
to the preceding question (Cohen & Crabtree, 2006).

1. Are the leaders of the healthcare system effective? Follow-up probing question:
   How about waste and efficiency of the healthcare system?
2. How satisfied are you with the health service delivered in the hospitals and clinics across the country? Follow-up probing question: Is the service provided
   timely? Is it of high quality?
3. Are there enough HCPs in the country? Follow-up probing question: Do you
   have plans to emigrate abroad to work?
4. Is the healthcare system adequately financed? Follow-up probing question: Are
   medication, vaccines, and needed primary equipment readily available?
5. What can you say about waste and honesty in the operations of the healthcare system?
6. What can you say about the level of cooperation among the HCPs? Follow-up
   probing questions: Do other professionals seek your opinion during clinical
   decisions? What are the challenges of the health information system in the
   country?
7. Do you have any other opinions to share on the healthcare system's strengths and
   weaknesses?

As indicated above, additional follow-up questions were posed when necessary
to clarify any ambiguity in the HCPs' responses.

Results

Following the interview, the opinions expressed on the seven questions were com-
piled and analyzed for shared perspectives. The analysis produced seven major
themes represented in Fig. 11.2.

Ineffective Leadership

When the HCPs were asked whether the healthcare system leaders are effective,
they expressed diverse opinions. The quotes below represent the points of view
expressed by the participants interviewed.

Fig. 11.2 The seven major themes identified in the study

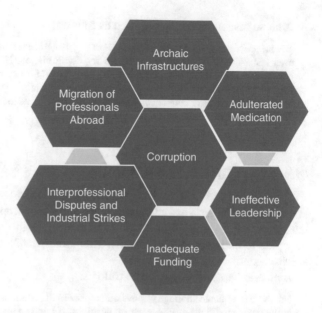

One of the physicians responded to the question as follows:

The healthcare system is in disarray and our leaders are not responsive to complaints... when we have no other means of getting our points across, we embark on industrial action. Buhari promised in 2015 during the campaign that he was going to ban the use of public funds by civil servant going abroad for treatment. He promised at the time, he was going to revamp our healthcare system. Six years later, we are still waiting; nothing .... Most importantly, our elected politicians (President and Governors) and appointed cabinet officers and head of government parastatals) need to vigorously fight corruption and promote ethical and good governance for the healthcare system to survive. (Respondent #1)

A nurse had this to say in response to the question:

It depends on the hospital. There are few hospitals in the country with good administrators, and the establishments are well-managed. Others have lousy and incompetent administrators who are only interested in getting rich. (Respondent #2)

Corruption

When the HCPs were asked about the waste and level of honesty in the operation of the healthcare system, they expressed diverse opinions.

A radiographer had this to say:

No, the leaders of the government hospitals, ministry of health are all doctors who always behave like they know it all. Most of them are greedy and corrupt. (Respondent #10)

A nurse responded to the question as follows:

You are in Nigeria, my brother; there are no angels here, everybody wants to survive, and even Buhari expects something in return for doing his job. He gives no s...t about the healthcare system. If he has a headache, he flies abroad for treatment. Why can he not use the money for his multiple trips overseas to equip the clinic at Aso Rock or one of our teaching hospitals? We have competent consultants and specialists in Nigeria who can treat him. (Respondent #9)

Migration of Professionals Abroad

When asked if Nigeria has adequate HCPs, and the concept of interdisciplinary collaboration has taken hold in the hospital setting., with the follow-up questions, if they plan to emigrate abroad to work The participants' responses to the questions are divergent:

A physiotherapist responded as follows:

No, there is an acute shortage of physiotherapists in the country, but the government is not hiring people to fill the available vacant positions. If I find an opportunity abroad, I will not hesitate to take the offer. (Respondent #5)

One of the physicians had this to say:

Not enough healthcare workers in the country. The consultants are leaving the country anywhere there is a better career opportunity, even South Africa, Ghana, and Namibia. Interdisciplinary teamwork is new in the country. No collaboration in patient care in my hospital. We only refer patients to other departments. (Respondent #3)

A pharmacist responded to the question as follows:

Pharmacists' demand is higher than the number produced in the university; therefore, there is a shortage. I have no plan to leave the country. No interdisciplinary teamwork, we operate within our disciplines. (Respondent #6)

Inadequate Financing

When participants were asked if the healthcare system is currently adequately financed, they were all of the opinion that the health sector is underfunded.

A physician responded to the question as follows:

No, health care is only funded at 5–7% of the annual budget. Consequently, many of our tertiary hospitals are in a terrible state with no essential diagnostic and treatment equipment. (Respondent #4)

A pharmacist responded as follows:

No. ...We need money to update our facilities and to expand the resources to accommodate more patients. In some of our wards, patients sleep on the floor because the hospital is overcrowded. I understand the annual budget allocation to health is below what the WHO recommends. The government should try and do better. (Respondent #12)

A medical laboratory scientist had this to say in response to the question:

Absolutely, no…When we provide our inventory needs at the beginning of every fiscal year, they come back to tell us there is no fund to buy what we need. (Respondent #7)

Archaic Infrastructures

When asked if the patients and HCPs have access to appropriate resources needed to deliver high-quality care, the participants' responses were very similar in describing their challenges.

A physiotherapist had this to say:

My profession is a hands-on discipline that utilizes sophisticated equipment for treatment. All our major electrotherapy equipment is imported. When they break down, we do not have much to offer our patients. It is very frustrating and demoralizing. (Respondent #8)

A radiographer responded as follows:

The new imaging devices are limited in the country. Only a few teaching hospitals have MRI and CT scan machines, and they are out of service frequently because of the epileptic power surge. They are costly to maintain because frequently, a technician from abroad have to come to a repair them. (Respondent #4)

A medical laboratory scientist had this to say:

The equipment needed to make an accurate diagnosis of the condition is not available, or the machine has broken down and no money to repair it. (Respondent #15)

When the HCPs were asked to describe the health information system's challenges, they shared similar points of view.

A nurse responded:

We need high-speed computers in our hospitals at all levels to promote efficiency and accuracy. (Respondent #3)

A medical laboratory scientist responded as follows:

Our health system at the federal level needs to develop robust medical intelligence and surveillance systems to inform our leaders about any impending and emerging diseases. (Respondent #7)

The pharmacist had this to say:

The country lags in information technology and communication in health care. In many university teaching hospitals across the country, the medical records are still manually processed, and patient records are often compromised. (Respondent #2)

Adulterated Medications

When asked if the patients have access to drugs and vaccines, the participants' responses were very similar in describing their challenges.

A pharmacist stated:

Only a few generic drugs are produced in the country. Access to authentic prescribed medication is one thing, but the major problem is the fake drugs from India and China. Vaccine's supply is adequate, but storage is a problem because of the unreliable power supply. (Respondent #14)

A nurse responded by saying:

Nigeria is the world capital for fake drugs. You cannot trust any medication you buy in private chemists and even in hospital pharmacy.... It is chalk you are taking ooo, my brother. (Respondent #13)

When asked how satisfied they are with the health service delivered in the country, the participants all expressed strong dissatisfaction with the system. The following responses are typical.

A physician responded to the question as follows:

...What service? I don't know of any Nigerian who is satisfied with our healthcare system. The poor state of our hospitals and clinics is real, and that is why the three pillars on which the health service hinges has broken down. Every patient now self-refers to the tertiary hospitals for treatment of the least consequential ailment that can be effectively managed at the community health centers. (Respondent #4)

A pharmacist responded as follows:

Many people die needlessly in this country because their diseases are not diagnosed early and later found to be too late. As an HCP, I am not satisfied with the quality of service that I receive in our teaching hospital. (Respondent #6)

Interprofessional Disputes and Industrial Strikes

When the study participants were asked if there is cooperation among the HCPs in their hospital, the following opinions were uniformly shared.

A physiotherapist had this to say:

Only when referring patients to our department do doctors talk to us. Most of the doctors are too proud to respect other professionals' input to patient care. (Respondent #12)

A medical laboratory scientist asserted:

The majority of the strikes are due to conflicts between pharmacists and physicians, nurses and physicians, laboratory scientists and pathologists, radiographers and radiologists, and between optometrists and ophthalmologists. (Respondent #14)

Only three of the 15 study participants at the end of the interview volunteered additional information on the healthcare system's strengths and weaknesses. One complained about "lack of coordination in the health system," another participant blurted out "unreliable electricity supply and bad roads," and the third person expressed concerns on "climate change, environmental pollution, and sanitary conditions of the hospitals in the country."

Discussion

This qualitative investigation uncovers the barriers to the delivery of affordable and high-quality healthcare services in the country. The study participants' recurrent shared views include ineffective leadership, corruption, lack of modern infrastructure, adulterated medications, inadequate funding, migration of professionals abroad, interprofessional disputes, and industrial strikes. These shared views corroborate the findings in the systematic review by Ephraim-Emmanuel et al. (2018) and the opinions expressed in review and critique articles on the Nigerian healthcare system by various analysts (Fajola et al., 2007; Tam 2015; Ogbebo, 2015; Orekunrin, 2015; Okpani & Abimbola, 2015; FMH, 2016; Ajao, 2017; Julius, 2017; Lopez, 2019; Asakitikpi, 2019; Scott-Emuakpor, 2010; Welcome, 2011).

Because corruption was a shared experience among all the study participants, an in-depth search of the literature was conducted on the PubMed and open access databases using the keywords "Nigeria," "corruption," and "health sector" to identify the source and scope of the problem in Nigeria. Four empirical-based studies and several media reports were identified, and the significant findings will be discussed here. Garuba and associates (2009) evaluated the perceived level of transparency and potential vulnerability to corruption in the registration, procurement, inspection, and distribution essential areas of the Nigerian pharmaceutical industry. The findings revealed an overall score of 7.4 out of 10, suggesting a marginally vulnerable system to corruption. The weakest permeable areas for the crime were in drug registration and inspection of ports. The absence of conflict-of-interest guidelines was the most glaring deficiency that can limit the declaration of corrupt practices. Additional contributing factors are the weak monitoring and evaluation processes, inconsistency in the documentation of procedures, and failure to make documentation available to the public.

Corruption is endemic in all the facets of Nigerian life, including the health sector, and is widely reported in the print media, both local and foreign. Abba-Aji and associates (2020) investigated how the top 10 Nigerian print media cover corruption in the health sector between 2016 and 2018. The *Punch* newspaper reported the highest number of corruption-related news—the NHIS attracted the most coverage, followed by the FMH. Corruption was predominantly framed as a political issue, and most of the content was episodic and focused on the details of the cases without reporting on the underlying causes. The reporting mainly attributed the cause of corruption to a lack of accountability, and enforcement was the most recommended solution.

During President Muhammadu Buhari's visit to the United States in 2015, Obama administration officials informed him that a former Nigerian minister stole $6 billion (£3.8 billion) of public money. Buhari requested the US government to help recover ₦150 billion from foreign bank accounts that was stolen over the last 10 years. US government officials described the corruption during the rule of the People's Democratic Party as momentous (BBC, 2015). The Economic and Financial Crimes Commission revealed in 2015 that leaders who steered the state's affairs between 1960 and 2005 stole $20 trillion from the Nigerian treasury. The commission clarified that in the year 2000 alone, $100 billion was stolen. Paying off the external debt that was only $33 billion at the time dwarfs the money stolen by the country's leadership (Ajayi & Ifegbayi, 2015).

The respected Associated Press and Reuters in the United States reported in 2016 that between 2006 and 2013, fifty-five Nigerians stole $6.8 billion (1.35 trillion Naira, at the exchange rate of 150 Naira to $1). The federal government allocated part of the stolen money to buy weapons to fight Boko Haram's six-year Islamist uprising. Analysts estimated that the stolen money could conveniently build 36 hospitals or provide education from the primary to the university level for 4000 children (Associated Press and Reuters, 2016). The world-renowned *Economist* reported in 2016 that £100 billion of illicit funds enter Britain every year, and African leaders hide and move stolen funds by setting up anonymous fake businesses and bank accounts (The Economist, 2019; Ojo, 2019).

In 2017, the Swiss government seized from President Sani Abacha's family $700 million from the total $4 billion he stole while in power. Abacha ruled the country for 5 years until his death in 1998. In the same year, 2017, another $480 million was seized by the US government and the United Nations Office on Drugs and Crime from the estimated $400 billion stolen from the Nigerian treasury between 1960 and 1999 (Monks, 2017).

In 2019, the former UK Prime Minister David Cameron described Nigeria as a "fantastically corrupt" nation. He based his assessment on the 2016 reports that revealed that $582 billion was stolen from Nigeria since independence. The report indicated that N11 trillion was diverted from the power sector alone since 1999, and the leaders and politicians laundered N1.3 trillion public funds between 2011 and 2015. United Kingdom's International Corruption unit confiscated £76 million ($117 million) loot from Nigeria since 2006. Worldwide, £791 million laundered money from Nigeria was frozen (Ojo, 2019). In 2019, the Nigerian government confirmed that $400 billion was looted through corrupt practices, and $40 million worth of jewelry was seized from former Minister of Petroleum Resources, Diezani Alison-Madueke (Nwezeh & Shittu, 2019). Considering all this mischief, yes, indeed, Nigeria is a "fantastically corrupt" nation.

Ezeibe and associates (2020) investigated the impact of political distrust on the spread of the coronavirus disease 2019 (COVID-19) pandemic in Nigeria by interviewing 120 educated Nigerians purposively selected from four heavily infected states—Lagos, Oyo, Kano, and Rivers, and the Federal Capital Territory. Again, the findings revealed that political corruption is a driver of large-scale political distrust and undermines public compliance with government protocols. The doubt limits the outcomes of government responses to the pandemic and facilitates the spread of the virus. The authors recommended improving government accountability in the public sector to build public trust and compliance with COVID-19 preventive measures to curtail the virus' community spread.

Corruption in the health sector is not limited to Nigeria. Globally, about $455 billion of the $7.35 trillion spent on health annually is lost to fraud and corruption. Besides, the Organisation for Economic Co-operation and Development (OECD) estimates that 45% of the people worldwide believe the health sector is corrupt or very corrupt (National Academies of Sciences, Engineering, and Medicine, 2018). Corruption in health care takes different forms: bribery of HCPs, regulators, and public officials, unethical research, diversion/theft/overpricing of medicines and medical supplies, adulterated/fake medications, fraudulent or overbilling for health services, absenteeism, unofficial payments, and embezzlements (Parmar, 2015). In addition, government officials misuse their discretionary powers to license services and products and accredit healthcare facilities. Thus, theft and fraud within the FMH and the state ministries of health impede efficient healthcare delivery and contribute to the overall low quality of care.

In Nigeria, the top five corrupt practices that negatively impact the delivery of high-quality health care are unreported absenteeism from work, procurement-related fraud, under-the-counter payments, health financing-related crime, and employment-related bribery (Onwujekwe et al., 2018, 2019, 2020; Ogbaa, 2017; Ibenegbu, 2018; Tormusa & Idom, 2016; International Medical Travel Journal, 2014). Formula and Idom, in 2016, averred that absenteeism from work is the most prevalent type of corruption in the health sector. Fortunately, it is easy to curtail by having a clock-in and out monitoring system in all the health facilities. The challenge for healthcare CEOs is that the other four corrupt practices are more challenging to resolve. For example, procurement-related fraud is problematic because many collaborators such as pharmaceutical sales representatives, physicians/dentists, auditors, and pharmacists are involved. Likewise, employment-related corruption is challenging to manage in public facilities as the ministry of health and not the establishment is responsible for hiring personnel. Many of whom are unqualified and unethical.

In secondary and primary healthcare facilities, patients often make under-the-table payments to obtain unauthorized medicines and to have their service expedited. Public education of patients about the dangers of using illegal drugs and regular audits of financial accounts and decentralized distribution of pharmaceuticals would curtail this illicit practice. Other corrupt practices include overbilling patients, irregular payments to the National Health Insurance Scheme, provision of unnecessary services, and issuing fake receipts by clerical staff. Publishing the price of health services, using an electronic payment system, and installing suggestion boxes in strategically located positions within the facilities would substantially decrease these corrupt practices (Tormusa & Idom, 2016).

Apart from corruption, incompetent leadership is one of the factors preventing high-quality healthcare delivery in the country. Many healthcare system leaders are oblivious to the challenges in the healthcare system, particularly the impacts of the migration of professionals abroad. For example, Nigeria's Minister of Labor and Employment, Dr. Chris Ngege, did not fully comprehend the ramifications of this problem on the health system when he declared that he was unconcerned about the migration of Nigerian physicians to other countries because the country had more than enough to spare (Rine, 2019). As a physician with over two decades of work experience who rose to the deputy director position in the FMH before his political career, Dr. Ngege was expected to be more astute about the short- and long-term impacts of mass emigration on the Nigerian health system that is one of the world's most inefficient and worst health outcomes (Ighobor, 2017, WHO, 2000, 2010).

One of the study participants' shared views, in addition to corruption, is the persistent industrial action in the health sector. The study participants indicated that the industrial strikes are due to disagreements over salary levels, complaints about the deplorable conditions of service, non-and-selective implementation of service schemes, and non-adherence to the legislated scope of clinical practice. Industrial strikes often lead to many unnecessary deaths as patients flee from public health facilities to private clinics and hospitals. The poor management of the crises by government bureaucrats at federal and state levels further compounds the problem. The allied health professionals who participated in the study alleged that government bureaucrats often fail to address the core complaints until matters fester to a point where they resort to industrial protests, and the leadership at the federal and state levels usually takes the medical profession's side during arbitration, rather than serving as a neutral arbitrator.

Two presidential commissions have intervened in the past with the hope of solving the industrial crises among the different health professional groups and their unions but to no avail. To break the deadlock, the federal government should constitute an impartial arbitration panel charged with resolving industrial strikes. The arbitration committee members should be experienced men and women of impeccable character who have training in conflict resolution and a well-respected society. The panel should quickly identify the cause(s) of the industrial strike and bring feuding parties together to resolve the crises effectively. The leaders of all the professional groups and union leaders should come to the negotiation table with an open mind and "give-and-take" disposition, respect for the professional practice oath, and their patient's interest. All parties should be encouraged to come to the negotiation with a no-victor-no-vanquished spirit (Lambo, 2019).

Conclusion

The solution to having a high-quality healthcare system is to address the seven themes identified in this chapter. The reforms should start by appointing visionary leaders based on merit and not tribalism, curtailing corruption, robust healthcare funding, refurbishing the dilapidated hospitals, and purchasing state-of-the-art equipment. Additionally, the government must improve the welfare and conditions of service of the healthcare workers to prevent the brain drain phenomenon. The government must establish an arbitration commission, consisting of persons of high integrity, to promptly investigate complaints before it festers and lead to industrial strikes. The National Agency for Food and Drug Administration and Control must do a better job in monitoring the production and distribution of medication in the country.

Case Study

Use the seven questions in the methodology section of this chapter to interview a health professional in your discipline. Compare the responses from your interview with the findings presented in the Results section. Highlight differences in the seven major themes identified (see Fig. 11.2).

References

Abba-Aji, M., Balabanova, D., Hutchinson, E., & McKee, M. (2020). How do Nigerian newspapers report corruption in the health system? *International Journal of Health Policy Management, 14*. [online]. Available at: https://pubmed.ncbi.nlm.nih.gov/32610718/. Accessed 26 Dec 2020.

Ajao, T. D. (2017, November 26). Nigeria's first University of Medical Sciences. *Vanguard.* [online]. Available at: https://www.vanguardngr.com/2017/11/nigerias-first-university-medical-sciences/. Accessed 26 Feb 2020.

Ajayi, O., & Ifegbayi, B. (2015). $20trn stolen from Nigeria's treasury by leaders – EFCC. Vanguard Newspaper. [online]. Available at: https://www.vanguardngr.com/2015/03/20trn-stolen-from-from-nigerias-treasury-by-leaders-efcc/. Accessed: 26 Dec 2020.

Asakitikpi, A. E. (2019). *Healthcare coverage and affordability in Nigeria: An alternative model to equitable healthcare delivery.* [online]. Available at: https://www.intechopen.com/books/universal-health-coverage/healthcare-coverage-and-affordability-in-nigeria-an-alternative-model-to-equitable-healthcare-delive. Accessed 23 Dec 2020.

Associated Press and Reuters. (2016). Nigerian minister claims $6.8bn of public funds stolen in seven years. *Guardian.* [online]. Available at: https://www.theguardian.com/world/2016/jan/19/nigerian-minister-claims-68bn-of-public-funds-stolen-in-seven-years; https://www.vanguardngr.com/2015/03/20trn-stolen-from-from-nigerias-treasury-by-leaders-efcc/amp/. Accessed 26 Dec 2020.

Balogun, J. A. (2020). Chapter 9: Reforming Nigeria's health care education system. In *Healthcare education in Nigeria: Evolutions and emerging paradigms.* Routledge Publication. [online]. Available at: https://www.routledge.com/9780367482091. Accessed 23 Dec 2020.

BBC. (2015). *Nigerian former minister 'stole $6bn of public money.* [online]. Available at: https://www.bbc.com/news/world-africa-33689115. Accessed 26 Dec 2020.

Cohen, D., & Crabtree, B. (2006). Qualitative research guidelines project: Unstructured interviews. *Robert Wood Johnson Foundation.* [online]. Available at: http://www.qualres.org/HomeUnst-3630.html. Accessed 16 Oct 2020.

Ephraim-Emmanuel, B. C., Adigwe, A., Oyeghe, R., & Ogaji, D. S. T. (2018). Quality of healthcare in Nigeria: A myth or a reality. *International Journal of Research Medical Sciences, 6*, 2875–2881. [online]. Available at: https://www.msjonline.org/index.php/ijrms/article/view/5173. Accessed 28 Dec 2020.

Ezeibe, C. C., Ilo, C., Ezeibe, E. N., Oguonu, C. N., Nwankwo, N. A., Ajaero, C. K., & Osadebe, N. (2020). Political distrust and the spread of COVID-19 in Nigeria. *Global Public Health, 15*(12), 1753–1766. [online]. Available at: https://pubmed.ncbi.nlm.nih.gov/33019916/. Accessed 26 Dec 2020.

Fajola, A. O., Ogbimi, R. N., Oyo-Ita, A., Mosuro, O., Mustapha, A., Umejiego, C., Fakunle, B., & Uduma, C.. (2007). *Innovative approaches to healthcare delivery in resource-limited settings: Lessons from Nigeria.* [online]. Available at: https://www.onepetro.org/conference-paper/SPE-183622-MS. Accessed 10 Oct 2020.

Federal Ministry of Health. (2016). *National health policy 2016: Promoting the health of Nigerians to accelerate socio-economic development.* [online]. Available at: https://extranet.who.int/countryplanningcycles/sites/default/files/planning_cycle_repository/nigeria/draft_nigeria_national_health_policy_final_december_fmoh_edited.pdf. Accessed 10 Oct 2020.

Garuba, H. A., Kohler, J. C., & Huisman, A. M. (2009). Transparency in Nigeria's public pharmaceutical sector: Perceptions from policy makers. *Global Health, 29*(5), 14. [online]. Available at: https://pubmed.ncbi.nlm.nih.gov/19874613/. Accessed 26 Dec 2020.

Ibenegbu, G. (2018). *What are the problems facing healthcare management in Nigeria?* [online]. Available at: https://www.legit.ng/1104912-what-the-problems-facing-healthcare-management-nigeria.html. Accessed 10 Oct 2020.

Ighobor, K. (2017). Diagnosing Africa's medical brain drain: Higher wages and modern facilities are magnets for Africa's health workers. *Africa Renewal.* [online]. Available at: https://www.un.org/africarenewal/magazine/december-2016-march-2017/diagnosing-africa%E2%80%99s-medical-brain-drain. Accessed 16 Oct 2020.

International Medical Travel Journal – IMTJ. (2014). *Nigeria spends $1 billion on outbound medical tourism.* [online]. Available at: https://www.imtj.com/news/nigeria-spends-1-billion-outbound-medical-tourism/. Accessed 10 Oct 2020.

Julius. (2017). *Nigeria healthcare system: The good and the bad.* [online]. Available at: http://www.visitnigeria.com.ng/nigeria-healthcare-system-the-good-and-the-bad/. Accessed 16 Oct 2020.

Koce, F., Randhawa, G., & Ochieng, B. (2019). Understanding healthcare self-referral in Nigeria from the service users' perspective: A qualitative study of Niger state. *BMC Health Services Research, 19*, 209. [online]. Available at: https://doi.org/10.1186/s12913-019-4046-9. Accessed 16 Oct 2020.

Koce, F. G., Randhawa, G., & Ochieng, B. (2020). A qualitative study of health care providers' perceptions and experiences of patients bypassing primary healthcare facilities: A focus from Nigeria. *Journal of Global Health Reports, 4*, e2020073. [online]. Available at: https://doi.org/10.29392/001c.14138. Accessed 16 Oct 2020.

Lambo, E. (2019). Managing inter professional disharmony in Nigeria's health sector for health security. *A presentation at the 55th annual scientific conference and workshop of the Association of Medical Laboratory Scientists of Nigeria*, Abuja, September 5, 2019.

Lopez, O. (2019, September 19). Nigeria's health care system on the mend: Reducing bureaucracy and improving vaccine storage have helped health experts better respond to disease outbreaks. *US News and Report.* [online]. Available at: https://www.usnews.com/news/best-countries/articles/2019-09-19/nigeria-slowly-improving-its-health-care-system. Accessed 10 Oct 2020.

Monks, K. (2017). *Switzerland to return $321 million of stolen money to Nigeria.* [online]. Available at: https://www.cnn.com/2017/12/06/africa/switzerland-returns-abacha-funds/index.html. Accessed 26 Dec 2020.

National Academies of Sciences, Engineering, and Medicine. (2018). *Crossing the global quality chasm: Improving healthcare worldwide*. The National Academies Press. [online]. Available at: https://www.nap.edu/catalog/25152/crossing-the-global-quality-chasm-improving-healthcare-worldwide. Accessed 10 Oct 2020.

Nwezeh, K., & Shittu, H. (2019). *Nigeria: U.S.$400 billion looted from treasury – Govt.* [online]. Available at: https://allafrica.com/stories/201909130041.html. Accessed 26 Dec 2020.

Ogaji, D. (2016). What does quality mean to the patients? An exploration of the expectations of patients for primary health care in Nigeria. *The Nigerian Health Journal, 16*(4). http://www.tnhjph.com/index.php/tnhj/article/view/257. Accessed 26 Dec 2020.

Ogbaa, M. (2017). *A Nigerian story: How healthcare is the offspring of imperialism and corruption.* [online]. Available at: https://www.theelephant.info/features/2017/11/16/a-nigerian-story-how-healthcare-is-the-offspring-of-imperialism-and-corruption/. Accessed 10 Oct 2020.

Ogbebo, W. (2015). *The many problems of Nigeria's health sector.* [online]. Available at: https://infoguidenigeria.com/problems-of-nigeria-health-sector-and-possible-solutions/. Accessed 10 Oct 2020.

Ojo, J. (2019). *The $582bn stolen from Nigeria since independence.* [online]. Available at: https://punchng.com/the-582bn-stolen-from-nigeria-since-independence/. Accessed 26 Dec 2020.

Okpani, A. I., & Abimbola, S. (2015). Operationalizing universal health coverage in Nigeria through social health insurance. *Nigeria Medical Journal, 56*(5), 305–310. [online]. Available at: https://www.ncbi.nlm.nih.gov/pmc/articles/PMC4698843/citedby/. Accessed 27 Dec 2020.

Onwujekwe, O., Agwu, P., Orjiakor, C., McKee, M., Hutchinson, E., Mbachu, C., Odii, A., Ogbozor, P., Obi, U., Ichoku, H., & Balabanova, D. (2019). Corruption in Anglophone West Africa health systems: A systematic review of its different variants and the factors that sustain them. *Health Policy and Planning, 34*(7), 529–543. [online]. Available at:https://academic.oup.com/heapol/article/34/7/529/5543565. Accessed 10 Oct 2020.

Onwujekwe, O., Odii, A., Mbachu, C., Hutchinson, E., Ichoku, H., Ogbozorf, P. A., Agwu, P., Obi, U. S., & Balabanova, D. (2018). Corruption in the Nigerian health sector has many faces: How to fix it. *University of London.* [online]. Available at: https://ace.soas.ac.uk/wp-content/uploads/2018/09/Corruption-in-the-health-sector-in-Anglophone-W-Africa_ACE-Working-Paper-005.pdf. Accessed 10 Oct 2020.

Onwujekwe, O., Orjiakor, C. T., Hutchinson, E., McKee, M., Agwu, P., Mbachu, C., Ogbozor, P., Obi, U., Odii, A., Ichoku, H., & Balabanova, D. (2020). Where do we start? Building consensus on drivers of health sector corruption in Nigeria and ways to address it. *International Journal of Health Policy Management, 9*(7), 286–296. [online]. Available at: https://pubmed.ncbi.nlm.nih.gov/32613800/. Accessed 26 Dec 2020.

Orekunrin, O. (2015). *Nigeria's healthcare problems: A three-pronged solution.* [online]. Available at: [online]. Available at: https://politicalmatter.org/2015/07/11/10769/. Accessed 10 Oct 2020.

Parmar, H. (2015, September 8). *Healthcare business challenges in Nigeria.* [online]. Available at:https://www.linkedin.com/pulse/healthcare-business-challenges-nigeria-hemraj-parmar-mba/. Accessed 10 Oct 2020.

Rine, R. (2019). Nigeria's life expectancy in 2019: Matters arising. *TNV. The Nigerian Voice.* [online]. Available at: https://www.thenigerianvoice.com/news/277752/nigerias-life-expectancy-in-2019-matters-arising.html. Accessed 16 Oct 2020.

Scott-Emuakpor, A. (2010). The evolution of healthcare systems in Nigeria: Which way forward in the twenty-first century. *Nigeria Medical Journal, 17*(51), 53–65. [online]. Available at: http://www.nigeriamedj.com/text.asp?2010/51/2/53/70997. Accessed 3 Feb 2020.

Tam, A. A. (2015). Healing the ills in the ailing Nigerian health system. *The Guardian.* [online]. Available at: https://guardian.ng/features/healing-the-ills-in-the-ailing-nigerian-health-system/. Accessed 16 Oct 2020.

The Economist. (2019). *African Kleptocrats are finding it tougher to stash cash in the West.* [online]. Available at: https://www.economist.com/middle-east-and-africa/2019/10/10/african-kleptocrats-are-finding-it-tougher-to-stash-cash-in-the-west. Accessed 19 Mar 2021.

Tormusa, D. O., & Idom, A. M. (2016). The impediments of corruption on the efficiency of health-care service delivery in Nigeria. *Journal of Health Ethics, 12(1).* [online]. Available at: https://aquila.usm.edu/ojhe/vol12/iss1/3/. Accessed 26 Dec 2020.

Uzochukwu. (n.d.). AIDS, the surgeon general, and the politics of public health. Everett Koop. *The C. Everett Koop Papers.* [online]. Available at: https://profiles.nlm.nih.gov/spotlight/qq/feature/aids. Accessed 16 Oct 2020.

Uzochukwu, B. S. C., Okeke, C., & O'Brien, N., et al. (2020). Health technology assessment and priority setting for universal health coverage: A qualitative study of stakeholders' capacity, needs, policy areas of demand and perspectives in Nigeria. *Global Health, 16*, 58. [online]. Available at: https://doi.org/10.1186/s12992-020-00583-2. Accessed 16 Oct 2020.

Welcome, M. O. (2011). The Nigerian health care system: Need for integrating adequate medical intelligence and surveillance systems. *Journal of Pharmacy and Bioallied Sciences, 3*(4), 470–478. [online]. Available at: https://www.ncbi.nlm.nih.gov/pmc/articles/PMC3249694/. Accessed 10 Oct 2020.

WHO (2000). *The world health organization's ranking of the world's health systems, by rank.* [online]. Available at: https://photius.com/rankings/world_health_systems.html. Accessed 10 Oct 2020.

WHO (2010). Economic analysis and evaluation team. Department of Health Systems Governance and Financing. [online]. Available at: https://www.who.int/choice/cost-effectiveness/inputs/country_inpatient_outpatient_2010.pdf?ua=1.

Chapter 12
The Political and Economic Reforms Needed to Achieve Universal and High-Quality Health Care in Nigeria

Learning Objectives

After reading this chapter, the learner should be able to:

1. Discuss the blueprint of Nigeria's Vision 20:2020 national economic plan.
2. Discuss the politics of state creation in Nigeria.
3. Describe the evolution of the local government system in Nigeria.
4. Discuss the current state of the Nigerian nation.
5. Analyze the controversies on census data manipulation and revenue allocation at the federal, state, and local government levels.
6. Trace the history of the sudden wealth in Nigeria and the economic woes that followed.
7. Discuss the wasteful spending and corruption is a major barrier to universal and high-quality health care in Nigeria.
8. Appraise the assets of the consequential Nigerian presidents after General Yakubu Gowon.
9. Discuss the controversy on who is considered the best head of state that Nigeria ever had.
10. Argue the need for political and economic restructuring to attain universal and high-quality health care in Nigeria.
11. Defend the statement that money is the "mother milk" of an efficient health system and provide specific recommendations that will adequately fund Nigeria's health system.

Introduction

Nigeria is a federal republic with a unitary constitutional arrangement. The central government wields enormous and dominant powers and controls the revenues and most natural resources, especially oil and natural gas. The country generates about 70% of its revenues from oil sales. The income accrues in the federation account and is allocated monthly to the states and the local governments by a federal executive body named the Revenue Mobilization, Allocation, and Fiscal Commission. Nearly 70% of the oil and gas revenue comes from its southern region (Ola-David, 2018). The blueprint of Nigeria's Vision 20:2020 national economic plan was conceived in 2006 by President Olusegun Obasanjo and launched amidst fanfare in September 2009 by President Umaru Yar'Adua's administration. The goal of the economic plan was for Nigeria to become one of the 20 top economies in the world by increasing the gross domestic product (GDP) from US$212 billion as of 2008 to at least US$900 billion by 2020. Sadly, on January 1, 2020, the goal was not met as the country's GDP ranked 28th globally with worse socioeconomic conditions than ever before.

Critics following the launch of the Vision 20:2020 in 2009 lamented that Nigeria joining the top 20 economies is inconsequential, as it would not provide for citizens' basic life needs. They affirmed that Nigeria should not anchor its development plan on the gross development plan (GDP) because it does not impact current realities on the ground (Onyenekenwa, 2011; Onyeji, 2020). Many Nigerian scholars affirmed that the Vision 20:2020 economic plan is Utopian and a colossal blunder of misplaced priority. The country's economic malaise is fueled by corruption, insecurity, epileptic power supply, antiquated infrastructure, and weak governance institutions. These challenges make the national financial goal's broader objectives out of reach (Onyenekenwa, 2011; Onyeji, 2020). During a visit to Nigeria in 2018, Bill Gates observed that the Vision 20:2020 economic plan did not address Nigerians' unique needs as it prioritizes physical capital over human capital. He charged the leaders to invest in the people, which is the most precious resource (Onyeji, 2020).

Due to poor performance and high costs, most Nigerians have given up on public healthcare establishments (Alagboso, 2020). Instead, the elites receive their health care at private hospitals/clinics or travel outside the country. The annual expense on medical tourism is between $1 and $1.5 billion (Ajimotokan, 2019; Onyenucheya, 2018; Basiru et al., 2018; NOIPolls, 2017; Okafor, 2017; Makinde, 2016; VOA, 2019; Punch, 2016; International Medical Travel Journal, 2014; Ajobe et al., 2013). A survey of 1000 Nigerians in 2018 to gauge the level of confidence in the nation's health system revealed that a whopping 44% of the respondents "did not feel confident at all," 30% felt "somewhat confident," and only 26% of the respondents felt "confident" in the health system. The above findings contrast with Taiwan and South Korea, where 80% of their population is satisfied with the healthcare system (Wu et al., 2010; Kwon et al., 2015).

Quality health care is a strong determinant of economic growth, and high-income countries worldwide rank their health sector highly in their budgeting. Nigeria's health system is at the bottom of most global health outcome indices, yet the health sector budget does not receive the attention it rightfully deserves. Healthcare spending in Nigeria has never risen to 10% of the GDP, and over 95% of the population are uninsured (Awosusi et al., 2015; Ifijeh, 2015; NOIPolls, 2017; Amu et al., 2018; Aregbeshola & Khan, 2018).

Adequate financing is the "mother's milk" needed to achieve the universal health care (UHC) recommended by the United Nations (UN) under the sustainable development goals, part of goal number three (UN, 2015, Global Compact, 2021. Aka put it poignantly, affirming that the four hallmarks of an efficient health system are "good laws, adequate funding, health care as a human right rather than a privilege, and good politics" (Aka, 2020). Moreover, the government cannot deliver UHC on a shoestring budget. Every country gets the type of health service they pay for, and Nigeria is no different. Therefore, a well-reasoned strategic plan is needed to achieve UHC by 2030.

Since independence, successive democratic and military governments in Nigeria have made great strides in building hospitals and health centers but neglect human capital. Starting with the first colonial plan in 1945 to President Muhammadu Buhari's most recent 2018–2022 National Strategic Health Development Plan, many health plans have been developed (Scott-Emuakpor, 2010; Essien & Yakubu, 2018), but UHC remains an illusion. The health system's disorders are reflective of the proverb: "a person who fails to plan is planning to fail." The health system problems remain unsolvable despite the many health plans implemented because they lacked coordination and continuity. Within each of the different administrations, the strong influence of politics on healthcare development leads to policy inconsistency. Each successive administration has its own "interest" and health policies, which are often not aligned with the initial national health plans.

The widely held dogma that insanity is doing the same thing repeatedly and expecting a different result is the basis of this chapter's argument. The nation cannot continue to engage in the scuttle and uncoordinated solutions to address the healthcare system's challenges and expect a positive outcome. The overwhelming consensus of health analysts and scholars is that the healthcare system is in a crisis and needs an urgent solution (Parmar, 2015). In 2016, President Muhammadu Buhari's government launched a plan to achieve 30% health insurance coverage by 2020, but this goal did not materialize, and UHC remains an illusion.

This chapter impugned Nigeria's relevance among the top 20 economies when it has one of the world's worst healthcare and educational systems (World Health Organization—WHO, 2000, 2010; Knoema, 2018; Psacharopoulos, n.d.). The health system challenges call for drastic measures focused on revamping the economy to provide the robust funding needed to implement universal and high-quality health care. This author infers that the health system is presently on life support, and the previously adopted piecemeal and patchwork solutions will not achieve the desired goal. This chapter has dual overarching objectives focusing on the political and economic reforms needed to achieve universal and high-quality health care in Nigeria.

Developmental Challenges and Budget Priorities

The health system of any country influences its ability to participate effectively in the global economy. In 2020, Nigeria's average life expectancy was 55.8 years, representing a World Life Expectancy ranking of 178 (Worldometer, 2020). Approximately 44% of Nigerians live in extreme poverty, and the country surpassed India at the bottom of the extreme poverty ranking (Akinyele & Otto Abasiekong, 2018). Sadly, less than 5% of the population has access to affordable health care (Awosusi et al., 2015; Ifijeh, 2015; NOIPolls, 2017; Amu et al., 2018; Aregbeshola & Khan, 2018). The aforementioned depressing statistics explain why Nigeria has not evolved into an economically independent country (Akinyele & Otto Abasiekong, 2018). After all, a malnourished and sick person will not have the stamina and capacity to be productive.

Although Nigeria, in recent years, has made some progress in socioeconomic terms, human capital development remains weak due to underinvestment. In 2018, Nigeria ranked 152 of 157 countries in the World Bank's human capital index. The country faces many developmental challenges, including reducing the dependency on oil and diversifying the economy, addressing insufficient infrastructure, building strong and effective institutions, addressing its perpetual governance problems, and stifling the corrupt and wasteful public financial management system. These pre-existing structural challenges have left the economy vulnerable to the coronavirus disease 2019 (COVID-19) outbreak and its consequences. The World Bank (2020) best diagnosed Nigeria's developmental challenges as follows:

> Inequality, in terms of income and opportunities, remains high and has adversely affected poverty reduction. The lack of job opportunities is at the core of the high poverty levels, regional Inequality, and social and political unrest. Without the COVID-19 shock (the counterfactual scenario), about 2 million Nigerians were expected to fall into poverty in 2020 as population growth outpaces economic growth. With COVID-19, the recession is likely to push an additional 5 million Nigerians into poverty in 2020, bringing the total newly poor to 7 million this year.

With the multiple developmental challenges discussed above, it is now convincing to infer that Nigerian "Giant of Africa" braggadocio is no longer justified, particularly when over 44% of the population live in extreme poverty and 95% have no access to health care. In a global economy, every progressive nation's primary goal is to develop an accessible, affordable, and high-quality healthcare system. For decades, Nigeria has failed to allocate enough funds to achieve the United Nations' stated goal that every country provides access to health care for all its citizens. For this reason, on April 27, 2001, African Heads of State held a meeting at Abuja and pledged to devote at least 15% of their annual budget to health care—a landmark event often referred to as the "Abuja Declaration" (WHO, 2011). None of the Nigerian governments has met the Abuja pledge because UHC is not ranked number one on the budget priorities. Healthcare spending in Nigeria has never risen to 10% of the GDP. In 2016, only ₦262 billion was allocated to health, representing 6% of the total budget. Many other African countries, such as Rwanda, Botswana, Niger, Malawi, Zambia, and Burkina Faso, expended 15.8–18% of their GDP on health care (Fig. 12.1).

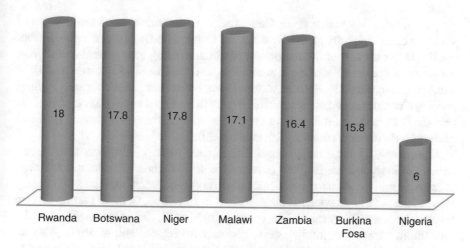

Fig. 12.1 Health budget allocation in 2016 (as a percentage of the total budget) in selected African countries. (Source: CIA, 2017)

In 2018, the amount allocated to health rose to ₦ 340.5 billion. Still, it represented only 3.9% of the total budget. This dismal level of funding cannot cater to the myriad healthcare challenges bedeviling the nation, including malnutrition, ongoing outbreaks of diseases, cancers, typhoid fever, malaria, and other primary healthcare concerns. In the most recent (2020) budget, President Buhari indicated his top four priorities: fiscal consolidation, investment in essential infrastructure, rewarding private-sector entrepreneurship, and developing social investment programs (Channels Television, 2019a). Contrast the hazy budget goals of Buhari to the Rwandan government's top four priority goals, which explicitly focus on fortifying the healthcare system, investing in agriculture and livestock, developing social protection coverage, and increasing jobs through investment in public works and support to all establishments impacted by the COVID-19 pandemic (Taarifa, 2020).

Evolution of States in Nigeria

In 1914, following the amalgamation of the Southern and Northern protectorates by Frederick Lugard, Nigeria became a new nation. However, with the promulgation of Richard's Constitution in 1949, the country was carved out into three regions—northern, eastern, and western. Each part is composed of a diversity of ethnic groups. However, the Yoruba, Igbo, and Hausa-Fulani were numerically and politically the dominant ethnic groups in the three regions. The creation of the three regions led to fears of domination and agitations for more by ethnic minorities in the various parts of the country (Ota et al., 2020).

In reaction to such agitations, the British colonial regime set up the Henry Willinks Commission in 1958 to study the fears of the ethnic minorities and ways to allay such fears. Surprisingly, the Commission did not recommend the creation of states for ethnic minority groups. Instead, the Commission held that the government could address the fear of domination by institutionalizing human rights principles, establishing special development authorities, and the sustained implementation of democratic practices. However, at various times, both Nnamdi Azikiwe and Obafemi Awolowo recommended creating states during the colonial era. Azikiwe argued the new states be based on the existing provinces, while Awolowo advocated ethnicity as the criteria for state creation (Ota et al., 2020).

Nigeria was a federal nation consisting of three regions (northern, western, and eastern) at independence in 1960. Barely six years of democratic rule then followed decades of military dictatorship. Major General Aguiyi Ironsi was the first military Head of State, but following his assassination in July 1966, General Yakubu Gowon became the new military ruler of the country. On May 27, 1967, Gowon dissolved the four (northern, western, mid-western, and eastern) regions and created a 12-state structure governed by military governors. Between 1967 and 1970, Odumegwu Ojukwu attempted to secede as Biafra during the Nigerian civil war. Ojukwu was born in Zungeru and studied at Oxford (1952–1955) before joining the Nigerian army and reached the rank of lieutenant-colonel by 1966. He was appointed the military governor of the eastern region after the January 15, 1966, coup, in which he did not participate. However, he refused to accept Gowon's leadership after the second coup of 1966, accusing Gowon of suppressing the Ibo people. He declared the eastern region independent, and the bloody Biafran war (1967–1970) ensued. The federal troops defeated Ojukwu's forces, and on January 11, 1970, he sought political asylum in the Ivory Coast. He returned to Nigeria in 1982 after a pardon. However, he was unsuccessful in his bid to resume a political career. After the 1983 coup, Ojukwu was imprisoned, released in 1984, and retired (Oxford University Press, 1993).

On February 3, 1976, General Murtala Mohammed reconfigured the administrative structure into 19 states, and relocated the federal capital from Lagos to Abuja. On September 23, 1987, General Ibrahim Babangida reconfigured the administrative structure into 21 states and subsequently reconfigured it into 30 states on August 27, 1991 (Cahoon, n.d.). On October 1, 1996, General Sanni Abacha reconfigured the administrative structure into a 36-state structure (Fig. 12.2).

In Nigeria, the creation of states has hitherto been by fiat based on political considerations under four military dictators (Yakubu Gowon, Murtala Mohammed, Ibrahim Babangida, Sanni Abacha). Coincidentally, the four military dictators are from the north. The states were created arbitrarily, not based on population. For example, by the 2016 census, Kano and Lagos' states have 15,076,892 and 12,000,598 people, respectively, while Nasarawa and Bayelsa have only 2,523,395 and 2,277,961, respectively. Critics assert that the military created the states in favor of the northern region, which disproportionally has more states (Cahoon, n.d.; Ota et al., 2020). For instance, in 1967, Gowon created from the north additional states (Benue-Plateau, Kano, North Central, North-Eastern, Kwara, and the North-Western States). In contrast, the former western region had only the Western and Lagos States and partly Kwara State. The former eastern region had three states—East

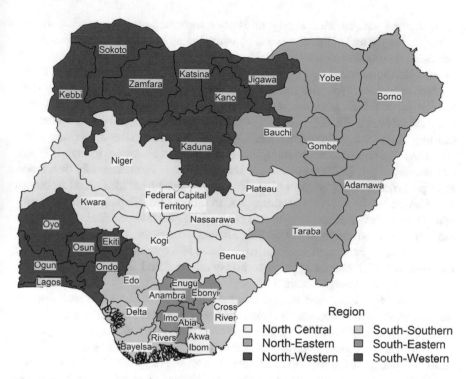

Fig. 12.2 Nigeria's 36-state structure. (Color signifies geopolitical region.). (Source: Reprinted from Upfill-Brown et al. (2014). Figure 2. https://doi.org/10.1186/1741-7015-12-92, distributed under the terms of the Creative Commons Attribution License (https://creativecommons.org/licenses/by/4.0/))

Central, Rivers, and South-Eastern States. Ota and associates (2020) argued that Gowon created Rivers and South-Eastern States specifically to break the Igbo dominance by turning them into a minority in the former eastern region.

Similarly, in 1976, Murtala Mohammed created seven states within the former northern region, three states in the former western region, and only two states in the former eastern region. The military regimes of Ibrahim Babangida and Sani Abacha sustained the trend of favoring the north in 1987, 1991, and 1996, respectively (Ota et al., 2020). Today, out of the 36 states, the Hausa-Fulani Muslim north has 14 states, and in addition the ethnic minorities in the north have five states. The Yoruba have six states with stakes in two states, and the Igbo have five states, which is just one state more than the ethnic minorities in the former eastern region.

The four military rulers anchored state creation on the need to bring governance closer to the grassroots and to allay the fears of ethnic minorities over the overbearing influence of their ethnically more dominant neighbors. The civilian government created the mid-western region in 1963 from the western region. Furthermore, provinces, which were a legacy of colonial and protectorate times, remained until 1976, when the military government of General Murtala Mohammed abolished them.

Additional state creation in Nigeria is often instigated by the elite, desperate to ensure economic and political survival by whipping up emotions and hysteria on the perceived domination by people considered outsiders or non-indigenes. Proponents of state creation argued that more states would engender development and check regional economic disparities and ensure equality in both political participation and the sharing of federal government resources. The opponents of state creation, such as President Shehu Shagari, argued that more states would impede development by draining the federal government's limited resources and encouraging laziness at the state level and conspicuous consumption among mega contractors (Shagari, 1996). Ota and associates (2020) contend that state creation is an unnecessary distraction from government tasks because of the unending competition for federal resources based on ethnically defined constituencies. In other words, opponents of state creation believe that such an exercise will continue to generate centrifugal challenges rather than engendering nation-building, national integration, unity, and patriotism. In particular, the federal administrative structure is responsible for the agitation of more states, which creates more financial burden on it and less attention on issues relating to national development.

A pertinent question often asked is whether the creation of states positively impacts the vast majority of Nigerians. Ota and associates (2020) contend that the creation of states psychologically benefited the masses, but it is the elites who occupy juicy political offices and get multi-million contracts. The truth of the matter is the creation of states has not significantly improved poverty alleviation. Materially, the social and economic conditions of the masses have either stagnated or worsened because of corruption by the elites, which makes resource development and better quality of life for most Nigerians a mirage. As a result, the rich continued to get richer, while the poor are getting poorer. Moreover, the states continue to depend on the federal government to allocate financial resources. This reliance trend negatively impacts the states' finances as they are not capable of tapping into other revenue streams.

Although the federal government allocates less than half of national revenue to the state and local governments, this largesse has not resulted in good public services or more accountability at the state and local government levels. A 2018 performance-based rating of states based on poverty diminution, access to electricity, business promotion, and raising local revenue showed Lagos at the top and Yobe at the bottom (Egbejule, 2018). Lagos has evolved from a symbol of urban disorder to a widely cited example of effective African governance. The civilian administration of Lateef Kayode Jakande (1979–1983), Bola Ahmed Tinubu (1999–2007), and Babatunde Raji Fashola (2007–2015) successfully overhauled the waste collection systems, regulated buses, contained extortion by youth gangs, multiplied the state tax revenues, used the resources to restore basic infrastructure, and expanded the public services and law enforcement. Furthermore, the three administrations increased municipal investments in housing, schools, and transportation (Gramont, 2015). Lagos is a model for other states and an example that development can flourish in Nigeria under visionary and pragmatic leaders.

Evolution of the Local Government System

In Nigeria, the origin of the local government system is traced to the Native Authority Ordinance of 1916, which the British colonial government passed ostensibly to leverage the existing traditional administrative systems in the regions. Thus, the ordinance was the first legal framework to operationalize a strategy of indirect rule. However, the local government system met some resistance from the east and west regions because of its perceived anti-democratic thrust—it did not fit well with the existing traditional administrative procedures in the two regions. Nonetheless, the ordinance lasted until 1946, when the Richard constitution created the new regional assemblies. By 1949, the House of Assembly in the east provided a forum for debates and led to the Local Government Ordinance of 1950, which set the scene for a democratic system of local government.

By 1954, democratic values had permeated the local government system in the east, west, and northern regions. As a result, each had absolute control over the administrative type, structure, and functions. Although the 1950 ordinance introduced democratic values in local governance—but also marked the beginning of federal and regional dominance over local government administration—this situation is evident throughout colonial rule to contemporary Nigeria (Abdulhamid & Chima, 2015).

The modern local government system started in 1976 under General Murtala Mohammed's administration with the primary goal to bring government to the grassroots level. For the first time, a single system of local government administration was attained nationally, and the financial system was restructured by providing statutory allocations of revenue from the Federation Account—with fixed proportions of federal and each state's revenue allocated to the local government. General Murtala Mohammed administration reform also protected local government revenue from state encroachment and defined several potential sources of revenue sources for local governments, including property, street lighting and community taxes, and poll tax; and fines and fees from the court, motor/forest parks, market, regulated premises, birth registrations fees, and public advertisement, etc. The local government administration and politicians were given a free hand to operate with little or no interference from the state authorities—their only responsibility is to advise, assist, and guide. Under the 1976 reforms, traditional rulers were also protected from party politics.

In 1988, General Ibrahim Babangida introduced the civil service reforms at the local government level. The reforms professionalized services by creating mandatory departments (personnel, finance, supply, etc.) and officers (councilors, secretary, treasurer, auditor-general for local government). The reform also clearly defined the functions of the Local Government Service Commission and sets guidelines for staffing, monitoring of local government activities (Abdulhamid & Chima, 2015).

At the state level, the ministry of local government and chieftaincy affairs, or bureau of local government affairs, is responsible for administering state-level acts governing local authorities. Local government exists in a single-tier across all 36 states. The number of local government authorities (LGAs) had risen steadily from 301 in 1976 to 774 and six area councils in 1999, yet the clamor for creating more LGAs has not abated. Also, over 500 new LGAs are considered by various state governments (Ukiwo, n.d.). Following the 2015 local elections, only 9.8% of councilors and 3.6% of chairpersons were female. All revenue collected is pooled in the federal account and split across the three levels of government. The core functions of the LGAs include preschool, primary, and adult education, primary health care, town planning, roads and transport, and waste disposal (Country profile, 2019).

Unfortunately, the LGAs have failed to meet the expectation of Nigerians. President Olusegun Obasanjo noted in 2003 that the creation of LGAs had not brought government and development closer to the people (Ukiwo, n.d.). Instead, the LGAs have produced absentee chairpersons only seen at council headquarters when the monthly Abuja Allocation arrives. They instantaneously vamoose with their standby jeeps and mobile police escorts after overseeing the sharing of the national cake among the relevant stakeholders. Consequently, LGA chairmanship has become one of the most sought-after elective positions after the presidency and governorship. This situation prompted most state governors to intervene using legal and political strategies to domesticate local governments. Sadly, the governors abused their authority when the Economic and Financial Crimes Commission (EFCC) alleged in 2006 that 31 out of 36 state governors have tampered with local government council funds (Ukiwo, n.d.).

The evolution of LGAs has been fraught with many controversies. The 1979 constitution vested the power to create new LGAs and councils on the national assembly, state, and local government councils. The process is cumbersome and complicated to achieve under a democratic government. This contentious provision in the 1999 constitution rocked the nation when six states—Lagos, Ebonyi, Katsina, Nassarawa, Niger, Yobe—exercised their constitutional powers to create new local government areas. The most celebrated of the six cases was in 2002, when the governor of Lagos State, Bola Ahmed Tinubu, carved out 37 new local government areas. President Olusegun Obasanjo clamped down on the states in April 2004 and announced that no allocation from the Federation Account should be released to the local government councils of the six states mentioned earlier. Obasanjo's action provoked a constitutional crisis and raised many fundamental questions about whether he acted lawfully to stop the Federation Account's statutory allocation to these states (Okafor, 2012).

The Supreme Court of Nigeria noted that the federal government has no power to suspend or withhold any period whatsoever; the statutory allocations are due and payable to the Lagos State government. The Chief Justice further ruled that the 57 newly created local government areas are constitutional, even though they were inchoate. The Court ordered the federal government to release the withheld fund to the Lagos state government for onward distribution to the 20 local government councils. Sadly, President Obasanjo refused to release the fund, arguing that the 37 new local government areas were unconstitutional (Okafor, 2012).

Many legal scholars consider President Obasanjo's action to be wrong, illegal, contemptuous, and a clear manifestation of executive lawlessness. The proper course of action for Obasanjo, many jurists argued, would have been to challenge the constitutionality of the new local government areas. However, he undermined the rule of law and overheated the polity. The attitude of Obasanjo depicts double standards and bias against Lagos State because he did not withhold the statutory allocations to other states that created new local government areas. They changed the names of the local government areas to "Development Areas." Lagos State did the same, yet Obasanjo treated the case differently (Okafor, 2012).

Globally, primary health care serves as the first point of contact for patients at communal levels, facilitating easy access to medical treatment and is the most efficient and cost-effective way to achieve universal health care. In Nigeria, the 36 states are responsible for providing secondary healthcare services in general hospitals, while the local governments coordinate primary healthcare delivery (Adebisi et al., 2020). However, of the three arms of government, the local government is the least funded. The first casualty of a decline in oil revenue has always been the defunding of primary health care, followed by education. As a result, Nigeria has not been able to efficiently implement primary health care, the backbone of the health system. Sadly, Nigeria still lags in allocating sufficient funding for primary healthcare services. The lag explains the deplorable conditions in some of the health facilities in the rural areas.

The Politics of Population Census and Revenue Allocation Formula

Nigeria is undoubtedly one of the world's more prominent federal republics, which has undergone considerable political restructuring to achieve true federalism. However, Nigeria's federalism has suffered from reliable data needed for educational and health systems planning and setting priorities for infrastructural development and nation building. The population of Nigeria has been a contentious issue since colonial times. The first noted enumeration of the population was conducted in 1911 but only covered a region of the country. A nationwide count occurred in 1921 but suffered from inadequate enumerators and was widely boycotted because of the perception that it would lead to higher taxes. Tax riots and a locust invasion marred the 1931 census, and the Second World War prevented the 1941 count. Eventually, it was conducted in 1952 (Akinyemi, 2020).

Post-independence, the census was conducted in 1962, 1963, 1973, 1991, and 2006 (Fawehinmi, 2018). Commenting on the shenanigans and census data manipulation, Fawehinmi (2018) opined that each state consistently maintained its exact share of the population across two censuses, 15 years apart. An aborted military coup rattled the military high command of General Ibrahim Babangida. It hastened the relocation of the federal capital from Lagos to Abuja in December 1991, right after the government completed the census. The population of Abuja rose from 0% of the total in 1991 to 1% in 2006. A group or someone within President Olusegun Obasanjo's administration made up the difference by decreasing Abia State to 2% in 2006 from 3% in 1991. Every other state remained unchanged.

The census figures in Nigeria were all beset with various challenges based on staffing and logistical shortages, undue political interference, and manipulation of data. The population is a critical criterion used in the allocation of revenue to the states. Hence, the incentive to inflate population figures to get more federal government resources. The shenanigans around the census cut through to the heart of the chaos and corruption in the country. Ordinary Nigerians do not trust official census data. This situation necessitates government officers and civil society appeal to international organizations for technical and financial assistance with the census. This embarrassing situation makes it imperative to reflect on the past challenges to ensure the next census is fair and accurate.

Attempts to conduct the census since 2006 did not materialize due to cost and lack of political will by successive democratic governments. Nevertheless, Nigeria will have to hold a census at some point; the question is whether the politicians can lay down weapons and allow a credible count to occur. In 2020, President Muhammadu Buhari approved ₦10 billion ($26 m) to prepare for a new census. The funding is for demarcating enumeration areas and is scheduled to be completed in 2021 (Akinyemi, 2020).

The pertinent question is the relevance of census data to the health and well-being of Nigerians. Nnaemeka and Okwudili, in 2019, explored the nexus between population census, democracy, and nation building. The challenges they identified inter-alia include building a solid institution for democracy, equitable distribution of amenities, justice, and equality of life for all Nigerians, among other issues. They contend that the over politicization of population census is a significant challenge for national unity. Thus, the politicians must avoid the politicization of the census to pave the way to obtain reliable data needed for nation planning. The achievement of this goal would put Nigeria on the right path toward sustainable development.

Both pre- and post-independence, the formula for revenue allocation—the primary driver for census manipulation—is characterized by controversy. Each government level—federal, state, and local—wants to have a sizeable share of the national cake. Since independence, the military governments promulgated several decrees and commissions to provide a revenue allocation formula to meet the aspiration of the stakeholders to have a fair share of allocation from the Federal account. The 1980 Okigbo Presidential Commission on revenue allocation recommended the following formula: federal government, 55%; state government, 35%; and local government, 10%. Like other revenue allocation formulas proposed post-independence, the public perceived Okigbo's recommendation with skepticism and disagreement (Lukpata, 2013).

The thorniest issue under General Ibrahim Babangida's regime was the issue of revenue allocation. Babangida had to review the revenue allocation strategy four times during his eight-year rule from 1985 to 1993. Under Babangida, the revenue allocation formula stood at federal government at 55%, state government at 32.5%, and local government at 10%. Allocation to the oil mineral-producing states and general ecological problems stood at 1.5% and 1%, respectively. From 1994 to 1998, General Sani Abacha's regime adopted the following formula: federal government at 48.5%, state government at 24%, local government at 20%, and special fund at 7.5%.

President Olusegun Obasanjo's (1999–2007) proposed revenue mobilization, allocation, and fiscal commission formula is as follows: federal government at 41.3%, state government at 31%, and local government at 16%. Not satisfied with Obasanjo's recipe, the southern governors proposed the following formula for revenue allocation: federal government at 36%, state government at 36%, local government at 25%, federal capital at 1%, and ecology at 2% (Lukpata, 2013). From 2000 to 2010, the nation adopted the "vertical allocation" formula based on the Presidential Executive order under President Olusegun Obasanjo: federal government at 52.68%, state government at 26.72%, and local government at 20.60%.

After 2010, the subsequent governments adopted the "horizontal allocation" formula that captured some priority factors: equality at 40%, population at 30%, land-mass/terrain at 10%, internally generated revenue at 10%, and social development factor, 10%. The government broke down the social development factor into 4% for education, 3% for health, and 3% for water.

Given the poor state of education, power supply, and limited clean water in the country, it is doubtful that there was any "priority" consideration in the budget for these infrastructures. It is conceivable that the allocated funds were embezzled and ended up in the bureaucrats' foreign bank accounts. Critics deplored the use of landmass, and terrain as a "special" factor for revenue allocation was designed purposefully to favor the northern states. Today, Nigeria is still searching for an acceptable formula for revenue allocation to satisfy the competing interests of all stakeholders (Cahoon, n.d.; Ota et al., 2020).

The State of the Nigerian Nation

The constant political and economic stresses, lack of progress in the education and health sectors, multiple violent conflicts and insecurity, and the escalated divisive rhetoric by politicians have renewed the debate on power and resource sharing. This situation has led several well-meaning citizens to call on Buhari's administration to restructure the Nigerian state. The arguments for and against restructuring is an ongoing and a contentious issue in the literature (Campbell, 2017; Ahmad el-Rufai, 2017; Ola-David, 2018; Yauri, 2018; Dapo-Asaju & Bamgbose, 2019; Bablola & Onapajo, 2019; Othman et al., 2019; Dan-Azumi et al., 2019; Abutudu, 2010).

The recent call for restructuring reignites the tension and instability of the Nigerian state since independence. Kinnan and associates (2011) adroitly described the political landscape as a "country that has been governmentally unstable. Ruled by corrupt elites who have shown an enormous reluctance to relinquish power, sometimes unto death, it has no history of majority governance or even national agreement on any major issue." Moreover, the country remains crisscrossed by many stress cracks and fissures resulting from the ethnic and religious cleavages spanning the six geopolitical zones. Many analysts posit that Nigeria will likely split into dozens or even hundreds of independent nations if sufficiently stressed (Kinnan et al., 2011).

The nascent insecurity challenges that bewildered the entire country, with Fulani herders incessantly engaged in killing farmers, destroying farmlands, raping women, and displacing people from their lands, shifted the debate from restructuring to succession. Many prominent groups and traditional rulers indicted the federal government for aiding and abetting the criminal herdsmen and failing to arrest and prosecute them. The crisis reignited the demand for the Biafra Republic and new agitation to create the Oduduwa Republic and the Kwararafa Republic (Ajeluorou, 2020; SaharaReporters, 2021).

History of Nigeria's Sudden Wealth and the Aftermath Economic Woes

A brief review of the history of how Nigeria suddenly became rich, and the excesses of past leaders are worth discussing here. Petroleum was first discovered in 1956 and is the primary source of revenue and foreign exchange. Nigeria joined the Organization of Petroleum Exporting Countries in 1971. The cartel imposed an oil embargo in 1973, which resulted in the price of oil skyrocketing four times over. Nigeria suddenly and startlingly became an energy force and affluent. The Naira's strength even dwarfed the US dollar, with ₦1.00 trading for $1.60 by 1976. Since the late 1970s, there have been cyclical increases and declines in oil sales revenues with untold hardship when prices fall. After paying off Paris Club in December 2006, Nigeria's external debt was only $3.5 billion. The thought was that paying the foreign debt would free up cash for capital expenditure and usher in an economic boom and development. Unfortunately, the external debt creeps back up after years of lower oil prices, excessive spending, defense of the exchange rate, and a lot of stolen wealth by politicians (Ojieh, 2016). The country is somewhat back full circle. The external debt at the beginning of 2015 was $9.7 billion but ballooned to $27 billion in December 2019—a 16-year high. President Muhammadu Buhari's government accrued most of the debts during the first four years of his administration, and the foreign reserves also dropped by $2.36 billion in 2019 (Nairametrics, 2020).

Nigeria operates a mono-social economy, with 85% of its revenue derived from oil and gas exports (Olamide et al., 2019). Without a doubt, the country ranks among the most richly endowed nations of the world in natural, mineral, and human resources. It has various untapped renewable and non-renewable resources. Solar energy, the most underutilized renewable resource, remains untapped, and the vast reserves of natural gas produced with crude oil are yet to be utilized fully. The economy was healthy and vibrant in the 1950s when agriculture accounted for over 70% of the employment opportunities (Uzonwanne, 2015).

The agriculture sector, which accounts for 26.8% of the GDP and two-thirds of employment, has witnessed years of mismanagement, inconsistent and poorly conceived government policies, neglect, and the lack of necessary infrastructure. The country has 19 million cattle, the largest in Africa, but no longer a primary exporter of cocoa, groundnuts (peanuts), rubber, and palm oil. In the last two decades, the agricultural sector experienced extremely low productivity because of the reliance on antiquated farming methods. The overall agricultural production rose by 28% during the 1990s, but per capita output increase by only 8.5% during the same decade (Suberu, 1998).

Sadly, the production in the agriculture sector has failed to keep pace with the exploding population growth, and the country no longer exports food but relies on imports to feed the nation. Given this untenable situation, there is an urgent need to diversify the economy's various sectors to attain substantial economic growth. Specifically, the government must diversify the mono-cultural economy based on oil revenue by promoting agriculture and agro-based industries, solid minerals, energizing local technology, and innovation. Also, the government must incentivize the vibrant private sector to harness the youth's energies to deliver the promise of the future. Additionally, renewed national efforts are needed to improve subsistence farming's productivity by using emerging technologies such as agroforestry and nitrogen-fixing trees, multiple cropping, improved genetic material, and crop biotechnology.

Suberu and associates (1998) linked the economic woes to spending spree culture, looting, lawlessness, and indiscipline—the modus operandi in national life. In diagnosing the country's financial status and future, Olamide et al. (2019) opined that corruption poses a genuine obstacle to diversification because the assets that the government should divert to different economic sectors are upset by unlawful practices. The politicians and government establishments are against diversification but prefer to maintain the status quo. The decline of revenue from oil, the explosion of foreign debts, and interest service obligations will handicap any progress toward UHC and inhibit any meaningful future capital developments at the federal and state levels. Any robust revenue from oil in the future is bleak because of the global popularity of the electric car and the increased solar energy utilization.

Wasteful Spending and Corruption: Barriers to Universal and High-Quality Health Care

Since independence, most of Nigeria's leaders have been wasteful and unable to harness the natural resources to provide UHC. Still, they live a sumptuous lifestyle and engage in extravagant spending. A brief review of how previous Nigerian leaders have wasted the resources and botched the implementation of UHC is worth discussing here.

It is well-established that between 20% and 40% of all health resources are wasted (Abuja Declaration, 2011). The secret to UHC is through restructuring and diversification of the economy. The interplay of corruption and politics plays a critical complementary role in ensuring that the earmarked fund is not reallocated to the other sectors. Wasteful spending is one of the dominant disconcerting vileness within the Nigerian state governance. Corruption is a social virus prevalent in the polity from colonial times to the present day. Ejovi and associates (2013) presented a poignant historical analysis and inferred that the "phenomenon of corruption attains a distinct and higher stage of development during the nine years of Gowon's administration." For example, throughout General Yakubu Gowon's nine-year military rule (1966–1975), the defense ministry overshot approved budgets by several million pounds sterling, spending without going through the executive council and every year consistently ignored the Auditor-General queries on the vast unauthorized and illegal expenditures. The subsequent military governments also exhibited a total lack of budgetary discipline and financial accountability (Ejovi et al., 2013). Many analysts contend that Gowon is not corrupt but could not control his governors and ministers. His lack of authority over his subordinates opened the floodgate for the grand scale corruption in Nigeria.

The "Father Christmas" foreign policy by General Gowon lavishly spent money on other nations worldwide as a show of generosity. Like Prime Minister Abubakar Tafawa Balewa (1912–1966), Gowon maintained an autocratic control of foreign policy and personalized decision-making without consultation with the Supreme Military Council. His successor, General Murtala Mohammed, after a successful coup d'état, accused Gowon of insensitivity to responsible opinion due to his never-ending pursuit of personal adulation (Ojieh, 2016). From the information available in open access literature (Ojieh, 2016), Gowon spent ₦5,235,440 in gifts to foreign nations within 3 years, from 1972 to 1975. In the 1970s, the exchange rate for ₦1 = $1.65 (USD). As of January 11, 2021, $1.00 USD = ₦475. In 2021 monetary value, the gift amount doled out by Gowon to other countries would be more than sufficient in making UHC a reality in Nigeria.

General Gowon also awarded an unspecified number of scholarships to students from the Gambia, Sudan, Guinea, Uganda, Liberia, and Kenya, to study in African universities. Shortly before the coup d'état that removed him from office, Gowon made Nigeria forego its right to receive the entitled financial dividends from the African Development Bank and instead gave it to less endowed African countries.

In 1973, Gowon provided foreign aid to help develop Papua and New Guinea and rescued the United Kingdom from its financial obligations in Jamaica to the tune of £20 million. He even extended his generosity to his foreign friends and other countries outside Africa. In May 1975, Gowon paid the civil servants' salaries in Grenada and Guyana and helped balance their recurrent budgets to prevent bankruptcy, even though, at that time, Granada has no diplomatic relationship with Nigeria (Ojieh, 2016).

The waste of the nation's resources and opulent lifestyle was taken to a new height at the peak of the oil boom when General Gowon proclaimed to foreign reporters on October 1, 1974, that Nigeria is a well-endowed country whose challenge is how to expend the wealth (Olayinka, 2014; Ojieh, 2016; Alake, 2018). General Gowon also spent the sudden wealth on eccentric construction projects for the Second World Black and African Festival of Arts and Culture (FESTAC '77) extravaganza held in Lagos for 17 days. The cultural jamboree cost over $300 million in the 1970s dollar. Nigeria hosted 17,000 artists from 55 African nations, the Americas, Europe, Canada, and the Islands to celebrate African culture. Why did Gowon engage in esoteric projects and foreign spending sprees when Nigerians were hungry and malnourished, have no access to free health care, and lacked clean water, reliable electricity, and tarred roads? No other leader of a country will behave like a drunken sailor in managing the public funds. Alake (2018) stirringly described Gowon's administration as corrupt and laid down an unmaintainable country. Gowon's military governors and civilian acolytes lacked vision and selfishly looted the treasury. The trend of entitlement to the nation's wealth festered into near-incurable corruption, laying the foundation for the country's ditch until today.

Alhaji Shehu Shagari (1979–1983) was the first civilian leader to take office under a presidential constitution modeled after the United States under a 19-state administrative structure. Cowell (2018) described Shagari as a likable but not particularly formidable candidate with the presidency imposed on him. Slumping oil prices and endemic corruption blighted Shagari's administration. Legg (2019) described Shagari's presidency as corrupt and marked by deep divisions between the Muslims in the north and Christians in the south. Shagari also became president at an inopportune time when oil—Nigeria's primary source of revenue—experienced a global decline with no funds to support his campaign promise to improve the standard of living.

Shagari took several bold steps to strengthen the economy by cutting spending, increasing import duties, and expelling over two million African workers in 1983 (Lawal, 1983). Expelling Africans from Nigeria is an unexpected development, given that Gowon, just a decade earlier, was dolling out money worldwide. Notwithstanding, Shagari won re-election in a bitterly contested election in 1983 and was removed in a coup on New Year's Eve by General Muhammadu Buhari. In a speech to the nation after the coup, Buhari accused Shagari of being incompetent and influenced by a few corrupt politicians holding onto the nation's wealth with a firm commitment to stay in power in perpetuity (Legg, 2019; Cowell, 2018). Some high officials in Shagari's administration were accused of corruption. One of them, Umaru Dikko, Mr. Shagari's campaign manager, fled to the United Kingdom (Cowell, 2018). Shagari was arrested and held under house arrest for 3 years and later cleared of corruption by a judge but banned from politics (Cowell, 2018; Legg, 2019).

Oluokun (2012) noted that Goodluck Jonathan (2007–2011) took the culture of waste a notch higher during his tenure as president. During his tenure, Jonathan wasted the $180 billion earnings from oil and gas, import duties, and taxes. He depleted the excess crude account to less than $1 billion, and the reserves were down to about $35 billion. Jonathan's administration was noted for large traveling contingents, indiscriminate setting up of committees, substantial budgetary allocations to the Presidential Villa, and stealthily conducted media campaigns. The administration was also known for a large number of government ministers and presidential aides—over 40 ministers and excessive and redundant special assistants and advisers.

In 2012, Jonathan was widely condemned for proposing to spend ₦477 million for foodstuffs and catering materials supplies, ₦293 million for refreshment and meals, and ₦45.4 million for kitchen equipment in his office and home. His Vice-President, Namadi Sambo, also proposed ₦20.8 million for refreshment and N104 million for meals and ₦6.2 million for cooking fuel. Jonathan also allocated N280 million for two Mercedes Benz armored S-guard vehicles and ₦239 million for assorted cars added to the presidential fleet. Billions from two federal government accounts were turned into a slush fund by the Jonathan administration (Oluokun, 2012).

Like Gowon, Jonathan was impervious to the looting within his cabinet and rejected the assertion that his administration was corrupt. In 2015, the American and British officials reported that Jonathan's Petroleum Minister Diezani Alison-Madueke organized a diversion of $6 billion (₦1.2 trillion) from the federal treasury (Sotubo, 2015). She was charged for the $20 billion missing from the National Petroleum Commission and accused of awarding multi-billion contracts without due process, recklessly spending government funds, money laundering, and wasting billions inappropriately on private jets. Oluokun (2012), a critic of Jonathan, opined that it is unfortunate that Nigerians elected an extravagant man who left the country broke because his political party (People's Democratic Party, PDP) has drained the treasuries, the foreign reserve, and excess crude and the stabilization accounts. Because of Jonathan's administration, Nigerians were forced to pay for their driver's licenses and plate numbers and even spend ₦145 for a liter of gas. Unfortunately, nothing has changed in the wasteful spending by the leaders of the country.

Even though President Muhammadu Buhari campaigned to curb corruption and waste, his administration is not different from his predecessors. Some analysts contend Buhari is weak and public trust in his government is in decline, coupled with a growing perception of lacking political inclusion. As a result, the standard of living for an average Nigerian has plummeted, and the country has become more divided and less secure (Olurounbi, 2021; Igwe, 2020).

Nigeria emulates the US government operations despite its meager economic and military powers. All previous and incumbent Nigerian Presidents like to compete in the social league they do not belong to. Air Force One marks the American presidency's luxury; Nigeria also purchased a Boeing 737NG BBJ and called it "Eagle One." Most countries cannot afford a private jet for their leader. The United Kingdom purchased its first jet for the Prime Minister in 2016. Before then, the United Kingdom was the only G20 leader without an aircraft.

As President, Buhari maintained a fleet of planes: Boeing 737NG BBJ, Gulfstream V-SP, a Gulfstream 550, two Falcon 7Xs, a Dornier Do 228, and three A139 helicopters. Boeing 737NG BBJ plane is a custom-built executive aircraft with additional fuel tanks for the extended flight, and it is compliant with the European Union noise regulations. It can land in all countries, unlike the aircraft used by former President Olusegun Obasanjo. Boeing 737NG BBJ plane has a master bedroom, a washroom with showers, a conference/dining area, and a living area and can comfortably seat 25–50 passengers. Is this grandiosity and display of luxury by the Nigerian President necessary in a country rated as the world's poverty capital?

With pressure from the public to fulfill his campaign promise to cut down on waste, President Buhari eventually, in 2016, sold the two Falcon 900s, a GIV-SP, and GII and reallocated the Citation Bravo and Hawker 800 to the air force (BBC, 2016). Although Buhari campaigned on a strong anti-corruption message and austere lifestyle, the cost of running the statehouse in Abuja has surged, with millions of investment in line items repeated from previous years, such as the "installation of electrical lighting and fittings." As of 2016, the government spends more on maintaining the presidential fleet than what is allocated to any federal university. Between 2013 and 2015, the government spent $72.3 million on maintaining the presidential jet (Kazeem, 2015). From 2011 to 2020, about ₦73.3 billion was set aside for the presidential fleet. The budgeting includes utilities, materials and supplies, maintenance services, training, and financial charges such as insurance. The maintenance cost of the presidential aircraft averaged ₦7 billion in the last 10 years. The highest allocation for the fleet was ₦22 billion by President Goodluck Jonathan's administration. In 2017, Buhari's government daily spent £4000 to park the presidential aircraft when he was in London for one of his many medical trips (Nda-Isaiah, 2017).

In 2019, the opposition party bemoaned Buhari's budget proposal as deceptive duplication, packed with false performance indicators and fraudulent and incomprehensible expenditure projections that create opportunities for looting the national treasury (Channels Television, 2019b). Also, the opposition party accused Buhari's government as grossly corrupt and depleted the foreign reserves to $41,852 billion—an all-time low—and accumulated substantial external and domestic debts and kept the exchange rate high at ₦360 to $1USD.

In January 2020, President Buhari drew angry criticism for allowing his daughter to use the presidential jet to Bauchi state for a private school assignment (Alfa Shaban, 2020). The trip's cost and the bad precedents it set for future Presidents are concerning (Emeka, 2020). In anger, a civil rights lawyer, Jiti Ogunye, rebuked Buhari's administration for using the presidential jet to conduct private business (Kabir, 2020). He noted that the office of the President's appurtenance has no provisions in the law that criminalizes the use of the President's jet by family members. The former Chairman of the National Human Rights Commission and a lawyer, Chidi Odinkalu, berated Buhari's administration, which marketed itself as having integrity, for crossing the line of virtue to criminality (Kabir, 2020). Similarly, the Centre for Social Justice in Abuja criticized the 2020 budget for containing about ₦150.07 billion expenditures that are ill-considered, imprudent, fatuous, and prodigal (Onuba, 2019).

During his first term in office, President Muhammadu Buhari spent a whopping 404 days (28% of his time in office) in 33 countries on four continents (Table 12.1). He spent 217 days in the United Kingdom receiving medical treatment and attending Commonwealth Heads of State and Government meetings and stayed 41 days in

Table 12.1 Countries visited by President Buhari during his first term in office

Serial No.	Countries	Total number of days stayed
1	United Kingdom	217
2	United States	41
3	France	14
4	China	13
5	Jordan	8
6	UAE, Morocco, Germany, and South Africa (7 days each)	28
7	Saudi Arabia	6
8	India, Chad, Kenya, Turkey, Poland, and Malta (5 days each)	30
9	Senegal, Ethiopia, Mauritania, the Netherlands, Togo, and Republic of Benin (4 days each)	24
10	Côte d'Ivoire, Iran, and Equatorial Guinea (3 days each)	9
11	Cameroon, Ghana, Niger, Gambia, Egypt, and Qatar (2 days each)	12
12	Mali and Sudan (1 day each)	2
Total	**33**	**404[a]**

Source: (Alechenu et al., 2019)

[a]About 28% of his four years (1460 days) in office was spent in foreign land

the United States and met with President Barack Obama and President Donald Trump and participated in the 70th, 71st, 72nd, and 73rd sessions of the United Nations General Assembly. On the other hand, Buhari did not visit any country in South America during his first term (Alechenu et al., 2019).

President Muhammadu Buhari's trip to the United Kingdom in March of 2021 caused an outrage. He was criticized widely for leaving the country even during the coronavirus pandemic when medical doctors were on industrial strike to protest against working conditions and nonpayment of salary arrears (Michael, 2021). His critics' recurring question is, "What is wrong with Nigeria that Buhari does not like and runs away from?" His overseas trips consist of several cabinet members, and the trips cost hundreds of thousands of dollars. Indeed, Buhari is an extravagant and wasteful manager of the national treasury. The president of many wealthy nations has not traveled as much as President Buhari. He escapes to foreign land whenever it is convenient for him to do so, under the guise of medical check-ups or attending meetings to promote Nigeria. Buhari and his minions are globetrotters living off the taxpayers' blood, sweat, and tears. Many analysts contend that he must cut back on foreign trips and use the money to develop the decrepit health system (Onuba, 2019; Daily Sabah, 2021). It would serve the nation better if he stayed at home and govern the country he was constitutionally elected to run.

President Buhari's global trip record makes him one of the most traveled world leaders while in office. He joined the ranks of Bharrat Jagdeo of Guyana (Kaieteur News, 2009) and Indonesia ex-President Abdurrahman Wahid, colloquially known as Gus Dur. Wahid traveled to 80 countries while in office for less than 20 months—from 1999 to 2001. Among the most traveled world leaders of all time include Pope

John Paul II. During his reign from 1978 to 2005, he made 104 foreign trips to 129 countries in 27 years. He logged more than 1,167,000 km even though he had Parkinson's and a failed assassination on his life (Rome Reports, 2017). Besides the Pope, Queen Elizabeth II also traveled to 120 countries in 68 years. US Secretary of State Hillary Clinton took American culture and diplomacy to 112 nations in 8 years. Recep Tayyip Erdogan visited 93 countries in 17 years as prime minister (2003–2014) and president (2014–) (Quora Inc., 2020).

Assets of Wealthy Nigerian Presidents

The assets of the consequential Nigerian Presidents after Gowon are worth discussing here. General Ibrahim Babangida (nicknamed by the press as "evil genius" "Maradona"), during his military rule from 1985 to 1993, laundered between $12 and $14 billion from the oil revenue during the 1992 Gulf War. To date, Babangida has not provided any valid account for the windfall, which disappeared mysteriously. Given the polity's lack of accountability, Babangida is considered an "untouchable" and remained a free man. His wealth is invested through several proxies of wealthy friends. His mansion at Minna is worth multi-million dollars and owns over 20 buildings in Nigeria and 42 real estate investments in different parts of the world. He owns 65% of the Fruitex International limited in London and 24% of Globacom, the second largest telecommunication company in Nigeria (Nigerian Finder, 2021b).

Upon his death in 1998, Sani Abacha was worth between $3 and $5 billion (Nsehe, 2011). The Nigerian government uncovered over $3 billion in foreign personal and proxy bank accounts in Jersey, Switzerland, Luxembourg, and Liechtenstein. Following negotiations between the Abacha family and the Nigerian government, his first son, Mohammed, returned $1.2 billion to the government in 2002 (Nsehe, 2011). In 2014, the US Department of Justice forfeited $480 million of Abacha's money—to the Nigerian government. The Abacha family laundered more than $267 million (£210 million in British pounds) in a Jersey account (Omojuwa.com, 2019). President Olusegun Obasanjo's net worth is over $1.5 billion. His assets are from farming and educational ventures and oil blocks, worth 6.5% of its total primary oil production, marketing, and distribution (Nigerian Finder, 2021a). Nigerianinfofinder.com named him the wealthiest Nigerian politician with a net worth of $1.8 billion (Ojo, 2021).

Over the years, President Goodluck Jonathan has been very secretive and reluctant to declare his assets. In 2007, Yar'Adua forced him to declare his assets publicly. On assumption of office, he reported it at ₦295,304,420 but refused to update it during his tenure as the president publicly. In 2014, a website ranked Jonathan the sixth richest President in Africa with a net worth of $100 million (Celebritynetworth.com, 2014). He was outraged by the publication and demanded the article be taken down. Indeed, the account on the website was suspended. In 2014, Sahara Reporters estimated Jonathan's net worth at ₦21 billion ($127 million)—the exchange rate in 2014 was ₦164 for 1$. In the same year, in 2014, the Constative.com website estimated Jonathan's net worth at over $500 million (Falae, 2017). In 2021, Jonathan's net worth is estimated at $10 million (Celebritynetworth.com, 2021). His successor, Muhammadu Buhari, is one of Nigeria's most influential public personalities with $80 million (Ikeru, 2020, Glusea.com, 2021). The net worth of Nigeria's top politicians in 2021 was estimated by the Glusea.com website (2021) as follows: Ibrahim Babangida ($5 billion), Sa'adu Abubakar ($4 billion), Bola Tinubu ($4 billion), Atiku Abubakar ($1.8 billion), Olusegun Obasanjo ($1.6 billion), and Rochas Okorocha ($1.5 billion).

Clearly, Nigeria's poverty and health inequality are not due to a shortage of resources but to corruption, wasteful spending, misallocation, and misappropriation of funds by the political elite unable to relate to the average citizen's struggle (Oxfam International, 2020). The past and current Nigerian leaders' ability to effectively manage the economy do not instill any confidence. The latest tempestuousness to hit the public revenue is the global recession that precipitated a sharp decline in oil prices and devaluation of the Naira (₦). The USD exchange rate to the Nigerian currency was ₦475 on January 11, 2021—a 1.06% rise for USD to Naira exchange rates for the year (NgnRates.com, 2021). The decline in the economic fortune is due to the continued fall in oil prices from the headwinds arising from the global COVID-19 crisis and the tension between the United States and Saudi Arabia—the world's two largest oil producers (Adesoji, 2020). The relevant question is, "What is the immediate and long-term plan for achieving universal and high-quality health care in Nigeria?"

Who Is Nigeria's Greatest President?

Nigerians continue to debate their president's performance, especially with the country's recent myriad of security challenges and escalation of poverty (Legit TV, 2017). From the opinions expressed in two available national polls, President Olusegun Obasanjo (1999 to 2007) is considered the "best" president in the history of the country (Legit TV, 2017; Elutidoye, 2020). He is credited for assembling one of the most productive cabinets and advisers—El-Rufai, Okonjo Iweala, Frank Nweke Jr., Bayo Ojo, and Bola Ige, among others. He pooled resources from all political parties to form a government of national unity. Unlike Buhari, he gave equal representation to all parts of the country in his cabinet and security cabinet.

Obasanjo's enthusiasts attribute his achievements, particularly in the health sector, for appointing brilliant technocrats such as Professor Eyitayo Lambo as health minister and Professor Friday Okonofua as a health adviser. Obasanjo also assembled an effective economic team that doubled the growth rate to 6%, and 13% derivation was paid to oil-producing states. The foreign reserves grew from $4 billion in 1999 to $43.5 billion by December 2006, even after repaying $14 billion to the Paris and London club. He left $60bn in the national treasury, the highest ever in the history of Nigeria even though, under him, it was not when oil prices were highest in history (Elutidoye, 2020).

Obasanjo is also credited for stabilizing the nascent democracy, solidifying the middle class, and encouraging Nigerians in Diaspora to return home to contribute to national development. Under Obasanjo, Nigeria's image abroad improved, national pride was high, and the country hosted many international sporting events.

In addition, the government had a sense of purpose and helped end the wars in Sierra Leone and Liberia (Elutidoye, 2020).

Obasanjo's supporters consider him progressive and visionary and often reference, among other things, his initiation of the NHIS in 2000 and the presidential library and hotel infrastructure edifice that he built at Ota—a library is one of the hallmarks of every modern American president. Obasanjo's government gave birth to many new institutions, including the EFCC, Independent Corrupt Practices Commission (ICPC), and the Niger Delta Development Commission (NDDC). However, the feat that Obasanjo is most acclaimed for was the Global System for Mobile Communications, launched in 2001—although it was never his original idea. Another progressive initiative that Obasanjo inaugurated includes the National Economic Empowerment Development Strategy (NEEDS). In 2005, after the take-off of the NEEDS, the moribund banking system was successfully consolidated from 89 Nigerian banks to 25. Other innovative initiatives launched are the State Economic Empowerment Development Strategy (SEEDS) and the Local Economic Empowerment Development Strategy (LEEDS). The latter successfully moved the digital telephone base through privatization and deregulation from below one million in 1999 to over 38 million by 2007 (Elutidoye, 2020).

Unlike Buhari, who refused to accept that the Fulani herdsmen are terrorizing other tribes even when the herdsmen are the fourth most deadly terrorist group globally, Obasanjo never allowed the Northern warlocks to control the military. Thus, Boko Haram bandits were not violent until Obasanjo left office. Obasanjo ensured equal distribution of armory among the regions against the Buhari's administration that used Boko Haram as an excuse for moving most armory and military arsenal back to the North (Legit TV, 2017).

Nevertheless, an unprecedented level of corruption marred Obasanjo and his cabinet members, including Atiku. Still, his admirers argue that Obasanjo is a fierce corruption crusader, and his fight against corruption, unlike Buhari's, was not one-sided; it was never fought on one end and fed on the other end.

Besides Murtala Mohammed (who ruled from July 30, 1975, to February 13, 1976) and Umaru Yar'Adua (who ruled from May 29, 2007, to May 5, 2010), whose tenure as president was short lived, Yakubu Gowon is widely acclaimed as the least corrupt of all past Nigerian leaders who served for more than 3 years in office. While Gowon never owned a decent home while in office (from August 1, 1966, to July 29, 1975) and decades after his tenure, several of his ministers and military governors looted the national treasury (Legit TV, 2017). Gowon is a gentleman to the core and too timid about removing his corrupt lieutenants from office even after intense pressure from the public.

Critics assert that the privatization of Transcorp became a piggy bank for Obasanjo and his minions (Legit TV, 2017; Elutidoye, 2020), and the power sector investment was an endless feast for Obasanjo and his loyalists. Since none of the Nigerian presidents ever declared their assets after leaving office, the amount reported earlier from different sources is speculative.

Civil organizations and critics bemoaned Obasanjo's regime for his authoritarian instincts and absolute disregard for democratic precepts. His critics describe his presidency as a gangster democracy because his opposition was consistently tyrannized (Legit TV, 2017; Elutidoye, 2020). He even canvassed for a third term in office against the tenets of the constitution. Many of his opponents were scared of his hooliganism as the leaders of the Movement for the Actualization of the Sovereign State of Biafra and O'odua People's Congress were detained perpetually. Within his party, Obasanjo ditches the dissenting voices and senate leaders like robes at a dress rehearsal. The EFCC became Obasanjo's wand of punishment and persecution of his perceived enemies.

The Political Reforms Needed to Achieve Universal and High-Quality Health Care

The workforce of a healthy and well-educated nation is always more productive and economically independent (WHO 2017a; WHO, 2020). As is the case in Nigeria, having an educated workforce is insufficient to attain economic independence when the workers have no access to health care. Following an in-depth analysis of the relationship between politics and health, Bambra and associates (2005) conclude that health is profoundly political, and individual social groups always have better healthcare access than others do. The social determinants of health are acquiescent to political intervention and legislative action or inaction. This chapter opines that the reform of the health system should take center stage in the negotiation concerning the country's future. The restructuring of the Nigerian administrative architecture is the first step needed to achieve UHC. That said, a brief discussion of the economic viability of the states is warranted here since it is the basis for the political reforms argument in this chapter.

For over a decade, several budget-tracking analyses have consistently revealed that only a few of the 36 states in the country are economically viable. The most recent budget-tracking assessment in 2020 showed that only six states (Lagos, Ogun, Rivers, Kwara, Kaduna, and Enugu) are financially viable. The insolvent states—Katsina, Kebbi, Borno, Bayelsa, and Taraba—have high recurring costs with internally generated revenue far below 10% of their revenue from the federation government (Agbakwuru, 2020). In 2019, only four states (Lagos, Rivers, Akwa Ibom, and Kano) were viable. Several states (Delta, Bayelsa, Ebonyi, Sokoto, Jigawa, Yobe, Cross River, Imo, Kogi, etc.) had huge recurrent expenditures and operated "bogus" budgets (Ewepu, 2019; Guardian, 2019; PMNews, 2019).

In 2018, only ten (Lagos, Ogun, Rivers, Kwara, Edo, Kano, Enugu, Ondo, Kaduna, Delta) of the 36 states were economically viable, and 17 were insolvent (PMNews, 2019). In 2017, eight states (Lagos, Ogun, Rivers, Edo, Kwara, Enugu, Kano, and Delta) were financially solvent while Bauchi, Yobe, Borno, Kebbi, and Katsina were insolvent (PRNigeria, 2017). Between 2010 and 2012, ten Southern states (Lagos, Rivers, Delta, Edo, Oyo, Ebonyi, Akwa Ibom, Cross Rivers, Ogun, and Enugu) had dominant economic activity. Eight of the ten least solvent states were from the North (Atuanya & Augie, 2013). The majority of the viable states are in the Southwestern region, including the oil-producing areas. Overall, most of the insolvent states were created between 1976 and 1996.

Only a few states and local governments in Nigeria provide up to 30% of their planned expenditures from internally generated revenue. Between 1990 and 1994, the statutory allocation from the federal account constituted over 70% of the states' revenues, while internally generated revenues accounted for only 17.8%, and the balance was by special (discretionary) grants from the federal government. The situation has not changed, even today (Suberu, 1998). In 2018, the Nigerian economy accrued $30.1 billion (₦1.103 trillion) as internally generated revenue, and over 70% of that amount came from the south, and the north's contribution remains abysmally low. Yet, the north takes at least 65% when internally generated revenues are disbursed to states and local government areas (BusinessDay, 2019; Ota et al., 2020). As a result of this inequity, Ota and associates (2020) assert that "the north owns Nigeria just like a slave owner owns his slaves."

Many of the insolvent states are so impoverished that they cannot pay their employees' salaries and cannot balance their budget for several consecutive years. It is unlikely the insolvent states will ever become financially independent of the federal government. An unsolvable state serves no useful political purpose because it defeats state creation's stated primary reason—to bring government closer to the grassroots. Moreover, an insolvent state is a liability to the federal government. No meaningful development can occur in an insolvent state. A decade is a lifetime in any nation's development, and it is high time to call a spade a spade and take decisive action against the insolvent states. From the aforementioned economic realities, this chapter advocates that the federal government dissolve the insolvent states and invest the revenue accrued in strengthening the national health insurance scheme (NHIS). Specifically, the country's administrative architecture should revert to the 12-state structure to achieve overall financial viability.

The Nigerian population is growing at an astronomical rate (United Nations Population Fund, n.d.). This concerning developmental challenge will further increase competition for the limited financial resources among the viable states.

Authority and Roles of the Federal and State Governments in the New Dispensation

In the new 12-state structure proposed, the central government should be less powerful but not rendered weak. It should retain its core functions in defense, national security, health care, transportation (managing the main express roads, railways, and aviation), foreign affairs, and central banks. The state and local governments should manage the intrastate and local roads, police, and education. This chapter proposes the devolution of the central powers, advocates for more resources and greater autonomy to the states and local governments. The federal government should garner 60% of the revenue from the natural resources in all states, and 40%

of the natural resources' revenue should be reallocated to state and local governments. The rationale for the recommendations will be discussed next.

Both education and health care are human right issues. In 1948, the United Nations General Assembly proclaimed the "inalienable rights" for every human being entitled to free elementary school education, while technical, professional, and higher education equally accessible to all based on merit (Global Partnership for Education, 2017). The right to health means access to free healthcare services without suffering financial hardship. The inalienable right also includes access to nutritious foods, safe drinking water and sanitation, adequate housing, and safe working conditions (WHO, 2017b). According to the United Nations, the right to free health care begins at birth and terminates at the end of life. In contrast, the right to free education is only at the early stage of life (Global Partnership for Education, 2017). Given that the spread of diseases knows no state or regional boundaries, healthcare provision requires coordination at the national level and should be one of the federal government's core functions.

Since independence, the country's pace of economic and educational development varies; some states are more assertive and deliberate in funding higher education. The chapter advocates that each state should be allowed to set educational priorities, and the federal universities, polytechnics, and the colleges of education returned to the states. The existence of the controversial Joint Admissions and Matriculation Board becomes irrelevant, as each university will be responsible for setting admission criteria. The transition of education to state and private control is not a radical idea since many states currently have private universities and at least one federal university and other higher learning institutions. The recommendation is consistent with practice in the United States where the only national institutions of higher learning are the military academies, the Haskell Indian Nations University, and Southwestern Indian Polytechnic Institute for Native Americans (Harris, 2018).

Another reason for returning education to state and private control is the recent ugly politics surrounding the appointments of chief executives at universities. In the early years of university education in the country, the appointment of Vice-Chancellors (VCs) is based on merit without ethnic consideration. For example, the University of Ibadan routinely appoints non-Yoruba as the VC—Professor Kenneth Onwuka Dike (1960–1967), Professor Oritsejolomi Thomas (1972–1975), and Professor Tekena Tamuno (1975–1979). Today, the academy has become tribal enclaves where only "natives" are welcomed to apply for the VC's position, even in federal government-owned universities. The traditional rulers in the institution's jurisdiction are now the power brokers in the selection of VCs.

In August 2020, leaders of a socio-cultural group in Ibadan appealed to President Muhammadu Buhari to appoint one of their own as the VC and Chief Medical Director of the University of Ibadan (Adelakun, 2020). I doubt this odious and brazen request can happen in any other country. Sadly, the zoning of the VC and Chief Medical Director's positions to indigenes abound in several of the other federal universities. The management of the university system reflects the decay and disorders in the larger society. The health and education systems are mangled in corruption, tribalism, and mediocrity, as in every aspect of Nigerian life (Onu, 2019).

The need for local control of the country's security arrangement has become a contentious issue following the violent rise and resilience of the Boko Haram—a jihadist group—in the Lake Chad basin and the upsurge in the Fulani herdsmen kidnapping. Both problems pose enormous humanitarian and governance challenges. As a solution, this chapter advocates decentralizing the federal police system and allowing each state and local government to manage their security. The concept of local policing is not new, and the advantages are well-documented in the literature (Owusu-Bempah, 2016). The literature consensus is that the benefits of local policing outweigh the use of federal police to maintain law and order. The local community often sees federal police as "occupant force." The return to local policing has the potential to address the insecurity problem in the country. Adequate security in the country will provide a conducive environment for foreign entrepreneurs to return to invest and create jobs.

A vexing political problem that has bedeviled the nation, and indirectly the healthcare system, is power sharing at the federal level. The governance and leadership of the country since independence are not distributed evenly across the country. The North has dominated and unwilling to share power with the other regions. Many critics pose the fairness question: Why have the eastern states not produce a President after Nnamdi Benjamin Azikiwe served as the first President of Nigeria from 1963 to 1966? This chapter advocates for constitutional amendments to guarantee the rotation of the presidency along the six geopolitical zones to solve the leadership conundrum and limit term in office for all political positions, including the presidency, to 5 years.

Another political reform needed to build trust and strengthen national unity is to have a constitutional amendment that will allow Nigerians to become an indigene of a state, with all rights, if they were born or reside in the state continuously for 5 years. The legislatures should enact laws to abolish the quota system in employment and create a level plan field for all citizens. The federal government should take over the oil rigs corruptly acquired by the elites, as the natural resources belong to the Nigerian people. The federal government must allocate more funds and human resources to strengthen the national security apparatus to address the Boko Haram and Fulani herdsmen crises—both are a threat to the country's sovereignty.

Economic Reforms Needed to Achieve Universal and High-Quality Health Care

The constitution of Nigeria was modeled after the US system but has several aberrant differences that make the democracy unaffordable in the hands of greedy Nigerian politicians. The United States, with a population of 328.2 million, has only 15 federal departments (ministries). In contrast, Nigeria, with 206 million people, has 28 federal ministries and overpaid legislators. The average legislators' pay in Nigeria is more than 50 times the GDP per capita (Kazeem, 2015). This situation is concerning, particularly when the minimum wage is $90 per month, with most

Nigerians living on less than $2.00 (£1.51) per day. In 2018, the national assembly passed only 106 bills out of the 1063 it reviewed in 4 years. Still, Nigerian legislators earn a whopping $480,000 (£361,610) annually. Although their monthly salary is only $2000 (£1512), they receive an additional guaranteed expense allowance of $35,720 (£27,000) per month (Lovemoney.com, 2019). Because of the exorbitant salary in the executive and legislative arms of government, many well-meaning Nigerians have previously called for a constitutional amendment to fix their wages at a reasonable level.

The "do-nothing" Nigerian legislators are the second-highest paid globally, outpacing Japan, New Zealand, United Kingdom, and South Africa (Table 12.2). The legislators in the United States receive $174,000 (£131,109), which ranks fifth in the

Table 12.2 Legislators' pay in different countries in 2018

Ranking	Country	$	£
1	Singapore	888,428	669,323
2	Nigeria	480,000	361,610
3	Japan	274,000	206,495
4	New Zealand	196,300	150,000
5	United States	174,000	131,109
6	Australia	141,330	108,380
7	Italy	143,352	108,038
8	Germany	133,279	100,439
9	Canada	130,710	100,335
10	Austria	117,903	90,271
11	Norway	108,907	82,010
12	Ireland	106,389	80,441
13	The Netherlands	104,076	79,098
14	United Kingdom	102,364	77,379
15	Denmark	100,587	75,762
16	France	98,647	74,307
17	Belgium	97,549	73,441
18	Russia	93,330	69,999
19	Finland	89,317	67,577
20	Sweden	86,556	65,476
21	South Africa	75,280	57,035
22	Kenya	73,200	55,395
23	Switzerland	66,000	50,000
24	Portugal	55,455	42,000
25	Spain	37,965	27,750
26	Turkey	33,630	25,470
27	Poland	31,480	23,853
28	Czech Republic	30,884	23,276
29	Hungary	28,000	21,216
30	China	22,000	16,662
31	India	17,424	13,188

Sources: (Lovemoney.com, 2019; Campbell, 2018)

world, and the parliamentarian in the United Kingdom earns $105,000 (£77,379) yearly (Lovemoney.com, 2019; Campbell, 2018). India's legislators, an emerging economy country, are paid only $17,424 (£13,188).

In Nigeria, politics is not a selfless enterprise but an opportunity to loot the nation's treasury. Legislators' compensation in Nigeria is so attractive that there is a general understanding that service in the national assembly is a moneymaking venture. The position is rotated among the different ethnic groups, regions, and religions. This well-entrenched shared belief system may explain why more than 60% of legislators following every national election are new. This author believes that only Nigerians genuinely interested in serving will run for political office if the compensation is similar to other countries.

The take-home pay for the legislators in Nigeria is three times greater than the executive arm's compensation. Under the constitution, the legislatures, not the executive arm of government, have the "power of the purse." The expression he who pays the piper calls the tune exemplifies the House of Representatives' audacity in awarding themselves an unconscionable salary and perks that the country can no longer afford. There are 360 members in the lower chamber of the national assembly—the House of Representatives—and 109 senators in the upper chamber. The United States has 100 senators and 435 congressmen/women. The 12-state structure proposed will reduce senators from 109 to 24 and the House of Representatives members from 360 to 120.

The current economic misery, level of poverty, and the projected gloomy revenue earning from oil necessitate cuts in expenditure. The government can achieve this goal in various ways. First, the federal government should reduce the 28 federal ministries to 14. Second, the legislators' take-home pay should be fixed at the same level as India ($17,424)—after all, the Nigerian politicians, in droves, travel to India for their health care. Furthermore, the cut should be extended to the executive arm of government.

An economic reform that can improve Nigerians' overall health and quality of life is to invest in providing a reliable power supply, ban the importation of power generators, and invest in solar energy generators. Also, the federal and state governments should provide access to clean water nationwide and build good roads to link rural and urban centers to allow farmers easy access to sell their products. The legislatures should enact laws to enforce a balanced budget at federal and state levels. Also, all external loans should only be used for credible capital projects and curb frivolous projects.

Another government sector worthy of reforming is the pension package and perks that governors and senators award themselves. As of January 2021, more than 20 former senators are receiving pensions as ex-governors and deputy governors. Also, many of the states have extraordinary benefits. The Akwa Ibom state law stipulates that ex-governors and deputy governors receive a pension equivalent to the incumbent's salaries. The perks also include a new official vehicle and a utility vehicle every 4 years; one personal staff, a cook, chauffeurs, and security guards for the governor at ₦five million per month and ₦2.5 million for the deputy governor. In River state, their law provides full basic annual salaries for the ex-governor and his deputy, one residential house for the former governor in any state in the country: one residential home within the state for the deputy governor, three vehicles for the ex-governor every 4 years, and two for the deputy every 4 years. The Lagos state government assigned the ex-governor a house in Lagos (estimated at ₦500 million) and Abuja (₦700 million). Besides, he also receives six new vehicles replaced every 3 years, a furniture allowance at 300% of annual salary paid every 2 years, and a ₦30 million pension annually for life (Anyaegbuna, 2020).

No country in the world does a government retiree get these outrageous benefits for serving 4 or 8 years in office. To prevent double-dipping, it makes sense that all politicians and retired military officers serving as a senator or appointed as a minister forfeits all pensions from the government while in office. In self-preservation mode, Nigerian legislators are not interested in reforming the system by enacting laws to curtail their eye-catching benefits. However, the Nigerian people must demand a referendum to change these spectacular pensions and services that are unsustainable.

The take-home pay of the executive arm of government also deserves scrutiny to ensure it is consistent with other similarly situated countries worldwide. Singapore, the United States, Canada, and Germany offer their President the highest compensation. Not surprising, their health system is among the best in the world. On the other hand, Cuba, which has one of the world's best health systems, pays its leader a paltry $360 per year. In 2020, the Nigerian President and Vice-President received a salary of ₦14 million ($39,037) and ₦12 million ($33,460), respectively (Table 12.3). Apart from the salary, the President also received an allowance pay of ₦35 498,519 ($100,382). His total take-home pay in 2020 was ₦49,498,519 ($139,419).

Other perks for the President not quantified monetarily include a personal assistant, special assistant, domestic staff, constituency, vehicle fueling/maintenance, entertainment, recess, newspaper/periodicals, utilities, houses maintenance, security, furniture, wardrobe allowances, including accommodation, duty tour, healthcare allowances, and an unspecified estacode allowance (Current School News Editorial Staff, 2020). The estacode allowance is open to abuse and often turned to

Table 12.3 The budgeted salary and allowances for the Nigerian President and Vice-President in 2020

Serial #		President	Buhari	Vice- President	Osinbajo
		₦	US$	₦	US$
1	Salary	14,000,000	39,037	12,000,000	33,460
	Allowances				
2	Hardship	1, 757,350		1,515,786	
3	Consistency	8, 786,762		7, 578,931	
4	Gratuity	10, 544,115		9, 094,717	
5	Leave	351, 470		303,157	
6	Vehicle	14, 058,820		12, 126,290	
7	Total allowances	35,498,519	100,382	30,618,882	86,440
	Grand total take-home pay	**49,498,517**	**139,419**	**42,618,882**	**119,900**

Source: (Current School News Editorial Staff, 2020)

be a personal "piggy bank." The Vice-President also received a total allowance of ₦30,618,882 ($86,440), and his total take-home pay is ₦42,618,882 ($119,900). Both the President and the Vice-President receive an estacode allowance and the "regular entitlements and benefits" that are not quantified in pecuniary terms. The federal government needs to clarify these unspecified entitlements and benefits.

Salaries of the Highest-Paid Heads of Government and Judiciary Around the World

The salary of the highest-paid heads of government in Africa and worldwide is presented in Table 12.4. Some African leaders (Cameroon, Morocco, South Africa, Algeria, and Equatorial Guinea) are not accountable to anyone and have turned politics into a profitable venture despite the lack of development in the country that they govern.

The head of government published salaries in several countries are mirages and should be viewed with skepticism because the "allowance" perks double or triples

Table 12.4 The highest-paid heads of government in Africa and around the world

Serial #	African Countries*	President	$	Other Countries*	$
1	Cameroon	Paul Biya	610,002	Singapore	1,442,000
2	Morocco	King Mohammed VI	480,000	United States	400,000
3	South Africa	Jacob Zuma	200,411	Canada	290,000
4	Algeria	Abdelaziz Bouteflika	168,000	Germany	268,448
5	Equatorial Guinea	Teodoro Obiang Nguema Mbasogo	150,000	United Kingdom	215,980
6	Kenya	Uhuru Kenyatta	132,000	South Korea	211,320
7	Somalia	Mohamed Abdullahi	144,000	Taiwan	180,000
8	Comoros	Azali Assoumani	115,000	Finland	141,367
9	Democratic Republic Congo	Joseph Kabila	110,000	Russia	136,000
10	Namibia	Hage Geingob	109,900	Colombia	134,676
11	Libya	Abdullah al-Thani	105,000	Barbados	110,499
12	Côte d'Ivoire	Alassane Ouattara	100,000	Brazil	102,524
13	Rwanda	Paul Kagame	85,000	India	84,500
14	Ghana	John Dramani Mahama	76,000	Cuba	360
15	Egypt	Abdel Fattah el-Sisi	70,400	Bulgaria	79,000
16	Zambia	Edgar Lungu	65,000	Haiti	3782
17	Botswana	Ian Khama	66,713		
18	Gabon	Ali Bongo Ondimba	65,000		
19	Malawi	Peter Mutharika	42,000		
20	Zimbabwe	Emmerson Mnangagwa	18,000		

Sources: (Nwabugo, 2020; African Ranking, 2016; Business Daily, 2017; Dzaferovic, 2018; Hodgson, 2017; MoTiNews, 2020)

the published salary amount. The Nigerian president and Vice-President's annual salary reduced by 50% to align it with other countries' heads of government. Their income will now be $69,710 for the president and $59,950 for the Vice-President. The take-home pay for the Nigerian president will rank the 21st highest paid in the world, ahead of the Italian head of government, who earns $64,861 per year. The salary of the highest-paid judiciary worldwide is worth mentioning here.

The UK judiciary in 2009 was the highest-paid in the world ($299,943), followed by Ireland ($270,891), Australia ($264,510), New Zealand ($211,900), France ($212,891), and the United States at $203,000 (Posner et al., 2009). In Europe, Switzerland, England, Wales, Scotland, Ireland, and Norway were at the top of the list in 2014 (Arnett, 2014).

This chapter also investigates the take-home pay of the Nigerian judiciary. The judiciary earns the least salary among the three arms of government in Nigeria. During the first two decades after independence, the pay for the high court judges was generous. They received an average of $100,000 per year. Ostein (1998) explained that the natives inherited the position and compensation rates when the expatriates departed. Eventually, discrimination and grievances emerged among the native elites. They demanded the entirety of colonial privileges that include subsidized rentals, car allowances, and a free airline ticket to England for vacation. By the 1990s, following the initiation of the structural adjustment program launched by General Ibrahim Babangida's military administration and the unintended decline of the currency exchange rate, the judges' compensation took a downward spiral to what it is today.

The wages of the 1067 judges who served at federal and state courts remained static for 12 years and were only raised slightly in 2019. In 2018, the Chief Justice of the federation's annual salary was a minuscule ₦3,353,973 ($9352), and his counterparts on the bench and the president of the court of appeal received ₦2,477,110 ($6907). The in-kind compensation, domestic staff, housing allowances, and vehicle loan are not available but estimated at $50,000 per year, consistent with the executive arm allowance (Isah, 2019). The judiciary take-home pay is estimated at $59,352 for the Chief Justice and $56,907 for the Court of Appeal. Conservatively, the executive arm's benefit was two times greater than the judiciary, and legislatures earned eight times more than the bench. The judges should keep their current annual $56,907 salary to have an independent and corrupt-averse judiciary.

Cost Analysis of the Proposed Economic and Political Reforms

Eliminating inefficiencies, corruption, and waste in government spending and curtailing the unreasonable pension and gratuities for retired politicians will generate more than adequate funds to make UHC a reality. An analysis will be presented next to support the above thesis. In 2020, the National Assembly passed a $35 billion budget, but the funding has a 1.52% ($7.2 billion) deficit of the estimated GDP (Al Jazeera, 2019). From the approved budget, $4.38 billion will be needed to achieve the Abuja pledge of funding health care at 15% of the budget (WHO, 2011). The federal government can obtain adequate funds for the NHIS to implement UHC by banning medical tourism, curtailing wasteful spending, and corruption (Punch, 2018).

In a landmark study published in 2017, Oxfam International asserted that $20 trillion was stolen from the treasury by public office holders between 1960 and 2005. This amount is more than the United States' $18 trillion GDP in 2012. With the substantial decline in oil revenue, Nigerian's democracy is unsustainable because of the pervasive corruption and egregious salary and benefits awarded to government legislators and the executive arm. The federal government should take decisive action and make the appropriate cuts in these sectors to prevent the country from going into bankruptcy and eventually a failed state.

In 2020, the country's external debt and foreign exchange reserve stood at $41 billion and $39 billion, respectively. The federal budget was ₦10.59 trillion, or $29.2 billion (Budgit, 2020; Eboh, 2020). The defense budget was ₦975 billion ($5.0 billion) and represents 9.2% of the federal funding—the largest of any ministry. The defense budget is large because the armed forces (army, navy, coast guard, and air force) have over 310,000 active personnel and 89,000 reserve personnel. The military alone has over 6000 officers and 150,000 soldiers. Military spending in 2018 was 0.507% of the GDP—the Nigerian armed forces in 2018 ranked 42 out of 138 nations worldwide (World Bank, 2018; The GlobalFirepower.com, 2020). On the other hand, the allocation for health in 2020 was ₦464 billion ($2.4 billion), representing only 4.4% of the federal budget, about 50% of the defense budget. The amount earmarked for education represents 6.7% (₦706 billion—$3.6 billion), while humanitarian affairs and police represent 4.2% (₦445 billion—$2.3 billion), and 3.9% (₦410 billion—$2.3 billion) of the budget, respectively (Budgit, 2020). The government should trim the defense budget by 25%. Although this recommendation will generate approximately $1.25 billion, it is controversial because the Nigerian military is considered under-armed and often outgunned by the Fulani herdsmen and Boko Haram bandits. Because of the current insecurity in the country, many military tacticians argue this is not the time to cut the defense budget.

As presented in Table 12.5, the savings from the executive arm, legislators, and the ministry of defense cuts will produce $3.31 billion of the $4.38 billion needed to provide universal and high-quality health care. The total savings did not include the $1–1.5 billion annually spent on medical tourism and anticipated revenue from curtailing wasteful spending and graft. The proposed decrease in states and ministries and salary cuts will make democracy affordable with adequate money to fund UHC.

Given that President Buhari's administration did not meet the 30% health insurance coverage goal at the end of 2020, the government must set a new aspirational NHIS goal. The government must protect the citizens from impoverishment and bankruptcy due to illness or high out-of-pocket expenses. As the former Director-General of the WHO, Margaret Chan, succinctly put it, "no one in need of health-care … should risk financial ruin as a result" (Chan, 2010). It is noteworthy that many health analysts and scholars have previously called for sacrifices to salvage the country from its economic doldrums. For example, a grassroots campaign in 2015 demanded cuts in legislators' compensation, but the effort failed because of

Table 12.5 Estimated annual savings from the cuts in benefits

Serial #	Office	Actuals under the 36 states structure			Projections under the 12 states structure				
		N	Salary ($)	Total ($)	Recommendation	N	Salary ($)	Total	Savings
1	President	1	139,419	139,419	Half pay	1	69,710	69,710	69,710
2	Vice President	1	119,900	119,900	Half pay	1	59,950	59,950	59,950
3	Legislators	435	480,000	208,800,000	2× Indian legislature's salary = ($34,848)	84[a]	34,848	2,927,232	205,872,768
4	Judiciary	1067	56,907	60,719,769	Same pay	1067	56,907	60,719,769	–
5	Defense								$1.25 billion
	Total			269,779,088				63,776,661	$3.31 billion
6	Medical tourism								$ 1–$1.5 billion

Source: (Current School News Editorial Staff, 2020)

[a]Under the 12-state structure proposed, there will be five members in the House of Representatives and two senators in each state = 60 members of the House of Representative and 24 senators

apathy. Surprisingly, not enough Nigerians were livid that their public officers are overpaid, while most citizens wallow in extreme poverty (Kazeem, 2015). In 2018, the Emir of Kano, Sansui Lamed Sansui II, advocated for a 50% cut in the legislators' and ministers' salaries (Akhaine, 2018).

Lessons from Other Countries

To curtail the ostentatious lifestyle that Nigeria can no longer afford, President Buhari must learn from the leaders of other countries. For example, in 2013, Malawi's Joyce Banda sold the only presidential aircraft for $15 million within a year in office. Also, Mexico's populist President sold the Boeing 787 Dreamliner purchased by his predecessor. Critics lampooned Buhari for keeping eight presidential air fleets - a departure from his campaign promise. The maintenance cost in 2021 rose to ₦12.55 billion - a 190% increase in four years (Punch Editorial, 2020). Several economic pundits assert that Nigeria cannot afford more than one presidential aircraft, and the remaining seven should be sold.

Similarly, Nigeria has many valuable lessons from Rwanda—an African country with only 12.3 million people. Mr. Paul Kagame became the sixth President of Rwanda in 2000 when his predecessor, Pasteur Bizimungu, resigned. Historically, Rwanda's healthcare system was of low quality, but on the assumption of office, Mr. Paul Kagame made health care the top priority of his administration. He declared his assets and cut his salary by 90% from $100,000 to $7000 a month, sympathizing with the poor, and canceled the lavish ceremonies marking their independence. He also slashed the extravagant cost of parliamentary dinners and added the allocation to public hospitals' budgets. Following a transparent audit of the mining sector, he dismissed the minister of mines and froze several British mining companies' assets under-reporting. Similarly, officials at Rwandan missions abroad were required to document their travels. He proceeded to terminate the appointment of 10,000 officials holding false credentials (Wade, 2018).

Mr. Kagame implemented a universal healthcare system that provides health insurance coverage through a network called *Mutuelles de Santé*. In 2008, health insurance became mandatory, and by 2010, over 90% of the population was covered, and by 2012 about 96% were insured. He boosted healthcare spending in 2013 to 6.5% of the GDP. This development was a significant increase compared with 1.9% in 1996 (AboutRwanda.com, n.d.; USAID, 2016; WHO, 2019). Today, Rwanda offers a cost-efficient healthcare system for its entire population, and life expectancy has doubled. In the last decade, HIV, TB, and malaria fatalities dropped by 80% each. The maternal mortality rate decreased by 60%; children's annual deaths also declined by 63%. Coupled with a 35% surge in population and control of diseases, it saw a marked rise in economic growth. Per capita GDP increased to $580, while millions of Rwandans stepped out of poverty. Rwanda has made progress on many of the SDGs, especially around poverty reduction, education, health, and access to basic infrastructure (Ndagijimana, 2020).

Today, every Rwandan has universal health insurance that provides adequate health care with minuscule out-of-pocket expenses. The country spends very little money—$55 per person per year—effectively on health care by adopting centralized planning and research and development strategy and prioritizing health as its development pillar (Staff Reports, 2013). For example, the ministries were encouraged to collaborate on cross-cutting issues, such as HIV and cardiovascular disease prevention, because they are interlinked in their progress. In addition to building clinics and hospitals, the Rwandan government trained 45,000 community HCWs to provide home care and psychosocial support to individuals with HIV. Furthermore, qualified professionals provide primary care to sustain and improve health (Crigler, 2021). The health system's financing strategies in Rwanda and Cuba are the best adaptable and fitting to improve Nigeria's low insurance coverage.

If the Rwandan President, Mr. Paul Kagame, can slash his compensation by 90% from $100,000 to $7000 a month, it is not too much of a sacrifice for the Nigerian President and politicians to take a pay cut. Mr. Kagame cut his pay to infuse a new ethical standard and transparency into his country's political landscape (Wade, 2018). For a start, the Nigerian President can cut the salary and generous allowances provided to the executive and legislative arms as previously recommended. Rwanda, with one of Africa's best health systems, in 2020, pays its President $85,000 per year (Nwabugo, 2020). Nigeria, with one of the worst health systems in the world (WHO, 2000, 2010), should under no circumstance pay its leaders more than the Rwandan President. Specifically, the President and Vice-President's pay and allowance should be reduced in half to $69,710 and $59,950, respectively, and the annual estacode allowance fixed at $5000 per year.

Conclusion

Health care is universally political, and power is exercised over it as part of a broader economic and social system. Consequently, Nigeria will not achieve UHC by 2030 as recommended by the UN under SDG 3 (Good Health and Well-being), described more comprehensively in Chap. 13. To achieve this goal, the government must subsequently, as a priority, commit at least 15% of the annual budget to the health sector and develop innovative financing strategies to boost the revenue of the NHIS. Additionally, the Nigerian government should consult with US and European leaders to repatriate the money laundered by previous military leaders and politicians and use the windfall to develop healthcare infrastructures.

Achieving UHC will not be easy, as those benefitting from the existing dysfunctional system would like to maintain the status quo. Changing the system will require political awareness and struggle. Concerned human rights groups and non-governmental organizations must get off the fence and demand the government to make health care the number one budget priority. Most importantly, progressive Nigerians must organize and run for elective offices in large numbers and pressure their political party to adopt the recommendations presented in this chapter. The greediness, corruption, and bold manner in which Nigerian politicians migrate from one party to another with impunity are concerning. Their behavior underscores the thesis that politics can be played without principle and bring to the fore Mahatma Gandhi's dictum that "politics without principle" is one of the "seven social sins." Undoubtedly, Nigeria must elect a purposeful and visionary leader who can marshal the presidential powers to achieve the transformational changes advocated in this chapter. Preferably, the President should pursue the implementation of the reforms presented through the legislative process. However, the executive action order, available in the constitution, can help achieve some low-hanging fruit proposals. If the executive order fails, the President should mount a vigorous campaign to pressure the legislators to pass a constitutional amendment to accomplish the recommendations put forward in this chapter.

Case Study

Specify one area of the administrative operations of the Nigerian healthcare system engulfed in corruption or waste and discuss the tangible reforms that you will implement to curtail the problem.

References

Abutudu, M. (2010). Federalism, political restructuring, and the lingering national question. In *Governance and politics in post-military Nigeria* (pp. 23–60). Palgrave Macmillan. [online]. Available at: https://link.springer.com/chapter/10.1057/9780230115453_2. Accessed 16 Oct 2020.

Abdulhamid, O. S., & Chima, P. (2015). Local government administration in Nigeria: the search for relevance. *Commonwealth Journal of Local Governance, 18*, 4850. [online]. Available at: https://doi.org/10.5130/cjlg.v0i18.4850. Accessed 16 Jun 2021

AboutRwanda.com. (n.d.). *Rwanda's health*. [online]. Available at: http://www.aboutrwanda.com/rwandas-health/. Accessed 22 Jul 2021.

Adebisi, Y. A., Umah, J. O., Olaoye, O. C., Alaran, A. J., Sina-Odunsi, A. B., et al. (2020). Assessment of health budgetary allocation and expenditure toward achieving universal health coverage in Nigeria. *International Journal of Health Life Science*. [online]. Available at: https://sites.kowsarpub.com/ijhls/articles/102552.html. Accessed 24 May 2021.

Adelakun, A. (2020). Ibadan elders want Ibadan vice-chancellor. August 6, *Punch*. [online]. Available at: https://punchng.com/ibadan-elders-want-ibadan-vice-chancellor/. Accessed 16 Oct 2020.

Adesoji, B. S. (2020). *CBN pays $4.45 billion external debt to World Bank, others in 2-month*. [online]. Available at: https://nairametrics.com/2020/03/24/cbn-pays-4-45-billion-external-debt-obligation-to-world-bank-others-in-2-month/. Accessed 16 Oct 2020.

African Ranking. (2016) *Top 15 highest paid African Presidents 2017*. [online]. Available at: http://www.africaranking.com/highest-paid-african-presidents/. Accessed 19 Mar 2021.

Agbakwuru, J. (2020). Only 6 states viable, as Katsina made N8bn but got N136bn federal allocation. *Vanguard*. July 27. [online]. Available at: https://www.vanguardngr.com/2020/07/only-6-states-viable-as-katsina-made-n8bn-but-got-n136bn-federal-allocation/amp/. Accessed 16 Oct 2020.

Ahmad el-Rufai, N. M. (2017). Next-generation Nigeria: What is restructuring and does Nigeria need it? Paper presented on September 21 at Chatham House. *The Royal Institute of*

International Affairs. [online]. Available at: https://www.chathamhouse.org/sites/default/files/publications/research/2017-09-21-What-is-restructuring-and-does-Nigeria-need%20it.pdf. Accessed 20 Apr 2021.

Ajeluorou, A. (2020). We cannot unitarise security if we want a liveable Nigeria, says Fayemi. *The Guardian*. [online]. Available at: https://guardian.ng/politics/we-cannot-unitarise-security-if-we-want-a-liveable-nigeria-says-fayemi/. Accessed 20 Apr 2021.

Ajimotokan, O. (2019). Korea jostles for slice of Nigeria's $1B medical tourism spending. *This Day*. March 21. [online]. Available at: https://www.thisdaylive.com/index.php/2019/03/21/korea-jostles-for-slice-of-nigerias-1b-medical-tourism-spending/. Accessed 16 Oct 2020.

Ajobe, A. T., Alhassan, A., Chung, S., Leonard, J., & Ahmad, R. (2013). Nigeria: How Nigerians spend billions on medical tourism. *Daily Trust*. [online]. Available at: https://allafrica.com/stories/201301071129.html. Accessed 10 Oct 2020.

Aka, C. (2020). Genetic counseling and preventive medicine in Bosnia and Herzegovina. *California Western International Law Journal*, *50*(2), Article 2. [online]. Available at: https://scholarlycommons.law.cwsl.edu/cwilj/vol50/iss2/2. Accessed 10 Oct 2020.

Akhaine, S. (2018). *Slash legislators', ministers' pay by half, Sanusi tells Buhari*. [online]. Available at: https://guardian.ng/news/slash-legislators-ministers-pay-by-half-sanusi-tells-buhari/. Accessed 10 Oct 2020.

Akinyele, B., & Otto Abasiekong, O. (2018). #EndPoverty: 9 ways Nigeria should address poverty. *Proshare Economy*. [online]. Available at: https://www.pro-shareng.com/news/Nigeria%20Economy/-EndPoverty-9-Ways-Nigeria-Should-Address%2D%2DPoverty/42284#:~:text=Investment%20in%20infrastructure%20is%20one,activities%20and%20empower%20more%20Nigerians. Accessed 22 Dec 2020.

Akinyemi, A. I. (2020). Nigeria's census has always been tricky: Why this must change. *The Conversation*. [online]. Available at: https://theconversation.com/nigerias-census-has-always-been-tricky-why-this-must-change-150391. Accessed 17 Jun 2021.

Alake, M. (2018). Find out about the twisted legacy of the great black festival. *Pulse.ng*. [online]. Available at: https://www.pulse.ng/gist/festac-77-find-out-about-the-twisted-legacy-of-the-great-black-festival/205nmc3.amp. Accessed 16 Oct 2020.

Alfa Shaban, A. (2020). *Private use of presidential jet by Buhari's daughter gets Nigerians sparring*. *AfricanNews*. [online]. Available at: https://www.africanews.com/2020/01/14/privateuse-of-presidential-jet-by-buhari-s-daughter-gets-nigerians-sparring//. Accessed16 Oct 2020.

Al Jazeera. (2019). *Nigeria's parliament passes record budget for 2020*. Dec 5. [online]. Available at: https://www.aljazeera.com/ajimpact/nigeria-parliament-passes-record-budget-2020-191205181608971.html. Accessed 16 Oct 2020.

Alagboso, C. (2020). FMC Ebute Metta is restoring Nigeria's confidence in public health centres. *Nigeria Health Watch*. March 24, [online]. Available at: https://nigeriahealthwatch.com/fmc-ebute-metta-is-restoring-nigerias-confidence-in-public-health-centres/#.XyRncyhKg2x. Accessed 16 Oct 2020.

Alechenu, J., Akinkuotu, E., & Aworinde, T. (2019). Buhari spends one year, 39 days abroad in three years, 10 months. *Punch NG*. [online]. Available at: https://punchng.com/buhari-spends-one-year-39-days-abroad-in-three-years-10-months/. Accessed 16 Apr 2021.

Amu, H., Dickson, K. S., Kumi-Kyereme, A., & Darteh, E. K. M. (2018). Understanding variations in health insurance coverage in Ghana, Kenya, Nigeria, and Tanzania: Evidence from demographic and health surveys. *PLoS ONE*, *13*(8), e0201833. [online]. Available at: https://journals.plos.org/plosone/article?id=10.1371/journal.pone.0201833. Accessed 10 Oct 2020.

Anyaegbuna, V. O. (2020). *Buhari is not a problem*. [online]. Available at: https://www.nairaland.com/6154107/buhari-not-problem. Accessed 16 Oct 2020.

Aregbeshola, B. S., & Khan, S. M. (2018). Predictors of enrolment in the national health insurance scheme among women of reproductive age in Nigeria. *International Journal of Health Policy Management*, *7*(11), 1015–1023. [online]. Available at: https://www.ncbi.nlm.nih.gov/pmc/articles/PMC6326643/. Accessed 10 Oct 2020.

Arnett, G. (2014). Scottish judges are the highest paid in Europe. *The Guardian*; October 5. [online]. Available at: https://www.theguardian.com/news/datablog/2014/oct/09/scottish-judges-are-the-highest-paid-in-europe. Accessed 16 Oct 2020.

Atuanya, P., & Augie, B. (2013) How viable are Nigerian states? *NewsWireNGR*. [online]. Available at: https://newswirengr.com/2013/12/09/how-viable-are-nigerian-states/. Accessed 16 Oct 2020.

Awosusi, A., Folaranmi, T., & Yates, R. (2015). *Nigeria's new government and public financing for universal health coverage.* [online]. Available at: https://www.thelancet.com/journals/langlo/article/PIIS2214-109X(15)00088-1/fulltext. Accessed 16 Oct 2020.

Bablola, D., & Onapajo, H. (2019). New clamour for "restructuring" in Nigeria: Elite politics, contradictions, and good governance. *African Studies Quarterly, 18*(4).

Bambra, C., Fox, D., & Scott-Samuel, A. (2005). Towards a politics of health. *Health Promotion International, 20*(2), 187–193. [online]. Available at: https://academic.oup.com/heapro/article/20/2/187/827479. Accessed 16 Oct 2020.

Basiru, S., Oluyemi, J., Abdulateef, J., & Atolagbe, E. (2018). Medical tourism in Nigeria: Challenges and remedies to healthcare system development. *International Journal of Development and Management Review, 13*(1), 223–238.

BBC. (2016). Nigeria to sell two presidential jets 'to cut waste. *Africa Service*. [online]. Available at: https://www.bbc.com/news/amp/world-africa-37562169. Accessed 16 Oct 2020.

Budgit. (2020). *2020 approved budget analysis.* [online]. Available at: https://yourbudgit.com/wp-content/uploads/2020/03/2020-Budget-Analysis.pdf. Accessed 16 Oct 2020.

BusinessDay. (2019). Business Day, Newspaper, May 16.

Business Daily. (2017). *The highest and lowest paid African presidents.* [online]. Available at: https://www.businessdailyafrica.com/news/The-highest-and-lowest-paid-African-presidents/539546-4129430-cbmf8iz/index.html. Accessed 19 Mar 2021.

Cahoon, B. (n.d.). *Nigeria states.* [online]. Available at: https://www.worldstatesmen.org/Nigeria_federal_states.htm. Accessed 14 Jun 2021.

Campbell, J. (2017). Arguments for the restructuring of Nigeria. June 14. *Council on Foreign Relations.* [online]. Available at: https://www.cfr.org/blog/arguments-restructuring-nigeria. Accessed 16 Oct 2020.

Campbell, J. (2018). Uproar over parliamentary salaries in Nigeria, again. *Africa in Transition.* Council on Foreign Relations. [online]. Available at: https://www.cfr.org/blog/uproar-over-parliamentary-salaries-nigeria-again. Accessed 26 Jul 2021.

Celebritynetworth.com (2014), *Richest African Presidents,* 2014. [online]. Available at: http://www.richestlifestyle.com/cgi-sys/suspendedpage.cgi. Accessed 16 Oct 2020.

Celebritynetworth.com (2021). *Goodluck Jonathan net worth:$10 Million.* [online]. Available at: https://www.celebritynetworth.com/richest-politicians/presidents/goodluck-jonathan-net-worth/. Accessed 21 Nov 2021.

Central Intelligence Agency (CIA). (2017). *The world factbook.* [online]. Available at: https://www.cia.gov/library/publications/the-world-factbook/geos/tw.html. Accessed 10 Oct 2020.

Chan, M. (2010). Message from the Director-General, *in* World Health Organization, *The World Health Report: Health Systems Financing: The Path to Universal Coverage.* WHO, Geneva.

Channels Television. (2019a). Top four priorities of the 2020 budget. *Channels Television*, October 8. [online]. Available at: https://www.channelstv.com/2019/10/08/top-four-priorities-of-the-2020-budget/. Accessed 16 Oct 2020.

Channels Television. (2019b). Budget 2020: We dare Buhari to make Presidency's allocation public – PDP. *Channels Television,* October 8. [online]. Available at: https://www.channelstv.com/2019/10/08/budget-2020-we-dare-buhari-to-make-presidency-allocation-public-pdp/. Accessed 16 Oct 2020.

Country profile. (2019). *Nigeria: The local government system.* [online]. Available at: http://www.clgf.org.uk/default/assets/File/Country_profiles/Nigeria.pdf. Accessed 17 Jun 2021.

Cowell, A. (2018). *Shehu Shagari, Nigerian President during '80s oil crisis, dies at 93.* [online]. Available at: https://www.nytimes.com/2018/12/29/obituaries/shehu-shagari-dead.html. Accessed 25 Jan 2021.

Crigler, L. (2021). *Rwanda's community health worker progam.* [online]. Available at: https://chwcentral.org/rwandas-community-health-worker-progam/. Accessed 21 Nov 2021.

Current School News Editorial Staff. (2020). *Nigeria's President salary structure 2020 – current monthly earnings of Buhari and Osinbajo.* July 14. [online]. Available at: https://www.currentschoolnews.com/job/nigerias-presidential-salary/. Accessed 16 Oct 2020.

Daily Sabah. (2021). *Nigerian President Buhari's London medical trips cause outrage.* [online]. Available at: https://www.dailysabah.com/world/africa/nigerian-president-buharis-london-medical-trips-cause-outrage. Accessed 19 Apr 2021.

Dan-Azumi, J., Jega, A., & Egwu, S. (2019). The challenge of re-federalizing Nigeria: Revisiting recent debates on political re-structuring. *Journal of Political Science Public Affairs, 7,* 353. [online]. Available at: https://www.researchgate.net/publication/334431619_The_Challenge_of_Re-Federalizing_Nigeria_Revisiting_Recent_Debates_on_Political_Re-Structuring. Accessed 16 Oct 2020.

Dapo-Asaju, H. S., & Bamgbose, O. J. (2019). The quest for restructuring the Nigerian nation: Myth or reality? The role of libraries in amplifying the debate. *International Journal of Legal Information, 47*(1), 13–21. [online]. Available at: https://doi.org/10.1017/jli.2019.9. Accessed 16 Oct 2020.

Dzaferovic, A. (2018). *Infographic: What are the monthly salaries of Presidents in the region.* [online]. Available at:http://www.sarajevotimes.com/infographic-monthly-salaries-presidents-region/. Accessed 19 Mar 2021.

Eboh, C. (2020). *Nigeria's president submits revised 2020 budget to parliament.* [online]. Available at: https://www.reuters.com/article/nigeria-budget-idUSL8N2DA6Q9. Accessed 16 Oct 2020.

Egbejule, E. (2018). Nigeria: The state of the states *The Africa Report.* [online]. Available at: https://www.theafricareport.com/571/nigeria-the-state-of-the-states/. Accessed 16 Jun 2021.

Ejovi, A., Mgbonyebi, V. C., & Akpokighe, O. R. (2013). Corruption in Nigeria: A historical perspective. *Research on Humanities and Social Sciences, 3*(16), 19–26. [online]. Available at: https://core.ac.uk/download/pdf/234673673.pdf. Accessed 21 Jan 2021.

Elutidoye, G. (2020). Who is considered the best head of state that Nigeria ever had? *Quora.* [online]. Available at: https://www.quora.com/Who-is-considered-the-best-head-of-state-that-Nigeria-ever-had. Accessed 21 Jun 2021.

Emeka, N. (2020). *12 things to know about Buhari's presidential plane.* [online]. Available at: https://autojosh.com/buhari-presidential-plane/. Accessed 16 Oct 2020.

Essien, G., & Yakubu, H. (2018). Nigeria launches new national health security plan. *VON.* [online]. Available at: https://www.von.gov.ng/nigeria-launches-new-national-health-security-plan/. Accessed 16 Oct 2020.

Ewepu, G. (2019). Nigeria: 2020 Budget – Only 4 States Are Viable in Nigeria - Report. October 29. *Vanguard.* [online]. Available at: https://www.vanguardngr.com/2019/10/only-4-states-are-viable-in-nigeria-report/. Accessed 16 Oct 2020.

Falae, V. (2017). *Is Goodluck Jonathan's net worth revealed?* [online]. Available at: https://m.scoopernews.com/2017/12/12/is-goodluck-jonathan-net-worth-revealed/454027. Accessed 16 Oct 2020.

Fawehinmi, F. (2018). *The story of how Nigeria's census figures became weaponized.* [online]. Available at: https://qz.com/africa/1221472/the-story-of-how-nigerias-census-figures-became-weaponized/. Accessed 17 Jun 2021.

Global Partnership for Education. (2017). *3 things to know about education as a human right.* [online]. Available at: https://www.globalpartnership.org/blog/3-things-know-about-education-human-right. Accessed 16 Oct 2020.

Global Compact. (2021). *UHC2030's mission is to create a movement for accelerating equitable and sustainable progress towards universal health coverage (UHC).* [online]. Available at: https://www.uhc2030.org/our-mission/; https://www.uhc2030.org/fileadmin/uploads/uhc2030/

Documents/About_UHC2030/mgt_arrangemts___docs/UHC2030_Official_documents/ UHC2030_Global_Compact_WEB.pdf. Accessed 27 May 2021.

GlobalFirepower.com. (2020). *Nigeria military strength (2020)*. [online]. Available at: https:// www.globalfirepower.com/country-military-strength-detail.asp?country_id=nigeria. Accessed 16 Oct 2020.

Glusea.com (2021). *Muhammadu Buhari net worth. Top 10 richest politicians in Nigeria. Glusea. com*. [online]. Available at: https://www.glusea.com/muhammadu-buhari-net-worth/. Accessed 27 June 2021.

Gramont, D. D. (2015). *Governing Lagos: Unlocking the politics of reform*. [online]. Available at: https://carnegieendowment.org/2015/01/12/governing-lagos-unlocking-politics-of-reform-pub-57671. Accessed 16 Jun 2021.

Guardian. (2019) Do we need unviable 32 states? *Editorial Board*. November 19. [online]. Available at: https://guardian.ng/opinion/do-we-need-unviable-32-states/. Accessed 16 Oct 2020.

Harris, A. (2018). *George Washington's broken dream of a national university*. [online]. Available at: https://www.theatlantic.com/education/archive/2018/09/founders-national-university/571003/. Accessed 18 Jan 2021.

Hodgson, C. (2017). *Richest royals: what Europe's royal families get from their taxpayers – Business Insider*. [online]. Available at: https://www.businessinsider.com/richest-royals-what-europes-royal-families-get-from-their-taxpayers-2017-7?r=UK&IR=T. Accessed 19 Mar 2021.

Ifijeh, M. (2015). Only five percent of Nigerians are covered by health insurance. *This Day Newspaper*. November 12. [online]. Available at: http://allafrica.com/stories/201511121412. html9. Accessed 16 Oct 2020.

Igwe, U. (2020). *Five years on: Are Nigerians better or worse under President Buhari?* [online]. Available at: https://blogs.lse.ac.uk/africaatlse/2020/10/01/five-years-on-nigerians-better-worse-under-president-buhari-development/. Accessed 19 Apr 2021.

International Medical Travel Journal. (2014). Nigeria spends $1 billion on outbound medical tourism. *International Medical Travel Journal*. May 22. [online]. Available at: https://www.imtj. com/news/nigeria-spends-1-billion-outbound-medical-tourism/. Accessed 16 Oct 2020.

Ikeru, A. (2020). *Muhammadu Buhari biography and net worth*. [online]. Available at: https:// austinemedia.com/muhammadu-buhari-biography-and-net-worth/. Accessed 10 Oct 2020.

Isah, A. (2019). Nigeria: Concerns as judges' salaries remain static for 12 years. *AllAffairs*. May 6. [online]. Available at: https://allafrica.com/stories/201905060102.html. Accessed 16 Oct 2020.

Kabir, A. (2020). *Use of private jet by Buhari's daughter: What the law states*. [online]. Available at: https://www.premiumtimesng.com/news/headlines/372286-use-of-private-jet-by-buharis-daughter-what-the-law-states.html. Acccssed 16 Oct 2020.

Kaieteur News. (2009). *The most travelled world leader?* [online]. Available at: https://www.kai-eteurnewsonline.com/2009/10/27/the-most-travelled-world-leader/. Accessed 16 Apr 2021.

Kazeem, Y. (2015). *Nigeria has some of the world's highest paid lawmakers and this start-up wants to slash their pay*. [online]. Available at: https://qz.com/africa/417192/nigeria-has-some-of-the-worlds-highest-paid-lawmakers-and-this-start-up-is-trying-to-slash-their-pay/. Accessed 23 Jan 2020.

Kinnan, C. J., Gordon, D. B., DeLong, M. D., Jaquish, D. W., & McAllum, R. S. (2011). *Failed State 2030: Nigeria—A Case Study*. [online]. Available at: https://media.defense.gov/2017/ May/05/2001743001/-1/-1/0/OP_0067_KINNAN_ET_AL_FAILED_STATE_2030. PDF. Accessed 18 Jan 2021.

Knoema. (2018). *Adult (15+) literacy rate*. [online]. Available at: https://knoema.com/atlas/ Nigeria/topics/Education/Literacy/Adult-literacy-rate?mode=amp. Accessed 16 Oct 2020.

Kwon, S., Lee, T., & Cy, K. (2015). *Republic of Korea health system review*. 5 (4). Manila: World Health Organization, Regional Office for the Western Pacific. [online]. Available at: http:// www.searo.who.int/entity/asia_pacific_observatory/publications/hits/hit_korea/en/. Accessed 10 Oct 2020.

Lawal, S. (1983). *Ghana must go: The ugly history of Africa's most famous bag.* [online]. Available at: http://atavist.mg.co.za/ghana-must-go-the-ugly-history-of-africas-most-famous-bag. Accessed 25 Jan 2021.

Legg, P. (2019). Shehu Shagari obituary. *The Guardian, US Edition.* [online]. Available at: https://www.theguardian.com/world/2019/jan/09/shehu-shagari-obituary. Accessed 25 Jan 2021.

Legit TV. (2017). *Who is Nigeria's greatest president ever?* [online]. Available at: https://www.youtube.com/watch?v=wZgfXEgvwYU. Accessed 21 Jun 2021.

Lovemoney.com. (2019). *This is what politicians get paid around the world: Parliamentarians' pay in different countries.* March 29. LoveMoney. [online]. Available at: https://www.love-money.com/gallerylist/65052/this-is-what-politicians-get-paid-around-the-world. Accessed 16 Oct 2020.

Lukpata, V. I. (2013). Revenue allocation formulae in Nigeria: A continuous search. *International Journal of Public Administration and Management Research, 2*(1). [online]. Available at: https://rcmss.com/2013/1ijpamr/Revenue%20Allocation%20Formulae%20in%20Nigeria_%20A%20Continuous%20Search.pdf. Accessed 19 Jun 2021.

Makinde, O. A. (2016). Physicians as medical tourism facilitators in Nigeria: Ethical issues of the practice. *Croatian Medical Journal, 57*(6), 601–604. [online]. Available at: https://www.researchgate.net/publication/312147016_Physicians_as_medical_tourism_facilitators_in_Nigeria_Ethical_issues_of_the_practice. Accessed 10 Oct 2020.

Michael, J. (2021). Buhari heads to UK for medical treatment as doctors strike erupts at home. *The Africa Report.* [online]. Available at: https://www.theafricareport.com/76967/nigeria-buhari-heads-to-uk-for-medical-treatment-as-doctors-strike-erupts-at-home/. Accessed 19 Apr 2021.

MoTiNews. (2020). *Pravind Jugnauth's salary vs other world leaders.* [online]. Available at: https://moti.news/news/pravind-jugnauths-salary-vs-other-world-leaders. Accessed 19 Mar 2021.

Nairametrics. (2020). *Nigeria's foreign debt has breached a 15-year trigger.* [online]. Available at: https://nairametrics.com/2020/04/11/nigerias-foreign-debt-has-breached-a-15-year-trigger/. Accessed 16 Oct 2020.

Ndagijimana, U. (2020). *Strategies for delivering on the sustainable development goals: Some lessons from Rwanda.* [online]. Available at: https://www.brookings.edu/blog/africa-in-focus/2020/01/20/strategies-for-delivering-on-the-sustainable-development-goals-some-lessons-from-rwanda/. Accessed 14 Jun 2021.

Nda-Isaiah, J. (2017). *Nigeria: Presidency denies spending £4000 daily on presidential aircraft.* [online]. Available at: https://allafrica.com/stories/201706300031.html. Accessed 16 Oct 2020.

NgnRates.com. (2021). *Dollar to Naira black market rate.* [online]. Available at: https://www.ngnrates.com/market/exchange-rates/us-dollar-to-naira/black-market. Accessed 16 Jan 2021.

Nigerian Finder. (2021a). *Ibrahim Babangida: Net worth.* [online]. Available at: https://nigerian-finder.com/ibrahim-babangida-net-worth/. Accessed 21 Jan 2021.

Nigerian Finder. (2021b). *Olusegun Obasanjo: Net worth.* [online]. Available at: https://nigerian-finder.com/olusegun-obasanjo-net-worth/. Accessed 21 Jan 2021.

Nnaemeka, M. C., & Okwudili, V. A. P. (2019). *The politics of population census: Challenge to democracy and nation-building in Nigeria since 1960.* [online]. Available at: https://www.researchgate.net/publication/337994137_The_Politics_of_Population_Census_Challenge_to_Democracy_and_Nation_Building_in_Nigeria_since_1960. Accessed 17 Jun 2021.

Nsehe, M. (2011). Who were Africa's richest dictators? *Forbes.* [online]. Available at: https://www.forbes.com/sites/mfonobongnsehe/2011/11/08/who-were-africas-richest-dictators/?sh=76d56d22170. Accessed 21 Jan 2021.

NOIPolls. (2017). *Emigration of Nigerian medical doctors: Survey report.* [online]. Available at: https://noi-polls.com/2018/wp-content/uploads/2019/06/Emigration-of-Doctors-Press-Release-July-2018-Survey-Report.pdf. Accessed 10 Oct 2020.

Nwabugo, O. (2020). 20 highest paid African Presidents for 2020. *AnswersAfrica.com.* [online]. Available   at: https://answersafrica.com/20-highest-paid-african-presidents-for-2015.html. Accessed 16 Oct 2020.

Ojieh, C. O. (2016). Extraneous Considerations to the Personality Variables in Foreign Policy Decision-Making: Evidence from Nigeria. [online]. *Ufahamu: A Journal of African Studies,*

39(2), 197–226. https://doi.org/10.5070/F7392031111. Retrieved from https://escholarship. org/uc/item/4pt5j44w. Accessed 18 Jan 2021.

Ojo, E. (2021). *Obasanjo – Biography, life story and net worth of Baba of Africa.* [online]. Available at: https://www.entrepreneurs.ng/obasanjo-biography. Accessed 21 Jan 2021.

Okafor, J. (2012). Constitutional challenges of creating new local government areas in Nigeria. *Commonwealth Journal of Local Governance.* [online]. Available at: https://epress.lib.uts.edu. au/journals/index.php/cjlg/article/view/2692. Accessed 16 Jun 2021.

Oluokun, A. (2012). Goodluck Jonathan: The wasteful President -*TheNEWS Magazine.* [online]. Available at: https://es-la.facebook.com/nasirelrufai/posts/goodluck-jonathan-the-wasteful-president-thenews-magazineposted-august-6-2012-by/10151986311755128/. Accessed 23 Jan 2021.

Olurounbi, R. (2021). *Nigeria: Buhari's legacy is one of 'missed opportunities and inaction' says analyst.* [online]. Available at: https://www.theafricareport.com/73266/nigeria-buharis-legacy-is-one-of-missed-opportunities-and-inaction-says-analyst/. Accessed 19 Apr 2021.

Onu, N. (2019). My greatest disappointment in academia was the tribalism- Prof. Ikenna Onyido. *The Nation.* [online]. Available at: https://thenationonlineng.net/my-greatest-disappointment-in-academia-was-the-tribalism/. Accessed 15 Apr 2021.

Okafor, P. (2017). Nigeria loses $1bn annually to medical tourism — Omatseye. *Vanguard.* August 23. [online]. Available at: https://www.vanguardngr.com/2017/08/nigeria-loses-1bn-annually-medical-tourism-omatseye/. Accessed 10 Oct 2020.

Ola-David, T. (2018). The need for restructuring Nigeria's political system. November 2. *The Oxford University Politics blog.* [online]. Available at: https://blog.politics.ox.ac.uk/the-need-for-restructuring-nigerias-political-system/. Accessed16 Oct 2020.

Olamide, F., Kalu, A E., Solomon, O. A., & Obamen, J. (2019). Economic diversification and national development in Nigeria: Challenges and prospects. *International Journal of Mechanical Engineering and Technology, 10*(8), 98–108. [online]. Available at: https://ssrn. com/abstract=3445930. Accessed 16 Oct 2020.

Olayinka, C. (2014). Nigeria: At 80 Gowon explains - 'Nigeria's problem is not money, but how to spend it. *Guardian.* [online]. Available at: https://allafrica.com/stories/201410202349.html. Accessed 16 Oct 2020.

Omojuwa.com. (2019). *U.S. to seize U.S.$480 million of Abacha's loot.* [online]. Available at: http://omojuwa.com/2014/08/u-s-to-seize-u-s-480-million-of-abachas-loot/. Accessed 22 Jul 2021.

Onuba, I. (2019). 2020 budget contains N150bn wasteful expenditure. *Punch NG.* [online]. Available at: https://punchng.com/2020-budget-contains-n150bn-wasteful-expenditure/. Accessed 22 Jul 2021.

Onyeji, E. (2020). Analysis: Why Nigeria's vision 20:2020 was bound to fail. *Premium Times*; January 19. [online]. Available at: https://www.premiumtimesng.com/news/top-news/373321-analysis-why-nigerias-vision-202020-was-bound-to-fail.html. Accessed 16 Oct 2020.

Onyenekenwa, C. E. (2011). Nigeria's Vision 20:2020-issues, challenges, and implications for development management. *Asian Journal of Rural Development, 1*, 21–40. [online]. Available at: https://scialert.net/fulltext/?doi=ajrd.2011.21.40. Accessed 16 Oct 2020.

Onyenucheya, A. (2018). Reversing medical tourism in Nigeria. *The Guardian.* October 25. [online]. Available at: https://guardian.ng/features/reversing-medical-tourism-in-nigeria/. Accessed 10 Oct 2020.

Ostein. (1998). A study of the compensation of Nigerian judges since independence. *Current Issues in Development* (Centre for Development Studies, University of Jos), *2*(2):1–21. [online]. Available at: https://papers.ssrn.com/sol3/papers.cfm?abstract_id=1458559. Accessed 16 Oct 2020.

Ota, E. N., Ecoma, C. S., & Wambu, C. G. (2020). Creation of states in Nigeria, 1967–1996: Deconstructing the history and politics. *American Research Journal of Humanities and Social Sciences, 6*(1), 1–8. [online]. Available at: https://www.arjonline.org/papers/arjhss/v6-i1/5.pdf. Accessed 22 Jul 2021.

Othman, M. F. B., Osman, N. B., & Mohammed, I. S. (2019). The restructuring Nigeria: The dilemma and critical issues. *Journal of Business and Social Review in Emerging Economies, 5*(1), 79–98. [online]. Available at: https://www.researchgate.net/publication/335925475_The_ Restructuring_Nigeria_The_Dilemma_and_Critical_Issues. Accessed 16 Oct 2020.

Owusu-Bempah, A. (2016). *Review of the roots of youth violence: Literature reviews. Volume 5. Community policing strategies. Centre of Criminology, University of Toronto.* [online]. Available at: http://www.children.gov.on.ca/htdocs/English/professionals/oyap/roots/volume5/ preventing03_community_polcing.aspx.

Oxfam International. (2020). *Nigeria: extreme inequality in numbers.* [online]. From the report published in 2017 titled Inequality in Nigeria: Exploring the drivers. Summary available at: https://www.oxfam.org/en/nigeria-extreme-inequality-numbers. Accessed 16 Oct 2020.

Oxford University Press. (1993). *Chukwuemeka Odumegwu Ojukwu.* [online]. Available at: https:// www.oxfordreference.com/view/10.1093/oi/authority.20110803100247727.   Accessed   16 Jun 2021.

Parmar, H. (2015). *Healthcare business challenges in Nigeria.* September 8. [online]. Available at: https://www.linkedin.com/pulse/healthcare-business-challenges-nigeria-hemraj-parmar-mba/. Accessed 10 Oct 2020.

PMNews. (2019). *Nigeria: Only 10 states economically viable, 17 insolvent – Viability Index report.* May 13. [online]. Available at: https://www.pmnewsnigeria.com/2019/05/13/nigeria-only-10- states-economically-viable-17-insolvent-viability-index-report/. Accessed 16 Oct 2020.

Posner, E., Choi, S. J., & Gulati, G. M. (2009). Are judges overpaid? A skeptical response to the judicial salary debate. *University of Chicago. Journal of Legal Analysis, 47.* [online]. Available at: https://chicagounbound.uchicago.edu/journal_articles/2928/. Accessed 16 Oct 2020.

PRNigeria. (2017). ASVI 2017: States generate N931bn, only 8 economically viable, 17 states are insolvent. *Nigeria Press Release.* [online]. Available at: https://prnigeria.com/2018/04/29/ asvi-2017-states-generate-n931bn/. Accessed 16 Oct 2020.

Psacharopoulos, G. (n.d.). Nigeria perspective: Education. *Copenhagen Consensus Center.* [online]. Available at: https://www.copenhagenconsensus.com/publication/nigeria- perspective-education. Accessed 16 Oct 2020.

Punch. (2016). Nigeria spends $1bn annually on medical tourism. *Punch,* October 14. [online]. Available at: https://punchng.com/nigeria-spends-1bn-annually-medical-tourism/. Accessed 16 Oct 2020.

Punch. (2018). How the 36 states can be viable. September 25. *Punch Editorial.* [online]. Available at: https://punchng.com/how-the-36-states-can-be-viable/. Accessed 16 Oct 2020.

Punch. (2020). *Editorial: Repercussions of wasteful government spending.* [online]. Available at: https://punchng.com/repercussions-of-wasteful-government-spending/. Accessed 23 Jan 2021.

Quora Inc. (2020). *Who were the most-traveled world leaders of all time?* [online]. Available at: https://www.quora.com/Who-were-the-most-traveled-world-leaders-of-all-timew.quora.com/ Who-were-the-most-traveled-world-leaders-of-all-time. Accessed 16 Apr 2021.

Rome Reports. (2017). *The traveling Pope: 104 international trips to 129 countries.* [online]. Available   at: https://www.romereports.com/en/2014/04/24/the-traveling-pope-104- international-trips-to-129-countries/. Accessed 16 Apr 2021.

SaharaReporters. (2021). *Why we are not for Oduduwa republic — Late Frederick Fasehun's OPC faction.* [online]. Available at: http://saharareporters.com/2021/04/12/why-we-are-not- oduduwa-republic-%E2%80%94-late-frederick-fasehuns-opc-faction#:~:text=The%20agita- tion%20for%20the%20Oduduwa%20Republic%20is%20popular,displacing%20people%20 from%20their%20lands%20in%20the%20South-West. Accessed 16 Apr 2021.

Scott-Emuakpor, A. (2010). The evolution of healthcare systems in Nigeria: Which way forward in the twenty-first century. *Nigerian Medical Journal, 17*(51), 53–65. [online]. Available at: http:// www.nigeriamedj.com/text.asp?2010/51/2/53/70997. Accessed 3 Feb 2020.

Shagari, S. (1996). *The time for muddling through is over.* Presentation at the Usman Dan Fodio University, Sokoto, on January 13.

Sotubo, M. (2015). Ex-minister might have personally supervised stealing of $6bn. [online]. Available   at: https://www.pulse.ng/news/local/diezani-ex-minister-might-have-personally- supervised-stealing-of-dollar6bn-video/edxh0m1. Accessed 16 Oct 2020.

StaffReports.(2013).*Rwanda'shealthcaresystem:ALessonfortheworld*.BorgenMagazine;February 25. https://www.borgenmagazine.com/rwandas-health-care-system-a-lesson-for-the-world/

Suberu, R. (1998). States creation and the political economy of Nigerian federalism. In K. Amuwo, A. Agbaje, R. Suberu, & G. Héraul (Eds.), *Federalism and political restructuring in Nigeria*. Spectrum Books Ltd.

Taarifa. (2020). 2020/21 Budget: Government outlines key priorities for fiscal year. *Taarifa*. [online]. Available at: https://taarifa.rw/2020-21-budget-government-outlines-key-priorities-for-fiscal-year/. Accessed 16 Oct 2020.

The Abuja declaration. (2011) Ten years on. WHO. [online]. Available at: https://www.who.int/healthsystems/publications/abuja_declaration/en/. https://www.who.int/healthsystems/publications/abuja_report_aug_2011.pdf?ua=1. Accessed:16 October 2020.

The World Bank. (2020). *Nigeria: Overview*. [online]. Available at: https://www.worldbank.org/en/country/nigeria/overview. Accessed 18 Jan 2021.

Ukiwo, U. (n.d.). *Creation of local government areas and ethnic conflicts in Nigeria: The case of Warri, Delta state*. [online]. Available at:https://citeseerx.ist.psu.edu/viewdoc/download?doi=1 0.1.1.119.5294&rep=rep1&type=pdf. Accessed 17 Jun 2021.

UN. (2015). *The 17 sustainable development goals (SDGs) Department of Economic and Social Affairs Sustainable Development)*. [online]. Available at: https://sdgs.un.org/goals. Accessed 27 May 2021.

United Nations Population Fund. (n.d.). *Sexual and reproductive health*. [online]. Available at: https://www.unfpa.org/sexual-reproductive-health. Accessed 16 Oct 2020.

Upfill-Brown, A. M., Lyons, H. M., Pate, M. A., et al. (2014). Predictive spatial risk model of poliovirus to aid prioritization and hasten eradication in Nigeria. *BMC Medicine, 12*, 92.

USAID – United States Agency for International Development. (2016). *African strategies for health*. [online]. Available at: http://www.africanstrategies4health.org/uploads/1/3/5/3/13538666/country_profile_-_rwanda_-_us_letter.pdf. Accessed 22 Jul 2021.

Uzonwanne, M. C. (2015). Economic diversification in Nigeria in the face of dwindling oil revenue. *Journal of Economics and Sustainable Development*. [online]. Available at: https://www.researchgate.net/publication/273882540_Economic_Diversification_in_Nigeria_in_the_Face_of_Dwindling_Oil_Revenue. Accessed 16 Oct 2020.

VOA. (2019). *Nigeria losing $1B annually to medical tourism, Authorities say*. May 10. [online]. Available at: https://www.voanews.com/africa/nigeria-losing-1b-annually-medical-tourism-authorities-say. Accessed 10 Oct 2020.

Wade, A. (2018). *Portrait of the good African president*. [online]. Available at: https://www.kapitalafrik.com/2018/07/11/portrait-of-the-good-african-president/. Accessed 16 Oct 2020.

WHO. (2000). *The world health organization's ranking of the world's health systems, by rank*. [online]. Available at: https://photius.com/rankings/healthranks.html. Accessed 10 Oct 2020; https://photius.com/rankings/world_health_systems.html. Accessed 10 Oct 2020.

WHO. (2010). Telemedicine in the member states: Opportunities and developments. Report on the second global survey on eHealth. *Global Observatory for eHealth series* - Volume 2. [online]. Available at: http://www.who.int/goe/publications/goe_telemedicine_2010.pdf. Accessed 16 Oct 2020.

WHO. (2011). *The Abuja declaration: Ten years on*. [online]. Available at: https://www.who.int/healthsystems/publications/abuja_declaration/en/; https://www.who.int/healthsystems/publications/abuja_report_aug_2011.pdf?ua=1. Accessed 16 Oct 2020.

WHO. (2017a). *Health is a fundamental human right*. [online]. Available at: https://www.who.int/mediacentre/news/statements/fundamental-human-right/en/#:~:text=The%20right%20to%20health%20for,them%2C%20without%20suffering%20financial%20hardship.&text=That's%20why%20WHO%20promotes%20the,in%20the%20practice%20of%20care. Accessed 16 Oct 2020.

WHO. (2017b). *Health workforce. Achieving the health-related MDGs. It takes a workforce*. [online]. Available at: http://www.who.int/hrh/fig_density.pdf?ua=1. Accessed 16 Oct 2020.

WHO. (2019). *Rwanda: the beacon of universal health coverage in Africa*. [online]. Available at: https://www.afro.who.int/news/rwanda-beacon-universal-health-coverage-africa. Accessed 22 Jul 2021.

WHO. (2020). *Health and development*. [online]. Available at: https://www.who.int/hdp/en/. Accessed 16 Oct 2020.

World Bank. (2018). *Nigeria – Military expenditure (% of GDP)*. [online]. Available at: https://tradingeconomics.com/nigeria/military-expenditure-percent-of-gdp-wb-data.html#:~:text=Military%20expenditure%20(%25%20of%20GDP)%20in%20Nigeria%20was%20reported%20at,compiled%20from%20officially%20recognized%20sources. Accessed 16 Oct 2020.

Worldometer. (2020). *Nigeria demographics*. [online]. Available at: https://www.worldometers.info/demographics/nigeria-demographics/. Accessed 16 Jan 2021.

Wu, T. Y., Majeed, A., & Kuo, K. N. (2010). An overview of the healthcare system in Taiwan. *London Journal of Primary Care* (Abingdon), *3*(2):115–119. [online]. Available at: https://www.ncbi.nlm.nih.gov/pmc/articles/PMC3960712/. Accessed 10 Oct 2020.

Yauri, N. M. (2018). *A political economy of Nigeria's restructuring debate*. Paper presented at the Nigeria Institute of Management (Chartered) colloquium on structure and organizational performance: The case of Nigeria held at Chris Abebe Auditorium, Management House, Plot 22, Idowu Taylor Street, Victoria Island, Lagos. Wednesday, 23rd May.

Chapter 13
Reimagining the Nigerian Healthcare System to Achieve Universal and High-Quality Health Care by 2030

Learning Objectives

After reading this chapter, the learner should be able to:

1. Discuss the reforms needed to achieve universal health care in Nigeria.
2. Describe the reforms that are needed to bring about a high-quality healthcare system in the country.
3. Discuss specific recommendations to address the governance and leadership challenges within the healthcare system.
4. Describe specific guidance to curtail the brain drain phenomenon among healthcare professionals in the country.
5. Proffer specific proposals that will ensure access to essential medications/vaccines and uninterrupted operation of critical diagnostic and therapeutic equipment in the nation's tertiary hospitals in the country.
6. Provide specific recommendations to address the health information system challenges in the country.

Introduction

Nigeria is a country endowed with natural resources, yet millions live in abject poverty. As of 2020, Nigeria has the highest number of people living in abject poverty worldwide, with 86.9 million living on less than $1 (₦381) a day. Also, the country is among the top 10 countries in the "misery index" category. Compared to the situation in high-income countries, the overwhelming majority of Nigerians are underfed and poor (Onyenekenwa, 2011). The poorest people in the country are among the poorest in Africa, while the wealthiest control much of the luxury and resources (Cool Geography, 2015). About 40.1% of Nigeria's population lived in poverty—an

© The Author(s), under exclusive license to Springer Nature Switzerland AG 2021
J. A. Balogun, *The Nigerian Healthcare System*,
https://doi.org/10.1007/978-3-030-88863-3_13

individual is considered poor when they have available less than ₦137,400 ($361) per year (Varrella, 2020a).

Poverty in the country is both state- and sector-based and is more pervasive in the north. In 2000, Kano and Kogi accounted for nearly one-third of the country's most deprived. Almost 90% of the core poor are farmers, while 58% of the urban dwellers live in poverty. By 2019, Sokoto and Taraba states had the highest number of people living below the poverty line. The lowest poverty rates are in the South and Southwestern states. Lagos state's poverty rate is 4.5%, the lowest rate in the country. The problem is at a crisis level because of the challenge of inequality. On average, the wealthiest Nigerian earns 150,000 times more in a year from their wealth than the lowest 10% of the population for their essential consumption (Onyeji, 2020).

By the fourth quarter of 2020, the country's unemployment rate continued to deteriorate. It stood at 33.3% or 23.2 million of the 70 million people who should be working, but cannot find a job. The underemployment rate—people who work less than 20 hours a week—is also high at 22.8% (Nwokoma & Ekeanyanwu, 2021). As a result of the high level of unemployment and violence due to insecurity, many Nigerians have lost hope. Past efforts that focused on poverty reduction, such as the well-funded Family Economic Advancement Program launched in 1997 by General Sani Abacha, only had a marginal impact because of poor program design/implementation and corruption (Obinne, 1999).

A survey of 1000 Nigerians in 2018 to gauge the level of confidence in the nation's health system revealed a whopping 44% of the respondents "did not feel confident at all," 30% felt "somewhat confident," and only 26% of the respondents felt "confident" in the health system. The lack of confidence was higher in public health institutions than in private establishments (Alagboso, 2020). Another survey study conducted by the Pew Research Center found that almost half of the Nigerian adults were desirous of leaving the country in the next five years (Nevin & Omosomi, 2019). Another survey study in 2017 by NOIPolls, a public opinion and research organization based in Abuja, reported that 90% of Nigerian physicians are dissatisfied with the health system and plan to seek job opportunities abroad (NOIPolls, 2017). The findings from these two studies from Nigeria is reflective of the poor state of the health system, lack of national pride, dwindling hope, and despair in the land. The findings mentioned earlier contrast with studies from Taiwan and South Korea, where 80% of the population are satisfied with their healthcare system (Wu et al., 2010; Kwon et al., 2015).

The overwhelming majority of Nigerians have abjured the public healthcare system, and those who can afford it often opt to receive their health care at private establishments or travel outside the country. The annual expense on medical tourism is between $1 and $1.5 billion (Ajimotokan, 2019; Onyenucheya, 2018; Basiru et al., 2018; NOIPolls, 2017; Okafor, 2017; Makinde, 2016; VOA, 2019; Punch, 2016; International Medical Travel Journal, 2014; Ajobe et al., 2013). Unfortunately, the global travel restrictions due to the coronavirus disease 2019 (COVID-19) pandemic did not constrain the elite and politicians' junketing ambitions. They seem not to have learned the necessity of committing the needed resources to upgrade the healthcare system.

Although successive Nigerian governments since independence have developed a panoply of national health plans starting with the first colonial plan in 1945 and the most recent 2018–2022 National Strategic Health Development Plan (Scott-Emuakpor, 2010; Essien & Yakubu, 2018), universal health care (UHC) remains a mirage in the country. The goal has been elusive, in part, because of the patchwork incremental approach adopted. The widely held dogma that "the definition of insanity is doing the same thing repeatedly and expecting a different result" is the basis of the argument in this chapter. The nation cannot continue to engage in piecemeal solutions to address the healthcare system's challenges and expect positive health outcomes.

Nigeria's healthcare system is one of the most inefficient and worst health outcome indices globally (WHO, 2000, 2010). Muhammad et al. (2017) deftly describe the health system as "weak while its management is ineffective and inefficient." In addition, tangible development in the health sector is hampered by corruption, waste, the continued deterioration of the physical facilities, rampant incidences of industrial strikes, limited access to clean water, and environmental air pollution (OECD, 2002). The human resources in the urban and rural areas are distributed unequally. For example, over 70% of the physicians are in urban areas where only 48% of the population lives, leaving 52% of the population who live in the rural area at the mercy of inadequate health personnel (Muhammad et al., 2017).

Nigeria has the second-largest HIV/AIDS incidence in the world, accounting for 9% of the global HIV infections, and the country bears the worst burden of malaria, accounting in 2018 for 25% of all cases and nearly 19% of all malaria fatalities worldwide (Rine, 2019; AXA.com, 2019). Despite these appalling health indices, less than 5% of Nigerians have access to health care (Awosusi et al., 2015; Ifijeh, 2015; NOIPolls, 2017; Amu et al., 2018; Aregbeshola & Khan, 2018). The formal economic sector employers account for almost all the Nigerians with health insurance enrollees (Onasanya, 2020).

These multidimensional challenges are compounded by inconsistent economic policies, socio-political factors, and limited institutional capacity to provide efficient responses at a population level (Muhammad et al., 2017). Lack of political will and government commitment, particularly during military rule, has worsened the fragile health sector. Successive governments have, on many occasions, heightened their commitment to the health sector. Unfortunately, the rhetoric is not met with tangible and enduring actions, particularly in health system financing (Muhammad et al., 2017). This author posits that the health system is presently on life support, and the previously adopted patchwork solution will not lead to UHC anytime soon. The "patient" requires a holistic and comprehensive treatment premised and modelled on best practices from different health systems worldwide. The word "reimagining" used in this chapter's title underscores the need for a total overhaul of the health system's structures and operations with every conceivable idea considered in the rebuilding of the new health system.

In 2014, a presidential summit on UHC, hosted by President Goodluck Ebele Jonathan, was held in Abuja. The presidency agreed that "Nigeria is not where it ought to be in terms of UHC with other Nations in the same development bracket." After the conference, the communiqué released reaffirmed that health care is a fundamental human right and the government's responsibility to provide good health for all citizens (WHO, 2014). Five years after the summit, Onwujekwe et al. (2019) opined that UHC has been an illusion in the country due to budgetary constraints, inadequate financial protection for the poor, shortage and uneven distribution of healthcare workers, varying quality of healthcare services, poor service coordination, weak referral system, and the variable utilization of health services.

In 2015, all 193 member states of the United Nations agreed on the sustainable development goals (SDGs) adopted in New York and set out an ambitious plan for a safer, fairer, and healthier world by 2030 (UN, 2015). UHC was included in the 17 SDGs and presents an opportunity for the Nigerian government to promote a comprehensive and coherent healthcare approach, focusing on strengthening the health systems. Recognizing that achieving UHC requires coordinated efforts across multiple sectors and developing strong, sustainable, and equitable health systems, a global organization tagged UHC2030 was formed with the mission to provide a platform where the private sector, civil society, international organizations, academia, and governmental organizations can collaborate to create a movement for accelerating equitable and sustainable progress towards UHC and strengthen health systems at global and country levels. WHO and the World Bank provides secretariat support to UHC2030 and facilitate coordination under the umbrella of UHC2030 at global, regional, and country levels, working with other signatories, as needed (Global Compact, 2021). Due to a lack of political will, Nigeria did not achieve the eight United Nations Millennium Development Goals (MDGs) and has made little or no progress toward implementing the 17 SDGs.

In 2016, President Muhammadu Buhari's government launched a plan to achieve 30% health insurance coverage by 2020. Still, this goal did not materialize, and the health system has not improved. Several reviews and critique articles explaining why UHC remained a pipe dream in the country have been published, including the analyses presented in Chap. 5. Drawing on these reports and the qualitative study findings in the preceding section, this chapter presents the roadmap needed to attain UHC in Nigeria by 2030—consistent with SDG #3 (UN, 2015; Global Compact, 2021). Furthermore, this chapter offers a blueprint for achieving high-quality health care, and the recommendations are in two parts: Part I proposes the reforms necessary to achieve UHC by 2030, and Part II discusses the comprehensive plan that will usher in high-quality health care in Nigeria.

The Pathway to Universal Health Care in Nigeria

From the literature reviewed, this chapter proposes five key factors that forestall the implementation of UHC in Nigeria. The five factors are presented in Fig. 13.1.

The key recommendations needed to address the five factors (Fig. 13.1) that hinder the implementation of UHC are discussed next.

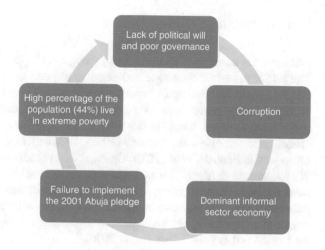

Fig. 13.1 Barriers against achieving universal health care in Nigeria

Lack of political will and poor governance

Corruption

Dominant informal sector economy

Failure to implement the 2001 Abuja pledge

High percentage of the population (44%) live in extreme poverty

Elect Leaders Committed to Universal Health Care

With the enormous human resources at home and in the diaspora, a competent and uncorrupted leader can transform Nigeria into a nation like Singapore—an impoverished country with only a $500 per capita income back in 1965. Today, their education and healthcare systems are the envy of the world. Singapore is one of the model health systems showcased in Chap. 10 of this publication. Singapore achieved the inexplicable feat through a national plan created by their leaders based on three simple vision commitments—MPH: meritocracy, pragmatism, and honesty. The Singaporean government intentionally makes leadership appointments based on merit and fiercely fights corruption (Mahbubani, 2017).

Singapore achieved UHC through a hybrid financing system. Its health system has attained extraordinary feats in delivering high-quality service at an affordable low out-of-pocket expense by the consumers (Tikkanen et al., 2020). An enthused scholar from the United States described how Singapore was able to attain its global stature, as follows: "Singapore has three compelling qualities woven into the country's fabric that has enabled it to achieve outstanding successes in so many areas, healthcare included" (Brookings.edu, 2017). The nation is united, and the leaders recognize talents and establish national priorities consistently. The lack of "MPH" is Nigeria's bane. Nigeria has abundant human talents, but they rarely bloom on its shores due to a political system fraught with corruption and waste. This author chronicled the extraordinary achievements of Nigerian healthcare academics in the diaspora (Balogun, 2020).

From Singapore's experience, the take-home lesson is the need for a stable democratic government led by a charismatic and visionary leader committed to UHC. To achieve this goal, Nigerians must vote in a political party that is committed to health care as the number one budget priority. The president of that party can use the office's bully pulpit to achieve the political and economic reforms discussed in Chap. 12. Equally important, the country needs an honest and capable health minister and competent chief executive officers at the federal and state hospitals who are committed to "MPH" philosophy.

Stifle Corruption

Corruption is a sure path that will destroy Nigeria if appropriate action is not taken. The author discussed the scope and negative impacts of health sector corruption in Chaps. 11 and 12. The top five corrupt practices that negatively impact the delivery of high-quality health care in Nigeria are unreported absenteeism from work, procurement-related fraud, under-the-counter payments, health financing-related crime, and employment-related bribery (Onwujekwe, Agwu, et al., 2019; Onwujekwe, Ezumah, et al., 2019; Onwujekwe et al., 2018; Ogbaa, 2017; Ibenegbu, 2018; Tormusa & Idom, 2016). In addition, corruption erodes public trust in government programs and perpetuates inequalities and discontent, particularly among the poor and vulnerable population. Several empirical studies revealed that the poor and vulnerable population disproportionally doles out the highest proportion of their income on bribes (The World Bank, 2020).

Moreover, because they are powerless to complain, they are often preyed upon. Every stolen or misdirected fund deprives the poor of equal life opportunities and prevents the government from investing in human capital. Employment opportunities must be made available for the youths, particularly women, to eliminate extreme poverty by 2030 and boost shared wealth for the lowest 40% of the population (The World Bank, 2020).

The work setting in Nigeria is informal—lateness and absenteeism are pervasive unethical behaviors that are not taken seriously. Public employees often make personal telephone calls lasting more than an hour when on duty. Some employees are absent from work for weeks, and their salary is still paid in full at the end of the month. Unfortunately, an average Nigerian cannot see the aforementioned detestable work behaviors as corruptive acts. Notably, corruption is not only about bribes, but it extends to any form of dishonesty or criminal offense committed by a person or organization entrusted with a position of authority or abuse of power for private gain. The areas, types, and negative impacts of corruption in the health sector are summarized in Table 13.1. Corruption affects the country's image globally. Hence, citizens must comprehend the various types of crime and their impact on the health system and develop the intelligent senses needed to nip it in the bud (Tormusa & Idom, 2016).

Corruption in the health sector has a disproportionate pernicious effect on the vulnerable population—the poor, people living with disabilities, and the elderly (Eshemokha, 2021). They are shortchanged when resources are wasted or in short supply. The impact increases healthcare costs and reduces access to critical health care by people who need the services most. Corruption in the pharmaceutical and medical equipment industry manifests in the form of fraud and kickbacks, bribes to speed up the process for drug registration and certification of products, fake drugs allowed on the market, under-the-counter payments for medication, theft/diversion of drugs/supplies and equipment for personal use/resale. The corruption mentioned above drives up prices and leads to the delivery of substandard equipment or adulterated drugs (World Bank, 2020).

Table 13.1 Types and effects of corruption in the health sector

Serial #	Area or process	Type of corruption and problem	Negative impact
1	Provision of healthcare services	Diversion of patients by HCPs to private clinics. HCPs use public facilities to treat private patients, collection of fees from patients for services, theft, diversion of budget allocations to other units, and unreported absenteeism from work	HCPs not available to provide service, leading to low-quality service and unmet needs; high costs of health care, patients sell assets to pay for costly care and loss of faith in the health system. Elites travel abroad for service and the poor result to African traditional medicine
2	Distribution of drugs and supplies	Diversion of government drugs and supplies in the hospital by HCPs to their private clinics and resale of medication and supplies	Lower utilization of resources, patients do not receive quality treatment and make under-the-table payments to obtain medication and often fail to complete treatment, leading to anti-microbial drug resistance
3	Regulation of services, facilities, and HCPs	Kickbacks to speed the process of drug registration, inspection, or certification of goods/HCPs	Fake drugs allowed on the market; marginal vendors permitted to bid
4	Building and repairs of health establishments	Kickbacks and contractors fail to perform and not held accountable.	Inflated cost, low-quality and shoddy construction work, biased distribution of infrastructure, favoring kinsmen, resulting in inequities in access to health care
5	Purchase of equipment and pharmaceutics including monitoring of product's quality	Bribes, collusion, or bid rigging during procurement, lack of incentives to choose low cost and high-quality vendors, unethical drug promotion, and vendors fail to deliver goods	High cost, inappropriate or duplicative drugs/equipment, substandard equipment/drugs, inequities due to inadequate funds left to meet needs
6	Education of HCPs	Political influence and nepotism to secure admission to healthcare education programs, and on the job training	Employment of incompetent HCPs, public loss of faith in an unfair system
7	Clinical research	Pseudo clinical trials funded by pharmaceutical companies with no informed consent, manipulation and unethical practice during data collection	Violation of patients' rights, selection biases, and inequities in research

Sources: (Tormusa & Idom, 2016; Onwujekwe, Agwu, et al., 2019; Onwujekwe, Ezumah, et al., 2019; Onwujekwe et al., 2018; Ogbaa, 2017; Ibenegbu, 2018; and Muhammad et al., 2017)

Health sector corruption is noticeable in various forms ranging from health financing crime to self referral of patients in public hospitals to private clinics, and diversion of drugs and equipment in public hospitals to private clinics. Corruption can also evince itself by diversion of budget allocations and lack of informed consent before starting a research study, unethical data collection including manipulation/falsification of data, employment-related bribery, failure to wait for a turn while on the service line, failure to report absenteeism from work, malpractice, and referrals of patients to private clinics (Eshemokha, 2021). There is no silver bullet for fighting corruption. If it is simple to wipe it out, Nigeria would have found a solution because of its pervasiveness in the country. Unfortunately, bribe-givers and takers are always on the lookout for ingenious solutions to beat the system. That said, what are the strategies to manage health sector corruption? It can be detected through internal and external audits, reports by concerned citizens, investigative journalists, whistle-blowers, modern technology (blockchain, smartphone applications, and open data web platforms), and through asset and interest declarations (UNODC, 2020). The health organizations at the three levels of government can make progress in fighting corruption by implementing the following recommendations:

1. Reform all major health institutions by focusing on improving financial management and strengthening auditors' power to curb corruption.
2. Promote transparency and access to financial information at all health establishments. Public access to information will increase administrators' and boards' responsiveness.
3. Support employees' demand for anti-corruption initiatives and empower them to hold health institution administrators accountable. This recommendation will break the cycle of impunity. Civil society organizations and journalists can assist in uncovering corrupt acts in the health sector.
4. Close international loopholes in the global financial system to prevent money laundering and forestall hiding the proceeds of looted state assets (Transparency International, 2016).
5. Dismantle institution red tapes to enable employees to initiate formal complaints about an ongoing corruptive act through the organization's Ombudsman.
6. Sanction—The organization must initiate appropriate sanctions following the detection of corruption. Sanction is a critical preventive component of any effective anti-corruption effort. The organization's Ombudsman must investigate and recommend appropriate disciplinary action. Administrative progressive disciplinary action (Indiana University, 2020) is an appropriate sanction for minor offenses such as failure to report absenteeism or cut-in service line. However, egregious crimes such as bribes, kickbacks, theft, and diversion of hospital drugs/supplies and equipment for personal use/resale should receive the ultimate punishment—termination of appointment and prosecution.
7. The organizations' anti-corruption initiatives must be monitored using advanced technologies to apprehend, analyze, and publicly share information to prevent, detect, and deter corrupt behaviors (The World Bank, 2020). Ongoing regular monitoring and evaluation are needed to determine the effectiveness of the organization's anti-corruption initiatives and any need for modification as the situations change (Hunja, 2015).
8. Enact legislation to make white-collar crimes, forgery of international passport, birth, and educational certificates a crime punishable for up to 3 years in jail.

Additionally, the health institutions must demonstrate transparency and accountability to enhance taxpayers' confidence in their willingness to improve the health sector. Furthermore, taxpayers must have access to budget information and implementation documents and audit reports of health institutions. Finally, to attract much-needed funds from local and international foundations and donors, health institutions must present their case factually, communicating their challenges and opportunities with credible evidence data.

Curtailing corruption requires determined efforts from people of conscience to fight the vested parties' interests. Promoting transparency and accountability is typically part of eliminating corruption, but it is not the whole story. It will promote good governance, but stiffer deterrent penalties against corruption are needed. Furthermore, the President must acquire the political will to fight corruption that has evaded every fabric of society. The judiciary, legislators, and cabinet officers must lead by example. The President must ensure the legislation requiring government officers to declare their assets on the resumption of office is enforced. Also, the President must appoint an independent ethics board to enforce the law, monitor the assets and sources of public officers' income, and re-invigorate the anti-corruption legislation.

Rwanda's exemplary health system, based on a strong sanction and public mobilization against corruption, and effective alignment of resources from internal and external sources, including effective use of such funds, offer essential lessons to resuscitate Nigeria's healthcare system (Awosusi et al., 2015). Rwanda's health-system reforms are discussed in greater detail in Chap. 12.

Demand for the Implementation of the 2001 Abuja Declaration Pledge, Supplemented by Innovative Financing Schemes

Healthcare financing is the revenue generation process from sources that include the government (primary) source at federal, state, and local levels. Secondary sources are revenue generated from out-of-pocket payments (OOP), taxes (indirect and direct), co-payment, health investments, voluntary prepayments, mandatory prepayment accumulated in a pooled fund, and external funding from the donors (Adebisi et al., 2020). Several internal and external stakeholders in the health sector are key players in the financing of health care. The internal actors include the Federal Ministry of Health (FMH) and its departments at federal, state, local government levels, the private sector, civil organizations, community partners, and academia. The external stakeholders include the Ministry of Finance, Ministry of Budget and National Planning, the Budget Office, National Assembly, Federal Inland Revenue Service, Customs, Central Bank, Accountant General Office, and Auditor General Office (Onwujekwe, Ezumah, et al., 2019).

Although the WHO (2008) considers health financing fundamental to health systems' ability to maintain and improve human welfare, the Nigerian government has not taken this issue seriously. At a conference in Abuja on April 27, 2001, African leaders pledged to allocate at least 15% of their annual budget to the health sector

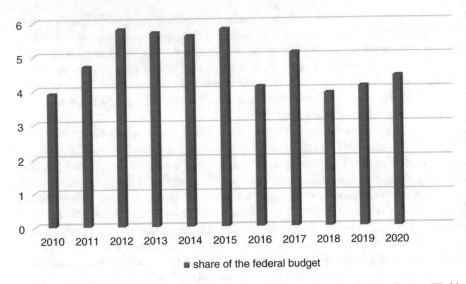

Fig. 13.2 Percentage share of the health budget in the last 10 years (2010–2020). (Source: World Bank, 2021)

(Biegon, 2020). For over two decades after the pledge, most African countries have yet to comply. Only four African countries (Zambia, Malawi, Liberia, and Rwanda) have met the 15% health budget allocation. Nigeria has never achieved this goal. In the past 10 years, Nigeria has not allocated up to 6% of its annual budget to health (Fig. 13.2).

To finance UHC in Nigeria, Okpani and Abimbola (2015) proposed a social insurance model that encouraged the states to set up and manage their insurance schemes. They argued that the model presents a unique opportunity for rapidly scaling up enrollment in the National Health Insurance Scheme (NHIS). On the other hand, Onwujekwe, Ezumah, et al. (2019) described six major models for healthcare financing in Nigeria. They include: (1) government budget using general tax revenue, (2) direct out-of-pocket payments, (3) social insurance program implemented by the National Health Insurance Scheme (NHIS), (4) funding from local and international organization donors, (5) demand-side financing through conditional cash transfers, and (6) community-based health insurance.

Adebisi and associates (2020) contend that healthcare financing in Nigeria is obtained mainly from pooled (direct and indirect taxation, budgetary allocation, and donor funding) and unpooled (OOPs in the form of payment for medical products such as bed-nets or condoms and services) sources. The latter source contributes over 70% of total health expenditure in Nigeria. The extreme reliance on out-of-pocket expenses creates a significant barrier to health services access and leaves many within the population exposed to impoverishment. OOPs that are above 40% is catastrophic health payment. Consequently, Nigeria faces a disproportionate distribution in health system financing.

The mechanisms that countries use to finance their healthcare system are an essential determinant for achieving UHC. Uzochukwu et al. (2015) discussed the persistent and significant weakness of the NHIS financing systems due to low public spending, very high levels in OOP expenditures (one of the highest in the world), and impoverishment due to healthcare costs and increased incidence of catastrophic health spending. Across the health systems in Nigeria, spending is distributed disproportionately with regional inequity in expenditure.

Because health care is not affordable and accessible to large segments of Nigerians, it is inescapable that public reforms must occur. Reform efforts should minimize waste in the supply of services and separate primary healthcare services from hospital services. Private outpatient clinics that offer general health care (both preventive and curative, including minor surgeries), and prenatal care must be encouraged and financially incentivized by the government. Hospitalization, which costs more than twice the average cost of outpatient care, and unnecessary services utilization, should be minimized. Given the potential for higher productivity and better quality of care, group private medical practices, rare in the country, should be encouraged instead of solo practices.

Tax avoidance and inefficient tax collection from the informal sector economy are significant roadblocks that the government should tackle to improve local revenue generation. For example, Lagos state successfully increased its monthly internally generated revenue from N600 million to N20 billion between 2000 and 2010. The other states should adopt the Lagos state example and expand fiscal space and prioritize health investments at the national level. Furthermore, the federal government can generate additional funds by imposing a tax on tobacco and alcohol products, which pose a health risk, impose progressive levies on telephone calls or mobile telephone purchases, tariffs on air tickets, foreign exchange transactions, and luxury goods.

The federal government could cut the enormous budget for fuel subsidies and launch an aggressive nationwide campaign to educate Nigerians on the cost and life-saving benefits of health insurance coverage. In addition, creating an appropriate business climate will incentivize foreign investors to infuse capital into the health sector. However, this prospect is unrealistic because of the onslaught of violence by the Boko Haram terrorists and Fulani herdsmen bandits and the occasional disruption of oil operations in the Niger Delta, among a legion of other problems that make the country unattractive to international entrepreneurs.

Additionally, the federal government should create competition between the government and private hospitals. Such an approach will moderate healthcare costs and promote efficiency. The federal government should recognize only private group practice, and they should be reimbursed for their services. The government should establish an agency to develop the necessary monitoring process to prevent fraud and abuse. The agency should be charged with registering private group practice and creating a licensure and accreditation body. Health facilities' regulators should visit every group of private practice annually to monitor compliance with the regulations. The agency should develop reimbursement fee schedules for healthcare providers, ambulance services, clinical laboratory services, durable medical equipment, prosthetics, orthotics, and supplies. Similarly, they should create a comprehensive fee schedule to pay providers/suppliers based on the fee-for-service and face-to-face interaction between the patient and the healthcare provider. They should also set the treatment reimbursement rate on a flat fee for each medical diagnosis.

Another private health system reform recommendation is that only physicians/dentists with advanced training of 2–3 years in a practice specialty are registered to own private clinical practice. Such graduate-level medical education, in addition to stricter control over hospital licensure, would improve outcomes of care. Some critics affirmed that the current five-year residency program is unduly too long and needs rethinking. Strengthening regulation by mandating private health facilities to annually report the number and types of health facilities, including staff and medical technologies, will go a long way toward achieving greater control and reliable data on the private sector's activities. The information will enable health planners to identify underserved regions and effectively monitor the impact of public policy on health sector development. Thus, professional regulatory agencies should be adequately equipped in terms of technical personnel and information technology.

Another issue that warrants consideration to achieve adequate control of the private sector is decentralizing the complaints and disciplinary processes to regional and lower levels. Failure to perform inspection internally could well compel consumers to seek "control" through the courts. In the end, this situation would not serve the interest of either the consumer or the provider. Finally, the private sector's expanding contribution to socioeconomic development and the opportunities for the rapid extension of services to underserved populations should be encouraged by policymakers. Concerted efforts should be made by both the government and the banks to actively influence the private health sector's development by granting loan assistance and tax concessions to control healthcare professionals' (HCPs) training and distribution (Ogunbekun et al., 1999).

In Nigeria, health financing mechanisms are presently not operating optimally due to political, socioeconomic, cultural, and human factors. The deployment of the varying financing mechanisms is not evidence-based data-driven. Resources are not allocated efficiently and equitably, and waste is prevalent. The risk protection coverage mechanisms are deficient and often benefit the elite class. None of the means effectively protects consumers from catastrophic health expenditure (Onwujekwe, Ezumah, et al., 2019). To address these issues at federal, state, and local government levels, authorities should invigorate the NHIS and explore concerted efforts to increase public funding of health alongside other options such as public-private partnerships and international development assistance to lessen high OOP expenses by consumers.

The low uptake of the NHIS is due to poor public awareness by the younger people, stereotypic ideas regarding the government's role in funding the nations' health care, cultural beliefs about health insurance attracting ill-health, and insufficient trust in governance (Onasanya, 2020). Therefore, increased public awareness through conversation around health insurance using the media to deliver communication packages on health insurance that are sociodemographic targeted will go a long way in addressing low health insurance uptake.

The Internet and social media are used widely in Nigeria. About 59% (113.3 million) of the population use mobile Internet, and many also use social networks and messaging applications. About 41% of Nigerians use Facebook and WhatsApp. Adults between 18 and 34 years of age account for between 34% and 80% of the primary social media site users (Onasanya, 2020). Thus, social media will be an attractive platform for health maintenance organizations (HMOs) to disseminate information about health insurance. The oral word-of-mouth marketing strategy will be more effective in reaching Nigerians in the informal economic sector with low levels of education or access to social media technology and who have no formal financial education. Leveraging the social networks of the different demographic and economic categories is expected to yield high gains in health insurance enrolment (Onasanya, 2020).

Reform the Informal Sector Economy

One of the primary reasons that make UHC still an illusion in Nigeria is the low uptake of the NHIS. Low- and medium-scale entrepreneurs are leery of registering their workers in the NHIS as mandated by the law, which requires workers to pay 7.5% of the premium and the employers to match the 7.5% of the premium. Unfortunately, most entrepreneurs in the country encourage the workers not to enroll in the NHIS because it is profitable for both parties not to be invested in the program. The motive behind the backdoor practice is the perception that the NHIS would not guarantee access to high-quality health care because of the historical experiences associated with insurance programs in the country. Pension schemes, life assurance, house, and education insurance programs introduced in the 1960s and early 1970s were a fraud, as the brokers did not process claims.

The historical antecedents significantly impact public perception about government-run insurance's dependability (Asakitikpi, 2019). Three critical transformation changes are needed from the government for the workers to gain trust in the NHIS:

1. The workers must perceive there is fairness in the country's tax system.
2. Government-run programs must be reliable and efficiently managed.
3. The funds collected are not diverted to other government programs but used for the purpose for which they are meant.

The informal sector's size and negative impact on the NHIS are discussed in more detail in Chap. 5 of this publication. The informal sector economy in Nigeria ranges from 47% to 67%, accounting for 56% of the gross domestic product (GDP). Annually, 56% of potential tax revenue is lost to informality. The estimated tax revenue loss in 2018 alone was ₦3.5 trillion. Workers employed in the informal economy are mostly uninsured with a high health insurance dropout rate (Umeh, 2018). Evidence from other studies revealed that no country had achieved UHC with voluntary health insurance (Awosusi et al., 2015). Therefore, the government must make NHIS compulsory by facilitating the amendment of the 1999 NHIS Act 35 and aggressively implement the amended NHIS Act passed by the Seventh National Assembly. The federal government should mandate that each state create a health insurance agency and develop innovative ways to generate revenue from formal and informal sectors. Addressing the multilayered challenges associated with the informal sector economy is key to the success of the NHIS. The following recommendations are proffered to address the informal sector economy debacle:

1. Streamline regulatory procedures by making it easier to register a business. When underground companies register, collecting taxes and enforcing regulation become easier. The reduced tax burden will incentivize informal businesses to operate formally. The collection of taxes from more informal small and mid-sized companies will enable governments to cut tax rates without reducing tax revenue while simultaneously breaking the tax evasion cycle.
2. Make the tax system more straightforward and less complex to understand. For example, calculating taxes based on physical characteristics, such as a store's square footage, rather than reported revenue, which is difficult to verify, will enhance compliance. Increasing the amount of taxes collected from small and mid-sized businesses will positively increase healthcare financing revenue (Farrell, 2004).
3. Launch an aggressive public education campaign on the informal sector economy's disadvantages and evils. The COVID-19 crisis underscored this need since workers in underground businesses cannot benefit from the lifeline social protection programs made available by the government.
4. Improve access to education by ensuring that students remain in school, complete their education, and offer ample technical and vocational training opportunities.
5. Enact policies to enhance financial inclusion by promoting expanded access to legitimate bank-based financial services. Lack of access to bank loans is a primary constraint for informal enterprises as it reduces productivity and economic growth.
6. Strengthen the use of digital platforms, including government-to-person mobile transfers. This development will contribute to inclusive growth by bringing financial investments to the poor and women and assisting small and medium-sized businesses to grow within the formal sector (Delechat & Medinal, 2020).

Eradicate Extreme Poverty

In June 2018, Nigeria had 86.9 million people living in extreme poverty—they represent 44% of the 195,874,683 citizens. Nigeria will become the world's third populous country in the world by 2050. As of June 2018, Nigeria surpassed India, a country with seven times its population, at the bottom of the extreme poverty ranking. The genesis of poverty lies in depriving a segment of society's access to basic human needs such as food, health care, sanitation, education, and assets, including housing. Resolving these basic needs generally lifts any population out of extreme poverty. Moreover, the fundamental link between abject poverty and human rights is disproportionately affected by many human rights violations. In 1987, it was

Joseph Wresinski who eloquently captured the nexus between human rights and extreme poverty with his gearing statement that wherever humans live in abject poverty, human rights are compromised, and to reinstate them is humanity's solemn obligation (Akinyele & Otto Abasiekong, 2018).

Although some progress has been made globally since 1987 in addressing human rights and extreme poverty, much remains to be done in Nigeria. The United Nations' SDG number three on UHC and end extreme poverty by 2030 can be achieved by addressing the following issues:

1. *Invest in girls' education*: Educate girls about economic returns and intergenerational social impact. Unfortunately, over ten million school-age children in Nigeria, around half of whom are girls, do not attend school. About 67% of the out-of-school children are from the northwest and northeastern states—the region is ravaged by the terror group, Boko Haram, affecting approximately 2.8 million schoolchildren.

2. *Support the NHIS*: Increased healthcare investment is a strong determinant of economic growth and a critical pathway to reducing poverty. To end poverty, the federal government must harness the demographic dividends by investing in health, education, and employment for young people. Nigerians are pushed into extreme poverty regularly because they faced financial hardship paying for unanticipated major health problems. To alleviate this conundrum, the NHIS needs robust funding from the federal government. Both the state and local governments must do their part in providing secondary and primary health care to their citizens. After all, health care is a human rights issue that every government is expected to make available to its citizen. Gerisch asserts this right when she eloquently states, "among all the rights to which we are entitled, health care may be the most intersectional and crucial. The very frailty of our human lives demands that we protect this right as a public good. Universal health care is crucial for the most marginalized segments of any population to live lives of dignity. Without our health, we—do not live, let alone live with dignity" (Gerisch, n.d.).

3. *Embrace technology and expand economic opportunities:* 18 million of Nigeria's labor force is without jobs, one of Africa's highest. Ending poverty will entail improving economic productivity and opportunities for all citizens. The government can achieve this goal by investing in human capital potential, creating jobs for women and young people, increasing access to capital, creating opportunities for rural dwellers, and fostering technological innovation. Nigeria ranks 152 (worst) out of 157 countries on the World Bank's *human capital index*. To address this concerning statistic, the government must train the youths—outside the formal school system or those who possess only a primary education—to develop new technical and vocational skills.

4. *Promote private sector partnerships:* Boosting entrepreneurial ecosystems (focusing on apprenticeships) through incentives are critical strategies the government can use to eradicate extreme poverty by galvanizing job creation and economic growth.

5. *Enhance access to microfinance*: Availability of bank loans and government grants and other social safety payouts to rural dwellers will bring the poor into the financial system and help government better develop healthcare services for the impoverished. Furthermore, the government's regulatory support for digital and mobile-based financial products and blockchain technologies' adoption can help bolster financial inclusion. Blockchain ledgers can help digital link identities with payments with the potential to reach workers in the informal sector. This transparent government regulatory support has the potential to plug corruption-related leakages in government disbursements to poverty-stricken citizens (Abdullahi, 2019). The Microfinance Banks' repositioning in the rural areas will increase access to capital through soft loans to a rising working class of youths ages 21–35 years living in rural areas.

6. *Review the national minimum wage:* In 2019, the minimum wage for federal workers was set at ₦30,000 ($77), but the monthly cost of living for an individual is about ₦43,200 and ₦137,600 for a family (Varrella, 2020b). With the inflation rate at over 11% and the purchasing power parity substantially reduced due to the global plummeting of oil prices, the minimum wage of ₦30,000 is insufficient to lift the workers out of extreme poverty. Consequently, a new salary review is needed to increase workers' purchasing power and their capacity to purchase health insurance coverage.

7. *Support gender equity:* Women empowerment is key to national development because it raises household incomes and improves the children's health and well-being. Economic empowerment will reduce poverty for future generations as well. The need to empower women is well articulated by former United States President Barack Obama when he asserted "we know from experience that nations are more successful when their women are successful" (The White House, 2015). To make Nigerian women successful, the government should make concerted efforts to promote women's participation in the economy, technology, and policymaking spaces.

8. *Promote administrative transparency*: By building strong institutions through transparency, federal allocations to the local governments will no longer be diverted by the state governors. This development will go a long way to reduce corruption and enable primary health care to be implemented successfully.

The Blueprint for High-Quality Health Care in Nigeria

Multiple reasons identified in the literature why the health system is not efficient and of low quality include the following: ineffective leadership, antiquated infrastructures, epileptic power supply, lack of access to clean water, interprofessional conflicts, brain drain effect leading to a shortage of personnel, absence of a centralized planning system needed for disease prevention, treatment, medical intelligence and surveillance, wrong policy priorities, lack of investment in facilities and prescription drugs, and poor management of the existing resources. The following are the comprehensive plan needed to usher in high-quality UHC in Nigeria.

Merge the University Teaching Hospitals, Federal Medical Centers, and Specialist Hospitals in All States

As of January 2021, there are 57 tertiary hospitals in the country—21 University Teaching Hospitals (UTHs), 23 Federal Medical Centers (FMCs), and 13 Specialist Hospitals. However, many health analysts and scholars worry about the low quality of care provided in many tertiary hospitals (Julius, 2017; Ogbebo, 2015; Orekunrin, 2015; Parmar, 2015; Onwujekwe et al., 2018; Adegoke, 2019). Most tertiary hospitals are in name only because previous leaders equate a tertiary hospital with the physical structure, without planning for an adequate workforce and the infrastructures needed to provide high-quality care.

There is the presumption on the part of the leaders that equipment and physical infrastructures are ageless, and they often fail to obtain a maintenance service agreement. Usually, funds are not provided to service equipment and maintain infrastructures. Once the equipment breaks down, they are often not replaced, and they become an artifact within the hospitals. Some of the tertiary hospitals even lack chemical reagents needed to run necessary diagnostic tests. Hospitals need state-of-the-art tools to make accurate diagnoses and provide effective treatments. Power supply from the national grid is unreliable—electricity is often interrupted while surgeons are at work. The unfathomable challenges mentioned above contribute to the low-quality care delivered in tertiary hospitals. The unacceptable condition is why the elites and politicians abandon the nation's tertiary hospitals for their treatment abroad.

As discussed in Chap. 5, Nigerian elites and politicians travel abroad specifically to receive cardiology, orthopedic, neurology, cancer treatments, cosmetic surgery, renal transplant surgery, and dialysis care. When the service delivery in the UTHs is of high quality as obtained in developed countries, there will be no need for the elites and politicians to seek health care in a foreign land. The $1–$1.5 billion spent annually on medical tourism will be paid to the UTHs. This development will shore up the finances of the tertiary hospitals and the NHIS.

Because of the aforementioned deplorable state of affairs in the tertiary hospitals in the country, this author recommends that the fragmented resources be consolidated by merging the FMCs and the Specialist Hospitals with the UTHs in each state. The federal government should designate each tertiary hospital a Center of Excellence in one of the seven clinical specialties mentioned above. There should be no duplication of specialty across the 12 states proposed in Chap. 12. The consolidation and specialization recommended will improve the tertiary hospitals' expertise and resources and make them economically viable and less dependent on the government. Additionally, it will enable tertiary hospitals to deliver high-quality health care. Long term, the federal government must fund all the tertiary hospitals to have:

1. Functional diagnostic tools that include *magnetic resonance imaging* and computed tomography scanner devices SPECT/CT, EEG (motorized thrombectomy), 3 Tesla MRI, and C-Arm Scan (Eke, 2020; Seven Hills Hospital, 2020).
2. The appropriate equipment needed to provide high-quality care. The following equipment is highly required: high-dose-rate brachytherapy, motorized throm-

bectomy system, Novalis Tx, Mevion S250 proton therapy system, shortwave diathermy, electrical stimulators, ultrasound, and laser bio-stimulators (Seven Hills Hospital, 2020).

3. An adequate number of qualified consultants and clinical specialists.

In the interim, the federal government should provide startup funds to refurbish the hospitals and invest in state-of-the-art diagnostic and therapeutic equipment. Each hospital must develop a maintenance culture to ensure equipment and other critical infrastructures are serviced regularly to prevent breakdown. Furthermore, the FMH must re-establish the functional roles of the three levels within the healthcare system to ensure that secondary and tertiary hospital systems are no longer used as primary healthcare centers. The physicians must ensure the patient referral process is enforced. Primary health care, which is the bedrock of the healthcare system, has crumbled due to administrative malfeasance.

The funneling of the local governments' allocations, in the past, from the federal government through the state has failed because state governors often withhold the funding and financially handicapped the implementation of primary care. Without funds, government impact cannot be felt at the grassroots. The recently enacted arrangement that allows the local governments to receive their funds directly from the federal government is a step in the right direction and must be implemented wholeheartedly by the federal government.

Train all Health Care Administrators in Conflict Resolution Strategies

The Nigerian health system is plagued by several disruptive labor actions arising from industrial activities embarked upon by HCPs and their unions on the one hand and against hospital administration or the FMH or State Ministry of Health on the other hand. The crises have become pronounced that it now negatively impacts the quality and continuity of patient care and the confidence in the health system. The nation needs to develop a culture of stability and continuity by building upon previous administration and leadership achievements without starting all over and reinventing the wheel. Precious efforts and time are wasted in the cyclic process. Training CEOs of hospitals and FMH or State Ministry of Health administrator is an effective strategy to stem the conflict's tide.

Conflict is a pervasive foe within the Nigerian healthcare system. Despite the recognized need for interdisciplinary work, only a small proportion of time is devoted by HCPs to genuine collaborative efforts. The health sector leadership at state and national levels should make every effort to prevent industrial strikes. The government should organize ongoing education seminars on negotiation and conflict management strategies for the health sector's chief executive officers. The healthcare team leader and administrator of large health organizations and systems must be astute at conflict management. The most typical conflict in healthcare teams and organizations is an intra- and inter-group misunderstanding, individual professionals' aberrant behaviors, poor communication, and unclear organizational structures. The leader must first identify the source of the disagreement and the central power players at the center of the dispute to diffuse the conflict effectively.

Usually, conflict develops from underlying latent issues, which often progress to perceived conflict (where the problem becomes apparent) and subsequently manifest the behavioral/action phase and, lastly, the aftermath of the battle. The leader can utilize any of the following approaches to creating a positive outcome for all feuding parties—compromise, accommodation, collaboration, bargaining/negotiation, mediation, facilitating communication, seeking consensus, and engendering vision to aid the conflict's resolution at all stages of its development. There are essential qualities that the leaders of healthcare teams, organizations, and systems must possess while managing a crisis-riddled and fast-changing practice landscape. The department or team leaders must be:

1. An independent thinker who is knowledgeable in the emerging healthcare market.
2. Passionate about meeting the needs of the followers.
3. A change agent for their organization.
4. Able to inspire team members.
5. Able to run a lean, high-quality organization.

Most importantly, the leaders must practice the following strategies to create harmony and prevent conflicts within a team:

1. Set some ground rules during the first and subsequent meetings to address what process will be taken to resolve disputes and inform the parties involved that their ideas are valid and not dismissed.
2. Understand destructive conflicts that develop when no resolution is in sight or the issue cannot be resolved. The leader must not slip into the fray but must try to recognize the ongoing team dynamics.
3. Resolve all conflicts as quickly as possible before it festers.
4. Understand the entire story and all parties' perspectives to address differences of opinions and prevent miscommunication or misunderstanding.
5. Make a compromise between parties a goal and must create harmony among followers.
6. Must avoid falling into a group thinking mentality that will suppress other members' views.
7. Must not try to change the team members' unique ideas and forms of expression, leading to resentment.
8. Propose alternatives by listing the benefits of other ideas, but ultimately must accept that followers may disagree with the resolution efforts' outcome (Dodson, 2017; Bunashe & Broder, 2015; Reddy, n.d.; Woodard, n.d.).

Invest in Electricity and Clean Water

No business, including the health sector, can thrive when there is no electricity. Health care cannot be delivered efficiently in darkness. Moreover, medication and vaccines are rendered useless when electricity is not reliable. The provision of clean water will prevent many of the endemic waterborne diseases—typhoid fever, cholera, giardia, dysentery, *Escherichia coli*, and hepatitis A Salmonella. The government should provide clean water and invest in solar and wind energies to replace fossil fuels—petroleum, coal, natural gas, and Orimulsion. Politicians and merchants sabotaging government efforts to provide dependable power supply nationwide should be considered the state's enemy and prosecuted.

Promote Telehealth and Mobile Health Van for Health Services Delivery

In the United States, mobile clinics represent an essential component of the health system serving vulnerable populations and promote high-quality care at a low cost. An estimated 1500 mobile clinics receive five million visits nationwide per year, bolstering prevention and chronic disease management (Hill et al., 2014). In a recent study, Malone and associates (2020) reported that mobile clinics provide 3491 visits annually, with 55% of the clients being women and 59% racial/ethnic minorities. Of the 146 clinics that reported insurance data, 41% were uninsured, while 44% had some form of public insurance. Prevention (47%) and primary care (41%) are the most common services of mobile clinics. About 33% are independent providers, 24% university-affiliated, and 29% are part of a hospital or healthcare system. About 52% of the mobile clinics receive financial support from philanthropy, and 45% receive federal funds (Malone et al., 2020). Coupling telehealth technology and mobile health clinics can drastically reduce personnel and capital costs (WHO, 2010). Investment in mobile clinics in Nigeria is ideal for serving rural areas and promoting high-quality care at a low price. The federal government should commit to training additional 500,000 community health workers and revamp the public health sanitation unit at the community level to ensure people no longer live in an unsanitary environment that breeds mosquitoes and waterborne diseases. Students in all the 44 College of Health Sciences and community health workers/auxiliary nurses should be trained by clinical faculty to acquire technical skills in e-health technology and the mobile health clinic.

Address the High Maternal and Perinatal Death

The MDGs—particularly MDG 4, 5, and 6, which focus on how to reduce child mortality, improve maternal health, and combat HIV/AIDS, malaria, and other diseases—were not met by the 2015 target date (United Nations Population Fund, n.d.). Concerted efforts are needed to scale-up women's education, improve newborn health, and promote universal access to reproductive health services, including health care that spans the life cycle. Similarly, a lot of work in reproductive health is needed, particularly in slowing HIV/AIDS spread, reducing maternal mortality, and improving family planning. Many developing countries are making a concerted effort in reaching their targets, but in Nigeria, the pace of development is slow; there are still significant needs and opportunities to do more.

Women in developing countries lose more disability-adjusted life years from maternal health-related causes than to any other reason. The unacceptable maternal mortality rate led the FMH in 2013 to recommend that all obstetric clinics periodically carry out maternal death reviews, surveillance, and response using the WHO protocol. The recommendation in 2013 by the WHO was updated by the FMH in 2016 to include perinatal death reviews and the program was re-branded as Maternal and Perinatal Death Surveillance and Response to underscore the equally high rates of stillbirth and neonatal and perinatal deaths. A recent finding by Professor Okonofua and his research team from the Women's Health and Action Research Centre at Benin City revealed that the hospital policymakers' proactive engagement is the most critical factor toward a successful outcome that can cause an immediate decline in maternal mortality ratio (Aikpitanyi et al., 2019). The strategy is to implement health education programs, improve HCPs' response to emergency obstetric care, establish an intensive care unit, and intensify blood donation drive. If implemented nationwide, the combined strategies will undoubtedly go a long way in curtailing the high maternal and perinatal deaths and improving health outcomes and quality of care.

Invest in Resources for People Living with Disabilities

The federal and state governments should ensure that people with mental disabilities arc institutionalized to receive psychiatric treatment and job training. Those with developmental, physical, and other forms of disabilities are housed in community-based habilitation facilities to receive vocational training (Joseph Rehabilitation Center, 2020). By establishing a Division of Medical Rehabilitation within the FMH, healthcare services for people living with disabilities can be better coordinated nationwide. The Division should also develop educational programs in medical sonography, medical social work, and rehabilitation counseling. These vocational careers are highly needed in the healthcare system, and they will nicely complement the existing medical rehabilitation disciplines currently offered in the universities. Drastic reforms, as discussed in Chap. 9, are required to enact legislation that will guarantee equal opportunities and learning accommodation for students with disabilities.

Slow Down Population Growth

The urbanite population has increased from 34.8% in 2000 to 46.9% in 2014, with an urbanization growth rate of 3.75%. At its current growth rate, Nigeria's population will surpass that of the United States by 2050. It would be the world's third most populous country after China and India by the end of the century, with 399 million people (United Nations Population Fund, n.d.). The growth rate is a vexing problem, mainly because of the dismal allocation of resources to the education and healthcare sectors. One good news is that the total fertility rate had dropped slightly from 5.7 in 2008 to 5.4 in 2019.

In the last decade, the country has witnessed low contraceptive practices that stayed static from 15% in 2008 and 15.1% in 2013 for all contraception methods. The rapid population growth can be attenuated using three strategies: health education, birth control, and government incentives. The famous dictum *"when you educate a woman, you educate a nation" is crucial* in reducing population growth. Studies have shown that women knowledgeable about family planning and childcare will have fewer children and better life quality (Gluck, 2012). Additionally, women need to have access to behavior modification health education and health care during pregnancy.

As the population continues to snowball, the health sector cannot meet the increased population growth, much less keep up with the emerging health dynamics that are equally co-occurring. More funding is urgently needed for family planning education, particularly among teenagers, to procure and distribute contraceptive commodities nationwide (Onigbinde et al., 2018). Because of the unrelenting youth bulge, the government at all levels should ensure sex education and family control methods are scaled up in school and health clinic settings nationwide and in the rural areas where most Nigerians live. Birth control methods, such as condoms, pills, and surgery, can prevent unwanted pregnancies and increase women's self-determination.

The government can also provide incentives, such as tax breaks, to parents to regulate family size. The incentives can be accompanied by raising parents' awareness about the advantages of a small number of children. It does not matter which method an individual chooses to reduce population growth. What matters most is the chance for the child to survive. An increase in children's life expectancy will result in lower population growth because parents will be assured that their children will survive, and quality is better than quantity. This line of thinking is consistent with the MDG 4 that aims to "reduce child mortality."

Curtail Industrial Strikes in the Health Sector

The health system in Nigeria is beset repeatedly by industrial actions by healthcare professionals (HCPs) agitating for better conditions of service. Low staff morale due to poor remuneration and a horrible work environment is a significant contributor to poor health outcomes (Ihekweazu, 2015). The intermittent labor strikes have caused untold sufferings and deaths of many patients across the nation. It has also forced some patients to seek care at private hospitals and clinics at a prohibitive cost that many could not afford. Ethically, the lockout embarked upon by HCPs is reprehensible because it is against the "first, do no harm" tenet of the Hippocratic Oath, to which they solemnly pledge (Greek Medicine, 2012).

Some infamously notable labor actions in the last decade include the 108-day work shutdown by the Association of Resident Doctors in the University College Hospital, Ibadan; five-month-long strike at Ladoke Akintola UTH Oshogbo; the two-month strike at the Psychiatric Hospital in Yaba; and the three-month-long strike at Federal Medical Centre in Owerri (Ihekweazu, 2015). In 2014, some public-sector hospitals also experienced lockdowns during the Ebola outbreak, leaving some patients without care. HCPs' industrial strike is a national menace that negatively affects the quality of healthcare services and the professional-patient relationship. Many ethicists assert that it is unsavory for HCPs to embark on strike because their role is specialized services. Unfortunately, genuine demands of improving work conditions are often rebuffed by non-perceptive administrators that, in some cases, include top officials like the health minister.

Hospital administrators and government representatives must negotiate in good faith and accede to HCPs' reasonable service demands to avert lockout. In light of the frequency of industrial strikes by HCPs, this author recommends that the government expand the National Human Rights Commission's mission to mediate labor disputes between the HCPs and the employers/State Ministry of Health and FMH. There is also the need for government officials to moderate their disposition during these mediations in the spirit of respectful dialogue and compromise, devoid of take-it-or-leave-it authoritarianism negotiation style.

Enhance Retention and Tracking of Healthcare Professionals

An adequate workforce is the cornerstone of a high-quality health system, but the shortage of HCPs impact work condition and performance and health outcome indices. To have an adequate workforce, retention of the existing HCPs should be of paramount concern. The recruitment and retention of HCPs require strategic planning for effective outcomes. Successful retention of HCPs begins with proper employment planning and ongoing evaluation of the negative organization factors in play — constraints in the hospital budget, poor remuneration, lack of practice autonomy, heavy workload, inflexible workshift, and limited career advancement opportunities —and address them. An aging workforce and shortage of HCPs often lead to staff burnout and shoddy work performance (Ogundipe et al., 2015).

The WHO's benchmark for optimal healthcare delivery stipulates one physician to every 600 people in the population. In 2019, there is one physician for every 5000 Nigerians—one of the highest rates in Africa. Aside from the national shortage of HCPs, their distribution is of concern since they are concentrated in the southern part. The inequity in the distribution is due to the lack of coordination of the public and private sector activities and pressures in the private sector, leading to shoddy quality work. In addition, the work environment has high attrition—mostly in the rural areas—and lack of planning, causing overproduction of some categories of HCPs and a shortage of others. These challenges are compounded further by the substantial increase in the migration of HCPs to other countries, the absence of an efficient and coordinated data collection system, and the explosion of medical tourism travel abroad (Global Health Workforce Alliance/WHO, n.d.).

To address these issues, the FMH, in 2011, partnered with the WHO and United States Centers for Disease Control and Prevention (CDC) to develop a functional human resources information system database to track HCPs' training, graduation, retirement, and exit from the country. At the time, the WHO representative in the country, Dr. Ruiz Gama Vaz, observed that the shortage and competence of HCPs posed the most significant challenges to the ability to deliver high-quality and affordable health services. The project was initiated in collaboration with the Carter Foundation in the United States. Still, the federal government did not address the dire shortage of HCPs in the country (Ogundipe et al., 2015. Moving forward, the FMH must reestablish this collaboration and provide technical support to professional regulatory bodies to put in place mechanisms that will allow for accurate tracking of the exits of HCPs beyond the current reliance on certificates of good standing. The data management systems must be based at the state ministries of the health and linked to healthcare education institutions. It must be integrated with the service delivery points, including the private sector, ports, and the professional regulatory bodies' registrar's computer system to ensure accurate tracking of the country's number of HCPs. Such a tracking system will facilitate health workforce planning.

In 2014, the number of physicians in Nigeria was estimated at 66,555, but the number currently employed is about 35% of the official number because the data have not been updated since 1963 (UK Home Office, 2018). As a best practice, the register of the professional regulatory bodies should be updated quarterly to capture exits from the country, retirements, and deaths of HCPs.

Migration abroad is one of the primary causes of HCPs shortage in the country. For example, Nigerian universities have produced 4748 bachelor's degree-prepared physiotherapists since the University of Ibadan first established a degree program in 1976 (Balogun et al., 2016a). Sadly, only 1000 of them are currently gainfully employed in the country (Okoghenun, 2015). The remaining 3748 physiotherapists have migrated to other countries due to unsatisfactory service conditions at home and because the federal and state governments do not create positions annually to employ new graduates. For example, in a 750-bed hospital where 70 physiotherapists are needed, only six are employed (Okoghenun, 2015). Here again, Nigeria universities are training physiotherapists for export to other countries when they are acutely in demand at home. The poor are the one suffering the HCPs shortage because the elites and politicians can afford to travel abroad for their medical rehabilitation. The private and public educational sectors must expand the number of students enrolled in the existing healthcare academic programs to meet the shortage of HCPs in the country.

Improve Work Conditions

A physician in the United States works, on average, 51 hours a week and on the average consults with 20 patients a day. Almost a quarter of the physician's time is spent on non-clinical and frustrating paperwork (Weber, 2019; Elflein, 2019). In

Nigeria, physicians attend to 100–150 per day, and it is common for physicians to be on call for up to 4 days working continuously (Ogundipe et al., 2015). Patients with chronic diseases (cancer, kidney failure, diabetes, asthma, stroke, and coronary heart disease) have problems accessing consultants. The shortage of HCPs contributes to many patients' deaths, low quality of patient care, low staff morale and retention, patient satisfaction, weaker practice standards, and loss of confidence in the health system. The high workload (patient to HCP ratio) is partly responsible for the frustration, stress, job burnout, poor attitude to work, workplace incivility, and higher staff turnover (Ogundipe et al., 2015). Consistent with practice in high-income countries, the federal government should abolish the forced retirement of HCPs and university lecturers based on an arbitrary age of 65 and 70 years, respectively (University World News, 2010). Continued employment should be based on performance and not age. Employees who demonstrate dedication, commitment, and exemplary performance should be incentivized to keep their appointment, especially in disciplines that the nation faces an acute shortage of personnel. University lecturers and HCPs should be allowed to continue to work as long as they can effectively perform their roles and responsibilities. The university system should annually evaluate professors in the three assessment domains—teaching, research, and service—and continue to retain those with satisfactory performance.

A survey of the senior management staff of health institutions conducted by NOIPolls in 2017 revealed massive discrepancies in the remuneration of HCPs on the same grade levels across the federal, state, and local governments. Poor service conditions, including low salaries and benefits, are the primary source of conflict between management and employees, often leading to industrial strikes (Oleribe, 2016; 2018; Adeloye et al., 2017). One of the common assertions often made without empirical evidence by medical and health professional associations and unions is that HCPs in the country are poorly paid compared to their counterparts worldwide. This author investigated this claim by obtaining salary data from the National Salaries, Income, and Wages Commission (2019) and employment and labor websites in the United States and the United Kingdom. The author obtained the salaries for consultant and resident physicians and dentists and entry-level wages for the other HCPs to compare the United Kingdom and United States data—the two preferred destinations for Nigerian HCPs. The data presented in Table 13.2 corroborates the speculation that Nigerian HCPs' salaries are dismal compared to their counterparts in the United Kingdom and the United States. For example, consultant physicians in the United States earn about ten times more than their counterparts in Nigeria and twice their peers in the United Kingdom. The salary differentials between the United States and Nigeria are even higher for some of the other health professions.

The cost of living and inflation, including the income tax rate, significantly influence workers' net pay in any country. These determinants of the workers' take-home pay vary widely across the globe. For example, in the United States, high-income HCPs are taxed between 15% and 33% of the gross pay. In the United Kingdom, the HCPs' income tax rate ranges from 0% to 45% based on income and region (Gov.UK, n.d.). In Nigeria, tax rates are scaled across income bands, ranging from 7% to 24% (Activpayroll Ltd., 2020). In South Korea, foreign nationals are

Table 13.2 Entry-level salary for primary healthcare professions in Nigeria, the United States, and the United Kingdom

Serial #	Profession	Nigeria (₦) (US$ equivalent)[a]	United States ($)[c]	United Kingdom [c] (£) (US$ equivalent)
	Physicians (Residents)	2,340,000-2,640,000 ($6047-6822)	62,297	37,191 (46,861)
1	Physicians (Consultants)	7,200,000 – 9,000,000 ($18,605-23,256)	203,450	77,913–105,042 ($98,170-132,352)
	Dentists (Residents)	2,160,000-3,360,000 ($5581-8682)	44,939	38,693 (48,753)
2	Dentists (Consultants)	7,200,000 – 9,000,000 ($18,605-23,256)	178,260	50,000–110,000 ($63,000–138,600) 79,860–107,668 ($100,624- 135,662)
3	Social worker	1,080,000-1,440,000 ($2791-3721)	50,470	47,243 ($59,526)
4	Dietician	1,320,000-1,800,000 ($3411-4652)	62,330	44,641 ($56,248)
5	Veterinarian	1,920,000-2,520,000 ($4961-6512)	104,820	40,000 ($50,400)
6	Clinical psychologists	1,980,000 ($5116)	80,370	37,570 ($47,338)
7	Pharmacists	1,980,000 – 3,600,000 ($5116-9302)	125,570	36,040 ($45,410)
8	Public environmental officer[d]	540,000-1,440,000 ($1395-3721)	71,360	33,015 ($41,599)
9	Optometrists	1,440,000-2,160,000 (3721–5581)	122,980	31,365 ($39,520)
10	Radiologic technologists/ Radiographers	1,860,000 ($4896)	63,120	31,228 ($39,347)
11	Public analysts	Not available	Not available	30,486 ($38,412)
12	Dental therapists	1,440,000 -2,160,000 ($3721–5581)	77,230	30,401 ($38,305)
13	Biomechanical engineers	1,080,000 -1,440,000 ($2791-3721)	91,410	28,558 ($35,983)
14	Physiotherapists	1,920,000-2,220,000 ($4961–5736)	90,170	28,293 ($35,649)
15	Occupational therapists	1,620,000 – 1,980,000 ($4186-5116)	86,210	27,860 ($35,104)
16	Audiologists	1,440,000 -2,160,000 ($3721–5581)	83,900	27,374 ($34,491)
17	Speech therapists	1,440,000 -2,160,000 ($3721–5581)	82,000	25,766 ($32,465)
18	Nurses	960,000 – 1,800,000 ($2480-4651)	77,460	24,969 ($31,461)
19	Prosthetist and Orthotists	1,200,000-1,680,000 ($3101-4341)	68,410	24,214 ($30,510)

Table 13.2 (continued)

Serial #	Profession	Nigeria (₦) (US$ equivalent)[a]	United States ($)[c]	United Kingdom[c] (£) (US$ equivalent)
20	Dieticians/Nutritionists	1,440,000-2,160,000 ($3721–5581)	62,330	24,020 ($30,265)
21	Medical lab. Technologists	1,860,000-2,160,000 ($4806-5581)	54,780	23,086 ($29,088)
22	Dispensing opticians	1,620,000-1,680,000($4186 -4341)	57,840	22,271 ($28,061)
23	Medical record clerk/ officers	1,044,000-1,500,000 ($2698-3876)	40,500	17,901 ($22,555)

aNational Salaries, Income and Wages Commission (2019). Consolidated health salary scale and consolidated medical salary scale circular. The Presidency, Federal Republic of Nigeria. Bureau of Labor and Statistics, 2018

bhttps://www.bls.gov/oes/current/oes_nat.htm#29-0000
https://www.bls.gov/ooh/healthcare/
https://www.payscale.com/research/US/Job
https://www.glassdoor.com/Salaries/resident-physician-salary-SRCH_KO0,18.htm
chttps://www.payscale.com/research/UK/Job
https://www.imgconnect.co.uk/news/2019/06/nhs-doctors-pay-scales-in-the-uk-explained/59#Typical%20NHS%20doctor%20salary%20in%20the%20UK
https://www.prospects.ac.uk/job-profiles/dentist#salary
https://www.healthcareers.nhs.uk/explore-roles/dental-team/roles-dental-team/dentist/pay-dentists

dThe wide range in salary is because some states are only able to implement a percentage of the recommended salary and environmental officers are mainly employed by the states

Exchange rate as of August 5, 2020: 1£ = 1.26 dollar; 387₦ = 1 dollars; 1$ = 0.80 British pound; 1$ = ₦387

The Nigerian currency against the United States dollar and the British pound is on a free fall in the world market. In the 1970s, the Naira and dollar were at par. The Nigerian currency devaluation started during the structural adjustment program implemented against the Nigerian people's wish in the late 1980s by General Ibrahim Babangida. The successive governments were unable to stabilize the currency, and the devaluation continues up till today

taxed at 20.9%, made up of 19% income tax, and 1.9% local income tax. The tax rate for Korean citizens varies from 6% to 38% (Expat.com, 2020), and in Singapore, it ranges from 0% to 20%. The tax collection system in communist Cuba is unsophisticated, and there is no personal income tax, no corporate tax, no value-added tax, and no sales tax. The tax system in Cuba discourages economic and job growth (Dominguez, 2015). It is plausible that the take-home pay of the HCPs in the United States may not be substantially different from the payment in the other countries after adjusting for the high federal, state, and municipal taxes and the high cost of living and education in the United States.

It is disconcerting that the HCPs are leaving the country to work abroad in large numbers. As of 2017, 51% of sub-Saharan African migrants in the United States were from Nigeria, Ethiopia, Ghana, and Kenya. There were 1.24 million Nigerians in the Diaspora in the same year (Pew Research Center, 2018; Nevin & Omosomi, 2019). The economic implications of the brain drain phenomenon are grave. For example, the cost of training physicians in the United Kingdom is about £269,527 for entry-level physicians and £564,112 for consultants. To train a physician in Nigeria, the government subsidizes the education up to N3,860,100. The countries that African physicians emigrate save a windfall. They save at least $621 million in Australia, $384 million in Canada, $2.7 billion in the United Kingdom, and $846 million in the United States, culminating to $4.55 billion. The United Kingdom had the highest number of African physicians and the most considerable savings (NOIPolls, 2017).

One of the typical pronouncements often made without empirical evidence by the Medical and Dental Consultants' Association of Nigeria (MDCAN) and Joint Health Sector Unions (JOHESU) is that their members earn lower wages than their counterparts worldwide (Alubo & Hunduh, 2017; Adinoyi, 2021). This claim has not been investigated previously. This chapter investigated this assertion by obtaining salary information for HCPs in Nigeria, Ghana, South Africa, United States, and the United Kingdom. For comparative purposes, the findings are summarized in Table 13.2.

The data revealed that consultant physicians in the United States earn about ten times more than their counterparts in Nigeria and twice their peers in the United Kingdom. The salary differentials between the United States and Nigeria are generally higher for the other health professions. The data also corroborates the speculation that Nigerian HCPs earn substantially lower—three to five times—than their counterparts in South Africa. Surprisingly, the wages in Ghana and Nigeria are comparable. The insecurity and chaos in everyday life, including the pervasive closure of schools and universities, are probably why Nigerians seek employment in Ghana and not for the financial reward (Adinoyi, 2021). The federal government must address the intractable security concerns and improve the welfare and conditions of service of HCPs to prevent the ongoing migration of Nigerians abroad.

Perhaps, it is not fair to compare Nigeria's salaries with high-income countries like the United States and the United Kingdom because of the high cost of living in developed nations. For example, physicians in the United States amass thousands of loans to pay for their medical education. Typically, a physician in the United States, on average, owes about $132,860 for 4 years of undergraduate education (Times Higher Education, 2020) and $150,224 to $248,776 for 4 years of medical education at public universities, and $242,660 to $248,444 at private institutions (Shemmassian Academic Consulting, 2019). Medical students in the United States often take 5–10 years' post-graduation to pay back their loans in full. On the other hand, the medical and dental education in Nigerian public institutions is subsidized heavily by the federal and state governments. The average educational debt following graduation does not exceed N357,900 ($2587). Some critics raised the question that if federal and state governments pay for the physicians' education in Nigeria, is it fair for them to earn the same as their peers in the United States? (NOIPolls, 2017) That said, this author believes that HCPs in the country deserve better wages than they currently earn.

With improved service conditions for HCPs in Nigeria, the brain drain phenomenon will be reduced substantially (Khan 2010, Adinoyi, 2021). Offering competitive compensation based on credentials will incentivize Nigerians in the Diaspora to return to their homeland and contribute to national development. Employers must also at least once annually provide continuing education opportunities for HCPs to acquire new knowledge and hone their clinical skills. Furthermore, the tertiary hospitals in the country should ramp up their research infrastructures and offer grant incentives to support faculty engaged in transformative research.

Foster Partnership with Nigerian Healthcare Professionals in the Diaspora

It is commendable that President Buhari's administration, in 2019, created the Diaspora Unit within the FMH to, among other things, coordinate and facilitate the activities of Nigerian HCPs in the Diaspora, develop programs that would enable HCPs in the Diaspora to transfer technical expertise, and keep track of Nigerian HCPs in the Diaspora and their activities in Nigeria (FMH, 2020). Sadly, three years after the FMH set these lofty goals in motion, no tangible progress has been made.

Also in 2019, Buhari's administration established the Nigerians in the Diaspora Commission (NIDCOM) to engage Nigerians abroad by making business and communication easy and to utilize Nigerians' human capital and material resources in the Diaspora toward Nigeria's overall socioeconomic, cultural, and political development (Dabiri-Erewa, 2019). Despite creating the NIDCOM and the Diaspora Unit within the FMH, there is still grave miscommunication between the government and professional organizations abroad. For example, the Nigerian Medical Association based in the United States, the United Kingdom, Germany, Canada, and South Africa, in 2020, accused the FMH of frustrating its efforts to improve health care in the country. The association alleged that they worked on a health initiative program designed to share their peers' skills for three years. The association's team planned to send 27 physicians and nurses in oncology, neurology, nephrology, and ophthalmology who had bought tickets and volunteered their time. Two weeks before the scheduled date, the health minister informed them that the project had been "suspended till further notice." The minister's communiqué did not state the reason for his decision (Owolabi, 2020). Mishandling of unique partnership opportunities like this, which is quite common, is disconcerting because of the acute shortage of HCPs and the significant expertise that the Diaspora HCPs can bring to the country. The ability of the FMH Diaspora unit in creating meaningful collaboration with organizations abroad remains to be seen.

It is an oxymoron to note that a crisis-free country will prevent many Nigerian HCPs from leaving their motherland (Omonijo et al., 2011). With adequate security and appropriate resources made available in the universities and the UTHs, most Nigerians in the Diaspora would relocate back home to contribute to national development (Balogun, 2020). They are also willing to collaborate with their colleagues and contribute to the health system's development. The Diaspora Unit within the FMH and the National Universities Commission (NUC) are well-positioned to facilitate such partnerships. The collaborations can foster innovative research in the various healthcare disciplines and drastically reduce the cases and astronomical cost of medical tourism in the country.

Promote the Production of Locally Produced Medical Equipment and Pharmaceuticals

The primary medical equipment and pharmaceutical products used in the health system are imported into the country at astronomical prices. The pharmaceutical sector is flooded with mixed and adulterated appurtenances because the National Agency for Food and Drug Administration and Control operation is weak and lacked the regulatory authority or willpower to act decisively. The agency rarely imposes fines and sanctions on errant vendors. The agency's internal controls need to be strengthened to prevent the importation and distribution of fake drugs.

The spending on medical equipment and pharmaceutical paraphernalia imported to the country contributes to the high cost of healthcare delivery. In 2013, the medical equipment market was $154 million and soared to $227 million in 2018. Foreign-owned companies such as Siemens (German) and General Electric (American) dominates the medical equipment market in the country (Orekunrin, 2015).

The advanced diagnostic and therapeutic medical equipment in the tertiary hospitals are dilapidated. Tragically, the hospitals lack technical experts to service the medical equipment. With every significant equipment breakdown or even minor glitches, technical personnel from abroad must be flown down by the UTHs' authorities at an astronomical cost to the nation. When the medical equipment is under repair, healthcare services in the affected facilities grind to a halt, and many patients die in the process.

Successive Nigerian governments have failed to take the manufacturing of medical equipment and pharmaceutical products seriously. There is an urgent need to train biomedical engineers and technologists to service the nation's health facilities' primary equipment. If implemented, this recommendation will conserve money and prevent unnecessary fatalities in the tertiary hospitals where the equipment is used. The NUC should adequately fund the biomedical engineering department in the universities to foster medical equipment development. Examples of locally produced medical equipment are the SureVent transport ventilator and the Embrace infant baby warmer. The SureVent transport ventilator manufactured locally costs only $700, compared to $30,000 for an imported ventilator. The Embrace infant baby warmer, used to keep newborn infants warm for hours, only costs $200, compared to the conventional baby incubator, which costs over $50,000 (Orekunrin, 2015).

In 2016, Michael Baggs, a student at Loughborough University in England, developed an ingenious device (Isobar Cooling Tank) that keeps the temperature of vaccines stable for up to 30 days, even in the blistering heat (Hrala, 2016). For decades, in Nigeria, vaccines worth millions of dollars were denatured in the rural health centers and clinics because the optimum storage temperature was not maintained. Why is this type of low technology not appealing to the country's engineers before now? The biomedical engineering and biomedical technology departments in the universities should use their knowledge to find solutions to domestic healthcare needs without depending solely on foreign vendors.

Ongoing collaboration should be encouraged between the biomedical engineers/ technologists and the HCPs, to pinpoint the medical equipment and pharmaceutical product needs within the healthcare system. The outcome of such collaboration should lead to the local invention of medical equipment and pharmaceutical paraphernalia; that will be a sizeable cost-saving measure within the healthcare system. Most importantly, HCPs should develop a culture of servicing the primary medical equipment periodically before breaking down. The realization of the above recommendations will stem the enormous cost of medical equipment and pharmaceutical products that is currently a significant drain on the already meager healthcare budget.

Invest in Medical Intelligence and Surveillance Systems to Improve Health Information Systems

The capacity of the electric power supply in the country is below 10%. The power supply is generally unreliable and seasonal, with better power availability in the rainy season than in the dry season (Popoola et al., 2011). The epileptic power supply leads to organization losses due to damaged equipment, production downtime, severe injuries, and even death (Awosope, 2014). Although there is a high demand for mobile phones, Nigeria has the largest number of people without Internet access in Africa, with 53% of subscribers lack reliable Wi-Fi connectivity (Menchaca, 2018; AXA.com (2019). Having an effective health information system is problematic without a reliable power supply and Internet connectivity. An effective health information system is critical for providing care in hospitals and instituting measures that promote wellness and prevent disease (Collins, 2015).

The nation's health system is poorly developed and lacks functional medical intelligence and surveillance systems to provide timely information to combat possible public health menace (Obansa & Orimisan, 2012). Adequate medical intelligence and surveillance systems could have averted many of the shortcomings in the healthcare system. Unfortunately, the previous efforts made to address security concerns did not positively affect the health system infrastructures (Welcome, 2011; Obansa & Orimisan, 2012). Because of the impact of ongoing insecurity threats on human health, the federal government should create a Rehabilitation Task Force at the national level to coordinate financial and medical assistance for the victims. The FMH should also develop robust and functional medical intelligence and surveillance systems to prevent, detect, and treat diseases using remote sensors technology. The electronic health records created should be interfaced with mobile technologies to share data online. The platform will provide an array of new healthcare solutions to prevent and treat diseases. The faculty in the Departments of Public Health at the universities must strengthen their curriculum to address the challenges of medical intelligence and surveillance systems (Rahim et al. 1987). The federal government must address the common threats to the healthcare system discussed more comprehensively in Chap. 3 of this book.

The educational curriculum of all health professions should teach students how to competently evaluate patients' state of health by performing age, gender, and culturally relevant screening. Patients with comorbid medical and psychiatric conditions should be referred to specialists for appropriate therapy and supportive services. The public health departments in the country should be funded to develop effective counseling methods and conduct health education campaigns to prevent chronic and emerging diseases.

To quantify health care delivery effectiveness nationally, the FMH should require secondary and tertiary hospitals to systematically monitor the quality of services provided, including the mortality rate of enrollees. The national data will enable each hospital to compare their results with similarly situated hospitals before making any operational changes. The FMH should calculate the economic impact of healthcare delivery and address the commercial distribution of services with an adequate capitation rate and regularly provide performance-based incentives to the hospitals. The FMH and tertiary hospitals should create a robust evidence-based research culture within their organization. Additionally, the federal government should produce an integrated circuit (a smart) card for all citizens. The card will store medical records and fosters efficient clinical documentation and processing of service claims by healthcare providers.

Update the Curricula of Healthcare Education Academic Programs

Despite the well-known critical shortage of healthcare professionals in Nigeria, many new graduates are unemployed. For example, it is estimated that about 40% of physicians trained in Nigeria are unemployed. It takes a year or two after the mandatory National Youth Service Corps program for physicians to get employment (Tyessi, 2019; Daily Trust, 2019). Similarly, it now takes an average of 8–16 months for newly qualified physicians to secure internship training positions. By the time the physicians complete the program, their provisional license has expired, and they conclude the internship without a permit to practice. In addition, many newly qualified physicians pass the primary exam, which qualifies them to start their residency program, but often fail to gain employment in the government recognized hospitals (Abubakar, 2019).

As of 2017, more than 2000 registered physiotherapists in Nigeria are not gainfully unemployed (Shuaibu, 2017). An online investigation conducteed between March 7, 2020, and April 8, 2020, by Egwuenu and Nshi on employment prospects reported that 3317 unemployed nurses responded to the survey. Among the respondents, 95% indicated they were willing to work in the rural community setting, 1% were unwilling to work in the rural environment, and 4% were undecided (Egwuenu & Nshi, 2020). The preponderance of the vacancy positions for HCWs in Nigeria is in private hospitals and they offer lower salaries (Tyessi, 2019; Daily Trust, 2019).

The unemployment of HCPs in Nigeria is "artificial" and not related to need, but the government's inability to fund earmarked vacancies. This situation triggers several unanswered questions and a symptom of a more significant problem due to endemic corruption in public life. This hideous situation is attributed to the systematic neglect due to underfunding of the tertiary hospitals, lack of coordination and planning by the FMH, and failure to implement a consistent health policy by the successive government (Federal Ministry of Health, 2016). Taxpayers' money is presently spent in training HCPs, only for them to be lured away by foreign countries because there is limited training infrastructure for them in the tertiary hospitals, coupled with inadequate incentives and appalling work conditions (Abubakar, 2019).

The NUC and professional regulatory boards should ensure the curricula of healthcare education programs are revised to include entrepreneurship contents. Such a curriculum will provide the graduates with the knowledge and skills on how to develop private practice and not depend on a government job. Furthermore, several scholars have advocated for the healthcare curricula in the Nigerian universities to include contents in management/administration, health economics, leadership, andragogy, and interdisciplinary team healthcare dynamics (Ojo & Akinwumi, 2015; Oleribe et al., 2016, 2017; Alubo & Hunduh, 2017; Balogun, 2017; Balogun, 2020, 2021a, 2021b, 2021c).

In the last decade, the government converted several general hospitals across the country to FMCs to increase tertiary hospitals that offer residency programs. Sadly, the government did not adequately fund the hospitals to hire the personnel needed to train the resident physicians. As a result, the hospitals now have beautiful edifices without the workforce needed to run them (Abubakar, 2019). To solve this myriad of problems would require a well-articulated health policy backed up by adequate funding and the political will to implement the health policy consistently. Furthermore, the government should set a target on the number of residents and house officers each tertiary hospital, FMCs, and other accredited hospitals can employ. Again, this plan should be adequately funds to achieve the target. Selected state-owned general hospitals in the country can be approved to offer joint residency programs in collaboration with the FMCs and tertiary hospitals.

Additionally, carefully selected private hospitals should be accredited by the National Postgraduate Medical College and the West African Postgraduate Medical College to offer postgraduate programs. The utilization of private hospitals will expand postgraduate program opportunities for physicians, improve the quality of health care provided to patients, and curtail the tide of the brain drain phenomenon facing the health sector. Implementing these recommendations will go a long way to decongest the tertiary hospitals where residency programs are offered and alleviate unemployment among HCPs.

Promote Transformative Research to Address Nigeria's Unresolved Developmental Health Challenges

Transformative research by design involves novel, innovative, and creative ideas. The findings can radically change existing knowledge, challenge current understanding, and provide pathways to new frontiers. Transformative discoveries leading to paradigm shifts can occur at scientific, personal, and sociological levels and often change cultural values and society at large (Trevors et al., 2012). Transformative research outcome typically causes controversies because it challenges entrenched assumptions and encompasses the big picture. A transformative research approach is best suited to solve Nigeria's unresolved developmental health challenges aligned with the SDGs. The challenges that are of topmost priority for transformative research include the ubiquitous issue of poverty, food insecurity, infectious diseases, maternal and child health, endemic noncommunicable diseases, gender inequality, energy insufficiency, and climate change (Anonymous, n.d.). To confront these issues, the federal government must address two pertinent questions. First, how can the country ensure that scientists focus on issues that provide solutions to local developmental challenges? Second, how can the findings from transformative inquiry lead to policy and industry collaboration and action? These two critical questions have, over the years, remained an enigma to both scientists and policymakers in the country. Okonofua (2019) poignantly diagnosed the problem by inferring that the preponderance of local research tends to focus on themes that describe a problem's nature rather than those that provide solutions to the developmental challenge.

Development-driven scientific inquiries are multidisciplinary in nature, and expensive since they require state-of-the equipment to implement them. Unfortunately, the Nigerian government has invested limited resources for such research work. For example, the African Union recommends that African countries spend 1% of their GDP on research and development (United Nations. Economic Commission for Africa., 2018). To date, only South Africa, Malawi, and Uganda have reached this goal. Aside from funding, other constraints in implementing innovative research include: (1) the depreciating appreciation for intellectual work, (2) implementation of scientific inquiries for personal career advancement, and (3) insufficient political demand for research findings.

Research productivity and timely dissemination are yardsticks for measuring the level of innovation within a health system. Health research is a global endeavor, and investigators increasingly recognize that their research efforts are enhanced by collaborating with colleagues in other multiple centers and countries and engaging in joint training of HCPs. Unfortunately, the research outputs from sub-Saharan Africa have not matched those from different parts of the world. A study conducted by the World Bank in 2014 revealed that although Africa constitutes 16% of the world's population, it produces only 1% of the global research outputs, with only 198 researchers/one million people in Africa, compared to 455 in Chile and 4500 in the United States and the United Kingdom (World Bank, 2014).

A study commissioned by the World Bank in 2014 estimated that sub-Saharan Africa will require an additional one million PhDs, especially those qualified to conduct cutting-edge research, if the continent meets up to half of the research momentum currently going on in the Western countries. The study also found that all African countries produce about 27,000 research publications annually, equivalent to the total number of papers generated in a small country such as the Netherlands. Three nations (Egypt, Nigeria, and South Africa) accounted for these publications in Africa. Most research publications in Africa now emanate from South Africa, Egypt, Nigeria, Algeria, Kenya, Morocco, and Tunisia. South Africa is the most research-productive country on the continent (World Bank, 2014).

For Nigeria to achieve sustainable support for high-quality research, the federal government must substantially increase research and development allocation to 1% of the GDP as recommended by the African Union. Despite the iteration by the NUC and the Tertiary Education Trust Fund (TETFund, 2020) for transformational research, the call has yet to find substantive support in the universities.

As the most populous country on the Africa continent, with the highest number of universities, Nigeria's research productivity is below par and unacceptable. In the 1970s, Nigerian universities and teaching hospitals significantly surpassed other African nations in human and fiscal resources, and in research productivity, quality and scientific impact. With the increased number of universities, specialist hospitals, and medical research centers in the country, this is no longer the case. The universities can turn around the declining academic standards by focusing on research activities that address local developmental challenges that improve citizens' quality of life. Unfortunately, in some universities, senior academics are promoted to professorial rank with low research output. Such professors are not able to train graduates who can conduct meaningful and impactful research in their discipline. University administrators should prod the government to fund ongoing capacity-building workshops and seminars in research methodology and biostatistics to address the problem.

Innovative intervention research that presents different facets of a given problem should be encouraged by the Nigerian government and funding agencies instead of descriptive studies seeking to identify a specific challenge. Transformational research that links investigators to industry partners and culminating in policy development must take center stage. Nigerian scientists, government health policymakers, and health organizations must use evidence-based research findings emanating from the country rather than those conducted abroad in decision-making to foster universal and high-quality health care. After all, universities, industries, and governments worldwide work together to promote economic and social development—a concept called the triple helix model (Okonofua et al., 2021). The difficulty in meeting this idea is due, in part, to researchers' inability to identify the correct approaches to achieve collaboration with industry partners and policymakers. Without further delay, the NUC should aim to bring scientists, technocrats, and industry partners together in a new collaborative effort that provides interaction starting with the research question's development phase until completion of the inquiry. The universities should take a leadership role in training young investigators in transformational inquiry methods, including strategic communication methods on the social media platform, to disseminate research findings to policymakers and industry audiences.

Expand Access to Essential Medicines and Vaccines

Healthcare institutions in Nigeria lack vital resources, including vaccines, medicines, and state-of-the-art equipment. Another critically needed healthcare reform is expanding access to essential drugs and vaccines necessary to keep the population in good health. Table 13.3 presents the top ten causes of death in Nigeria (US CDC, 2019), along with the medications and relevant modalities used to treat each condition.

The public hospitals can use the information presented in Table 13.3 to prioritize the drugs to procure. Within the next three years, the federal government, with private partnerships, should explore the production of these medications in the country.

Table 13.3 The top ten causes of death in Nigeria and the common medications and other modalities used for treatment

Ranking	Causes of death (US CDC, 2019)	Common medications and other modalities used to treat condition (WHO, 2019)	Source of information
1	Lower respiratory infections	β-lactams, fluoroquinolones, and gentamicin	Egbe et al. (2011)
2	Neonatal disorders	Preterm or low birthweight, of which 80% die within the first 7 day	Amadi and Kawuwa, (2017)
		Neonatal jaundice: phototherapy and exchange transfusion, A novel, low-cost canopy, medicinal plants, herbal concoctions, black soap, and water extract of unripe pawpaw	Olusanya et al. (2016)
		Neonatal sepsis: cefuroxime, cefepime, ceftriaxone, ofloxacin, and gentamicin	
		Neonatal mortality: neonates delivered by cesarean section had a higher relative risk of neonatal mortality compared with vaginal deliveries	Arowosegbe et al. (2017); Ezeh et al. (2014)
3	HIV/AIDS	Pre-exposure prophylaxis, or PrEP; *Truvada*	Adepoju (2020)
4	Malaria	Artemisinin combination therapy, artesunate, chloroquine and brands of sulphadoxine-pyrimethamine— – malareich, fansidar, maloxine	Uzochukwu et al. (2018)
5	Diarrheal diseases	Oral rehydration solution (ORS), intravenous fluids, ciprofloxacin, metronidazole, gentamicin	Efunshile et al. (2019)
		Oral rehydration solution (ORS), salt sugar solution (SSS), metronidazole, kaolin, tetracycline	Aguwa et al. (2010)
6	Tuberculosis	Rifampicin, isoniazid, pyrazinamide, and ethambutol	Oladimeji et al. (2021)
		Rifampicin, isoniazid, ethambutol, streptomycin	Otu et al. (2013)
7	Meningitis	Meningococcal vaccines, polysaccharide vaccines, serogroup C plain polysaccharide vaccines, conjugate vaccines, mass immunization with polysaccharide conjugate vaccines	Balarabe (2018)
		Antimicrobial chemoprophylaxis	
		Prophylactic drugs— – rifampicin, ciprofloxacin, ceftriaxone	
		Pediatric vaccinations: H. influenzae type b (Hib), meningococcal A conjugate vaccine (MenAfriVac), 10-valent pneumococcal conjugate vaccine (PCV10)	Tagbo et al. (2019)

Table 13.3 (continued)

Ranking	Causes of death (US CDC, 2019)	Common medications and other modalities used to treat condition (WHO, 2019)	Source of information
8	Ischemic heart disease	The typical causes of congestive cardiac failure (CCF) were hypertension (56.3%) and cardiomyopathy (12.3%). Chronic renal failure, rheumatic heart disease, and ischemic heart disease accounted for 7.8%, 4.3%, and 0.2% of CCF, respectively. The burden of CCF is mainly due to hypertension. Efforts should be geared toward prevention (hypertension awareness), detection, and treatment	Onwuchekwa and Asekomeh (2009)
		Antithrombotic agents (streptokinase), cardiac glycosides (Digoxin), antiarrhythmics, class I and class III (lidocaine, amiodarone), cardiac stimulants excluding cardiac glycosides (dopamine, epinephrine), vasodilators used in cardiac diseases (glyceryl trinitrate, isosorbide dinitrate), antiadrenergic agents, centrally acting (m,ethyldopa), arteriolar smooth muscle agents (hydralazine), low-ceiling diuretics (hydrochlorothiazide), (high-ceiling diuretics (furosemide, mannitol), potassium-sparing agents (spironolactone)	Wirtz et al. (2016)
9	Stroke	Diagnosis, pharmacotherapy, rehabilitation— – modification of risk factors. Effective treatment of hypertension, control of blood sugar, treatment of hyperlipidemia, and exercise	Ogungbo et al. (2005)
		Population strategy— – lifestyle modification— – reduction of salt in food and drink, management of hypertension; diabetes is a modifiable risk factor for stroke; management of atrial fibrillation; treatment of hyperlipidemia with statins is essential; treatment of transient ischemic attacks; carotid endarterectomy is a safe preventive procedure; thrombolytic therapy	
		Hypertension, hyperlipidemia, diabetes, and atrial fibrillation were prevalent among 83.7%, 26.5%, 25.6%, and 9.6% of patients with stroke, respectively	Alkali et al. (2016)
		The following list of medications is used in the treatment of stroke: Clopidogrel, Plavix, Aspirin, Bayer Aspirin, Aspir 81, Ecotrin, Alteplase, Activase	Drugs.com. (2020)
10	Cirrhosis	Conventional treatment involves managing symptoms and addressing complications of the disease— – procedures and medications to treat the viral hepatitis infection, control hypertension, and help reduce the build-up of toxins in the blood. A liver transplant remains the last resort "curative" treatment for liver damage and is not feasible in Nigeria	Keeney (2019)

Conclusion

Previous national healthcare policies on UHC were unsuccessful because the governments implemented their plans in isolation without addressing the underlying political and economic factors described in Chap. 12. Other countries' experiences revealed that it is difficult in a large informal sector economy like Nigeria to achieve UHC from contributory insurance schemes. Funding UHC will need a combination of federal funding at 15% of the GDP, supplemented by tax-based financing by the formal sector workers (at 15% of their salary collected through payroll deduction), private health insurance for the wealthy individuals (at 25% of the annual income), and state-managed social health insurance for the informal sector workers. The federal government should provide free health care to every child, Nigerian older than 65 years of age, persons with life-threatening chronic diseases including people living with disabilities, and workers who earn below the poverty line—less than ₦137,400 ($361) assets.

To increase the revenue stream for the NHIS, the federal and state governments should expand job opportunities for the unemployed and provide a job-training program for the youth. Failure to address extreme poverty is why previous healthcare reforms came up bootless. A citizen in search of the next meal will not be interested in purchasing health insurance coverage. For any impactful change to occur in the health sector, Nigerians must vote for the political party that campaigns on health care as the number one priority in their manifesto. Most importantly, the country must elect visionary and ethical leaders who have the country's interest at heart and usher in the long-anticipated UHC by 2030.

Case Study

The official website of the Federal Ministry of Health (FMH), when accessed on June 10, 2020, using a computer with an anti-virus protection software, provided a red screen indicating "dangerous webpage blocked" from navigation. Also, when the website was again accessed on July 16, 2021, the following response was obtained: "its security certificate expired 76 days ago. This may be caused by a misconfiguration or an attacker intercepting your connection." These blunders are concerning and embarrassing to the nation.

1. Discuss the impact of this incident on the image and influence of Nigeria at a global level.
2. What department/unit within the FMH should be held responsible for this aberrant situation?
3. What should be done to prevent this situation from happening in the future?

References

Abdullahi, S. A. (2019). Three things Nigeria must do to end extreme poverty. *The world economic forum COVID action platform.* [online]. Available at: https://www.weforum.org/agenda/2019/03/90-million-nigerians-live-in-extreme-poverty-here-are-3-ways-to-bring-them-out/. Accessed 22 Dec 2020.

Abubakar, S. A. (2019). *Unemployment among medical doctors.* [online]. Available at: http://www.gamji.com/article4000/NEWS4395.htm. Accessed 7 Jun 2021.

Activpayroll Ltd. (2020). *Nigeria payroll and tax: Overview.* [online]. Available at: htts://www.activpayroll.com/global-insights/nigeria. Accessed 10 Oct 2020.

Adebisi, Y. A., Umah, J. O., Olaoye, O. C., Alaran, A. J., Sina-Odunsi, A. B., et al. (2020). Assessment of health budgetary allocation and expenditure toward achieving universal health coverage in Nigeria. *International Journal of Health Life Science*; [online]. Available at: https://sites.kowsarpub.com/ijhls/articles/102552.html. Accessed 24 May 2021.

Adegoke, Y. (2019). Does Nigeria have too many doctors to worry about a 'brain drain'? *BBC* Africa, Lagos. April 25. [online]. Available at: https://www.bbc.com/news/world-africa-45473036. Accessed 16 Oct 2020.

Adeloye, D., David, R. A., Olaogun, A. A., Auta, A., Adesokan, A., Gadanya, M., Opele, J. K., Owagbemi, O., & Iseolorunkanmi, A. (2017). Health workforce and governance: the crisis in Nigeria. Human Resources for Health;15:32. [online]. Available at: https://human-resources-health.biomedcentral.com/articles/10.1186/s12960-017-0205-4#citeas. Accessed 16 Oct 2020.

Adepoju, P. (2020). *A breakdown of Nigeria's 2020 budget for health.* [online]. Available at: http://www.healthnews.ng/a-breakdown-of-nigerias-2020-budget-for-health/. Accessed 24 May 2021.

Adinoyi, S. (2021). *Insecurity, poor remuneration, bane of mass emigration of doctors, says MDCAN.* [online]. Available at: https://www.thisdaylive.com/index.php/2021/02/12/insecurity-poor-remuneration-bane-of-mass-emigration-of-doctors-says-mdcan/. Accessed 23 Jul 2021.

Aikpitanyi, J., Ohenhen, V., Ugbodaga, P., Ojemhen, B., Omo-Omorodion, B. I., Ntoimo, L. F. C., Imongan, W., Balogun, J. A., & Okonofua, F. E. (2019). Maternal death review and surveillance: The case of central Hospital, Benin City, Nigeria. *PLoS One, 19*(12), 14. [online]. Available at: https://www.ncbi.nlm.nih.gov/pmc/articles/PMC6922332/. Accessed 16 Oct 2020.

Ajimotokan, O. (2019). Korea jostles for slice of Nigeria's $1B medical tourism spending. *This Day.* March 21. [online]. Available at: https://www.thisdaylive.com/index.php/2019/03/21/korea-jostles-for-slice-of-nigerias-1b-medical-tourism-spending/. Accessed 16 Oct 2020.

Ajobe, A. T., Alhassan, A., Chung, S., Leonard, J., & Ahmad, R. (2013). Nigeria: How Nigerians spend billions on medical tourism. *Daily Trust.* [online]. Available at: https://allafrica.com/stories/201301071129.html. Accessed 10 Oct 2020.

Akinyele, B., & Otto Abasiekong, O. (2018). #EndPoverty:9 ways Nigeria should address poverty. *Proshare Economy.* [online]. Available at: https://www.proshareng.com/news/Nigeria%20Economy/-EndPoverty-9-Ways-Nigeria-Should-Address%2D%2DPoverty/42284#:~:text=Investment%20in%20infrastructure%20is%20one,activities%20and%20empower%20more%20Nigerians. Accessed 22 Dec 2020.

Alagboso, C. (2020). FMC Ebute Metta is restoring Nigeria's confidence in public health centres March 24, *Nigeria Health Watch.* [online]. Available at: https://nigeriahealthwatch.com/fmc-ebute-metta-is-restoring-nigerias-confidence-in-public-health-centres/#.XyRncyhKg2x. Accessed 16 Oct 2020.

Alkali, N. H., Bwala, S. A., Dunga, J. A., Watila, M. M., Jibrin, Y. B., & Tahir, A. (2016). Prestroke treatment of stroke risk factors: A cross-sectional survey in central Nigeria. *Annals of African Medicine, 15*(3), 120–125. [online]. Available at: https://www.ncbi.nlm.nih.gov/pmc/articles/PMC5402807/. Accessed 28 May 2021.

Aguwa, E. N., Aniebue, P. N., & Obi, I. E. (2010). Management of childhood diarrhea by patent medicine vendors in Enugu north local government area, Southeast Nigeria. *International Journal of Medicine and Medical Sciences, 2*(3), 88–94. [online]. Available at: https://www.shopsplusproject.org/sites/default/files/resources/Nigeria_Aguwa_Managementof DiarrheabyPPMVs_2010.pdf. Accessed 28 May 2021.

Alubo, O., & Hunduh, V. (2017). Medical dominance and resistance in Nigeria's healthcare system. *International Journal of Health Services, 47*(4), 778–794.

Amadi, H. O., & Kawuwa, M. B. (2017) Reducing early neonatal mortality in Nigeria—The solution. *IntechOpen.* [online]. Available at: https://www.intechopen.com/books/selected-topics-in-neonatal-care/reducing-early-neonatal-mortality-in-nigeria-the-solution.   Accessed 28 May 2021.

Amu, H., Dickson, K. S., Kumi-Kyereme, A., & Darteh, E. K. M. (2018). Understanding variations in health insurance coverage in Ghana, Kenya, Nigeria, and Tanzania: Evidence from demographic and health surveys. *PLoS ONE, 13*(8), e0201833. [online]. Available at: https://journals.plos.org/plosone/article?id=10.1371/journal.pone.0201833. Accessed 10 Oct 2020.

Anonymous. (n.d.). *Drought conditions and management strategies in Nigeria.* [online]. Available at   https://www.ais.unwater.org/ais/pluginfile.php/629/mod_page/content/6/Nigeria_EN.pdf. Accessed 28 Dec 2020.

Aregbeshola, B. S., & Khan, S. M. (2018). Predictors of enrolment in the national health insurance scheme among women of reproductive age in Nigeria. *International Journal of Health Policy and Management, 7*(11), 1015–1023. [online]. Available at: https://www.ncbi.nlm.nih.gov/pmc/articles/PMC6326643/. Accessed 10 Oct 2020.

Arowosegbe, A. O., Ojo, D. A., Dedeke, I. O., Shittu, O. B., & Akingbade, O. A. (2017). Neonatal sepsis in a Nigerian tertiary hospital: Clinical features, clinical outcome, aetiology and antibiotic susceptibility pattern. *Southern African Journal of Infectious Diseases, 32*(4), 127–131. [online].   Available   at: https://www.tandfonline.com/doi/citedby/10.1080/23120053.201 7.1335962?scroll=top&needAccess=true. Accessed 28 May 2021.

Asakitikpi, A. E. (2019). *Healthcare coverage and affordability in Nigeria: An alternative model to equitable healthcare delivery.* [online]. Available at: https://www.intechopen.com/books/universal-health-coverage/healthcare-coverage-and-affordability-in-nigeria-an-alternative-model-to-equitable-healthcare-delive. Accessed 16 Oct 2020.

Awosope, A. C. (2014). Nigeria electricity industry: Issues, challenges and solutions. *Public Lecture Series, 3*, 5–9. [online]. Available at: http://eprints.covenantuniversity.edu.ng/9474/1/ Prof%20Awosope%20Public%20Lecture%20%2838th%29.pdf. Accessed 16 Oct 2020.

Awosusi, A., Folaranmi, T., & Yates, R. (2015). *Nigeria's new government and public financing for universal health coverage.* [online]. Available at: https://www.thelancet.com/journals/langlo/article/PIIS2214-109X(15)00088-1/fulltext. Accessed 16 Oct 2020.

AXA.com. (2019). Nigeria: laying the groundwork for safe, quality healthcare. May 24. *AXA Magazine.* [online]. Available at: https://www.axa.com/en/magazine/nigeria-laying-the-groundwork-for-safe-quality-healthcare. Accessed 16 Oct 2020.

Balarabe, S. A. (2018). Epidemics of meningococcal meningitis in Northern Nigeria focus on preventive measures. *Annals of African Medicine, 17*(4), 163–167. [online]. Available at: https://www.ncbi.nlm.nih.gov/pmc/articles/PMC6330781/. Accessed 28 May 2021.

Balogun, J. A. (2017). The case for a paradigm shift in the education of health professionals in Nigeria. *Second distinguished university guest lecture, University of Medical Sciences, Ondo, Nigeria.* [online]. Available at: https://www.researchgate.net/publication/317387397_ The_case_for_a_paradigm_shift_in_the_education_of_healthcare_professionals_in_Nigeria. Accessed 23 Sep 2020.

Balogun, J. A. (2020). Healthcare education in Nigeria: Evolutions and emerging paradigms. *Routledge Publication.* [online]. Available at: https://www.routledge.com/9780367482091. Accessed 10 Feb 2020.

Balogun, J. A. (2021a). *Nigerian healthcare system: Roadmap to universal and high-quality healthcare.* Springer.

Balogun, J. A. (2021b). *Healthcare professionals in contemporary Nigeria: An interdisciplinary analysis*. Palgrave Macmillan.

Balogun, J. A. (2021c). Leadership of healthcare teams, organizations and systems: Implications for curriculum revision in medical education. In F. E. Okonofua, J. A. Balogun, & K. Odunsi (Eds.), *Contemporary obstetrics, and gynecology for developing countries*. Springer.

Basiru, S., Oluyemi, J., Abdulateef, J., & Atolagbe, E. (2018). Medical tourism in Nigeria: Challenges and remedies to healthcare system development. *International Journal of Development and Management Review, 13*(1), 223–238.

Biegon, J. (2020). *19 years ago today, African countries vowed to spend 15% on health*. [online]. Available at: https://africanarguments.org/2020/04/27/19-years-africa-15-health-abuja-declaration/. Accessed 16 Oct 2020.

Brookings.edu. (2017). *The Singapore healthcare system: An overview*. [online]. Available at: https://www.brookings.edu/wp-content/uploads/2016/07/affordableexcellence_chapter.pdf. Accessed 16 Oct 2020.

Bunashe, J., & Broder, L. (2015). *How leaders can best manage conflict within their teams*. [online]. Available at: https://www.entrepreneur.com/article/247275. Accessed 16 Oct 2020.

Collins, F. S. (2015). *Growing importance of health in the economy*. [online]. Available at: http://widgets.weforum.org/outlook15/10.html. Accessed 16 Oct 2020.

Cool Geography. (2015). *How economic development is improving the quality of life for the population*. [online]. Available at: http://www.coolgeography.co.uk/gcsen/EW_Nigeria_Quality_of_Life.php. Accessed 16 Oct 2020.

Dabiri-Erewa. (2019). A keynote speech by Hon. Abike Dabiri-Erewa, Chairman/CEO, Nigerians in the Diaspora Commission (NIDCOM) during the Maiden migration summit of Journalists International Forum for Migration (JIFORM) held at Merit House, Abuja. Available at: https://jiformalert.org/193/; https://www.vanguardngr.com/2021/05/fg-to-strengthen-ties-with-dias-pora-nigerians-minister/. Accessed 6 July 2021.

Daily Trust. (2019). *Nigeria: 40% of doctors unemployed in Nigeria – NMA*. [online]. Available at: https://allafrica.com/stories/201907190589.html. Accessed 7 Jun 2021.

Delechat, C., & Medinal, L. (2020). What is the informal economy? *International Monetary Fund*. [online]. Available at: https://www.imf.org/external/pubs/ft/fandd/2020/12/what-is-the-informal-economy-basics.htm. Accessed 22 Dec 2020.

Dodson, D. (2017). *What's the best leadership style for healthcare?* [online]. Available at: https://nchica.org/whats-the-best-leadership-style-for-healthcare/. Accessed 16 Oct 2020.

Dominguez, J. I. (2015). What you might not know about the Cuban economy. *Harvard Business Review*. [oneline]. Available at: https://hbr.org/2015/08/what-you-might-not-know-about-the-cuban-economy. Accessed 10 Oct 2020.

Drugs.com. (2020). *Medications for ischemic stroke*. [online]. Available at: https://www.drugs.com/condition/ischemic-stroke.html. Accessed 28 May 2021.

Efunshile, A. M., Ezeanosike, O., Nwangwu, C. C., König, B., Jokelainen, P., & Robertson, L. J. (2019). Apparent overuse of antibiotics in the management of watery diarrhoea in children in Abakaliki, Nigeria. *BMC Infectious Disease, 19*(1), 275. [online]. Available at: https://www.ncbi.nlm.nih.gov/pmc/articles/PMC6429783/. Accessed 28 May 2021.

Egbe, C. A., Ndiokwere, C., & Omoregie, R. (2011). Microbiology of lower respiratory tract infections in benin city, Nigeria. *Malaysia Journal of Medical Sciences, 18*(2), 27–31. https://www.ncbi.nlm.nih.gov/pmc/articles/PMC3216205/. Accessed 28 May 2021.

Egwuenu, & Nshi, G. I. (2020). Nigerian nurses and midwives unemployment survey. *International Journal of Research - Granthaalayah, 8*(6), 92–101. [online]. Available at: https://www.granthaalayahpublication.org/journals-html-galley/13_IJRG20_B06_3439.html. Accessed 7 Jun 2021.

Eke, C. (2020) Healthcare Resource Guide: Nigeria. Export.gov. [online]. Available at: https://2016.export.gov/industry/health/healthcareresourceguide/eg_main_092285.asp. Accessed: 28 Dec 2020.

Elflein, J. (2019). Number of patients U.S. physicians saw per day 2012-2018. Statista. [online]. Available at: https://www.statista.com/statistics/613959/us-physicans-patients-seen-perday/. Accessed: 10 Feb 2020.

Essien, G., & Yakubu, H. (2018). Nigeria launches new national health security plan. *VON*. [online]. Available at: https://www.von.gov.ng/nigeria-launches-new-national-health-security-plan/. Accessed 16 Oct 2020.

Eshemokha, U. (2021). *Prof. Elusoji UBTH surgeon, banned from practicing medicine for life*. [online]. Available at: https://nimedhealth.com.ng/2021/04/08/prof-elusoji-ubth-surgeon-banned-from-practicing-medicine-for-life/. Accessed 24 Apr 2021.

Expat.com. (2020). *The tax system in South Korea*. [online]. Available at: https://www.expat.com/en/guide/asia/south-korea/9639-tax-system-in-south-korea.html. Accessed 10 Oct 2020.

Ezeh, O. K., Agho, K. E., Dibley, M. J., et al. (2014). Determinants of neonatal mortality in Nigeria: Evidence from the 2008 demographic and health survey. *BMC Public Health, 14*, 521. [online]. Available at: https://doi.org/10.1186/1471-2458-14-521. Accessed 28 May 2021.

Global Compact. (2021). *UHC2030's mission is to create a movement for accelerating equitable and sustainable progress towards universal health coverage (UHC)*. [online]. Available at: https://www.uhc2030.org/our-mission/; https://www.uhc2030.org/fileadmin/uploads/uhc2030/Documents/About_UHC2030/mgt_arrangemts___docs/UHC2030_Official_documents/UHC2030_Global_Compact_WEB.pdf. Accessed 27 May 2021.

Hill, C. F., Powers, B. W., Jain, S. H., Bennet, J., Vavasis, A., & Oriol, N. E. (2014). Mobile health clinics in the era of reform. *The American Journal of Managed Care, 20*(3), 261–264. https://www.ajmc.com/view/mobile-health-clinics-in-the-era-of-reform. Accessed 10 Oct 2020.

Farrell, D. (2004). Boost growth by reducing the informal economy. *Asian Wall Street Journal*. [online]. Available at: https://www.mckinsey.com/mgi/overview/in-the-news/boost-growth-by-reducing-the-informal-economy#. Accessed 22 Dec 2020.

Federal Ministry of Health. (2016). *National health policy 2016: Promoting the health of Nigerians to accelerate socio-economic development*. [online]. Available at: https://extranet.who.int/countryplanningcycles/sites/default/files/planning_cycle_repository/nigeria/draft_nigeria_national_health_policy_final_december_fmoh_edited.pdf. Accessed 10 Oct 2020.

Federal Ministry of Health. (2020). *PPP/Diaspora unit*. [online]. Available at: https://www.health.gov.ng/index.php?option=com_content&view=article&id=133&Itemid=498. Accessed 10 Oct 2020.

Ifijeh, M. (2015). Only five percent of Nigerians are covered by health insurance. *This Day Newspaper*. November 12. [online]. Available at: http://allafrica.com/stories/201511121412.html9. Accessed 16 Oct 2020.

Gerisch, M. (n.d.). Health care as a human right. *Human Rights Magazine*; 43, 3: The state of healthcare in the United States. American Bar Association. [online]. Available at: https://www.americanbar.org/groups/crsj/publications/human_rights_magazine_home/the-state-of-healthcare-in-the-united-states/health-care-as-a-human-right/#:~:text=Among%20all%20the%20rights%20to,to%20live%20lives%20of%20dignity. Accessed 22 Dec 2020.

Greek Medicine. (2012). *The Hippocratic oath*. [online]. Available at: https://www.nlm.nih.gov/hmd/greek/greek_oath.html. Accessed 23 Sept 2020.

Global Health Workforce Alliance WHO. (n.d.). [online]. Available at: https://www.who.int/workforcealliance/countries/nga/en/. Accessed 10 Oct 2020.

Gluck, M. (2012). *How to stop population growth #Rural development*. [online]. Available at: https://www.eoi.es/blogs/marieglueck/2012/02/15/how-to-stop-population-growth-rural-development/. Accessed 10 Oct 2020.

Gov.UK. (n.d.). *Income tax rates and personal allowances in the UK*. [online]. Available at: https://www.gov.uk/income-tax-rates. Accessed 10 Oct 2020.

Hrala, J. (2016). *This new "refrigerator backpack" could help transport vaccines to remote areas. This could change countless lives*. [online]. Available at: http://www.sciencealert.com/this-refrigerator-backpack-could-help-us-transport-vaccines. Accessed 16 Oct 2020. https://web.archive.org/web/20130603030344/http://www.mdcnigeria.org/. Accessed 10 Feb 2020.

Hunja, J. (2015). *Here are 10 ways to fight corruption*. [online]. Available at: https://blogs.worldbank.org/governance/here-are-10-ways-fight-corruption. Accessed 22 Dec 2020.

Ibenegbu, G. (2018). *What are the problems facing healthcare management in Nigeria?* [online]. Available at: https://www.legit.ng/1104912-what-the-problems-facing-healthcare-management-nigeria.html. Accessed 10 Oct 2020.

Ihekweazu, C. (2015). Three reasons strike will continue in Nigeria's health sector. *Nigeria Healthwatch*. September 1, [online]. Available at: https://nigeriahealthwatch.com/three-reasons-strikes-will-continue-in-nigerias-health-sector/#.XxeOd8LCGuU. Accessed 23 Sept 2020.

International Medical Travel Journal. (2014). Nigeria spends $1 billion on outbound medical tourism. *International Medical Travel Journal*. May 22. [online]. Available at: https://www.imtj.com/news/nigeria-spends-1-billion-outbound-medical-tourism/. Accessed 16 Oct 2020.

Indiana University. (2020). *Progressive discipline*. [online]. Available at: https://hr.iu.edu/training/ca/progressive.html. Accessed 26 Dec 2020.

Joseph Rehabilitation Center. (2020). *Community housing services for persons with disabilities*. [online]. Available at: http://www.josephrehabilitationcenter.com/. Accessed 10 Oct 2020.

Julius. (2017). *Nigeria healthcare system: The good and the bad*. [online]. Available at: http://www.visitnigeria.com.ng/nigeria-healthcare-system-the-good-and-the-bad/. Accessed 16 Oct 2020.

Keeney, TA. (2019). Liver cirrhosis in Nigeria; Causes, treatment and natural remedies. *Businessday*. [online]. Available at: https://businessday.ng/health/article/liver-cirrhosis-in-nigeria-causes-treatment-and-natural-remedies/. Accessed 28 May 2021.

Khan, A. A. (2010). How to stop brain drain. *Dawn Newspaper*, October 28. [online]. Available at: https://www.dawn.com/news/875799/how-to-stop-brain-drain. Accessed 16 Oct 2020.

Kwon, S., Lee, T., & Cy, K. (2015). *Republic of Korea health system review*. 5 (4). Manila: World Health Organization, Regional Office for the Western Pacific. [online]. Available at: http://www.searo.who.int/entity/asia_pacific_observatory/publications/hits/hit_korea/en/. Accessed 10 Oct 2020.

Mahbubani, K. (2017). Why Singapore is the world's most successful society? *HuffPost News*. [online]. Available at. https://www.huffpost.com/entry/singapore-world-successful-society_b_7934988?guccounter=1&guce_referrer=aHR0cHM6Ly9zZWFFyY2gueWFob28uY29tLw&guce_referrer_sig=AQAAAE2KEzZpH971iTgZdgTSbbhg2TkNYtNuUd_egYpkGSqax0lZV__K07RX0vv-ivlAixk2LafIf78rhsQhih9RZRx_WBHzgbjngb5g7pCamYU8LmrAkyMvZbUsvtvOdzqqduL_Y44oPotIxArYqMuvbwezfNT552B1tnPkP_JeauPg. Accessed 26 Apr 2020.

Makinde, O. A. (2016). Physicians as medical tourism facilitators in Nigeria: Ethical issues of the practice. *Croatian Medical Journal, 57*(6), 601–604. [online]. Available at: https://www.researchgate.net/publication/312147016_Physicians_as_medical_tourism_facilitators_in_Nigeria_Ethical_issues_of_the_practice. Accessed 10 Oct 2020.

Malone, N. C., Williams, M. M., Smith Fawzi, M. C., et al. (2020). Mobile health clinics in the United States. *International Journal of Equity Health, 19*, –40. [online]. Available at: https://equityhealthj.biomedcentral.com/articles/10.1186/s12939-020-1135-7. Accessed 10 Oct 2020.

Menchaca, W. (2018). Crossroads: Top 10 facts about living conditions in Nigeria. September 23. *The Borgen Project*. [online]. Available at: https://borgenproject.org/cr. Accessed 16 Oct 2020.

Muhammad, F., Abdulkareem, J. H., & Alauddin Chowdhury, A. (2017). Major public health problems in Nigeria: A review. *Southeast Asia Journal of Public Health, 7*(1), 6–11.

Nevin, A. S., & Omosomi, O. (2019). Strength from abroad: The economic power of Nigeria's diaspora. *PricewaterhouseCoopers Limited*. [online]. Available at: https://www.pwc.com/ng/en/pdf/the-economic-power-of-nigerias-diaspora.pdf. Accessed 16 Oct 2020.

NOIPolls. (2017). *Emigration of Nigerian medical doctors: Survey report*. [online]. Available at: https://noi-polls.com/2018/wp-content/uploads/2019/06/Emigration-of-Doctors-Press-Release-July-2018-Survey-Report.pdf. Accessed 10 Oct 2020.

Nwokoma, N., & Ekeanyanwu, O. (2021). A third of Nigerians are unemployed: Here's why. *The Conversation US, Inc*. [online]. Available at: https://theconversation.com/a-third-of-nigerians-are-unemployed-heres-why-159262. Accessed 15 Jun 2021.

Obansa, S. A. J., & Orimisan, A. (2012). *Healthcare financing in Nigeria: Prospects and challenges*. [online]. Available at: https://www.researchgate.net/publication/283609489_Health_care_financing_in_Nigeria_Prospects_and_challenges. Accessed 10 Oct 2020.

Obinne, C. P. O. (1999). *The family economic advancement programme in Nigeria: A rural development approach*. Community Development Journal. Oxford University Press. 34(3), 252–254. [online]. Available at: https://www.jstor.org/stable/44257485.

OECD. (2002). *Nigeria*. [online]. Available at: https://www.oecd.org/countries/nigeria/1826208. pdf. Accessed 16 Oct 2020.

Ogbaa, M. (2017). *A Nigerian story: How healthcare is the offspring of imperialism and corruption*. [online]. Available at: https://www.theelephant.info/features/2017/11/16/a-nigerian-story-how-healthcare-is-the-offspring-of-imperialism-and-corruption/. Accessed 10 Oct 2020.

Ogbebo, W. (2015). *The many problems of Nigeria's health sector*. [online]. Available at: https://infoguidenigeria.com/problems-of-nigeria-health-sector-and-possible-solutions/. Accessed 10 Oct 2020.

Ogunbekun, I., Ogunbekun, A., & Orobaton, N. (1999). Private health care in Nigeria: Walking the tightrope. *Health Policy and Planning, 14*(2), 174–181.

Ogundipe, S., Obinna, C., & Olawale, G. (2015). Shortage of medical personnel: Tougher times ahead for Nigerians. 27 January. *Vanguard*. [online]. Available at: https://www.vanguardngr.com/2015/01/shortage-medical-personnel-tougher-times-ahead-nigerians-1/. Accessed 16 Oct 2020.

Ogungbo, B., Ogun, S. A., Ushewokunze, S., et al. (2005). How can we improve the management of stroke in Nigeria, Africa? *African Journal of Neurological Sciences, 24*(2). [online]. Available at: https://ajns.paans.org/how-can-we-improve-the-management-of-stroke-in-nigeria-africa/. Accessed 28 May 2021.

Ojo, T. O., & Akinwumi, A. F. (2015). Doctors as managers of healthcare resources in Nigeria: Evolving roles and current challenges. *Nigeria Medical Journal, 56*(6), 375–380.

Okonofua, F., Odubanjo, D., & Balogun, J. (2021). Assessing the triple helix model for research and development in sub-Saharan Africa. *The Proceedings of the Nigerian Academy of Science, 13*(2), 1–5. [online]. Available at: https://www.researchgate.net/publication/349194791_Assessing_the_triple_helix_model_for_research_and_development_in_sub-Saharan_Africa. Accessed 27 Apr 2021.

Okonofua, F. (2019). *IFA: A quintessential Nigerian patriot and academic icon*. A keynote address delivered at the commissioning of the Isaac Folorunso Adewole library of tomorrow (IFA-LoT) at the University of Ibadan on Saturday, November 16.

Okoghenun, J. (2015). Nigeria has only 1,000 physiotherapists, say experts. *Guardian Newspaper*. August 10. [online]. Available at: https://guardian.ng/news/nigeria-has-only-1000-physiotherapists-say-experts/. Accessed 3 Jun 2021.

Okpani, A. I., & Abimbola, S. (2015). Operationalizing universal health coverage in Nigeria through social health insurance. *Nigeria Medical Journal, 56*(5), 305–310. [online]. Available at: https://www.ncbi.nlm.nih.gov/pmc/articles/PMC4698843/citedby/. Accessed 27 Dec 2020.

Oladimeji, O., Adepoju, V., Anyiam, F. E., San, J. E., Odugbemi, B. A., Mpotte Hyera, F. L., Sibiya, M. N., et al. (2021). Treatment outcomes of drug susceptible tuberculosis in private health facilities in Lagos, South-West Nigeria. *PLoS One*. [online]. Available at: https://journals.plos.org/plosone/article?id=10.1371/journal.pone.0244581. Accessed 28 May 2021.

Oleribe, O. O., Ezieme, I. P., Oladipo, O., Akinola, E. P., Udofia, D., & Taylor-Robinson, S. D. (2016). Industrial action by HCWs in Nigeria in 2013–2015: An inquiry into causes, consequences and control—a cross-sectional descriptive study. *Human Resource Health, 14*(1), 46. [online]. Available at: https://www.ncbi.nlm.nih.gov/pmc/articles/PMC4962455/. Accessed 23 Sept 2020. Available at: https://pubmed.ncbi.nlm.nih.gov/27465121/. Accessed 16 Oct 2020.

Oleribe, O. O., Udofia, D., Oladipo, O., Ishola, T. A., Taylor-Robinson, S. D., Omisore, A. G., Adesoji, R. O., & Abioye-Kuteyi, E. A. (2017). Interprofessional rivalry in Nigeria's health sector: A comparison of doctors and other health workers' views at a secondary care center. *International Quarterly of Community Health Education*. [online]. Available at: https://doi.org/10.1177/0272684X17748892. Accessed 3 Feb 2020.

Oleribe, O. O., Udofia, D., Oladipo, O., Ishola, TA., Taylor-Robinson, SD. (2018). Healthcare workers' industrial action in Nigeria: A cross-sectional survey of Nigerian physicians. *Hum Resour Health*, 16: 54. [online]. Available at: https://www.ncbi.nlm.nih.gov/pmc/articles/PMC6192190/. Accessed: 16 Oct 2020.

Olusanya, B. O., Osibanjo, F. B., Mabogunje, C. A., Slusher, T. M., & Olowe, S. A. (2016). The burden and management of neonatal jaundice in Nigeria: A scoping review of the literature.

Nigeria Journal of Clinical Practice, 19, 1–17. [online]. Available at: https://www.njcponline. com/text.asp?2016/19/1/1/173703. Accessed 28 May 2021.

Onasanya, A. A. (2020). Increasing health insurance enrolment in the informal economic sector. *Jogh.org*;10 (1). [online]. Available at: http://www.jogh.org/documents/issue202001/jogh-10-010329.pdf. Accessed 29 May 2021.

Onigbinde, O., Samuel, A., Faleye, A., Olaleye, O., Jolayemi, T., Fauziyyah, A., Yusuf, R., & Omokhaye H. (2018). *Policy brief first quarter*. [online]. Available at: https://yourbudgit.com/wp-content/uploads/2018/04/Nigeria-Health-Budget-Analysis.pdf. Accessed 24 May 2021.

Onwuchekwa, A. C., & Asekomeh, G. E. (2009). Pattern of heart failure in a Nigerian teaching hospital. *Vascular Health Risk Management, 5*, 745–750. [online]. Available at: https://www.ncbi.nlm.nih.gov/pmc/articles/PMC2747392/. Accessed 28 May 2021.

Onwujekwe, O., Agwu, P., Orjiakor, C., McKee, M., Hutchinson, E., Mbachu, C., Odii, A., Ogbozor, P., Obi, U., Ichoku, H., & Balabanova, D. (2019). Corruption in Anglophone West Africa health systems: A systematic review of its different variants and the factors that sustain them. *Health Policy and Planning, 34*(7), 529–543. [online]. Available at: https://academic.oup.com/heapol/article/34/7/529/5543565. Accessed 10 Oct 2020.

Onwujekwe, O., Odii, A., Mbachu, C., Hutchinson, E., Ichoku, H., Ogbozorf, P. A., Agwu, P., Obi, U. S., & Balabanova, D. (2018). Corruption in the Nigerian health sector has many faces: How to fix it. *University of London*. [online]. Available at: https://ace.soas.ac.uk/wp-content/uploads/2018/09/Corruption-in-the-health-sector-in-Anglophone-W-Africa_ACE-Working-Paper-005.pdf. Accessed 10 Oct 2020

Onwujekwe, O., Ezumah, N., Mbachu, C., et al. (2019). Exploring effectiveness of different health financing mechanisms in Nigeria; what needs to change and how can it happen? *BMC Health Services Research, 19*, 661. [online]. Available at: https://bmchealthservres.biomedcentral.com/articles/10.1186/s12913-019-4512-4#citeas. Accessed 24 May 2021.

Okafor, P. (2017). Nigeria loses $1bn annually to medical tourism — Omatseye. *Vanguard*. August 23. [online]. Available at: https://www.vanguardngr.com/2017/08/nigeria-loses-1bn-annually-medical-tourism-omatseye/. Accessed 10 Oct 2020.

Omonijo, D. O., Obiajulu, A., Ugochukwu, N., & Ezeokana, J. (2011). Understanding the escalation of brain drain in Nigeria from poor leadership point of view. *Mediterranean Journal of Social Sciences, 2*(3), 434. [online]. Available at: https://www.researchgate.net/publication/260533114_Understanding_the_Escalation_of_Brain_Drain_in_Nigeria_From_Poor_Leadership_Point_of_View. Accessed 16 Oct 2020.

Onyeji, E. (2020). Analysis: Why Nigeria's vision 20:2020 was bound to fail. *Premium Times*, January 19. [online]. Available at: https://www.premiumtimesng.com/news/top-news/373321-analysis-why-nigerias-vision-202020-was-bound-to-fail.html. Accessed 16 Oct 2020.

Onyenekenwa, C. E. (2011). Nigeria's Vision 20:2020-issues, challenges, and implications for development management. *Asian Journal of Rural Development, 1*, 21–40. [online]. Available at: https://scialert.net/fulltext/?doi=ajrd.2011.21.40. Accessed 16 Oct 2020.

Onyenucheya, A. (2018). Reversing medical tourism in Nigeria. *The Guardian*. October 25. [online]. Available at: https://guardian.ng/features/reversing-medical-tourism-in-nigeria/. Accessed 10 Oct 2020.

Orekunrin, O. (2015). *Nigeria's healthcare problems: A three-pronged solution*. [online]. Available at: https://politicalmatter.org/2015/07/11/10769/. Accessed 10 Oct 2020.

Otu, A., Umoh, V., Habib, A., Ameh, S., Lawson, L., & Ansa, V. (2013). Drug resistance among pulmonary tuberculosis patients in Calabar, Nigeria. *Pulmonary Medicine*, 235190. [online]. Available at: https://www.hindawi.com/journals/pm/2013/235190/. Accessed 28 May 2021.

Owolabi, F. (2020). *Nigerian doctors in diaspora: How FG frustrated us when we offered to improve healthcare back home*. [online]. Available at: https://www.thecable.ng/.Xj4zmxti71k. whatsapp. Accessed 16 Oct 2020.

Parmar, H. (2015). *Healthcare business challenges in Nigeria*. September 8. [online]. Available at: https://www.linkedin.com/pulse/healthcare-business-challenges-nigeria-hemraj-parmar-mba/. Accessed 10 Oct 2020.

Pew Research Center. (2018). *At least a million sub-Saharan Africans moved to Europe since 2010.* [online]. Available at: https://www.pewresearch.org/global/2018/03/22/at-least-a-million-sub-saharan-africans-moved-to-europe-since-2010/. Accessed 16 Oct 2020.

Popoola, J. J., Ponnle, A. A., & Ale, T. O. (2011). Reliability worth assessment of electric power utility in Nigeria: Residential customer survey results. *Assumption University Journal of Technology, 14*(3), 217–224. [online]. Available at: https://pdfs.semanticscholar.org/aebf/71eb57b215257620cf13fef48dae838c1ba3.pdf. Accessed 16 Oct 2020.

Punch. (2016). Nigeria spends $1bn annually on medical tourism. *Punch,* October 14. [online]. Available at: https://punchng.com/nigeria-spends-1bn-annually-medical-tourism/. Accessed 16 Oct 2020.

Rahim, A. I. M., Abdeen, A. Z. E., Faki, B. A., Mustafa, A. E., & Nalder, S. (1987). Introducing training in primary health care programme management into the curriculum. *Medical Education, 21*(4), 288–292. [online]. Available at: http://onlinelibrary.wiley.com/doi/10.1111/j.1365-2923.1987.tb00365.x/abstract. Accessed 16 Oct 2020.

Reddy, K. (n.d.). *Strategies for conflict resolutions in teams.* [online]. Available at: https://content.wisestep.com/conflict-resolution-in-teams/. Accessed 16 Oct 2020.

Rine, R. (2019). Nigeria's life expectancy in 2019: Matters arising. *TNV. The ..* [online]. Available at: https://www.thenigerianvoice.com/news/277752/nigerias-life-expectancy-in-2019-matters-arising.html. Accessed 16 Oct 2020.

Scott-Emuakpor, A. (2010). The evolution of healthcare systems in Nigeria: Which way forward in the twenty-first century. *Nigerian Medical Journal, 17*(51), 53–65. [online]. Available at: http://www.nigeriamedj.com/text.asp?2010/51/2/53/70997. Accessed 3 Feb 2020.

SevenHills Hospital. (2020). [online]. Available at: http://www.sevenhillshospital.com/advanced-technologies.html. Accessed 2 Jan 2021.

Shemmassian Academic Consulting. (2019). *Tuition at every medical school in the United States.* [online]. Available at: https://www.shemmassianconsulting.com/blog/medical-school-tuition. Accessed 10 Oct 2020.

Shuaibu I. (2017), 2,000 Nigerian Physiotherapists Unemployed, Says Rufai. *This Day Newspaper.* [online]. Available at: https://www.thisdaylive.com/index.php/2017/04/23/2000-nigerian-physiotherapists-unemployed-says-rufai/. Accessed: 10 Feb 2020.

Tagbo, P. N., Bancroft, R. E., & Fajolu, I. (2019). Paediatric bacterial meningitis surveillance network, pediatric bacterial meningitis surveillance in Nigeria from 2010 to 2016, Prior to and during the phased introduction of the 10-valent pneumococcal conjugate vaccine. *Clinical Infectious Diseases, 69*(2), S81–S88. [online]. Available at: https://doi.org/10.1093/cid/ciz474. Accessed 28 May 2021.

Tertiary Education Trust Fund (TETFund, 2020). [online]. Available at: https://tetfund.gov.ng/. Accessed 10 October 2020.

Times Higher Education. (2020). *The cost of studying at a university in the United States.* [online]. Available at: https://www.timeshighereducation.com/student/advice/cost-studying-university-united-states. Accessed 10 Oct 2020.

Tormusa, D. O., & Idom, A. M. (2016). The impediments of corruption on the efficiency of health-care service delivery in Nigeria. *Online Journal of Health Ethics, 12*(1). [online]. Available at: https://aquila.usm.edu/ojhe/vol12/iss1/3/. Accessed 10 Oct 2020.

Transparency International. (2016). *How to stop corruption: 5 key ingredients.* [online]. Available at: https://www.transparency.org/en/news/how-to-stop-corruption-5-key-ingredients#. Accessed 22 Dec 2020.

Trevors, J. T., Pollack, G. H., Saier, M. H. Jr., Masson, L. (2012). Transformative research: definitions, approaches and consequences. *Theory Biosciences,* 131(2):117–123. [online]. Available at: https://www.ncbi.nlm.nih.gov/pmc/articles/PMC3990254/. Accessed: 31 May 2021.

Tyessi, K. (2019). *40% of doctors in Nigeria are unemployed, says FCT NMA president.* [online]. Available at: https://www.thisdaylive.com/index.php/2019/07/25/40-of-doctors-in-nigeria-are-unemployed-says-fct-nma-president/. Accessed 7 Jun 2021.

UK Home Office. (2018). *Country policy and information note Nigeria: Medical and healthcare issues Version 2.0.* [online]. Available at: https://www.justice.gov/eoir/page/file/1094261/download. Accessed 20 May 2021.

Umeh, C. A. (2018). *Challenges toward achieving universal health coverage in Ghana, Kenya, Nigeria, and Tanzania.* https://doi.org/10.1002/hpm.2610. [online]. Available at: Challenges toward achieving universal health coverage in Ghana, Kenya, Nigeria, and Tanzania - Umeh - 2018 - The International Journal of Health Planning and Management - Wiley Online Library. Accessed 24 Dec 2020.

UN. (2015). *The 17 sustainable development goals (SDGs) Department of Economic and Social Affairs Sustainable Development).* [online]. Available at: https://sdgs.un.org/goals. Accessed 27 May 2021.

United Nations Population Fund. (n.d.). *Sexual and reproductive health.* [online]. Available at: https://www.unfpa.org/sexual-reproductive-health. Accessed 16 Oct 2020.

United Nations Economic Commission for Africa. (2018). Towards achieving the African Union's recommendation of expenditure of 1% of GDP on research and development. Addis Ababa. [online]. Available at: https://repository.uneca.org/handle/10855/24306. Accessed: 16 Oct 2020.

UNODC. (2020). *Module 6: Detecting and investigating corruption.* [online]. Available at: https://www.unodc.org/e4j/en/anti-corruption/module-6/key-issues/detection-mechanisms%2D%2D-auditing-and-reporting.html. Accessed 26 Dec 2020.

US CDC. (2019). *US Centers for Disease Control and Prevention - Global Health - Nigeria.* [online]. Available at: https://www.cdc.gov/globalhealth/countries/nigeria/default.htm. Accessed 16 Jun 2021.

University World News. (2010). *Nigeria: Retirement age for professors rises to 70.* [online]. Available at: https://www.universityworldnews.com/post.php?story=20100827225301559. Accessed 16 Jun 2021.

Uzochukwu, BSC, Okeke, C, O'Brien, N. et al. (2018). Health technology assessment and priority setting for universal health coverage: a qualitative study of stakeholders' capacity, needs, policy areas of demand and perspectives in Nigeria. *Global Health,* 16, 58. [online]. Available at: https://doi.org/10.1186/s12992-020-00583-2. Accessed: 16 Oct 2020.

Uzochukwu, B., Ughasoro, M. D., Etiaba, Okwuosa, C., Envuladu, E., & Onwujekwe, O. E. (2015). Healthcare financing in Nigeria: Implications for achieving universal health coverage. *Nigeria Journal of Clinical Practice.* [online]. Available at: http://www.njcponline.com/text.asp?2015/18/4/437/154196. Accessed 10 Oct 2020.

Varrella, S. (2020a). Poverty headcount rate in Nigeria as of 2019, by state. *Statistica.* [online]. Available at: https://www.statista.com/statistics/1121438/poverty-headcount-rate-in-nigeria-by-state/#:~:text=An%20individual%20is%20considered%20poor,in%20Nigeria%20lived%20in%20poverty. Accessed 10 Oct 2020.

Varrella S, (2020b). *Monthly minimum wage in Nigeria 2018-2020.* [online]. Available at: https://www.statista.com/statistics/1119133/monthly-minimum-wage-in-nigeria/. Accessed 22 Dec 2020.

VOA. (2019). *Nigeria losing $1B annually to medical tourism, Authorities say.* May 10. [online]. Available at: https://www.voanews.com/africa/nigeria-losing-1b-annually-medical-tourism-authorities-say. Accessed 10 Oct 2020.

Weber, D. O. (2019). How many patients can a primary care physician treat? *The American Association for Physician Leadership.* [online]. Available at: https://www.physician-leaders.org/news/how-many-patients-can-primary-care-physician-treat. Accessed: 10 Feb 2020.

Welcome, M. O. (2011). The Nigerian health care system: Need for integrating adequate medical intelligence and surveillance systems. *Journal of Pharmacy and Bioallied Sciences, 3*(4), 470–478. [online]. Available at: https://www.ncbi.nlm.nih.gov/pmc/articles/PMC3249694/. Accessed 10 Oct 2020.

The White House. (2015). *The Peace We Seek: President Obama Speaks to the People of India.* [online]. Available at: https://obamawhitehouse.archives.gov/blog/2015/01/28/peace-we-seek-president-obama-speaks-people-india. Accessed 16 Jul 2021.

WHO. (2000) *The world health organization's ranking of the world's health systems, by rank.* [online]. Available at: https://photius.com/rankings/world_health_systems.html. Accessed: 10 Oct 2020.

WHO. (2008). *Health systems financing: toolkit on monitoring health systems strengthening.* [online]. Available at: http://www.who.int/health-info/statistics/toolkit_hss/EN_PDF_Toolkit_HSS_Financing.pdf. Accessed 10 Oct 2020.

WHO. (2010). Telemedicine in the member states: Opportunities and developments. Report on the second global survey on eHealth. *Global Observatory for eHealth series* - Volume 2. [online]. Available at: http://www.who.int/goe/publications/goe_telemedicine_2010.pdf. Accessed 16 Oct 2020.

WHO. (2014). *Presidential summit on universal health coverage ends in Nigeria.* [online]. Available at: https://www.afro.who.int/news/presidential-summit-universal-health-coverage-ends-nigeria. Accessed:16 Oct 2020.

WHO. (2019). *Access to medicines and vaccines: Report by the director-general.* [online]. Available at: https://apps.who.int/gb/ebwha/pdf_files/WHA72/A72_17-en.pdf. Accessed: 10 Oct 2020.

Wirtz, V. J., Kaplan, W. A., Kwan, G. F., & Laing, R. O. (2016). Access to medications for cardiovascular diseases in low-and middle-income countries. *Circulation, 133*(21), 2076–2085. [online]. Available at: https://www.ncbi.nlm.nih.gov/pmc/articles/PMC4880457/. Accessed 28 May 2021.

Woodard, R. (n.d.). *10 methods of resolving conflict in your project team.* [online]. Available at: https://www.brighthubpm.com/resource-management/95564-ten-ways-to-halt-conflicts-with-project-team-members/. Accessed 16 Oct 2020.

World Bank. (2014). *A decade of development in sub-Saharan African science, technology, engineering and mathematics research.* [online]. Available at: https://documents1.worldbank.org/curated/en/237371468204551128/pdf/910160WP0P126900disclose09026020140.pdf. Accessed 19 Mar 2021.

World Bank. (2020). *Combating corruption.* [online]. Available at: https://www.worldbank.org/en/topic/governance/brief/anti-corruption. Accessed 26 Dec 2020.

World Bank. (2021). *Current health expenditure (% of GDP).* [online]. Available at: https://data.worldbank.org/indicator/SH.XPD.CHEX.GD.ZS?locations=NG. Accessed 4 Jan 2021.

Wu, T. Y., Majeed, A., & Kuo, K. N. (2010). An overview of the healthcare system in Taiwan. *London Journal of Primary Care* (Abingdon), *3*(2): 115–119. [online]. Available at: https://www.ncbi.nlm.nih.gov/pmc/articles/PMC3960712/. Accessed 10 Oct 2020.

Chapter 14
Nigeria's Health System Response to the COVID-19 Pandemic and Lessons from Other Countries

Learning Objectives

After reading this chapter, the learner should be able to:

1. Contextualize the role of patients' satisfaction in judging the effectiveness of a healthcare system.
2. Compare and contrast the satisfaction of Nigerians with their health system with the rest of the world.
3. Describe the surveillance and laboratory testing capabilities to curb emerging diseases in Nigeria.
4. Apprise Nigeria's health system response to the COVID-19 pandemic
5. Discuss the challenges facing healthcare workers at the frontline of the COVID-19 crisis in Nigeria.
6. Describe and evaluate the success of the COVID-19 social welfare assistance program implemented by the Nigerian government.
7. Analyze the relationship between the COVID-19 diagnostic testing per capita (1 million/population) and the number of cases and death rate.
8. Discuss the impact of the national strategy (centralized vs. state/region) and COVID-19 death rate.
9. Identify the top five countries that handled the coronavirus crisis the best and the bottom five countries that performed the worst.
10. Discuss the common elements among nations that were successful and those that mismanaged the response to the COVID-19 pandemic.
11. Describe the COVID-19 vaccine developments and therapeutics.

© The Author(s), under exclusive license to Springer Nature Switzerland AG 2021
J. A. Balogun, *The Nigerian Healthcare System*,
https://doi.org/10.1007/978-3-030-88863-3_14

Introduction

In the last four decades, severe acute respiratory syndrome coronavirus 2 (SARS-CoV-2) is the deadliest virus after AIDS, which has claimed over 35 million lives. Coronavirus disease 2019 (COVID-19) was first reported in Wuhan, China, in December 2019 (Jarus, 2020). The COVID-19 pandemic exposes the global health systems' fragilities as many developed countries poorly handled the crisis (Mugwagwa et al., 2020).

At the onset of the COVID-19 outbreak, Singapore and South Korea's response was acclaimed as a model for other countries worldwide. Their health system was able to curtail the spread of the virus effectively, and they both recorded one of the lowest fatalities in the world (World Health Organization—WHO, 2020a; Moradi & Vaezi, 2020; Lin et al., 2020). The United States and South Korea had their first confirmed COVID-19 case on January 20, 2020. The United States' response was delayed, while South Korea was more aggressive in community testing, contact tracing, and quarantining those exposed. The delayed governmental response in the United States resulted in a relatively higher number of cases and death (per capita) compared to the rest of the world (Balogun, 2020).

Some health analysts attribute the success of South Korea to the responsiveness and adaptability of their health system. The response alert system adopted by South Korea consists of close monitoring of the outbreak globally and swift initiation of appropriate preventive measures. First, the government alerted the public on spreading the infection to other areas and quickly mobilized their response capabilities. Second, the South Korean research team developed a rapid screening test by January 31, 2020; the product was immediately made available in some health facilities. By February 7, 2020, all health establishments within the country had the test available (Moradi & Vaezi, 2020). On the other hand, due to bureaucratic delays at the Centers for Disease Control and Prevention (CDC) and the US Food and Drug Administration (FDA), it took the United States months to develop the first COVID-19 screening test.

Like the United States, Sweden also had a delayed response with a laissez-faire approach to the COVID-19 pandemic. They had more infected cases and deaths than its neighbors—Denmark, Norway, and Finland. Sweden's controversial herd immunity strategy adopted in response to the global crisis did not work. By June 18, 2020, Sweden recorded the highest number of cases and fatalities in Scandinavia. It had 37,000 confirmed cases when compared to its neighbors, Denmark, Norway, and Finland, with 12,000, 8000, and 7000, respectively. The three neighboring countries adopted a lockdown strategy and sealed their borders early. On a 7-day average between May 25 and June 2, 2020, Sweden recorded the most COVID-19 fatalities per capita in Europe. The mortality rate in Sweden was 5.29 deaths per million people compared to the United Kingdom, with 4.48 deaths per million, and ranked second in Europe (Habib, 2020).

Eleven months into the COVID-19 pandemic, many nations' health systems were overwhelmed and their leaders mismanaged the situation. This chapter sets out to determine the lessons Nigeria can learn from other countries worldwide that managed the COVID-19 problem effectively. The chapter analyzes the literature on patient's satisfaction with the healthcare system around the world and in Nigeria. It explores the challenges Nigerian healthcare workers faced at the frontline and the government's social welfare assistance programs. This chapter identifies the top five countries worldwide with the lowest coronavirus deaths and investigates their public health system. This chapter also highlights the common elements among successful nations and those that mismanaged the pandemic response and discusses COVID-19 vaccine developments and therapeutics.

Assessment of Patient Satisfaction with the Healthcare System

Satisfaction with the national health system varies widely between countries. Patient satisfaction is used as a proxy to judge the success of healthcare systems worldwide. Other outcome measures used to evaluate the health system's effectiveness are discussed in detail in Chaps. 2 and 10.

Global

Zhang and associates (2020) examined public satisfaction with the Chinese health system between 2013 and 2015. In the study, public satisfaction was defined as "being satisfied" if a respondent's rating of the healthcare system is over 70 out of 100 points. *In the* two years, *the average* satisfaction score ($N = 15,969$) was 68.5, and the 2015 satisfaction score is higher than 2013 by 3.5 points. The findings revealed disparities in public satisfaction with the health system in China. Specifically, the seniors ($OR = 1.19, p < 0.001$), rural dwellers ($OR = 1.23, p < 0.01$), and those in the higher socioeconomic status were more likely to be satisfied. Internal migrants with higher education are less likely to report satisfaction ($OR = 0.75, p < 0.001$). The total health expenditure (as a % of GDP and density of hospital beds) is positively associated with satisfaction ($OR = 1.13, p < 0.001$). The government's share in total healthcare spending had a moderately negative association with satisfaction ($OR = 0.97, p < 0.001$). The density of hospital beds was correlated positively with satisfaction in rural areas ($OR = 1.26, p \leq 0.01$). The Shanghai and Northeast regions were less likely to report being satisfied ($OR = 0.49, p < 0.001$; $OR = 0.71, p < 0.05$) and remained unchanged in 2015.

In 2020, Cosma and colleagues investigated Romanian patients' perception and satisfaction with the quality of their national health system. Of the 2305 respondents, 83% used the health system in the past 12 months, and 58% did not trust the system. Accommodation, food, and other facilities within the hospitals were perceived as being at a low level. About one-third of the respondents were unsatisfied and very unsatisfied concerning the overall impression of the Romanian health system. The findings revealed a significant correlation between confidence in the health system, age, gender, overall perception, age, and income ($p < 0.05$).

In 2019, the Independent Polling System of Society (IPSOS)—Canada's most prominent market research and public opinion polling firm—investigated the level of satisfaction with national health systems in 32 countries worldwide. The online survey occurred between November 22, 2019, and December 6, 2019, and the results were released in February 2020. The sample consists of 16,000 participants ranging in age between 16 and 74 years. Each survey participant was asked, "To what extent, if at all, are you satisfied with (country's) health system?" *Respondents rated their satisfaction on a continuum from "very/fairly satisfied," "neither satisfied nor dissatisfied," and "not very/not at all satisfied." The percentage of respondents that rated their health system "very/fairly satisfied" is reported next. In each country, the percentages do not add to 100% as the researchers did not include "don't know/refusal" responses in the data analysis.*

Citizens of Saudi Arabia (72%), Singapore (60%), Belgium (54%), the United Kingdom (53%), China (52%), India (51%), Australia (49%), France (47%), and Canada (46%) are the most satisfied with their country's health system. On the other hand, only 39% of Americans, 24% of South Africans, 15% of Brazilians, and 11% of Russians are satisfied with their healthcare system (Elflein, 2020).

Although the IPSOS did not include Nigeria in their evaluation, several investigations have examined the level of satisfaction with the Nigerian healthcare system. A review of the pertinent studies conducted in Nigeria from 2013 to 2021 is summarized in the next section.

Nigeria

Iloh and associates in 2013 assessed the satisfaction with healthcare quality received by patients without national health insurance attending a primary care clinic in a tertiary hospital in Umuahia between April 2011 and October 2011. The researcher used a five-point Likert scale questionnaire ranging in the continuum from 1 (lowest) to 5 (highest) to gauge patients' satisfaction with waiting time, patient-staff communication, patient-staff relationship, cost of care, hospital bureaucracy, and hospital environment. Patients who scored three points and above in each domain were considered satisfied, and below 3 points were dissatisfied. The patients' overall satisfaction score was 3.1. Specifically, the patients expressed satisfaction with staff relationship (3.9), staff communication (3.8), and hospital environment (3.6) and dissatisfaction with waiting time (2.4), hospital bureaucracy (2.5), and the cost of health care (2.6).

Also, in 2013, Adekanye et al. investigated the patients' satisfaction with the healthcare services at Federal Medical Centre, Bida. Overall, 79% of the patients ($N = 480$) were satisfied with the hospital services, and 78% had their expectations met. Specifically, satisfaction was highest (96%) at the maternity unit and lowest (73%) at the revenue department. The patients expressed concerns about waiting time, hospital ambiance, and personnel attitude/aptitude. The patients' satisfaction positively correlated with HCP's promptness, level of communication, relationship with patients, environmental cleanliness, and facilities' comfort. Cost of services and delay in obtaining services were negatively correlated with satisfaction. About 92% of the patients indicated they would recommend the facility to a friend.

In 2017, Osiya and associates compared the satisfaction with general practice care delivered at the University of Port Harcourt Teaching Hospital and the Aluu Comprehensive Health Center in Rivers State. A total of 1290 patients participated in the study and patients who received care at the comprehensive health center were significantly ($p < 0.01$) more satisfied with patient-physician communication, interpersonal mannerism, accessibility and convenience, technical quality, financial aspects of care, and general satisfaction than their counterparts at the University Teaching Hospital. However, there was no significant difference in the time spent during consultations in both centers ($p > 0.05$). Other predictors of satisfaction were younger age, male gender, married, higher education, and Muslim religious faith.

Bolarinde and colleagues in 2018 evaluated patients' satisfaction with the healthcare service at Abuja's public secondary hospitals. The patients interviewed rated the hospitals at a "high" satisfaction level. There was a significant positive correlation between patients' satisfaction and careful listening by healthcare workers, patients' perception of being valued and appreciated by hospital personnel ($p < 0.01$ and $p < 0.001$), respectively.

Similarly, in 2018, Potluri and Angiating investigated the quality of healthcare services provided at the Federal Medical Center, Yola. A total of 150 patients completed a structured questionnaire, and the majority of them expressed discontentment over the responsiveness of the HCP. Overall, 42% of the patients were neither satisfied nor dissatisfied with the services received, against 43% of dissatisfied patients. Also, using a five-point Likert scale satisfaction questionnaire, Umoke and associates, in 2020, investigated patients' satisfaction with healthcare quality in general hospitals in Ebonyi State. Overall, the 396 patients who participated in the study were satisfied with the quality of care. Satisfaction was highest with personnel empathy (3.12 ± 0.57) followed by service responsiveness (3.06 ± 0.63) and assurance (3.07 ± 0.63). The lowest satisfaction rating was on tangibility (2.57 ± 0.99). Patients expressed concerns relating to the neat appearance of personnel, waiting time, and hospital hygiene condition.

In 2021, Olamuyiwa and Adeniji evaluated patients' satisfaction with the quality of care at the National Health Insurance Scheme (NHIS) clinic at the University of Port Harcourt Teaching Hospital. The findings revealed that 51% of the study respondents ($N = 379$) were satisfied with the hospital facilities but were not satisfied with the long waiting time at the medical records, account, laboratory, and pharmacy departments. Overall, 76% of the patients were satisfied with the health care provided at the NHIS clinic. A significant correlation was found between treatment outcome and patient satisfaction (($p < 0.01$).

A cross-sectional study conducted at the beginning of the COVID-19 pandemic (between May 15, 2020, and May 21, 2020), by Oleribe and associates examined Nigerians' perception of the government handling of the crisis. About 99% of the study participants were aware of COVID-19, and 95% knew it is a viral disease. The study participants overall rated the government's response to the pandemic as "poor." Approximately 58% of the sample rated the President's Office as "poor," followed by communication rated as "poor" by 50% of the respondents. Public prevention messages received the highest good rating perception by 44% of the sample. Females and participants less than 40 years of age generally rated the governmental responses as "poor" (Oleribe et al., 2020). Despite the government's best efforts, many Nigerians perceive the management of the coronavirus crisis as concerning.

Based on the findings from the seven aforementioned studies that were reviewed, five salient conclusions are drawn. First, to improve consumer satisfaction with the health system, the federal government should set national targets for quality improvement and make national health insurance available for all Nigerians irrespective of their employment status (Iloh et al., 2013). Second, the waiting time needed to obtain services at the medical records, account, laboratory, and pharmacy departments in the secondary and tertiary hospitals should be monitored regularly and a quality assurance intervention instituted to improve the services provided (Adekanye et al., 2013; Olamuyiwa & Adeniji, 2021).

Third, the Federal Ministry of Health (FMH) must sensitize the healthcare workers in the secondary and tertiary hospitals on the need to utilize the primary healthcare centers as the first point of contact within the health system (Oleribe et al., 2020) and expand the private sector involvement in delivering healthcare services for individuals with coronavirus infection (Osiya et al., 2017).

Fourth, the FMH must develop a rigorous accreditation process for secondary and tertiary hospitals. Part of the accreditation standards must include the training of healthcare workers and support staff on effective communication and customer service skills (Adekanye et al., 2013; Potluri & Angiating, 2018). The standard must also mandate hospital management to use satisfaction surveys for planning and quality control improvement (Bolarinde et al., 2018) and monitor hospital environment cleanliness, structural deficits, and staff shortage (Olamuyiwa & Adeniji, 2021). Finally, the federal government must promote the public-private partnership to disseminate public health prevention information more effectively (Oleribe et al., 2020).

The sections that follow examine the human resources, surveillance and laboratory testing capabilities, and other critical infrastructure available in the country to manage emerging diseases.

Management of COVID-19 Crisis in Nigeria: Evaluation of Physical Resources and Human Capacity

Before the outbreak of COVID-19 in 2020, the Nigerian government fast-tracked the legislation and policy frameworks supporting the WHO's health regulations recommendation at the three government levels. Specifically, legislation that approved the establishment of the Nigeria Centre for Disease Control (NCDC) was already finalized. The center had been autonomous for over a full year before the onset of the pandemic. At the beginning of the COVID-19 crisis, the NCDC launched the "National Strategy to Scale-up Coronavirus Disease Testing." The plan includes expanding the NCDC's existing laboratory network by engaging private sector clinics and laboratories about antigen and antibody tests. The strategy ensures that every state establishes a molecular laboratory linked to the NCDC National Reference Laboratory. The laboratories serve as a state-level hub that is well-coordinated for other disease-specific laboratories for HIV and tuberculosis (Eke, 2020).

In 2017, WHO funded a study that evaluated Nigeria's capacity to prevent, detect, and respond to a natural disaster such as a COVID-19 pandemic (WHO, 2017). The mean score on the external indicators in the prevention category was only 1.9 across the 15 measures. This finding suggests the country has limited capacity to prevent biological, chemical, or radiation health risks. A mean score of 2.6 across the 13 indicators in the *detection* category indicates that the NCDC has acquired some capabilities to detect new health risks through real-time surveillance and laboratory capabilities to test the diseases. However, the sustainability of these capabilities is in doubt. The *response* category's performance had a mean score of 1.5 across the 20 indicators, suggesting the country has limited capacity to respond to a sudden health risk.

In a blog post on July 2, 2020, Dixit and associates confirmed that only 2500 samples could be tested. Because of the shortage of personnel and laboratory kits, testing was at 50% capacity. As of June 30, 2020, only 138,462 samples from a population of over 200 million were tested. In contrast, South Africa, with 58 million people, has already tested 1,630,008 samples. Realizing the depth of unpreparedness, President Buhari's government strengthened laboratory capacities in specimen shipping, transportation, referral, and inter-sectoral collaboration on emergency response (Dixit et al., 2020). There were only 350 ventilators and 350 ICU beds before the outbreak of the COVID-19 pandemic. By April 2020, 100 additional ventilators were acquired.

Nigeria's Health System Response to the COVID-19 Pandemic

The first COVID-19 case was confirmed in Nigeria on February 27, 2020, but the health system was unprepared at the time of the outbreak. An Italian employed in Nigeria who returned from Milan, Italy, to Lagos was the first case. His specimen was confirmed positive by the Virology Laboratory at the Lagos University Teaching Hospital—an affiliate of the NCDC Laboratory Network. On admission at the Infectious Disease Hospital in Yaba, the Italian was clinically stable, with no severe symptoms. Subsequently, the FMH assured the nation that they have the technical capacity to control the outbreak's spread and activated its National Emergency Operations Centre to respond and implement firm control measures in cooperation with Lagos State Health authorities (Ehanire, 2020).

By June 22, 2020, Lagos reported the highest number of cases (10,510 cases, 128 deaths), followed by Ogun (1870 cases, 33 deaths) and Oyo (1380 cases, 12 deaths). The three states accounted for about 54% of the total infection and 29% of the deaths. As of June 30, 2020, there were more than 100 confirmed cases each in 16 states—Ebonyi, Enugu, Imo, Oyo, Ogun, Kwara, Edo, Delta, Sokoto, Katsina, Kaduna Kano, Jigawa, Bauchi, Gombe, and Borno. As of December 30, 2020, Nigeria had 85,560 confirmed coronavirus cases, 1267 deaths, and 71,937 recoveries from the virus.

The number of COVID-19 cases and deaths in Nigeria (30th day of each month and February 28, 2020) from January to December are presented in Figs. 14.1 and 14.2, respectively.

In totality, the number of COVID-19 cases and mortality rate in Africa is relatively low compared to the rest of the world. In May 2020, WHO had estimated in the first year of the pandemic that 44 million people would be infected and 190,000 deaths expected in Africa. Several theories have been advanced for low cases and fatalities in Africa. Many analysts attributed it to the underreporting of the cases due to the low density of testing facilities. Thus, the actual burden of the disease remains murky in the absence of extensive testing infrastructure. Other scientists attribute it to the young age of the population. In Africa, where 60% of the people are under the age of 25, and the median age is 19.4 years, COVID-19 is more prevalent among the elderly over 60 years.

Another school of thought is that Africa's hot and humid climate interacts to heighten their personal effects (SciDev.Net, 2020). Some scientists attributed the low death rate in Africa to environmental, genetic, and spiritual factors or less fatal coronavirus variants. Ndubuaku and Watanabe (2020) posit that population density is a crucial factor in spreading the disease. In high-income countries where the pandemic is currently high, urbanites are packed in crowded spaces, vehicles, and stadia, accommodating 50,000 to 75,000 people close to one another. On the other hand, Ndubuaku and Watanabe (2020) argue Africans live in less crowded spaces

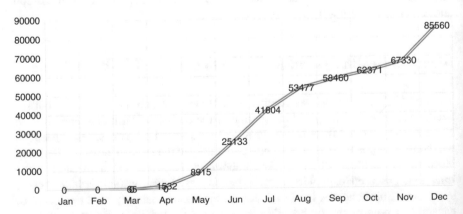

Fig. 14.1 The number of COVID-19 cases in Nigeria from January 30, 2020, to December 30, 2020. (Source: WHO, 2020b)

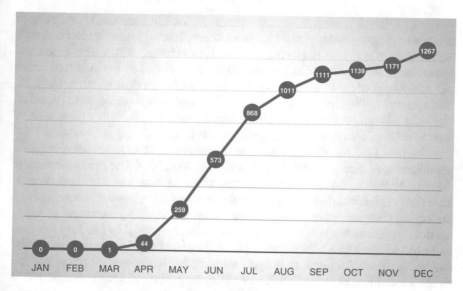

Fig. 14.2 The number of COVID-19 deaths in Nigeria from January 30, 2020, to December 30, 2020. (Source: WHO, 2020b)

and enjoy provincial lifestyles to relax. In Africa, most coronavirus cases are in the cities and fewer in rural areas. Other scientists have proposed genetic and immunological factors.

Healthcare Workers at the Frontline of the COVID-19 Crisis

Following the COVID-19 outbreak, the Nigerian government set up isolation centers across the country to test and treat patients who have contracted the virus. However, many sick individuals deliberately remained at home instead of going to the hospital because of the disease's stigma and phobia. Many of those who have access to hospitals often provide false medical information and travel history. Also, many people who tested positive deserted the isolation centers to seek treatment in private hospitals not equipped to manage COVID-19 cases (Onigbinde et al., 2020). The isolation centers around the country had personal protective equipment, but the health workers at other health establishments had limited supplies.

As of April 21, 2020, globally, more than 35,000 healthcare workers have contracted COVID-19 (WHO, 2020b). A WHO's report released on June 9, 2020, indicated over 800 healthcare workers have tested positive for coronavirus in Nigeria, and about 2100 in South Africa have contracted the virus. The number of infections among health workers in Nigeria represents only 6% of the cases and 19% in neighboring Niger—the highest infection rate in Africa. The health workers' infection rate as a percentage of the population cases in Liberia and Sierra Leone is about 12%.

The COVID-19 crisis was marred when physicians in Lagos and other parts of the country began a 3-day strike over inadequate personal protective kits and non-payment of hazard and inducement allowances (Presse, 2020). The scope and dimension of the health system's problems are exacerbated by the industrial action and adulterated drugs in the country. On the day of the industrial strike (July 13, 2020), over 32,500 coronavirus cases and 740 deaths nationwide were recorded. The virus has infected more than 800 health workers. Lagos, with a population of over 20 million, accounts for the majority of the fatalities.

As of June 17, 2020, the National Association of Resident Doctors confirmed ten physicians have died of COVID-19 (Mwai & Giles, 2020). The health workers in different hospitals, except those employed at the coronavirus treatment centers, embarked on industrial strikes on several occasions complaining of low pay and inadequate personal protective equipment. Subsequently, the government provided the frontline health workers with 2 months of hazard pay. And by late July, the government had spent 15.8 billion Naira ($42 million) on hazard compensation. Sadly, due to the economic downturn brought about by the low global oil prices and the national lockdown from the COVID-19 crisis, the government implemented a 43% cut in the primary healthcare budget (Mwai & Giles, 2020).

Comparatively, the COVID-19-related deaths among health workers in Nigeria are substantially less than in the United States. As of August 10, 2020, the United States had lost 922 healthcare workers (Kaiser Family Foundation, 2020), but only 14 deaths in Nigeria as of August 14, 2020 (Adepoju, 2020). The most remarkable migration of physicians abroad in search of greener pastures occurred even during the COVID-19 crisis. The incident is probably the most noteworthy migration of Nigerian physicians abroad searching for greener pastures since the 1980s. Amid an ongoing nationwide strike by resident physicians over nonpayment of salary, among other complaints, desperate Nigerian physicians, on August 24, 2021, stormed the Sheraton Hotels, Abuja, where a consultancy firm held interviews for those willing to work in the United Arab Emirates (Business Hallmark, 2021).

COVID-19 Social Welfare Assistance Program

The House of Representatives, on March 24, 2020, passed an *Emergency Economic Stimulus Bill* to provide 50% tax rebates to businesses to retain their employees. Although the Bill provided relief to formal sector businesses, 65% of the total GDP comes from the informal sector, but the Bill left over 90% of the workforce in the cold because the government has no means of reaching them. The government paid 20,000 Naira ($52) to the 11 million vulnerable workers in the formal economy registered with the National Social Register. The government pledged to increase the support to 3.6 million households. So far, the government financial outlay is a drop in the bucket since over 87 million Nigerians live on less than $1.90 a day. Getting the cash in the hands of the needy was a challenge since making electronic payments is challenging. Furthermore, the *Central Bank of Nigeria stimulus package* offers 3 million Naira credit to low-income families impacted by COVID-19, but the loan requires collateral and is with interest.

The extended lockdown in the Federal Capital Territory, Lagos and Ogun states, led to food insecurity among many families. Consequently, on April 1, 2020, the Federal Ministry of Humanitarian Affairs Disaster Management and Social Development vowed to provide food to vulnerable households in these states. Unfortunately, the pledges never reached the poor that needed food support, as the distribution system was marred by corruption and opaque accountability (Dixit et al., 2020).

The federal government projected that $330 million would be needed to procure medical equipment, personal protective equipment, and medicines in response to the COVID-19 crisis. The Nigerian state oil company pledged $30 million toward the COVID-19 efforts. The European Union contributed 50 million Euros to the basket fund to strengthen the COVID-19 response. The private sector established the Coalition against COVID-19 and collected over $72 million when the European Union launched the basket fund on March 26, 2020. The funds generated were used to purchase food and provide medical facilities and equipment in different countries.

Although the federal government provided health, social, and economic assistance to cushion the impact of the COVID-19 crisis, some of the measures adopted were abused by the citizens and bureaucrats in charge of implementing the policies. Overall, the assistance offered was not adequate to address the magnitude of the problem.

Comparative Analyses

The number of cases, fatalities, deaths/1 M population, and the number of diagnostic tests (1million/population) are now globally used to gauge the adaptability and effectiveness of health systems. A comparative analysis of Nigeria's COVID-19 related outcome performance data is presented in the remaining section of this Chapter.

COVID-19 Diagnostic Testing Per Capita (1 Million/Population)

On June 22, 2020, a global assessment was conducted to identify countries with robust COVID-19 diagnostic testing program. Gibraltar, Cayman Islands, and the United Arab Emirates were the top three countries with the highest number of screening tests per capita (1 million/population) (Table 14.1). Paradoxically, the majority of the nations with the highest screening tests per capita are from developing countries such as Gibraltar, Cayman Islands, United Arab Emirates, Bahrain, Falkland Island, Faeroe Islands, and Malta.

COVID-19 Cases and Deaths

As of June 16, 2020, the highest number of COVID-19 cases and fatalities are in the United States. With a population of 51.3 million, South Korea had 12,155 COVID-19 cases and 278 deaths, while the United States, with a population of 330.9 million in

Table 14.1 The top ten nations in the world with robust COVID-19 tests per capital as of June 22, 2020

Serial #	Country	COVID-19 tests/1 M population
1	Gibraltar	329,821
2	Cayman Island	310,041
3	United Arab Emirates	307,270
4	Bahrain	285,850
5	Falkland Island	282,221
6	Faeroe Islands	244,438
7	Luxembourg	238,732
8	Malta	200,885
9	Iceland	200,508
10	Denmark	159,520

Sources: (Worldometer, 2020a; Johns Hopkins University of Medicine, 2020)

the same period, had 2,202,776 cases and 119,001 deaths. With 5.8 *million people,* Singapore had 42,313 COVID-19 cases and 26 deaths (4 deaths/1 M population). Similarly, with a population of *23.8 million, Taiwan had* only 451 COVID-19 incidents and seven fatalities (0.3 deaths/1 M population), which constitutes one of the lowest in the world (Worldometer, 2020a). With 4% of the world population, the United States, as of June 30, 2020, had over 25% of the global COVID-19 cases, despite its high investment in health and sophisticated medical technology. The ineptness made the United States the laughingstock of the world (Andrew, 2020).

There is no relationship between the type of government (democratic and authoritarian) and effectiveness in responding to the COVID-19 crisis. Taiwan, South Korea, and Singapore managed the pandemic successfully without overwhelming their health system. Democratic nations such as Canada, Germany, and Finland that did not politicize the crisis and adopted a nation-wide implementation strategy rather than a patchwork approach had fewer COVID-19 cases and fatalities. In contrast, countries with leaders (United States, United Kingdom, Mexico, and Brazil) who had nonchalant, dismissive, and *lackadaisical* attitudes and downplayed the pandemic's seriousness had the highest cases and fatalities.

Available evidence revealed that countries with leaders who provide clear scientific information about the virus and model appropriate preventive behaviors, such as wearing masks in public and promoting handwashing and six feet social distancing, were more successful in building trust in government curtailing the spread of the COVID-19 virus.

Table 14.2 summarizes the critical COVID-19-related data for Nigeria and the six shining model health systems that were discussed in Chap. 10. Singapore, representing only 0.08% of the world population, is the least populated and smallest landmass of the six countries. The overwhelming majority (ranging from 78.3% in Cuba to 100% in Singapore) of the six countries are urban dwellers. Only 52% of Nigerians live in the metropolitan area (Worldometer, 2020b).

Table 14.2 COVID-19 indicators for Nigeria and six high-performing health systems as of June 22, 2020

Serial #	COVID-19 measures	Nigeria	United States	United Kingdom	S. Korea	Singapore	Taiwan	Cuba
1	Population (millions)	205,962,220	330,954,637	67,877,301	51,268,205	5,849,157	23,818,146	11,326,764
2	COVID-19 cases	20,244	2,384,864	305.289	12,438	42,313	451	2315
3	COVID-19 deaths	518	122,571	42,647	280	26	7	85
4	COVID-19 deaths/1 M population	4	416	660	6	4	0.3	8
5	COVID-19 recovered	6879	989,573	N/A[a]	10,881	35,590	438	2113
6	COVID-19 tests/1 M population	551	87,306	118,298	23,057	98,508	3296	13,138

Sources: (WHO, 2020b; Worldometer, 2020a)

[a]*N/A* Not available

As of June 22, 2020, the United Kingdom performed the highest number of COVID-19 diagnostic tests/1 M population *(118, 298),* followed by Singapore (98,508). Compared to the six model countries, the number of diagnostic tests and COVID-19 cases in Nigeria is dismal. Nigeria only conducted 551 tests/1 M population and had 20,244 cases. The COVID-19 deaths/1 M population is highest in the United Kingdom (660), followed by the United States (416).

The Top Five Countries that Handled the Coronavirus Crisis the Best

The global response to the COVID-19 pandemic bolsters the rationale to have federal control over the health system. As of August 3, 2020, nations such as South Korea, Singapore, Cuba, Australia, Finland, and India that adopted a centralized strategy had fewer fatalities. In contrast, countries such as the United States, Brazil, the United Kingdom, Germany, and Sweden that adopted a state-controlled strategy had more deaths (Worldometer, 2020a).

As of December 4, 2020, coronavirus had infected almost 64 million people worldwide, with approximately 1.5 million deaths. The introduction section of this chapter discussed the initial global response to the coronavirus crisis. From the start, some countries handled the COVID-19 problem better than others. Eleven months after the pandemic onset, more information is available in the literature on the virus' pathophysiology, transmissibility, and practical strategies to curtail the virus' spread. At the same time, the number of COVID-19 cases and deaths has shifted somewhat. On December 6, 2020, South Korea, widely praised for its aggressive testing and contact tracing procedures at the onset of the pandemic, had 31 new infections 1 day—the highest number of cases in the country in 9 months. South Korea had struggled in recent weeks as the total number of cases stands at 37,546 and 545 deaths. South Korea health minister, Park Neung-hoo, expressed genuine concern about the virus expanding nationwide if the government did nothing. The country's contact tracers worked long hours to get suspected carriers to quarantine, and at least 3 weeks restriction is under consideration.

A retrospective study conducted by Beth Howell on December 1, 2020, identified the countries that managed the pandemic the best and the worst. The findings of the study are summarized in Table 14.3.

The top five countries that handled the coronavirus crisis the best is Taiwan, New Zealand, Iceland, Singapore, Vietnam, and the nations (Table 14.3). The lessons that the rest of the world can learn from the top countries will now be discussed. Taiwan employed technology to trace suspected cases from the start, and if found positive, the individuals were quarantined in hotels. Based on the SARS outbreak in 2003, Taiwan strengthened its preparations, set up an infectious disease prevention network, and held annual drills in hospitals. They also maintained a stockpile of face masks, trained their medical personnel, and build up their laboratory capacity to handle any outbreaks (Howell, 2020).

Table 14.3 The top five countries in the world that handled coronavirus the best and the worst from January 1, 2020, to December 1, 2020

Ranking	Best Countries[a]				Worst Countries[b]			
	Country	Population	Number of cases	Number of deaths	Country	Population	COVID-19 cases	COVID-19 deaths
1	Taiwan	23,816,775	675	7	United States	331,002,651	13.54 million	268,045
2	New Zealand	4,822,233	25	25	Brazil	212,559,417	6.34 million	173,120
3	Iceland	341,243	26	26	India	1.37 billion	9.46 million	137,621
4	Singapore	5,850,342	29	29	Mexico	128,932,753	1.11 million	105,940
5	Vietnam	97,338,579	35	35	United Kingdom	67,886,011	1.63 million	58,545
	South Korea[c]	51,290,207	37,546	545	Global[##]	7,794,798,739	64.0 million	1.5 million

Sources: (Howell, 2020; Worldometer, 2021)
[a]Top five countries that handled coronavirus the best; [b]Top five countries that handled coronavirus the worst; [c]Measurements as of December 6, 2020
[##]Global measurements as of December 6, 2020

New Zealand's Ministry of Health wasted no time in preventing the spread of the virus by swiftly setting up the National Health Coordination Centre to respond to the pandemic and immediately issued an "infectious and modifiable diseases order" which mandates health practitioners to report any suspected cases. As early as early February 2020, the government imposed international travel restrictions. On March 23, 2020, authorities announced the country's commitment to an elimination strategy, and a complete national lockdown was imposed 3 days later, on March 26, 2020.

The Iceland government rushed into action early to curtail the virus' spread by hiring a team of contact tracers to track down people with positive tests and interview them to identify and quarantine people they came into contact with. The Icelanders were told to stay home, and they complied religiously. The government paid the full salary of those with positive tests as long as they complied with the "stay-at-home" order. Iceland's success story is attributed to the widespread testing, contact tracing, and quarantine procedures, including an emphasis on mask-wearing and social distancing strategies (Howell, 2020).

The experience of Singapore with SARS in 2003 gave it the upper hand in managing the COVID-19 virus. After the virus broke out in China, the government initiated an aggressive testing and tracing program, closed the borders, and provided ongoing clear public announcements on preventing the virus. Although the number of COVID-19 cases is relatively high, the number of fatalities was comparatively low. Most of the new cases are younger, and the low mortality rate was attributed to the population's average young age (36.7 years).

Following the outbreak, the government put Vietnam's emergency plan into action immediately. The first case was confirmed in Vietnam on January 23, 2020—months before other countries took any action. The government initially monitored travel restrictions by enforcing health checks at borders and later closed the border with China. At the same time, health officers scaled up the contact tracing process. At the end of January, schools shut down—again, months before other countries took action—for the Lunar New Year holiday and remained shut until mid-May 2020. In contrast, schools were not closed in the United States until the first week in March 2020 (Howell, 2020).

The Bottom Five Countries that Handled the Coronavirus Crisis the Worst

Now that we have discerned what works, it is pertinent to identify the common elements among the nations that mismanaged the coronavirus crisis. In ranking order, the countries that bungled the problem are the United States, Brazil, India, Mexico, and the United Kingdom (Table 14.3). President Donald Trump displayed a nonchalant attitude in the United States and continuously dished out misinformation about the pandemic. As far back as May 2018, Trump's medical and biodefense preparedness adviser, Luciana Borio, warned at a symposium that a flu pandemic was the number one health security threat to America. President Trump did not adequately prepare the nation. For four years, Trump's administration did nothing to address this concerning problem.

After President Trump dismantled the National Security Council's global health security office in 2019, Ms. Borio and other high-level experts resigned from his administration. The security office's closure is among many of the shortsighted administrative reversals of President Obama's national security policies. When asked at a news conference about his decision to disband the office, Trump, as usual, did not accept responsibility and refused to answer the legitimate question. He bristled and evaded the line of questioning (Shesgreen, 2020; Balogun, 2020). Akin to how he exited the United Nations Paris climate agreement, Trump also opted out of the WHO at the pandemic onset. He incessantly promoted Hydroxychloroquine® as a cure for the virus, despite research evidence showing otherwise. He even floated the idea of injecting disinfectant and a "powerful ultraviolet ray" as a cure for the disease. President Trump jettisoned the idea of wearing a face mask and conducted his campaign rallies unmasked and with no social distancing strategies which further enhances the spread of the virus. Stubbornly, he undermined the seriousness of the pandemic by making several ignorant proclamations at his press conference: "One day it's like a miracle, the virus will disappear." "I encourage all Americans to gather, in homes and places of worship, to offer a prayer of thanks to God for our many blessings" (Howell, 2020).

With over 800 Americans lost every day in October 2020, Trump was fully recovered from COVID-19 treatment and proudly traveled around the country and falsely proclaimed at his rallies prematurely that coronavirus disease is defeated. Most Americans, especially the senior citizens whose vote usually determines the American election outcome, knew he was lying to them. Indeed, they made him pay at the ballot box! He lost the election to Joe Biden because of the way he mismanaged the coronavirus crisis. Sadly, by December 15, 2020, 3000 Americans died every day from COVID-19, and fatality projections are bleak.

After nearly 100 days in office, 65% of Americans in a national poll ($N = 4423$) approved President Biden's handling of the coronavirus pandemic, and 55% supported his overall job performance. President Trump never achieved this high level of support during his 4 years in office (Kahn, 2021). In curtailing the pandemic, analysts praised Biden for having a detailed plan with a measurable set of objectives easily communicated with clear messages (Anderson, 2021a). Biden and his team emphasized wearing a mask and getting vaccinated not as a political statement but as the right thing to do. In sharp contrast to President Trump, Biden's administration leveraged the expertise of the CDC and FDA to help control the narrative of the pandemic. He empowered both the CDC and FDA by providing the resources needed to efficiently and expediently distribute vaccinations across the country.

Leading by example, Biden and his staffers wore face masks during public appearances and publicly received their vaccine dose, behaviors that Trump and his cabinet members refused to display in public. Biden's administration defined success in vaccine distribution as "100 million shots in 100 days"—a yardstick that an average American can use to measure success. The administration exceeded the goal set. Within 100 days in office, 290,692,005 vaccine doses were distributed and 79.4% (230,768,454) administered; 42.5% of the population had received at least one dose of the vaccine, and 28.9% were fully vaccinated (Anderson, 2021a). As of June 16, 2021, 375,186,675 vaccine doses were distributed in the United States, with 312,915,170 (83.4%) administered. Additionally, 175,053,401 Americans had received at least one dose of the vaccine, and 146,456,124 were fully vaccinated. This means 52.7% of the population had received at least one dose of the vaccine, and 44.1% were fully vaccinated. The Biden administration also set a goal to have 70% of Americans vaccinated by July 4, 2021 (Anderson, 2021b).

Brazil did not enforce a national lockdown policy despite having one of the world's highest coronavirus mortality rates. Like the United States, no centralized implementation strategy; each region and locality adopted varying measures, and compliance declined with time. President Jair Bolsonaro, like Trump, repeatedly played down the risks of the virus. He described it as a "little flu," and vaccination against the virus is only for his dog. He even joined anti-lockdown protests in the capital. Bolsonar's health minister resigned when Bolsonaro ignored his medical advice, and he sacked another minister for an undisclosed reason. Mass testing took a long time to start, and contact tracing never started. As a developing country with a poorly run universal and free health system, Brazilians are less likely to survive when hospitalized because of inadequate infrastructures. Masks and ventilators were in short supply at the peak of the crisis, and the shortages strained the health system. The situation culminated in severe delays in the admission of patients and testing. Because of cultural reasons, local administrators' deaths due to disease are underreported—family members object to the use of the word "coronavirus" to describe their loved ones (Howell, 2020).

India responded quickly to the COVID-19 outbreak by implementing surveillance as early as January 17, 2020, and enforced a strict lockdown policy when cases surged between March 24 and May 31, 2020. Unexpectedly, the prolonged lockdown effect impacted millions of low-income migrant workers. Their families faced hunger and illness because they did not receive any government assistance for over 45 days after the lockdown. More concerning, the health system was not adequately equipped and lacked funding to manage the outbreak, causing many patients to be turned away from the hospitals, especially when the virus engulfed India's rural areas. National testing is limited—in June 2020, testing was about 4100 people per million—compared with an average of over 29,000 tests per million globally.

As cases declined between September 2020 and February 2021, the Indian government ignored warnings of a second wave, even though scientists identified new homegrown B.1.617 variants in January. Scientists in the United Kingdom reported that the new variant is more lethal and 60% more transmissible between humans (Khan, 2021). Like most countries worldwide, Indian citizens completely let down their guard and assumed that the pandemic was over. COVID surveillance and control measures took a back seat. The apocalyptic explosion of COVID-19 cases in India is due to the enormous social gatherings during religious festivals, the reopening of public spaces, and the final "unlocking" of restrictions in December 2020.

Additionally, the crowded political events held before the elections played a significant part. As the number of cases surged, Prime Minister Narendra Modi, like President Trump, addressed election rallies in Kerala, Tamil Nadu, and Puducherry on March 30, 2021, with most of the audience not wearing a mask (Khan, 2021). Trump and Modi share some similarities, including a nativist governing philosophy and a strongman appeal. Perhaps their most significant commonality is their adherence to a familiar autocratic playbook adopted by other democratically elected leaders around the world (Serhan, 2020).

After the first wave, in January 2021, India increased its oxygen sales to other countries by a whopping 734% and sold 193 million doses of vaccines. Justifying the government's decision to export medical resources to other countries, a few weeks before the new surge, health minister Harsh Vardhan asserted that India was in the "endgame" of the COVID-19 pandemic. Subsequently, the healthcare system tackled other medical emergencies neglected during the first wave, and the dedicated COVID-19 facilities converted back to their previous functions. Suddenly, the situation changed. The sudden spike in coronavirus cases and the new variant overwhelmed the healthcare system with no hospital beds and no oxygen and medicines. The situation on the ground is precarious because India invests less than 2% of its GDP on health—significantly less than most of its peers. Brazil spends more than 9% of its GDP on health, and the United States spends nearly 18% (Frayer & Pathak, 2021).

By April 15 onward, India observed more than 200,000 cases daily, and many critically ill patients died due to oxygen shortages across the country (Bhowmick, 2021). On April 25, 2012, India broke the world record with 346,786 new cases and 2624 fatalities (Khan, 2021). Some analysts contend that fatalities are undercounted by at least two-thirds (Frayer & Pathak, 2021). The United States set the 1-day record of 300,669 new cases on January 8, 2021 (Bhowmick, 2021). As of April 30, 2021, with a population of 1.37 billion, India had almost 19 million COVID-19 cases, representing 1.4% of the total population—compared to more than 32 million, or 9.7%, of the United States population (Frayer & Pathak, 2021).

Like the United States and Brazil, Mexico is governed by an authoritarian leader who responded nonchalantly to the coronavirus crisis. President Andres Manuel López Obrador was against the closure of the borders or exercise caution at airports. Like Trump, Obrador is a denier of the virus. He once effusively asserted that the spirituality of the country would protect it from COVID-19. He pulled out two traditional medicine amulets and vouched the charms would protect him against the virus. He stated his administration would keep the status quo in managing the pandemic. Again, like Trump, Obrador is cynical about wearing a mask (Howell, 2020).

The high mortality rate in the United Kingdom is attributed to Prime Minister Boris Johnson's failure to grasp the pandemic's seriousness at the onset until he was infected. Five weeks after the first case was reported in the country, the Prime Minister announced that people go about their business as usual, to the surprise of many of his medical advisors (Howell, 2020). He reluctantly imposed a considerably relaxed lockdown after 285 people had passed away, but the government did not impose international travel restrictions until June! Amid the chaos, the health minister made the matter worse without ensuring that 25,060 patients were tested for coronavirus, allowing them to be discharged from NHS hospitals to nursing homes. The government decided to abandon contact tracing strategy in March at the pandemic's peak and failed to provide adequate protective wear for the frontline workers (Howell, 2020).

To protect jobs and support the economy, the government of the five top successful nations implemented robust financial support programs to help businesses and workers cope with the COVID-19 pandemic. For example, in New Zealand, full-time workers received $585.80 per week, while part-time workers received $350 per week during the national lockdown from March 11 to June 30, 2020. Workers, including contractors, self-employed, and people living with disabilities who need to stay away from work and cannot work from home, were also paid $585.80 per week for full-time workers and $350.00. Singapore allocated a stimulus package of $59.9 billion that is about 12% of its GDP. The government provided $4600 for all workers for 9 months and some stimulus packages and grants for businesses to help them manage the economic impacts of COVID-19. On the other hand, the United States, over 9 months, paid $600 for workers earning less than $75,000 per year.

While vaccination against the coronavirus significantly lags behind the United States' projection, the death toll continues to surge with ferocity. On the last day of President Trump in office, January 20, 2021, America's fatalities from coronavirus reached 400,000—a once-unthinkable number. One American dies from COVID-19 every 26 second. More Americans die of coronavirus each week than any other condition, ahead of heart disease and cancer (Stone, 2021). Compliance with long-term lockdown, which is necessary to curtail the virus's spread, is successful in countries that provide robust financial support for businesses and workers. The United States and New Zealand best exemplify this thesis. The United States represents only 4% of the world population but has 25% of the COVID-19 cases and deaths. In contrast, New Zealand has the lowest number of cases and fatalities (per capita) worldwide. The US Congress and President Trump spent months arguing over the amount of financial support to provide to workers. Unlike the United States, the New Zealand government acted swiftly in providing financial support that kept compliance with the lockdown high.

Overall, the number of COVID-19 cases and the mortality rate in Africa is surprisingly low compared to the rest of the world. In May 2020, WHO had projected that 44 million Africans would be infected and 190,000 dead in the first year of the pandemic. Several theories have been advanced for the unexpected low cases and fatalities in Africa. Many scientists attributed it to the underreporting of the cases due to the low density of testing facilities. Thus, the actual burden of the disease remains murky in the absence of robust testing infrastructure. Other scientists attributed the low cases and fatalities in Africa to the young age of the population. In Africa, COVID-19 cases affected mostly the elderly over 60 years; 60% of the people are under 25 years of age, and the median age is 19.4 years. Another theory is that Africa's hot and humid climate interacts to heighten their personal effects (SciDev.Net, 2020).

Ndubuaku and Watanabe attributed the low death rate in Africa to environmental, genetic, spiritual, and population density factors. They explain that in high-income countries where the pandemic is currently high, urbanites are packed in crowded spaces, vehicles, and stadia, accommodating 50,000 to 75,000 people close to one another. On the other hand, in general, Africans live in less crowded spaces and enjoy provincial lifestyles, where people can relax. In Africa, most coronavirus cases are in the cities, and fewer cases in rural areas (Ndubuaku & Watanabe, 2020). Other scientists have attributed the low cases and fatalities in Africa to immunological factor and posited a less contagious coronavirus variant on the continent.

COVID-19 Vaccine Development and Therapeutics

The global race to develop a safe and effective vaccine for COVID-19 is beginning to yield positive dividends. As of December 15, 2020, few vaccines are authorized, and some in developmental stages worldwide at the time of writing this chapter. A multinational mRNA-based vaccine (BNT162b2) was developed by Pfizer, BioNTech; Fosun Pharma is now authorized in the United Kingdom, the United States, Bahrain, Canada, and Mexico. China has also approved three inactivated vaccines developed by Sinovac, Wuhan Institute of Biological Products, China National Pharmaceutical Group (Sinopharm), and Beijing Institute of Biological Products. Russia has also authorized a non-replicating viral vector (Sputnik V). The Russians also developed a peptide vaccine (EpiVacCorona) at the Gamaleya Research Institute, Acellena Contract Drug Research, and Development and Federal Budgetary Research Institution State Research Center of Virology and Biotechnology. There are over ten other vaccines in phases two and three clinical trials. The most prevalent vaccine in phase three clinical trials is the mRNA-based vaccine (mRNA-1273) by Moderna developed at the Kaiser Permanente Washington Health Research Institute (Craven, 2020).

Aside from vaccine development, scientists worldwide are also in search of reliable therapeutics for coronavirus. There are several promising medications and treatments that have been making a buzz among scientists. In the United States, the FDA issued an emergency use authorization (EUA) on October 22, 2020, for the use of *remdesivir* (Veklury)—an antiviral product given by intravenous (IV) infusion in the hospital setting for patients ages 12 and older. The approval of remdesivir (Veklury)in the United States is controversial worldwide because the WHO does not recommend it for COVID-19 due to a lack of convincing empirical data supporting its effectiveness. Currently, remdesivir is under investigation in combination with other medications. Preliminary findings revealed that patients who received a combination of remdesivir and *baricitinib* (Olumiant) recovered 1 day faster than patients on remdesivir. Also, patients on combination therapy had a 30% higher probability of clinical improvement at day 15. However, patients who received both medications were also less likely to need ventilation or die on day 29 than patients who only received remdesivir (23% vs. 28%) (Tran, 2020).

Given this promising preliminary data, the FDA, on November 19, 2020, granted a EUA for remdesivir to be used in combination with baricitinib in the hospital setting for patients with COVID-19 who need extra oxygen or breathing support (Tran, 2020). In contrast to the aforementioned promising findings, a study funded by the WHO found that remdesivir had no significant effect on the death rate among hospitalized patients with COVID-19. The death rate was about 11% regardless of whether patients got remdesivir or not. Other RCT in the United States and China did not find remdesivir to be significantly beneficial (Tran, 2020).

Scientists found that patients in the hospital setting ($N = 2104$) on a low, daily dose of *dexamethasone* (administered either by mouth or IV injection)—a common corticosteroid (steroid) medication used to treat autoimmune conditions and allergic reactions—had a statistically significant lower death rate at day 28, compared to other patients ($N = 4321$) who did not get it (26% versus 23%, respectively). The dexamethasone treatment was not beneficial for patients with less severe symptoms but was most helpful for patients on a ventilator or oxygen therapy. A meta-analysis of seven RCTs found mortality rates to be lower in the hospital setting among patients on one of the three different corticosteroids—dexamethasone, hydrocortisone, or methylprednisolone—compared to patients who took none (32% vs. 40%).

The US FDA, on March 24, 2020, issued an Emergency Investigational New Drug (EIND) application to use *convalescent plasma* as a therapy for COVID-19. Scientists speculate that antibodies found in the convalescent plasma can help fight the coronavirus infection. A study from Mayo Clinic of over 35,000 hospitalized patients with COVID-19 given convalescent plasma at day 7 had a lower death rate within 3 days of diagnosis than the group who received it after four or more days. Death rates were also lower in patients who got convalescent plasma with higher antibody levels than plasma with lower antibody levels. The study design is weak because it lacked a control group (i.e., patients without convalescent plasma treatment), so it's unclear if the difference in mortality rates was actually due to the treatment or other factors. Based on this finding, on August 23, 2020, the FDA issued a EUA for convalescent plasma for patients with COVID-19 in the hospital setting. The National Institutes of Health (NIH) panel disagreed with the FDA's recommendation, stating the scientific evidence for convalescent plasma is insufficient. So far, the use of convalescent plasma for COVID-19 has also been inconclusive because studies from other parts of the world found no difference in clinical improvement and death rate between those who received convalescent plasma and the control.

Monoclonal antibodies (MABs) are made in the lab setting and used with the potential to fight off infections sooner. Two pharmaceutical companies in the United States—Eli Lilly and Regeneron—developed two types of MABs (bamlanivimab (LY-CoV555) and REGN-COV2, respectively) as therapeutics for COVID-19. They applied for EUAs in early October 2020, and the FDA issued EUAs for both medications in November 2020. Other companies around the world are pursuing long-acting antibody combination therapies—bamlanivimab (LY-CoV555) and REGN-COV2.

Without any empirical evidence, President Trump aggressively promoted *hydroxychloroquine and chloroquine* as a preventive agent for COVID-19. The two medications have routinely been used for decades to treat malaria in developing countries and the countries in the north for treating autoimmune disorders like rheumatoid arthritis and lupus. At the onset of the coronavirus crisis, a few studies suggested that hydroxychloroquine and chloroquine are beneficial in the hospital setting for treating mild cases of COVID-19. In contrast, several other researchers worldwide found them not to help prevent or treat COVID-19.

Azithromycin (Z-pak)—an antibiotic used to treat bronchitis and pneumonia—was shown to have some in vitro activity against influenza A and Zika but did not show a positive effect against the coronavirus that causes MERS. Combination therapy of azithromycin and hydroxychloroquine for patients with COVID-19 found 93% of the patients cleared the virus after 8 days, but the experimental design did not include a control group. There are concerns about this combination therapy's potentially severe side effects, and the NIH currently recommends against it for treating COVID-19.

Tocilizumab (Actemra) and other IL-6 inhibitors used to treat rheumatoid arthritis and juvenile idiopathic arthritis work by blocking interleukin-6 (IL-6), a protein involved in the natural immune responses. IL-6 is a cytokine (signaling protein) that alerts other cells to activate the immune system. Too much activation can cause an overactive severe immune system (a cytokine storm), a potentially fatal problem when the immune system goes chaotic and inflammation gets out of control.

Patients with COVID-19 can be at risk of cytokine storms as their body continues to ramp up their immune system to fight off the infection. By blocking IL-6, tocilizumab helps to calm down the immune system and manage the cytokine storms. Research on using tocilizumab started in France. The investigators found that patients on tocilizumab were less likely to require a ventilator or die. Another study from Italy reported that patients on tocilizumab had lower fatalities, but about the same proportion of patients from both groups needed ventilators.

On the other hand, tocilizumab was not beneficial for managing COVID-19 in early-stage pneumonia. Another phase three clinical trial by the manufacturer of tocilizumab also found that it does not help treat severe pneumonia in hospitalized patients with COVID-19. More extensive investigations have reported conflicting results attributed to the heterogeneity of the patients included in the studies. *Kevzara* (sarilumab), with a similar mechanism of action to tocilizumab, has been tested for COVID-19, but the preliminary findings were not promising. Compared to the placebo group, the patients on Kevzara with severe symptoms did worse, but those with more severe (critical) symptoms improved compared to the placebo group. The NIH is against the use of IL-6 inhibitors, such as tocilizumab or sarilumab, for treating patients with COVID-19.

Conclusion

Compared to the rest of the world, the number of COVID-19 cases and deaths in Africa is significantly lower than the projection of the World Health Organization at the onset of the pandemic. Paradoxically, the United States and the United Kingdom—the two nations perceived as the best prepared to manage a pandemic—had the highest cases and deaths. On the other hand, with low mortality rates, Vietnam and Iceland managed the crisis exceedingly well, after previously ranked poorly on the preparedness scorecard. At the beginning of the pandemic, South Korea did very well but did not rank in the top five countries 11 months later. Their authorities let their guards down, and the virus took advantage of the situation. Indeed, it is safe to say that timing is everything in concluding any nation's effectiveness in curtailing the virus's spread. The critical global lesson learned is that curtailing COVID-19 is a marathon race and not a sprint competition. The size and timeliness of the stimulus packages and grants provided to workers and businesses distinguished the effective nations from those that bungled the pandemic. The global financial support provided cushioned the economic impacts of the crisis, enhanced compliance with the lockdown order, and helped curtail the virus' spread. Countries with autocratic leaders who exhibited nonchalant attitudes failed miserably, with too many lives needlessly lost. As the more virulent variants of COVID-19 in India, Brazil, the United Kingdom, and South Africa emerge, the Nigerian government can deploy these valuable lessons to manage the continually evolving crisis.

Case Study

This case study will enable students to explore the practice of their profession in other countries. The students will select any country in the world and conduct an in-depth review of the status of the health discipline in that country by addressing the following issues:

1. Brief description of the country; including population and number of professionals in the discipline selected.
2. Type of healthcare system.
3. History of the health discipline in the country.
4. Entry-level education, competitiveness, number of schools, duration of the training, curriculum, internship, and license mechanism.
5. Professional autonomy and direct access opportunity.
6. Opportunities for post-professional training.
7. Demand for health discipline services; pay compared to other health professions.
8. How does the health discipline compare to other health professions in terms of professional status and esteem?

References

Adekanye, A. O., Adefemi, S., Okuku, A. G., Onawola, K. A., Taiwo, A. I., & James, J. A. (2013). Patients' satisfaction with the healthcare services at a north central Nigerian tertiary hospital. *Journal of the National Association of Resident Doctors of Nigeria, 22*(3), 218–224. [online]. Available at: https://www.researchgate.net/publication/258248219_Patients'_satisfaction_with_ the_healthcare_services_at_a_north_central_Nigerian_tertiary_hospital. Accessed 19 Jun 2021.

Adepoju, P. (2020). *On the frontline of Nigeria's coronavirus fight, health workers brace for inevitable.* [online]. Available at: https://www.devex.com/news/on-the-frontline-of-nigeria-s-coronavirus-fight-health-workers-brace-for-inevitable-97928. Accessed 16 Dec 2020.

Akunne, M. O., Okonta, M. J., Ukwe, C. V., et al. (2019). Satisfaction of Nigerian patients with health services: a protocol for a systematic review. *Systematic Review, 8,* 256. [online]. Available at: https://systematicreviewsjournal.biomedcentral.com/articles/10.1186/s13643-019-1160-z. Accessed 19 Jun 2021.

Anderson, M. (2021a). States ranked by percentage of COVID-19 vaccines administered: April 27. *Becker's Hospital Review.* [online]. Available at: https://www.beckershospitalreview.com/public-health/states-ranked-by-percentage-of-covid-19-vaccines-administered.html. Accessed 27 Apr 2021.

Anderson, M. (2021b). *States ranked by percentage of COVID-19 vaccines administered: June 17.* [online]. Available at: https://www.beckershospitalreview.com/public-health/states-ranked-by-percentage-of-covid-19-vaccines-administered.html. Accessed 19 Jun 2021.

Andrew, S. (2020). *The US has 4% of the world's population but 25% of its coronavirus cases.* [online]. Available at: https://www.cnn.com/2020/06/30/health/us-coronavirus-toll-in-numbers-june-trnd/index.html. Accessed 15 Dec 2020

Balogun, J. A. (2020). Lessons from the USA delayed response to COVID-19 pandemic. *African Journal of Reproductive Health, 24*(1). [online]. Available at: https://www.ajrh.info/index.php/ajrh/article/view/2063/pdf. Accessed 10 Oct 2020.

Bhowmick, N. (2021). *How India's second wave became the worst COVID-19 surge in the world.* [online]. Available at:https://www.nationalgeographic.com/science/article/how-indias-second-wave-became-the-worst-covid-19-surge-in-the-world. Accessed 27 Apr 2021.

Bolarinde, J. L., Agbla, S. C., Bola-Lawal, Q. N., Afolabi, M. O., & Ihaji, E. (2018). Patients' satisfaction with care from Nigerian federal capital territory's public secondary hospitals: A cross-sectional study. *Journal of Patient Experience, 5*(4), 250–257. [online]. Available at: https://www.ncbi.nlm.nih.gov/pmc/articles/PMC6295802/. Accessed 19 Jun 2021. Business Hallmark. (2021) Hundreds of Nigerian doctors set to emigrate to Saudi Arabia as country's health sector worsens. [online]. Available at: https://hallmarknews.com/hundreds-of-nigerian-doctors-set-to-emigrate-to-saudi-arabia-as-countrys-health-sector-worsens/ (Accessed: 23 November 2021)

Cosma, S. A., Bota, M., Fles, C., Morgovan, C., Văleanu, M., & Cosma, D. (2020). *Measuring patients' perception and satisfaction with the Romanian healthcare system.* [online]. Available at: https://www.mdpi.com/2071-1050/12/4/1612/pdf. Accessed 19 Jun 2021.

Craven, J. (2020). *COVID-19 vaccine tracker.* [Online]. Available at: https://www.raps.org/news-and-articles/news-articles/2020/3/covid-19-vaccine-tracker. Accessed 8 Jan 2021.

Dixit, S., Ogundeji, Y. K., & Onwujekwe, O. (2020). *How well has Nigeria responded to COVID-19?* [online]. Available at: https://www.brookings.edu/blog/future-development/2020/07/02/how-well-has-nigeria-responded-to-covid-19/. Accessed 16 Dec 2020.

Elflein, J. (2020). *Percentage of respondents worldwide who were satisfied with their country's national health system as of 2019, by country.* [online]. Available at: https://www.statista.com/statistics/1109036/satisfaction-health-system-worldwide-by-country/. Accessed 19 Jun 2021.

Ehanire, O. (2020). *First case of corona virus disease confirmed in Nigeria.* Nigeria Centre for Disease Control. [online]. Available at: https://ncdc.gov.ng/news/227/first-case-of-corona-virus-disease-confirmed-in-nigeria. Accessed 28 Dec 2020.

Eke, C. (2020). *Nigeria – Country commercial guide.* [online]. Available at: https://www.trade.gov/country-commercial-guides/nigeria-healthcare. Accessed 30 Dec 2020

Frayer, L., & Pathak, S. (2021). *India Is counting thousands of daily COVID deaths. How many is it missing?* [online]. Available at: https://www.npr.org/sections/goatsand-soda/2021/04/30/992451165/india-is-counting-thousands-of-daily-covid-deaths-how-many-is-it-missing. Accessed 30 Apr 2021.

Habib, H. (2020). Has Sweden's controversial COVID-19 strategy been successful? *British Medical Journal, 369,* m2376. [online]. Available at: https://www.bmj.com/content/369/bmj.m2376. Accessed 10 Oct 2020.

Howell, B. (2020). *The countries who've handled coronavirus the best – and worst.* [online]. Available at: https://www.movehub.com/blog/best-and-worst-covid-responses/. Accessed 12 Dec 2020.

GUP, I., Ofoedu, J. N., Njoku, P. U., GOC, O., Amadi, A. N., & Godswill-Uko, E. U. (2013). Satisfaction with quality of care received by patients without National Health Insurance attending a primary care clinic in a resource-poor environment of a tertiary hospital in eastern Nigeria in the era of scaling up the Nigerian formal sector health insurance scheme. *Annals of Medical Health Sciences Research, 3*(1), 31–37. [online]. Available at: https://www.ncbi.nlm.nih.gov/pmc/articles/PMC3634220/. Accessed 19 Jun 2021.

Iloh GUP, Ofoedu JN, Njoku PU, Okafor GOC, Amadi A, Godswill-Uko Eu. Satisfaction with quality care received by patients without National Health Insurance attending a primary care clinic in a resource-poor environment of a tertiary hospital in Eastern Nigeria in the era of scaling up the Nigeria formal sector health insurance. Annals of Medical and Health Sciences; 2013;3(1):31–37. [online]. Available at: scheme. file:///C:/Users/Admin/Desktop/Aka%20book%20review/87717-Article%20Text-217433-1-10-20130423.pdf (Accessed: 19 June 2021)

Jarus, O. (2020) 20 of the worst epidemics and pandemics in history. [online]. Available at: https://www.livescience.com/worst-epidemics-and-pandemics-in-history.html (Accessed: 18 December 2020)

Johns Hopkins University of Medicine. (2020). *Coronavirus resource center.* [online]. Available at: https://coronavirus.jhu.edu/. Accessed 22 Jun 2020.

Kahn, C. (2021). Biden fares better than Trump over his first 100 days. *Reuters/Ipsos poll.* [online]. Available at: https://www.reuters.com/world/us/after-100-days-americans-give-biden-high-marks-covid-19-response-economy-2021-04-27/. Accessed 27 Apr 2021.

Khan, A. (2021). Why does India have so many COVID cases? *Al Jazeera Media Network.* [online]. Available at: https://www.aljazeera.com/features/2021/4/25/why-does-india-have-so-many-covid-cases. Accessed 29 Apr 2021.

Kaiser Family Foundation. (2020). *Lost on the frontline.* [online]. Available at: https://khn.org/news/lost-on-the-frontline-health-care-worker-death-toll-covid19-coronavirus/. Accessed 2 Jan 2021.

Lin, C. F., Wu, C. H., & WU, CF. (2020). Reimagining the administrative state in times of global health crisis: An anatomy to the COVID-19 pandemic. *European Journal of Risk Regulation, 2,* 1–17. [online]. Available at: https://www.ncbi.nlm.nih.gov/pmc/articles/PMC7156569/. Accessed 10 Oct 2020.

Mugwagwa, J., Onyeka, O. V., & Shaxson, L. (2020) *Covid-19 shows why health and well-being should be an everyday target.* [online]. Available at: https://blogs.lse.ac.uk/africaatlse/2020/04/01/covid-19-why-health-well-being-everyday-target-health-system/. Accessed 23 Dec 2020.

Presse, A. F. (2020). Nigeria doctors launch latest strike amid pandemic. *Barron's AFP News.* July 13. [online]. Available at: https://www.barrons.com/news/nigeria-doctors-launch-latest-strike-amid-pandemic-01594634706. Accessed 16 Oct 2020.

Mwai, P., & Giles, C. (2020). *Coronavirus: How vulnerable are health workers in Nigeria.* [online]. Available at: https://www.bbc.com/news/world-africa-53013413. Accessed 16 Dec 2020.

Moradi, H., & Vaezi, A. (2020). *Lessons learned from Korea: Covid-19 pandemic.* [online]. Available at: https://www.researchgate.net/publication/340416184_Lessons_Learned_From_Korea_Covid-19_Pandemic. Accessed 10 Oct 2020.

Ndubuaku, V., & Watanabe, N. C. (2020). *Why is the coronavirus death rate in Africa quite low?* [online]. Available at: https://www.researchgate.net/post/Why-is-the-Corona-Virus-death-rate-in-Africa-quite-low. Accessed 16 Dec 2020.

OECD. (2002). *Nigeria.* [online]. Available at: https://www.oecd.org/countries/nigeria/1826208.pdf. Accessed 16 Oct 2020.

Oleribe, O., Ezechi, O., Osita-Oleribe, P., et al. (2020). Public perception of COVID-19 management and response in Nigeria: a cross-sectional survey. *British Medical Journal Open, 10*(10), e041936. [online]. Available at: https://bmjopen.bmj.com/content/10/10/e041936. Accessed 16 Dec 2020.

Olamuyiwa, T. E., & Adeniji, F. O. (2021). *Patient's satisfaction with quality of care at a National Health Insurance clinic at a tertiary center, South-South Nigeria*. [online]. Available at: https://journals.sagepub.com/doi/full/10.1177/2374373520981471. Accessed 19 Jun 2021.

Onigbinde, O. A., Babatunde, O., & Ajagbe, A. O. (2020). The welfare of healthcare workers amidst COVID-19 pandemic in sub-Sahara Africa: A call for concern. *Ethics in Medicine and Public Health, 15*, 100555. [online]. Available at: https://www.ncbi.nlm.nih.gov/pmc/articles/PMC7430272/. Accessed 30 Dec 2020.

Osiya, D. A., Ogaji, D. S., & Onotai, L. (2017). Patients' satisfaction with healthcare: Comparing general practice services in a tertiary and primary healthcare settings. *The Nigerian Health Journal, 17*(1). [online]. Available at: https://www.ajol.info/index.php/nhj/article/view/154264/143845. Accessed 19 Jun 2021.

Potluri, R. M., & Angiating, G. (2018). A study on service quality and customer satisfaction in Nigerian healthcare sector. *International Journal of Industrial Distribution and Business, 9*(12), 7–14. [online]. Available at: https://www.researchgate.net/publication/330022486_A_Study_on_Service_Quality_and_Customer_Satisfaction_in_Nigerian_Healthcare_Sector. Accessed 19 Jun 2021.

SciDev.Net. (2020). *Reasons for Africa's low COVID-19 rates revealed*. [online]. Available at: https://medicalxpress.com/news/2020-10-africa-covid-revealed.html. Accessed 16 Dec 2020.

Serhan, Y. (2020). *The Trump-Modi playbook*. [online]. Available at: https://www.theatlantic.com/international/archive/2020/02/donald-trump-narendra-modi-autocrats/607042/. Accessed 30 Apr 2021

Shesgreen, D. (2021). Gross misjudgment': Experts say Trump's decision to disband pandemic team hindered coronavirus response. *USA Today*. [online]. Available at: https://www.usatoday.com/story/news/world/2020/03/18/coronavirus-did-president-trumps-decision-disband-global-pandemic-office-hinder-response/5064881002/. Accessed 3 Apr 2020.

Stone, W. (2021). *As death rate accelerates, U.S. records 400,000 lives lost to the coronavirus*. [online]. Available at: https://www.npr.org/sections/health-shots/2021/01/19/957488613/as-death-rate-accelerates-u-s-records-400-000-lives-lost-to-the-coronavirus. Accessed 20 Jan 2021.

Tran, J. (2020). *The latest research on COVID-19 treatments and medications in the pipeline*. [online]. Available at: https://www.goodrx.com/blog/coronavirus-treatments-on-the-way/#:~:text=Remdesivir%20(Veklury)%20is%20currently%20the,remdesivir%20(Veklury)%20recovered%20faster. Accessed 8 Jan 2021.

Umoke, M., Umoke, P. C. I., Nwimo, I. O., Nwalieji, C. A., Onwe, P. O., Ifeanyi, N., & Olaoluwa, S. A. (2020). Patients' satisfaction with quality of care in general hospitals in Ebonyi State, Nigeria. *SAGE Open Medicine, 27*(8), 2050312120945129. [online]. Available at: https://pubmed.ncbi.nlm.nih.gov/32782795/. Accessed 19 Jun 2021.

WHO. (2017) *Half the world lacks access to essential health services, 100 million still pushed into extreme poverty because of health expenses*. [online]. Available at: https://www.who.int/news-room/detail/13-12-2017-world-bank-and-who-half-the-world-lacks-access-to-essential-health-services-100-million-still-pushed-into-extreme-poverty-because-of-health-expenses. (Accessed: 10 October 2020).

WHO. (2020a). *Rolling updates on coronavirus disease (COVID-19)*. Updated June 11. [online]. Available at: https://www.who.int/emergencies/diseases/novel-coronavirus-2019/events-as-they-happen. Accessed 10 Oct 2020.

WHO. (2020b). *Coronavirus disease (COVID-19) dashboard*. [online]. Available at: https://covid19.who.int/. Accessed 28 Dec 2020.

WHO. (2020c). *News Room. WHO calls for healthy, safe, and decent working conditions for all health workers, amidst COVID-19 pandemic*. [online]. Available at: https://www.who.int/news-room/detail/28-04-2020-who-calls-for-healthy-safe-and-decent-working-conditions-for-all-health-workers-amidst-covid-19-pandemic. Accessed 16 Dec 2020.

Worldometer. (2020a). *Countries in the world by population; Coronavirus report*. [online]. Available at: https://www.worldometers.info/coronavirus/#countries. Accessed 10 Oct 2020.

Worldometer. (2020b). [online]. Available at: https://www.worldometers.info/coronavirus/country/nigeria/#:~:text=Nigeria%20Coronavirus%3A%2073%2C374%20Cases%20and%201%2C197%20Deaths%20%2D%20Worldometer. Accessed 28 Dec 2020.

Worldometer. (2021). *Countries in the world by population.* [online]. Available at: https://www.worldometers.info/world-population/population-by-country/. Accessed 26 Jul 2021.

Zhang JH, Peng X, Liu, C, Chen, Y, Zhang, H, Iwaloye, OO. (2020) Public satisfaction with the healthcare system in China during 2013–2015: a cross-sectional survey of the associated factors. BMJ Open;10:e034414. [online]. Available at: https://bmjopen.bmj.com/content/10/5/e034414 (Accessed: 19 June 2021).

Zhang, J. H., Peng, X., Liu, C., Chen, Y., Zhang, H., & Iwaloye, O. O. (2020). Public satisfaction with the healthcare system in China during 2013–2015: A cross-sectional survey of the associated factors. *BMJ Open, 10*, e034414. [online]. Available at: https://bmjopen.bmj.com/content/10/5/e034414. Accessed 19 Jun 2021.

Index

A

Accommodation, 290, 291, 293
Activities of daily living (ADL), 308
Acupuncture, 158–161, 220, 221
Affordable Care Act (ACA), 40, 329
African traditional medicine (ATM),
        237, 266–270
Alma Ata Declaration, 106, 136
Aromatherapy, 180–187, 224
Ayurveda, 171–173, 223

B

Barriers, 345, 347, 353
Basic Health Services Scheme (BHSS), 106
Brain drain, 70
Burden of disease (BOD), 28, 29
Business ventures, 74, 75

C

Causes of death in the United States in
        2017, 144
Center for Research in Traditional
        Complementary and Alternative
        Medicine (CRTCAM), 215
Centers for Disease Control and Prevention
        (CDC), 112
Centers for Medicare and Medicaid
        Services, 34
Child and maternal mortality rates, 121
Children's Health Insurance Program
        (CHIP), 41
Chiropractic, 161–164, 221
Cirrhosis, 443

Classical osteopaths, 167
Climate change, 72, 73
Community-based rehabilitation, 136
Community Health Extension Workers
        (CHEWs), 137, 138
Community health workers, 137–139
Community physiotherapy scheme, 137
Complementary and alternative
        medicine (CAM)
    action and safety, 154
    acupuncture, 158–161, 220, 221
    aromatherapy, 180–187, 224
    Ayurveda, 171–173, 223
    chemical composition and toxicity, 154
    chiropractic, 161–164, 221
    classification of, 154–156
    evolution of, 214–217
    global demand, 193–195
    herbal medicine, 226, 228
    homeopathy, 176–180, 223, 224
    and integrative medicine, 157
    medical professions and
            occupations, 198–203
    naturopathy, 173–176, 223
    osteopathy, 164–168, 221, 222
    side effects, 154
    spirituality, 187–193, 224–226
    traditional Chinese medicine (TCM),
            169–171, 222
    treatment philosophy, 157, 158
    utilization, 195–197, 217–220
    and Western medications, 154
Complete care, 139
Conventional medicine private health
        care, 96–98

Corruption, 67, 68, 362, 368, 372
COVID-19, 364, 420, 456, 457
    cases, 466
    comparative analyses, 465, 466
    deaths, 466
    five countries, 468, 470–475
    global response, 468
    healthcare workers, 463, 464
    Nigeria, 460–463
    satisfaction, 457–460
    social welfare assistance program,
        464, 465
    therapeutics, 476, 477
    vaccine development, 475–477
Cranial osteopaths, 167
Cuba, 321, 322

D
"Decade of African Traditional Medicine"
        (2000-2010), 239
Diarrheal diseases, 442
Diaspora Nigerians, 74
Disability, 277
    activity limitations, 277
    burden, 284
    causes, 281
    classification, 279, 280
    consequences, 280
    dimensions, 281
    impairments, 277
    Nigeria, 285, 286
    participation restrictions, 277
    quality of life, PLWDs, 286, 287
    relevant protection laws, 288, 289
    scope, 282, 283
    types, 279
Disability-adjusted life years (DALYs), 284
Dismal health outcomes, 73
Donabedian model, 16, 35

E
Economic stresses, 373
Economy, 364
Electronic Medical Record technology, 75
Emergency medical services (EMS), 328
Emotional health, 17
Environmental health, 17
Environmental pollution, 72

F
Federal College of Complementary and
        Alternative Medicine (FEDCAM),
        215, 216
Federal Medical Centers, 92
Federal Ministry of Health (FMH),
        88–91, 93, 215
Federal Specialty Hospitals, 92
Federal Traditional Medicine Board Act's
        policies and guidelines, 213

G
General Ibrahim Babangida's
        administration, 64
Germ theory, 236
Gross development plan (GDP), 362
Gross domestic product (GDP), 419
Grossman's health demand model, 16, 24

H
Handicap, 281
Health care
    advances and innovations, 38–40
    biological characteristics, 18
    burden of disease (BOD), 28, 29
    components of, 17
    cultural factors, 21
    data collection, 37, 38
    definition, 16
    demographic factors, 18
    Donabedian model, 16, 35
    emotional health, 17
    environmental health, 17
    equity, 21
    global access to health care, 27, 28
    governance, leadership, and health
        information systems, 36
    Grossman's health demand model, 16, 24
    hand hygiene, 30–32
    HCAI, 32, 33
    healthcare financing models, 40–42
    health disparities, 19
    Health in All Policies, 22, 23
    health inequities, 20
    health information systems, 37
    health outcome measurement, 33–35
    health system performance, 36
    health systems financing, 37

healthy child development, 19
healthy equity, 19
high-quality care, 24
life expectancy, 29, 30
lifestyle and behaviors, 19
mental health, 17
physical environment, 18
physical health, 17
racism, 21
reproductive health, 17
social and economic conditions, 16
social and economic factors, 18
social health, 17
social policies, 21
socioeconomic factors, 20, 21
sound health, 18
spiritual health, 17
United Nations' Development
    Goals, 25–27
WHO's health and development, 25
workers' health status, 24
Healthcare organization, 88
Healthcare professionals (HCPs), 346, 428
Healthcare system structure
    government levels, 93
    organogram, 93
    PharmAccess Foundation, 94
    public primary healthcare facilities, 95
    tax-funded models, 95
    three-tier structure, 93
    triad delivery system, 94
Healthcare workers (HCWs), 300
Health financing, 330
Health in All Policies, 22, 23
Health outcome indicators, 61, 62
Health system in African Countries, 75–79
Health system, Nigeria
    comparative analyses, 325, 327–331
    Cuba, 321–325
    operational definitions, 300, 301
    performance indicators, 301–303
    Singapore, 315–318
    South Korea, 313–315
    Taiwan, 319, 320
    United Kingdom, 310, 312
    United States, 304, 307–310
    workforce supply, 303, 304
Herbalists, 257
Herbal medicine, 226, 228
HIV/AIDS, 442
Homeopathy, 176–180, 223, 224

I

Impairment, 278, 291
Impairments, Disabilities, and Handicaps
    (ICIDH), 280
Incessant industrial action, 71
Infant and maternal mortality rates, 143
Ischemic heart disease, 443
Itinerant and community physiotherapy
    programs, 136

J

*Journal of Homeopathic Ayurvedic
    Medicine*, 173
*Journal of the American Osteopathic
    Association*, 167

L

Laboratory capacity, 468
Lack of continuity, 69
Lagos Social Health Insurance, 63
Lagos University Teaching Hospital (LUTH)
    Cancer Center, 66
Leadership, 89, 422, 424
Leadership of Federal Ministry of
    Health, 100–109
Local government authorities (LGAs), 370
Low back pain (LBP), 281
Lower respiratory infections, 442

M

Malaria, 442
Manpower shortage, 335
Maternal and infant mortality rate, 117
Medical and Dental Council of Nigeria
    (MDCN), 90, 213, 214
Medical and surgical discoveries, 139–141
Medical rehabilitation, 278
Medical tourism, 69
Medicare, 40
Mega-churches in Nigeria, 227–228
Meningitis, 442
Mental health, 17
Michigan Health System, 186
Millennium Development Goals (MDGs), 118
Ministers of health, 101–104
Ministers of health in Nigeria, 107, 110
Monoclonal antibodies (MABs), 476
Multi-payer health system, 41

N

National Agency for Food and Drug
    Administration and Control
    (NAFDAC), 74–75, 253, 254
National Basic Health Services Scheme, 136
National Center for Complementary and
    Integrative Health (NCCIH), 172
National College of Natural Medicine
    (NCNM), 215
National Health Bill, 66
National Healthcare Development Plan, 52
National Health Insurance Scheme (NHIS),
    62–67, 416
National Health Interview Survey (NHIS), 177
National health plan, 117
National health policy, 136
National Health Service (NHS), 88
National Postgraduate Medical College of
    Nigeria (NPGMCN), 90
National Primary Healthcare Development
    Agency, 106, 108
Naturopathy, 173–176, 223
Neonatal disorders, 442
Nepotism and tribalism, 70
Nigeria, 346, 347, 350, 362, 363, 408, 410,
    458, 459
    blueprint, high-quality health care,
        423, 424
    budget priorities, 365
    conflict resolution strategies, 424, 425
    corruption, 413
    curtail industrial strikes, 428, 429
    developmental challenges, 364
    diaspora, 435
    economic reforms, 387–390
    economy, 4, 5
    electricity, 426
    ethnicity, 3, 4
    evolution of states, 365, 366, 368
    extreme poverty, 420–422
    federal governments, 386
    geography, 1–3
    healthcare professionals, 438, 439
    health system, 6, 7
    highest-paid head, 391, 392
    improve work conditions, 431, 433–435
    income inequality, 5, 6
    informal sector economy, 419
    instability, 373
    lessons from other countries, 395, 396
    local government system, 369–371
    medicines, 441
    natural resources, 407
    perinatal death, 426, 427
    pharmaceutical products, 436–438
    political reforms, 384, 385, 393
    presidents, 381–384
    primary medical equipment, 436
    promote telehealth, 426
    proposed economic, 392, 393
    religion, 4
    revenue allocation formula, 371–373
    slow down population growth, 428
    state governments, 385–387
    sudden wealth, 374, 375
    tracking, healthcare
        professionals, 429, 430
    transformative research, 440, 441
    universal health care, 375–381, 410–418
    vaccines, 441
Nigeria Centre for Disease Control
    (NCDC), 460
Nigeria Natural Medicine Development
    Agency (NNMDA), 215
Nigerian Baptist Convention, 226
Nigerian Council of Physicians of Natural
    Medicine (NCPNM), 215, 216
Nigerian Health Insurance program, 64
Nigerian Health System (2019–2021), 56–61
Nigerian herbal pharmacopoeia, 254
Nigerian Medical Association (NMA), 49
Nigerian National Health Conference, 70
Nigerians in the Diaspora Commission
    (NIDCOM), 435
Nigerian traditional medicine policy, 251–253
North Atlantic Treaty Organization (NATO)
    countries, 110

O

Osteopathic manipulative treatment
    (OMT), 167
Osteopathy, 164–168, 221, 222
Out-of-pocket payments (OOP), 315, 415, 416

P

People living with disabilities (PLWDs), 278,
    280, 282, 284, 286, 288, 290, 293
PharmAccess Foundation, 94
Philanthropy, 332–334
Physical health, 17
Population explosion, 73
Population's peculiar demographics, 70

Poverty, 408
"Primary Healthcare Under One Roof"
    plan, 55
*Promoting the Role of Traditional Medicine in
    Health Systems:A Strategy for the
    African Region*, 238
Public-private partnership model, 75
PubMed database, 118, 347, 353

Q

Qualitative investigation, 345, 346
    challenges, 345
    HCPs, 347
    medicines, 346
    methodology, 347, 348
    public health programs, 346
    results, 348–352
    vaccines, 346
Quality health care, 362
Quality of life, PLWDs, 289–293
Queen Elizabeth's administration, 50

R

Recommended Quality of Care
    Framework, 35
Regional Government of Lombardy, 177
Reproductive health, 17
Restructuring, 373, 374
Ribonucleic acid-based therapies, 40

S

Secretaries of US Department of Health and
    Human Services, 105–106
Secretary of health, 99
Severe acute respiratory syndrome coronavirus
    2 (SARS-CoV-2), 456
Singapore, 315
Single-payer health system, 40
Social commentator, 88
Socialized medicine payer system, 42
Socioeconomic inequities, 68, 69
Sound health, 18
South Korea, 313
Spiritual health, 17
Spirituality, 187–193
Stroke, 443
Surgeon general, 110–112
Sustainable development goal
    (SDG), 118
Swine flu (H1N1), 141–143

T
Taiwan, 318
Telehealth, 74
Traditional birth attendants, 257
Traditional Chinese medicine (TCM),
    169–171, 222
Traditional medical practitioners (TMPs), 47
Traditional medicine, 47
Traditional Medicine Council of Nigeria, 213
Traditional medicine practice (TMPs)
    African traditional medicine, 266–270
    bone setters, 258, 259
    common medicinal plants, 240–249
    definition, 235
    development of, 262, 263
    genesis of, 237, 238
    indications, 260
    ingredient dealers, 259
    NAFDAC, 253, 254
    Nigerian herbal pharmacopoeia, 254
    Nigerian traditional medicine
        policy, 251–253
    occupations, 256–258
    pharmaceutical products
        development, 264–266
    practitioners of therapeutic occultism,
        259, 260
    regulation and practice, 254–256
    rehabilitation, 259
    traditional psychiatrists, 259
    traditional surgeon, 258
    training and practice trends, 263, 264
    treatment approach, 261, 262
    treatment philosophies, 261
    utilization of, 236
    wild animal species, 249–251
    World Health Organization (WHO)
        role, 238–240
Traditional medicine private health
    care, 98–100
Transformative research, 439
Tuberculosis, 442
Two-tier health insurance coverage system, 41

U
United Kingdom's publicly-funded health
    system, 88
United States, 304
Universal health care (UHC), 117, 118,
    363, 409–411
University of Nigeria Teaching Hospital
    (UNTH), 139

University Teaching Hospitals, 91
U.S. Federal Trade Commission
     (FTC), 178

V
Vulnerabilities
     global health, 135
     limited access to essential medicines and
          vaccines, 130–132
     low-quality health service
          delivery, 120–124
     paltry health systems financing, 127–129

poor governance and ineffective
     leadership, 119–120
shortage of healthcare workforce,
     124–127
weak health information systems, 133–135

W
Weak surveillance system, 71
Western-style healthcare system
     1472-1960, 48–50
     1960-1990, 51–53
     1990-2018, 53–56